P9-DEC-106

CLINICIAN'S POCKET DRUG REFERENCE 2014

CLINICIAN'S POCKET DRUG REFERENCE 2014

EDITORS

Leonard G. Gomella, MD, FACS
Steven A. Haist, MD, MS, FACP
Aimee G. Adams, PharmD

www.eDrugbook.com
www.thescutmonkey.com

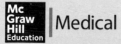

Medical

New York Chicago San Francisco Athens
London Madrid Mexico City Milan New Delhi
Singapore Sydney Toronto

Clinician's Pocket Drug Reference 2014

1 2 3 4 5 6 7 8 9 0   QLM/QLM   18 17 16 15 14 13

ISBN 978-0-07-182496-5
MHID 0-07-182496-0
ISSN 1540-6725

The book was set in Times by Cenveo® Publisher Services.
The editors were Catherine Johnson and Harriet Lebowitz.
The production supervisor was Catherine Saggese.
Project management was provided by Yashmita Hota, Cenveo Publisher Services.
Quad/Graphics Leominster was printer and binder.

This book is printed on acid-free paper.

CONTENTS

ix

PREFACE

We are pleased to present the 12th edition of the *Clinician's Pocket Drug Reference*. This book is based on the drug presentation style originally used in 1983 in the *Clinician's Pocket Reference*, popularly known as the Scut Monkey Book. Our goal is to identify the most frequently used and clinically important medications, including branded, generic, OTC, and herbal products. The book now includes more than 1400 generic product listings with the true number approaching 4000 entries when specific brand names are considered.

Our unique style of presentation includes key "must-know" facts of commonly used medications, essential for both the student and practicing clinician. The inclusion of common uses of medications rather than just the official FDA-labeled indications are based on supporting publications and community standards of care and have been reviewed by our editors and editorial board.

The limitations of difficult-to-read traditional package inserts have been recognized by the US Food and Drug Administration. Today, all newly approved medications provide a more user-friendly package insert. Although very useful, these summaries do not appear alongside similarly approved generic or "competing" similar products, and older medications may not have a newer user-friendly package insert.

It is essential that students and residents in training learn more than the name and dose of the medications they prescribe. Certain common side effects and significant warnings and contraindications are associated with almost all prescription medications. Although providers should ideally be completely familiar with the entire package insert of any medication prescribed, such a requirement is unachievable. References such as the *Physician's Desk Reference* and the drug manufacturer's web site make many package inserts readily available. While newly released medications often have a prominent presence and easy access to all their FDA approved data on the web, it is often not the case of older medications, OTC products, or generics. Likewise, encyclopedic information can be found on certain web sites as well and is occasionally needed when unique clinical situations arise. However, resources that identify the most common and essential facts are sometimes lacking. Our goal is to provide access to not only dosing but to these clinically significant facts and key data, whether for commonly prescribed brand name drugs, generics, or OTC products in this pocket-sized book format. Information contained within is meant for use by healthcare professionals who are already familiar with these commonly prescribed medications.

For 2014 we have added about 40 new drugs with hundreds of changes in other medications based on recent FDA actions and manufacturers, updates. These include deletions of discontinued brand names and compounds and many black box updates. Emergency cardiac care (ECC) guidelines for commonly used medications are based on the American Heart Association (*Circulation*. 2010; 122 [Suppl 3] http://circ.ahajournals.org/content/vol122/18_suppl_3/) and appear in summary cover tables in the back of the book.

Versions of this book are produced in a variety of electronic or eBook formats. Visit www.eDrugbook.com for a link to some of the electronic versions currently available. Additionally, this web site has enhanced content features such as a comprehensive listing of "look alike–sound alike" medications that can contribute to prescribing errors and other useful information related to medication prescribing.

Nursing versions of this book (*Nurses Pocket Drug Guide*) with a section of customized Nursing interventions is available and updated annually. An EMS guide based on this book (*EMS Pocket Drug Guide*) with enhanced content specifically for the field provider and emergency medical practitioners is also available. Information and links for these related publications are available on the web site www.eDrugbook.com.

We express special thanks to our spouses and families for their long-term support of this book and the entire Scut Monkey Project (www.thescutmonkey.com). The Scut Monkey Project, launched in 1979 at the University of Kentucky College of Medicine, is designed to provide new medical students and other health professional students with the basic tools needed when entering the world of hands-on patient care. Many other schools have adopted the concept of "students teaching students" over the years.

The contributions of the members of the editorial board and in particular, Harriet Lebowitz at McGraw-Hill and Yashmita Hota at Cenveo Publisher Services, are gratefully acknowledged. As a reader, your comments and suggestions are always welcome. Improvements to this and all our books would be impossible without the interest and continual feedback of our readers. We hope this book will help you learn some of the key elements in prescribing medications and allow you to care for your patients in the best way possible.

Leonard G. Gomella, MD, FACS

Philadelphia, Pennsylvania

Leonard.Gomella@jefferson.edu

Steven A. Haist, MD, MS, FACP

Philadelphia, Pennsylvania

Aimee G. Adams, PharmD

Lexington, Kentucky

MEDICATION KEY

Medications are listed by prescribing class and the individual medications are then listed in alphabetical order by generic name. Some of the more commonly recognized trade names are listed for each medication (in parentheses after the generic name) or if available without prescription, noted as **OTC** (over-the-counter).

> **Generic Drug Name (Selected Common Brand Names) [Controlled Substance]** BOX: Summarized/paraphrased versions of the "Black Box" precautions deemed necessary by the FDA. These are significant precautions, warnings, and contraindications concerning the individual medication. **Uses:** This includes both FDA-labeled indications bracketed by ** and other "off-label" uses of the medication. Because many medications are used to treat various conditions based on the medical literature and not listed in their package insert, we list common uses of the medication in addition to the official "labeled indications" (FDA approved) based on input from our editorial board **Acts:** How the drug works. This information is helpful in comparing classes of drugs and understanding side effects and contraindications. *Spectrum:* Specifies activity against selected microbes for antimicrobials **Dose:** *Adults.* Where no specific pediatric dose is given, the implication is that this drug is not commonly used or indicated in that age group. At the end of the dosing line, important dosing modifications may be noted (ie, take with food, avoid antacids, etc) *Peds.* If appropriate, dosing for children and infants is included with age ranges as needed **W/P (Warnings and Precautions):** [pregnancy/fetal risk categories, breast-feeding (as noted below)] Warnings and precautions concerning the use of the drug in specific settings **CI:** Contraindications **Disp:** Common dosing forms **SE:** Common or significant side effects **Notes:** Other key useful information about the drug.

CONTROLLED SUBSTANCE CLASSIFICATION

Medications under the control of the US Drug Enforcement Agency (DEA) (Schedules I–V controlled substances) are indicated by the symbol **[C]**. Most medications are "uncontrolled" and do not require a DEA prescriber number on the prescription. The following is a general description for the schedules of DEA-controlled substances:

Schedule (C-I) I: All nonresearch use forbidden (eg, heroin, LSD, mescaline).
Schedule (C-II) II: High addictive potential; medical use accepted. No telephone call-in prescriptions; no refills. Some states require special prescription form (eg, cocaine, morphine, methadone).
Schedule (C-III) III: Low to moderate risk of physical dependence, high risk of psychological dependence; prescription must be rewritten after 6 months or 5 refills (eg, acetaminophen plus codeine).
Schedule (C-IV) IV: Limited potential for dependence; prescription rules same as for schedule III (eg, benzodiazepines, propoxyphene).
Schedule (C-V) V: Very limited abuse potential; prescribing regulations often same as for uncontrolled medications; some states have additional restrictions.

FDA FETAL RISK CATEGORIES
Category A: Adequate studies in pregnant women have not demonstrated a risk to the fetus in the first trimester of pregnancy; there is no evidence of risk in the last two trimesters.
Category B: Animal studies have not demonstrated a risk to the fetus, but no adequate studies have been done in pregnant women.

or

Animal studies have shown an adverse effect, but adequate studies in pregnant women have not demonstrated a risk to the fetus during the first trimester of pregnancy, and there is no evidence of risk in the last two trimesters.
Category C: Animal studies have shown an adverse effect on the fetus, but no adequate studies have been done in humans. The benefits from the use of the drug in pregnant women may be acceptable despite its potential risks.

or

No animal reproduction studies and no adequate studies in humans have been done.
Category D: There is evidence of human fetal risk, but the potential benefits from the use of the drug in pregnant women may be acceptable despite its potential risks.
Category X: Studies in animals or humans or adverse reaction reports, or both, have demonstrated fetal abnormalities. The risk of use in pregnant women clearly outweighs any possible benefit.
Category ?: No data available (not a formal FDA classification; included to provide complete dataset).

BREAST-FEEDING CLASSIFICATION
No formally recognized classification exists for drugs and breast-feeding. This shorthand was developed for the *Clinician's Pocket Drug Reference*.

+	Compatible with breast-feeding
M	Monitor patient or use with caution
±	Excreted, or likely excreted, with unknown effects or at unknown concentrations
?/–	Unknown excretion, but effects likely to be of concern
–	Contraindicated in breast-feeding
?	No data available

ABBREVIATIONS

Δ: change
?: possible or uncertain
✓: check, follow, or monitor
↓: decrease/decreased
↑: increase/increased
≠: not equal to; not equivalent to
÷: divided
μM: symbol for micromolar
Ab: antibody, abortion
abbrev: abbreviation
Abd: abdominal
ABG: arterial blood gas
ABMT: autologous bone marrow transplantation
abn: abnormal
abx: antibiotics
ac: before meals (*ante cibum*)
ACE: angiotensin-converting enzyme
ACH: acetylcholine
ACIP: American College of International Physicians; Advisory Committee on Immunization Practices
ACLS: advanced cardiac life support
ACS: acute coronary syndrome, American Cancer Society, American College of Surgeons
ACT: activated coagulation time
Acts: Action(s)
ADH: antidiuretic hormone
ADHD: attention-deficit hyperactivity disorder
ADR: adverse drug reaction
ADT: androgen deprivation therapy
AED: anti-epileptic drug
AF: atrial fibrillation

AHA: American Heart Association
AKA: also known as
alk phos: alkaline phosphatase
ALL: acute lymphocytic leukemia
ALT: alanine aminotransferase
AMI: acute myocardial infarction
AML: acute myelogenous leukemia
amp: ampule
ANA: antinuclear antibody
ANC: absolute neutrophil count
antag: antagonist
APACHE: acute physiology and chronic health evaluation
APAP: acetaminophen [*N*-acetyl-*p*-aminophenol]
aPTT: activated partial thromboplastin time
ARB: angiotensin II receptor blocker
ARDS: adult respiratory distress syndrome
ARF: acute renal failure
AS: aortic stenosis
ASA: aspirin (acetylsalicylic acid)
ASAP: as soon as possible
AST: aspartate aminotransferase
ATE: arterial thrombotic event
ATP: adenosine triphosphate
attn: attention
atyp: atypical
AUB: abnormal uterine/vaginal bleeding
AUC: area under the curve
AV: atrioventricular
AVM: arteriovenous malformation
BBB: bundle branch block
BCL: B-cell lymphoma
BCP: birth control pills

bid: twice daily
bili: bilirubin
BM: bone marrow, bowel movement
↓BM: bone marrow suppression, myelosuppression
BMD: bone mineral density
BMI: body mass index
BMT: bone marrow transplantation
BOO: bladder outlet obstruction
BP: blood pressure
↓BP: hypotension
↑BP: hypertension
BPH: benign prostatic hyperplasia
BPM: beats per minute
BSA: body surface area
BUN: blood urea nitrogen
Ca: calcium
CA: cancer
CABG: coronary artery bypass graft
CAD: coronary artery disease
CAP: community-acquired pneumonia
caps: capsule
cardiotox: cardiotoxicity
CBC: complete blood count
CCB: calcium channel blocker
CCR5: human chemokine receptor 5; HIV attaches to the receptor to infect CD4$^+$ T cells
CDC: Centers for Disease Control and Prevention
CF: cystic fibrosis
CFCs: chlorofluorocarbons
CFU: colony-forming units
CHD: coronary heart disease
CHF: congestive heart failure
chol: cholesterol
CI: contraindicated
CIDP: chronic inflammatory polyneuropathy
CIWA: Clinical Institute Withdrawal Assessment Score; used to monitor EtOH withdrawal

CK: creatinine kinase
CLL: chronic lymphocytic leukemia
CML: chronic myelogenous leukemia
CMV: cytomegalovirus
CNS: central nervous system
combo: combination
comp: complicated
conc: concentration
cond: condition
cont: continuous
COPD: chronic obstructive pulmonary disease
COX: cyclooxygenase
CP: chest pain
CPP: central precocious puberty
CR: controlled release
CrCl: creatinine clearance
CRF: chronic renal failure
CRPC: castrate-resistant prostate cancer
CSF: cerebrospinal fluid
CV: cardiovascular
CVA: cerebrovascular accident, costovertebral angle
CVH: common variable hypergammaglobulinemia
CXR: chest x-ray
CYP: cytochrome P450 enzyme
D: diarrhea
d: day
DA: dopamine
DBP: diastolic blood pressure
D/C: discontinue
DDP-4: dipeptidyl peptidase-4
derm: dermatologic
D$_5$LR: 5% dextrose in lactated Ringer solution
D$_5$NS: 5% dextrose in normal saline
D$_5$W: 5% dextrose in water
DHT: dihydrotestosterone

DI: diabetes insipidus

DIC: disseminated intravascular coagulation

Disp: dispensed as; how the drug is supplied

DKA: diabetic ketoacidosis

dL: deciliter

DM: diabetes mellitus

DMARD: disease modifying antirheumatic drug; refers to drugs in randomized trials to decrease erosions and joint space narrowing in rheumatoid arthritis (eg, methotrexate, azathioprine)

DN: diabetic nephropathy

DOT: directly observed therapy (used for TB treatment)

DR: delayed release

DRESS: drug rash with eosinophilia and systemic symptoms

d/t: due to

DTap: Diptheria toxin

DVT: deep venous thrombosis

Dz: disease

EC: enteric coated

ECC: emergency cardiac care

ECG: electrocardiogram

ED: erectile dysfunction

EE: erosive esophagitis

eGFR: estimated glomerular filtration rate

EGFR: epidermal growth factor receptor

EIB: exercise-induced bronchoconstriction

ELISA: enzyme-linked immunosorbent assay

EL.U.: ELISA

EMG: electromyelogram

EMIT: enzyme-multiplied immunoassay test

epi: epinephrine

EPS: extrapyramidal symptoms (tardive dyskinesia, tremors and rigidity, restlessness [akathisia], muscle contractions [dystonia], changes in breathing and heart rate)

ER: extended release

ESA: erythropoiesis-stimulating agents

ESR: erythrocyte sedimentation rate

ESRD: end stage renal disease

ET: endotracheal

EtOH: ethanol

extrav: extravasation

fam: family

FAP: familial adenomatous polyposis

Fe: iron

FLP: fasting lipid profile

FMF: familial Mediterranean fever

FSH: follicle-stimulating hormone

5-FU: fluorouracil

Fxn: function

g: gram

GABA: gamma-aminobutyric acid

GBM: glioblastoma multiforme

GC: gonorrhea

G-CSF: granulocyte colony-stimulating factor

gen: generation

GERD: gastroesophageal reflux disease

GF: growth factor

GFR: glomerular filtration rate

GHB: gamma-hydroxybutyrate

GI: gastrointestinal

GIST: gastrointestinal stromal tumor

GLP-2: glucagon-like peptide-2

glu: glucose

GM-CSF: granulocyte-macrophage colony-stimulating factor

GnRH: gonadotropin-releasing hormone

G6PD: glucose-6-phosphate dehydrogenase

gtt: drop, drops (*gutta*)

GU: genitourinary

GVHD: graft-versus-host disease

h: hour(s)

H1N1: swine flu strain

HA: headache

HAE: hereditary angioedema

HBsAg: hepatitis B surface antigen

HBV: hepatitis B virus

HCL: hairy cell leukemia

HCM: hypercalcemia of malignancy

Hct: hematocrit

HCTZ: hydrochlorothiazide

HD: hemodialysis

HDL-C: high-density lipoprotein cholesterol

heme: hematologic

hep: hepatitis

hepatotox: hepatotoxicity

HFA: hydrofluroalkane chemicals; propellant replacing CFCs in inhalers

HFSR: hand-foot skin reaction

Hgb: hemoglobin

HGH: human growth hormone

HIT: heparin-induced thrombocytopenia

HITTS: heparin-induced thrombosis-thrombocytopenia syndrome

HIV: human immunodeficiency virus

HMG-CoA: hydroxymethylglutaryl coenzyme A

h/o: history of

HP: high potency

HPV: human papillomavirus

HR: heart rate

↑ HR: increased heart rate (tachycardia)

hs: at bedtime (*hora somni*)

HSCT: hematopoietic stem cell transplantation

HSV: herpes simplex virus

5-HT: 5-hydroxytryptamine

HTN: hypertension

Hx: history of

hypersens: hypersensitivity

IBD: irritable bowel disease

IBS: irritable bowel syndrome

IBW: ideal body weight

ICP: intracranial pressure

IFIS: intraoperative floppy iris syndrome

Ig: immunoglobulin

IGF: insulin-like growth factor

IHSS: idiopathic hypertropic subaortic stenosis

IL: interleukin

IM: intramuscular

impair: impairment

in: inches

Inf: infusion

inflam: inflammation

Infxn: infection

Inh: inhalation

INH: isoniazid

inhal: inhalation

inhib: inhibits, inhibitor(s)

Inj: injection

INR: international normalized ratio

Insuff: insufficiency

Int: international

intol: intolerence

Intravag: intravaginal

IO: intraosseous

IOP: intraocular pressure

IR: immediate release

ISA: intrinsic sympathomimetic activity

IT: intrathecal

ITP: idiopathic thrombocytopenic purpura

Int units: international units

IUD: intrauterine device

IV: intravenous

JME: juvenile myoclonic epilepsy

JRA: juvenile rheumatoid arthritis (SJIA now preferred)

jt: joint

K: klebsiella

K+: potassium

L&D: labor and delivery

LA: long-acting

LABA: long-acting beta₂-adrenergic agonists

LAIV: live attenuated influenza vaccine

LDL: low-density lipoprotein

LFT: liver function test

LH: luteinizing hormone

LHRH: luteinizing hormone-releasing hormone

liq: liquid(s)

LMW: low molecular weight

LP: lumbar puncture

LR: lactated ringers

LVD: left ventricular dysfunction

LVEF: left ventricular ejection fraction

LVSD: left ventricular systolic dysfunction

lytes: electrolytes

MAC: *Mycobacterium avium complex*

maint: maintenance dose/drug

MAO/MAOI: monoamine oxidase/ inhibitor

max: maximum

mcg: microgram(s)

mcL: microliter(s)

MDD: major depressive disorder

MDI: multidose inhaler

MDS: myelodysplasia syndrome

meds: medicines

mEq: milliequivalent

met: metastatic

mg: milligram(s)

Mg²⁺: magnesium

MgOH₂: magnesium hydroxide

MI: myocardial infarction, mitral insufficiency

mill: million

min: minute(s)

mL: milliliter(s)

mo: month(s)

MoAb: monoclonal antibody

mod: moderate

MRSA: methicillin-resistant *Staphylococcus aureus*

MS: multiple sclerosis, musculoskeletal

ms: millisecond(s)

MSSA: methicillin-sensitive *Staphylococcus aureus*

MTC: medullary thyroid cancer

MTT: monotetrazolium

MTX: methotrexate

MyG: myasthenia gravis

N: nausea

NA: narrow angle

NAG: narrow angle glaucoma

NCI: National Cancer Institute

nephrotox: nephrotoxicity

neurotox: neurotoxicity

ng: nanogram(s)

NG: nasogastric

NHL: non-Hodgkin lymphoma

NIAON: nonischemic arterial optic neuritis

nl: normal

NO: nitric oxide

NPO: nothing by mouth (*nil per os*)

NRTI: nucleoside reverse transcriptase inhibitor

NS: normal saline

NSAID: nonsteroidal anti-inflammatory drug

NSCLC: non-small cell lung cancer

NSR: normal sinus rhythm

NSTEMI: non-ST elevation myocardial infarction

N/V: nausea and vomiting
N/V/D: nausea, vomiting, diarrhea
NYHA: New York Heart Association
OA: osteoarthritis
OAB: overactive bladder
obst: obstruction
OCD: obsessive compulsive disease
OCP: oral contraceptive pill
OD: overdose
ODT: orally disintegrating tablets
oint: ointment
OK: recommended
ONJ: osteonecrosis of jaw
op: operative
ophthal: ophthalmic
OSAHS: obstructive sleep apnea/
    hypopnea syndrome
OTC: over-the-counter
ototox: ototoxicity
oz: ounces
PAT: paroxysmal atrial tachycardia
pc: after eating (*post cibum*)
PCa: cancer of the prostate
PCC: Prothrombin Complex
    Concentrate
PCI: percutaneous coronary
    intervention
PCN: penicillin
PCP: *Pneumocystis jiroveci* (formerly
    carinii) pneumonia
PCWP: pulmonary capillary wedge
    pressure
PDE5: phosphodiesterase type 5
PDGF: platelet-derived growth factor
PE: pulmonary embolus, physical
    examination, pleural effusion
PEA: pulseless electrical activity
PEG: polyethylene glycol
perf: perforation
PFT: pulmonary function test
pg: picogram(s)
PGE-1: prostaglandin E-1

PGTC: primary generalized
    tonic-clonic (PGTC)
Ph: Philadelphia chromosome
Pheo: pheochromocytoma
photosens: photosensitivity
PI: product insert (package label)
PID: pelvic inflammatory disease
pkg: package
PKU: phenylketonuria
plt: platelet
PMDD: premenstrual dysphoric
    disorder
PML: progressive multifocal
    leukoencephalopathy
PMS: premenstrual syndrome
PO: by mouth (*per os*)
PPD: purified protein derivative
PPI: proton pump inhibitor
PR: by rectum
PrEP: pre-exposure prophylaxis; a
    safer sex practice to reduce the risk
    of sexually acquired HIV-1 in adults
    at high risk
PRG: pregnancy
PRN: as often as needed (*pro re nata*)
PSA: prostate-specific antigen
PSVT: paroxysmal supraventricular
    tachycardia
pt: patient
PT: prothrombin time
PTCA: percutaneous transluminal
    coronary angioplasty
PTH: parathyroid hormone
PTSD: post-traumatic stress disorder
PTT: partial thromboplastin time
PUD: peptic ulcer disease
pulm: pulmonary
PVC: premature ventricular contraction
PVD: peripheral vascular disease
PWP: pulmonary wedge pressure
Px: prevention
pyelo: pyelonephritis

q: every (*quaque*)

q_h: every _ hours

qd: every day

qh: every hour

qhs: every hour of sleep (before bedtime)

qid: four times a day (*quater in die*)

q other day: every other day

QRS: electrocardiogram complex

QT: time from the start of QRS complex to the end of T wave on an electrocardiogram

QTc: QT interval on ECG

RA: rheumatoid arthritis

RAS: renin-angiotensin system

RBC: red blood cell(s) (count)

RCC: renal cell carcinoma

RDA: recommended dietary allowance

RDS: respiratory distress syndrome

rec: recommends

REMS: risk evaluation and mitigation strategy; FDA plan to help ensure that the drug's benefits outweigh its risks. As part of that plan, the company must conduct educational outreach

resp: respiratory

RHuAb: recombinant human antibody

RIA: radioimmune assay

RLS: restless leg syndrome

R/O, r/o: rule out

RPLS: reversible posterior leukoencephalopathy syndrome

RR: respiratory rate

RSI: rapid sequence intubation

RSV: respiratory syncytial virus

RT: reverse transcriptase

RTA: renal tubular acidosis

Rx: prescription or therapy

Rxn: reaction

s: second(s)

SAD: social anxiety disorder or seasonal affective disorder

SAE: serious adverse event

SBE: subacute bacterial endocarditis

SBP: systolic blood pressure

SCLC: small cell lung cancer

SCr: serum creatinine

SDV: single-dose vial

SE: side effect(s)

SGLT2: sodium glucose co-transporter 2

SIADH: syndrome of inappropriate antidiuretic hormone

sig: significant

SIRS: systemic inflammatory response syndrome/capillary leak syndrome

SJIA: systemic juvenile idiopathic arthritis

SJS: Stevens-Johnson syndrome

SL: sublingual

SLE: systemic lupus erythematosus

SLUDGE: mnemonic for: Salivation, Lacrimation, Urination, Diaphoresis, GI motility, Emesis

SMX: sulfmethoxazole

SNRIs: serotonin-norepinephrine reuptake inhibitors

SOB: shortness of breath

soln: solution

sp: species

SPAG: small particle aerosol generator

SQ: subcutaneous

SR: sustained release

SSRI: selective serotonin reuptake inhibitor

SSS: sick sinus syndrome

S/Sxs: signs & symptoms

stat: immediately (*statim*)

STD: sexually transmitted disease

STEMI: ST elevation myocardial infarction

subs: substances
supl: supplement
supp: suppository
susp: suspension
SVT: supraventricular tachycardia
SWFI: sterile water for injection
SWSD: shift work sleep disorder
Sx: symptom
synth: synthesis
synd: syndrome
Sz: seizure
tab/tabs: tablet/tablets
TB: tuberculosis
TCA: tricyclic antidepressant
TE: thromboembolic event
TEN: toxic epidermal necrolysis
TFT: thyroid function test
TG: triglycerides
TIA: transient ischemic attack
tid: three times a day (*ter in die*)
TIV: trivalent influenza vaccine
TKI: tyrosine kinase inhibitors
TMP: trimethoprim
TMP-SMX: trimethoprim-
    sulfamethoxazole
TNF: tumor necrosis factor
TOUCH: Tysabri Outreach Unified
    Commitment to Health
tox: toxicity
TPA: tissue plasminogen activator
TRALI: transfusion-related acute
    lung injury
tri: trimester
TSH: thyroid-stimulating hormone
TTP: thrombotic thrombocytopenic
    purpura
TTS: transdermal therapeutic system
Tx: treatment
UC: ulcerative colitis

UGT: uridine 5′
    diphosphoglucuronosyl transferase
ULN: upper limits of normal
uncomp: uncomplicated
URI: upper respiratory infection
US: United States
UTI: urinary tract infection
V: vomiting
VAERS: Vaccine Adverse Events
    Reporting System
Vag: vaginal
VEGF: vascular endothelial growth
    factor
VF: ventricular fibrillation
vit: vitamin
VKA: vitamin K antagonist
VLDL: very-low-density lipoprotein
VOD: venoocclusive disease
vol: volume
VPA: valproic acid
VRE: vancomycin-resistant
    Enterococcus
VT: ventricular tachycardia
VTE: venous thromboembolism
w/: with
WBC: white blood cell(s) (count)
WHI: Women's Health Initiative
WHIMS: Women's Health Initiative
    Memory Study
w/in: within
wk: week(s)
WNL: within normal limits
w/o: without
W/P: warnings and precautions
WPW: Wolff–Parkinson–White
    syndrome
Wt: weight
XR: extended release
ZE: Zollinger–Ellison (syndrome)

CLASSIFICATION (Generic and common brand names)

ALLERGY

Antihistamines

Azelastine (Astelin, Optivar)
Cetirizine (Zyrtec, Zyrtec-D)
Chlorpheniramine (Chlor-Trimeton)

Clemastine fumarate (Tavist)
Cyproheptadine (Periactin)
Desloratadine (Clarinex)
Diphenhydramine (Benadryl)

Fexofenadine (Allegra, Allegra-D, generic)
Hydroxyzine (Atarax, Vistaril)
Levocetirizine (Xyzal)
Loratadine (Alavert, Claritin)

Miscellaneous Antiallergy Agents

Budesonide (Rhinocort, Pulmicort)
Cromolyn sodium (Intal, NasalCrom, Opticrom)

Montelukast (Singulair, generic)

Phenylephrine, oral (Sudafed, others [OTC])

ANTIDOTES

Acetylcysteine (Acetadote, Mucomyst)
Amifostine (Ethyol)
Atropine, systemic (AtroPen Auto-Injector)
Atropine/pralidoxime (DuoDote Auto-Injector)
Centruroides (scorpion) immune F(ab')2 (Anascorp)

Charcoal, activated (Actidose Aqua, CharcoCaps, EZ Char, Kerr Insta-Char, Requa Activated Charcoal)
Deferasirox (Exjade)
Dexrazoxane (Totect, Zinecard)
Digoxin immune Fab (Digibind, DigiFab)
Flumazenil (Romazicon, generic)
Glucarpidase (Voraxaze)

Hydroxocobalamin (Cyanokit)
Iodine [potassium iodide] (Lugol's Solution, SSKI, Thyro-Block, ThyroSafe, ThyroShield) [OTC]
Mesna (Mesnex [oral], generic [inf])
Methylene blue (Urolene Blue, various)
Naloxone (generic)
Physostigmine (generic)
Succimer (Chemet)

1

ANTIMICROBIAL AGENTS

Antibiotics

AMINOGLYCOSIDES

Amikacin (Amikin)
Gentamicin, injectable (generic)

Neomycin sulfate (Neo-Fradin, generic)
Streptomycin (generic)
Tobramycin (Nebcin)

Tobramycin, inhalation (TOBI, TOBI Podhaler)

CARBAPENEMS

Doripenem (Doribax)
Ertapenem (Invanz)

Imipenem-cilastatin (Primaxin, generic)

Meropenem (Merrem, generic)

CEPHALOSPORINS, FIRST-GENERATION

Cefadroxil (Duricef, Ultracef)

Cefazolin (Ancef, Kefzol)

Cephalexin (Keflex, generic)

CEPHALOSPORINS, SECOND-GENERATION

Cefaclor (Ceclor, Raniclor)
Cefotetan

Cefoxitin (Mefoxin)
Cefprozil (Cefzil)

Cefuroxime (Ceftin [oral], Zinacef [parenteral])

CEPHALOSPORINS, THIRD-GENERATION

Cefdinir (Omnicef)
Cefditoren (Spectracef)
Cefotaxime (Claforan)
Cefpodoxime (Vantin)

Ceftazidime (Fortaz, Ceptaz, Tazidime, Tazicef)

Ceftibuten (Cedax)
Ceftriaxone (Rocephin)

CEPHALOSPORINS, FOURTH-GENERATION

Cefepime (Maxipime)

CEPHALOSPORINS, UNCLASSIFIED ("FIFTH-GENERATION")

Ceftaroline (Teflaro)

FLUOROQUINOLONES

Ciprofloxacin (Cipro, Cipro XR)
Gemifloxacin (Factive)
Levofloxacin (Levaquin, generic)

Moxifloxacin (Avelox)
Norfloxacin (Noroxin, Chibroxin Ophthalmic)

Ofloxacin (generic)

KETOLIDE
Telithromycin (Ketek)

MACROLIDES
Azithromycin (Zithromax)

Clarithromycin (Biaxin, Biaxin XL)

Erythromycin (E-Mycin, E.E.S., Ery-Tab, EryPed, Ilotycin)

Erythromycin and sulfisoxazole (E.S.P.)

PENICILLINS
Amoxicillin (Amoxil, Moxatag)

Amoxicillin and clavulanate potassium (Augmentin, Augmentin ES-600, Augmentin XR)

Ampicillin

Ampicillin/sulbactam (Unasyn)

Dicloxacillin (Dynapen, Dycill)

Nafcillin (Nallpen, generic)

Oxacillin (generic)

Penicillin G, aqueous (potassium or sodium) (Pfizerpen, Pentids)

Penicillin G benzathine (Bicillin)

Penicillin G procaine (Wycillin, others)

Penicillin V (Pen-Vee K, Veetids, others)

Piperacillin/tazobactam (Zosyn, generic)

Ticarcillin/clavulanate potassium (Timentin)

TETRACYCLINES
Doxycycline (Adoxa, Periostat, Oracea, Vibramycin, Vibra-Tabs)

Minocycline (Dynacin, Minocin, Solodyn)

Tetracycline (generic)

Tigecycline (Tygacil)

Miscellaneous Antibiotic Agents
Aztreonam (Azactam)

Clindamycin (Cleocin, Cleocin T, others)

Fosfomycin (Monurol)

Linezolid (Zyvox)

Metronidazole (Flagyl, MetroGel)

Mupirocin (Bactroban, Bactroban Nasal)

Neomycin topical (*See* bacitracin/neomycin/ polymyxin B, topical [Neosporin ointment]; bacitracin/neomycin/ polymyxin B/ hydrocortisone, topical [Cortisporin])

Nitrofurantoin (Furadantin, Macrobid, Macrodantin, generic)

Quinupristin/dalfopristin (Synercid)

Retapamulin (Altabax)

Rifaximin (Xifaxan)

Telavancin (Vibativ)

Trimethoprim (Primsol, generic)

Trimethoprim (TMP)/ sulfamethoxazole (SMX)

[Co-Trimoxazole, TMP-SMX] (Bactrim, Bactrim DS, Septra DS, generic)

Vancomycin (Vancocin, generic)

Antifungals

Amphotericin B (Fungizone)
Amphotericin B cholesteryl (Amphotec)
Amphotericin B lipid complex (Abelcet)
Amphotericin B liposomal (AmBisome)
Anidulafungin (Eraxis)
Caspofungin (Cancidas)
Clotrimazole (Lotrimin, Mycelex, others) [OTC]
Clotrimazole/ betamethasone (Lotrisone)

Econazole (Spectazole)
Fluconazole (Diflucan, generic)
Itraconazole (Onmel, Sporanox, generic Caps)
Ketoconazole, oral (Nizoral)
Ketoconazole, topical (Extina, Kuric, Xolegel, Nizoral A-D shampoo) [shampoo OTC]
Micafungin (Mycamine)
Miconazole (Monistat 1 combination pack, Monistat 3, Monistat 7)

[OTC], (Monistat-Derm)
Nystatin (Mycostatin, Nilstat, Nystop)
Oxiconazole (Oxistat)
Posaconazole (Noxafil)
Sertaconazole (Ertaczo)
Terbinafine (Lamisil, Lamisil AT, generic [OTC])
Triamcinolone/nystatin (Mycolog-II)
Voriconazole (Vfend, generic)

Antimycobacterials

Bedaquiline fumarate (Sirturo)
Dapsone, oral
Ethambutol (Myambutol, generic)

Isoniazid (INH)
Pyrazinamide (generic)
Rifabutin (Mycobutin)
Rifampin (Rifadin, Rimactane, generic)

Rifapentine (Priftin)
Streptomycin

Antiparasitics

Benzyl alcohol (Ulesfia)
Ivermectin, oral (Stromectol)

Ivermectin, topical (Sklice)
Lindane (Kwell, others)

Spinosad (Natroba)

Antiprotozoals

Artemether/lumefantrine (Coartem)
Atovaquone (Mepron)

Atovaquone/proguanil (Malarone)
Hydroxychloroquine (Plaquenil, generic)

Nitazoxanide (Alinia)
Tinidazole (Tindamax, generic)

Antiretrovirals

Abacavir (Ziagen)
Daptomycin (Cubicin)
Darunavir (Prezista)
Delavirdine (Rescriptor)
Didanosine [ddI] (Videx)
Efavirenz (Sustiva)
Efavirenz/emtricitabine/
  tenofovir (Atripla)
Etravirine (Intelence)
Fosamprenavir (Lexiva)
Indinavir (Crixivan)

Lamivudine (Epivir,
  Epivir-HBV, 3TC
  [many combo
  regimens])
Lopinavir/ritonavir
  (Kaletra)
Maraviroc (Selzentry)
Nelfinavir (Viracept)
Nevirapine (Viramune,
  Viramune XR, generic)
Raltegravir (Isentress)

Rilpivirine (Edurant)
Ritonavir (Norvir)
Saquinavir (Invirase)
Stavudine (Zerit, generic)
Tenofovir (Viread)
Tenofovir/emtricitabine
  (Truvada)
Zidovudine (Retrovir,
  generic)
Zidovudine/lamivudine
  (Combivir, generic)

Antivirals

Acyclovir (Zovirax)
Adefovir (Hepsera)
Amantadine (Symmetrel)
Atazanavir (Reyataz)
Boceprevir (Victrelis)
Cidofovir (Vistide)
Emtricitabine (Emtriva)
Enfuvirtide (Fuzeon)
Famciclovir (Famvir,
  generic)

Foscarnet (Foscavir,
  generic)
Ganciclovir (Cytovene,
  Vitrasert)
Oseltamivir (Tamiflu)
Palivizumab (Synagis)
Peginterferon alfa-2b
  (PegIntron)
Penciclovir (Denavir)

Ribavirin (Copegus,
  Rebetol, Virazole,
  generic)
Rimantadine (Flumadine,
  generic)
Telaprevir (Incivek)
Telbivudine (Tyzeka)
Valacyclovir (Valtrex,
  generic)
Valganciclovir (Valcyte)
Zanamivir (Relenza)

Miscellaneous Antiviral Agents

Daptomycin (Cubicin)
Pentamidine (Pentam
  300, NebuPent)

ANTINEOPLASTIC AGENTS

Alkylating Agents

Altretamine (Hexalen)
Bendamustine (Treanda)
Busulfan (Myleran,
  Busulfex)
Carboplatin (Paraplatin)
Cisplatin (Platinol,
  Platinol-AQ)

Oxaliplatin (Eloxatin,
  generic)
Procarbazine (Matulane)
Streptozocin (Zanosar)
Tapentadol (Nucynta)
Temozolomide
  (Temodar, generic)

Triethylenethiophos-
  phoramide (Thiotepa,
  Thioplex, Tespa,
  TSPA)

NITROGEN MUSTARDS

Chlorambucil (Leukeran)
Cyclophosphamide (Cytoxan, Neosar)
Ifosfamide (Ifex, generic)
Mechlorethamine (Mustargen)
Melphalan [L-PAM] (Alkeran, generic)

NITROSOUREAS

Carmustine [BCNU] (BiCNU, Gliadel)
Streptozocin (Zanosar)

Antibiotics

Bleomycin sulfate (generic)
Dactinomycin (Cosmegen)
Daunorubicin (Cerubidine)
Doxorubicin (Adriamycin, Rubex)
Epirubicin (Ellence)
Idarubicin (Idamycin, generic)
Mitomycin (Mitosol [topical], generic)

Antimetabolites

Clofarabine (Clolar)
Cytarabine [Ara-C] (Cytosar-U)
Cytarabine liposome (DepoCyt)
Floxuridine (generic)
Fludarabine phosphate (Fludara)
Fluorouracil [5-FU] (generic)
Fluorouracil, topical [5-FU] (Carac, Efudex, Fluoroplex, generic)
Gemcitabine (Gemzar, generic)
Mercaptopurine [6-MP] (Purinethol, generic)
Methotrexate (Rheumatrex Dose Pack, Trexall)
Nelarabine (Arranon)
Omacetaxine (Synribo)
Pemetrexed (Alimta)
Pralatrexate (Folotyn)
Romidepsin (Istodax)
Thioguanine (Tabloid)

Hedgehog Pathway Inhibitor

Vismodegib (Erivedge)

Hormones

Abiraterone (Zytiga)
Anastrozole (Arimidex)
Bicalutamide (Casodex)
Degarelix (Firmagon)
Enzalutamide (Xtandi)
Estramustine phosphate (Emcyt)
Exemestane (Aromasin, generic)
Flutamide (generic)
Fulvestrant (Faslodex)
Goserelin (Zoladex)
Histrelin acetate (Supprelin LA, Vantas)
Leuprolide (Eligard, Lupron, Lupron DEPOT, Lupron DEPOT-Ped, generic)
Megestrol acetate (Megace, Megace ES)
Nilutamide (Nilandron)
Tamoxifen
Triptorelin (Trelstar 3.75, Trelstar 11.25, Trelstar 22.5)

Immunotherapy

BCG [Bacillus Calmette-Guérin] (TheraCys, Tice BCG)

Interferon alfa (Roferon-A, Intron A)

Sipuleucel-T (Provenge)

Mitotic Inhibitors (Vinca Alkaloids)

Etoposide [VP-16] (Etopophos, Toposar, Vepesid, generic)

Vinblastine (generic)
Vincristine (Marqibo, Vincasar, generic)

Vinorelbine (Navelbine, generic)

Monoclonal Antibodies

Alemtuzumab (Campath relaunch as Lemtrada)
Belimumab (Benlysta)
Bevacizumab (Avastin)

Brentuximab vedotin (Adcetris)
Cetuximab (Erbitux)
Ipilimumab (Yervoy)

Ofatumumab (Arzerra)
Panitumumab (Vectibix)
Pertuzumab (Perjeta)
Trastuzumab (Herceptin)

Proteasome Inhibitor

Bortezomib (Velcade)

Taxanes

Cabazitaxel (Jevtana)
Docetaxel (Taxotere)

Paclitaxel (Abraxane, Taxol, generic)

Tyrosine Kinase Inhibitors (TKIs)

Axitinib (Inlyta)
Bosutinib monohydrate (Bosulif)
Cabozantinib (Cometriq)
Crizotinib (Xalkori)
Dasatinib (Sprycel)

Erlotinib (Tarceva)
Everolimus (Afinitor)
Imatinib (Gleevec)
Lapatinib (Tykerb)
Nilotinib (Tasigna)
Pazopanib (Votrient)

Regorafenib (Stivarga)
Sorafenib (Nexavar)
Sunitinib (Sutent)
Temsirolimus (Torisel)
Vandetanib (Caprelsa)

Miscellaneous Antineoplastic Agents

Aldesleukin [Interleukin-2, IL-2] (Proleukin)
Aminoglutethimide (Cytadren)
ʟ-Asparaginase (Elspar)

Carfilzomib (Kyprolis)
Cladribine (Leustatin)
Dacarbazine (DTIC)
Eribulin (Halaven)
Hydroxyurea (Droxia, Hydrea, generic)

Irinotecan (Camptosar, generic)
Ixabepilone (Ixempra Kit)
Letrozole (Femara)
Leucovorin (generic)
Mitoxantrone (generic)

Panitumumab (Vectibix)
Pemetrexed (Alimta)
Pertuzumab (Perjeta)
Pomalidomide (Pomalyst)
Rasburicase (Elitek)

Sipuleucel-T (Provenge)
Thalidomide (Thalomid)
Topotecan (Hycamtin, generic)

Tretinoin, topical [retinoic acid] (Retin-A, Avita, Renova, Retin-A Micro)
Ziv-Aflibercept (Zaltrap)

CARDIOVASCULAR (CV) AGENTS

Aldosterone Antagonists

Eplerenone (Inspra)

Spironolactone (Aldactone)

Alpha₁-Adrenergic Blockers

Doxazosin (Cardura, Cardura XL)

Prazosin (Minipress, generic)

Terazosin (Hytrin, generic)

Angiotensin-Converting Enzyme (ACE) Inhibitors

Benazepril (Lotensin)
Captopril (Capoten, others)
Enalapril (Vasotec)
Fosinopril (Monopril, generic)

Lisinopril (Prinivil, Zestril)
Moexipril (Univasc, generic)
Perindopril erbumine (Aceon, generic)

Quinapril (Accupril, generic)
Ramipril (Altace, generic)
Trandolapril (Mavik, generic)

Angiotensin II Receptor Antagonists/Blockers (ARBs)

Amlodipine/olmesartan (Azor)
Amlodipine/valsartan (Exforge)
Azilsartan (Edarbi)

Azilsartan and chlorthalidone (Edarbyclor)
Candesartan (Atacand)
Eprosartan (Teveten)

Irbesartan (Avapro)
Losartan (Cozaar)
Telmisartan (Micardis)
Valsartan (Diovan)

Antiarrhythmic Agents

Adenosine (Adenocard, Adenoscan)
Amiodarone (Cordarone, Nexterone, Pacerone)
Atropine, systemic (AtroPen Auto-Injector)
Digoxin (Digitek, Lanoxin, Lanoxicaps)

Disopyramide (Norpace, Norpace CR)
Dofetilide (Tikosyn)
Dronedarone (Multaq)
Esmolol (Brevibloc, generic)
Flecainide (Tambocor, generic)
Ibutilide (Corvert, generic)

Lidocaine, systemic (Xylocaine, others)
Mexiletine (generic)
Procainamide (generic)
Propafenone (Rythmol, Rhythmol SR, generic)
Quinidine (generic)
Sotalol (Betapace, Sorine, generic)

Beta-Adrenergic Blockers

Acebutolol (Sectral)
Atenolol (Tenormin)
Atenolol/chlorthalidone (Tenoretic)
Betaxolol (Kerlone)
Bisoprolol (Zebeta)
Carvedilol (Coreg, Coreg CR)

Labetalol (Trandate, Normodyne)
Metoprolol succinate (Toprol XL, generic)
Metoprolol tartrate (Lopressor, generic)
Nadolol (Corgard, generic)

Nebivolol (Bystolic)
Penbutolol (Levatol)
Pindolol (generic)
Propranolol (Inderal LA, Innopran XL, generic)
Timolol (generic)

Calcium Channel Antagonists/Blockers (CCBs)

Amlodipine (Norvasc)
Amlodipine/olmesartan (Azor)
Amlodipine/valsartan (Exforge)
Clevidipine (Cleviprex)
Diltiazem (Cardizem, Cardizem CD, Cardizem LA, Cardizem SR, Cartia XT, Dilacor XR, Diltia

XT, Taztia XT, Tiamate, Tiazac)
Felodipine (Plendil, generic)
Isradipine (DynaCirc, generic)
Nicardipine (Cardene, Cardene SR, generic)
Nifedipine (Adalat CC, Afeditab CR,

Procardia, Procardia XL, generic)
Nimodipine (generic)
Nisoldipine (Sular, generic)
Verapamil (Calan, Covera HS, Isoptin, Verelan, generic)

Centrally Acting Antihypertensive Agents

Clonidine, oral (Catapres)

Clonidine, transdermal (Catapres-TTS)
Guanfacine (Tenex)

Methyldopa (generic)

Combination Antihypertensive Agents

Aliskiren/amlodipine (Tekamlo)
Aliskiren/amlodipine/ hydrochlorothiazide (Amturnide)
Amlodipine/valsartan/ hydrochlorothiazide (Exforge HCT)

Lisinopril/ hydrochlorothiazide (Prinzide, Zestoretic, generic)
Olmesartan, amlodipine, hydrochlorothiazide (Tribenzor)

Olmesartan, olmesartan/ hydrochlorothiazine (Benicar, Benicar HCT)
Telmisartan/amlodipine (Twynsta)

Diuretics

Acetazolamide (Diamox)
Amiloride (Midamor)
Bumetanide (Bumex)
Chlorothiazide (Diuril)
Chlorthalidone
Furosemide (Lasix, generic)
Hydrochlorothiazide (HydroDIURIL, Esidrix, others)
Hydrochlorothiazide/amiloride (Moduretic)
Hydrochlorothiazide/spironolactone (Aldactazide)
Hydrochlorothiazide/triamterene (Dyazide, Maxzide)
Indapamide (Lozol)
Mannitol, intravenous (generic)
Metolazone (Zaroxolyn, generic)
Spironolactone (Aldactone, generic)
Torsemide (Demadex, generic)
Triamterene (Dyrenium)

Inotropic/Pressor Agents

Digoxin (Digitek, Lanoxin, Lanoxicaps)
Dobutamine (Dobutrex)
Dopamine (Intropin)
Epinephrine (Adrenalin, EpiPen, EpiPen Jr, others)
Inamrinone [amrinone] (Inocor)
Isoproterenol (Isuprel)
Midodrine (Proamatine)
Milrinone (Primacor, generic)
Nesiritide (Natrecor)
Norepinephrine (Levophed)
Phenylephrine, systemic (generic)

Lipid-Lowering Agents

Cholestyramine (Questran, Questran Light, Prevalite)
Colesevelam (WelChol)
Colestipol (Colestid)
Ezetimibe (Zetia)
Fenofibrate (Antara, Lipofen, Lofibra, TriCor, Triglide, generic)
Fenofibric acid (Fibricor, Trilipix, generic)
Gemfibrozil (Lopid, generic)
Icosapent ethyl (Vascepa)
Lomitapide (Juxtapid)
Mipomersen (Kynamro)
Niacin [nicotinic acid] (Niaspan, Slo-Niacin, Niacor, Nicolar) [OTC forms]
Niacin/lovastatin (Advicor)
Niacin/simvastatin (Simcor)
Omega-3 fatty acid [fish oil] (Lovaza)

Statins

Atorvastatin (Lipitor)
Fluvastatin (Lescol, generic)
Lovastatin (Mevacor, Altoprev)
Pitavastatin (Livalo)
Pravastatin (Pravachol, generic)
Rosuvastatin (Crestor)
Simvastatin (Zocor)

Statin/Antihypertensive Combinations

Amlodipine/atorvastatin
(Caduet)

Vasodilators

Alprostadil
[prostaglandin E₁]
(Prostin VR)
Epoprostenol (Veletri,
Flolan)
Fenoldopam (Corlopam,
generic)
Hydralazine (Apresoline,
others)
Iloprost (Ventavis)

Isosorbide dinitrate
(Dilatrate-SR, Isordil,
Sorbitrate, generic)
Isosorbide mononitrate
(Ismo, Imdur,
Monoket, generic)
Minoxidil, oral (generic)
Nitroglycerin (Nitrostat,
Nitrolingual,
Nitro-Bid Ointment,

Nitro-Bid IV,
Nitrodisc,
Transderm-Nitro,
NitroMist, others)
Nitroprusside
(Nitropress)
Treprostinil sodium
(Remodulin, Tyvaso)

Miscellaneous Cardiovascular Agents

Aliskiren (Tekturna)
Aliskiren/
hydrochlorothiazide
(Tekturna HCT)

Ambrisentan (Letairis)
Conivaptan (Vaprisol)
Dabigatran (Pradaxa)
Prasugrel (Effient)

Ranolazine (Ranexa)
Sildenafil (Viagra,
Revatio)

CENTRAL NERVOUS SYSTEM (CNS) AGENTS

Alzheimer Agents

Donepezil (Aricept)
Galantamine (Razadyne,
Razadyne ER)
Memantine (Namenda)

Rivastigmine (Exelon,
generic)

Rivastigmine,
transdermal (Exelon
Patch, generic)

Antianxiety Agents

Alprazolam (Xanax,
Niravam)
Buspirone (generic)
Chlordiazepoxide
(Librium) [C-IV]
Diazepam (Diastat,
Valium)

Doxepin (Sinequan,
Adapin)
Hydroxyzine (Atarax,
Vistaril, generic)
Lorazepam (Ativan,
others)

Meprobamate (generic)
[C-IV]
Oxazepam (generic)
[C-IV]

Anticonvulsants

Carbamazepine (Tegretol XR, Carbatrol, Epitol, Equetro)
Clonazepam (Klonopin)
Clobazam (Onfi)
Diazepam (Diastat, Valium)
Ethosuximide (Zarontin)
Ezogabine (Potiga)
Fosphenytoin (Cerebyx, generic)
Gabapentin (Neurontin, generic)
Lacosamide (Vimpat)
Lamotrigine (Lamictal)

Lamotrigine, extended-release (Lamictal XR)
Levetiracetam (Keppra, Keppra XR)
Lorazepam (Ativan, others)
Magnesium sulfate (various)
Oxcarbazepine (Oxtellar XR, Trileptal, generic)
Pentobarbital (Nembutal) [C-II]
Perampanel (Fycompa)

Phenobarbital (generic) [C-IV]
Phenytoin (Dilantin, generic)
Rufinamide (Banzel)
Tiagabine (Gabitril, generic)
Topiramate (Topamax, generic)
Valproic acid (Depakene, Depakote, Stavzor, generic)
Vigabatrin (Sabril)
Zonisamide (Zonegran, generic)

Antidepressants

MONOAMINE OXIDASE INHIBITORS (MAOIs)

Phenelzine (Nardil, generic)
Selegiline, oral (Eldepryl, Zelapar, generic)

Selegiline, transdermal (Emsam)

Tranylcypromine (Parnate)

SELECTIVE SEROTONIN REUPTAKE INHIBITORS (SSRIs)

Citalopram (Celexa)
Escitalopram (Lexapro, generic)
Fluoxetine (Gaboxetine, Prozac, Prozac Weekly, Sarafem, generic)

Fluvoxamine (Luvox CR, generic)
Paroxetine (Paxil, Paxil CR, Pexeva, generic)

Sertraline (Zoloft)

SEROTONIN-NOREPINEPHRINE REUPTAKE INHIBITORS (SNRIs)

Desvenlafaxine (Pristiq)
Duloxetine (Cymbalta)

Venlafaxine (Effexor, Effexor XR, generic)

TRICYCLIC ANTIDEPRESSANTS (TCAs)

Amitriptyline (Elavil)
Desipramine (Norpramin)

Doxepin (Adapin)
Imipramine (Tofranil, generic)

Nortriptyline (Aventyl, Pamelor)

MISCELLANEOUS ANTIDEPRESSANTS

Bupropion hydrobromide (Aplenzin)
Bupropion hydrochloride (Wellbutrin, Wellbutrin SR, Wellbutrin XL, Zyban)

Milnacipran (Savella)
Mirtazapine (Remeron, Remeron SolTab, generic)

Nefazodone (generic)
Trazodone (Oleptro, generic)
Vilazodone (Viibryd)

Antiparkinson Agents

Amantadine (Symmetrel)
Apomorphine (Apokyn)
Benztropine (Cogentin)
Bromocriptine (Parlodel)
Carbidopa/levodopa (Parcopa, Sinemet)
Entacapone (Comtan)

Pramipexole (Mirapex, Mirapex ER, generic)
Rasagiline (Azilect)
Rivastigmine, transdermal (Exelon Patch)
Ropinirole (Requip, Requip XL, generic)

Rotigotine (Neupro)
Selegiline (Eldepryl, Zelapar)
Tolcapone (Tasmar)
Trihexyphenidyl (generic)

Antipsychotics

Aripiprazole (Abilify, Abilify Discmelt)
Asenapine (Saphris)
Chlorpromazine (Thorazine)
Clozapine (Clozaril, FazaClo, Versacloz)
Haloperidol (Haldol, generic)
Iloperidone (Fanapt)
Lithium carbonate, citrate (generic)
Lurasidone (Latuda)

Olanzapine (Zyprexa, Zyprexa Zydis, generic)
Olanzapine, LA parenteral (Zyprexa Relprevv)
Paliperidone (Invega, Invega Sustenna)
Perphenazine (generic)
Pimozide (Orap)
Prochlorperazine (Compro, Procomp, generic)

Quetiapine (Seroquel, Seroquel XR, generic)
Risperidone, oral (Risperdal, Risperdal M-Tab, generic)
Risperidone, parenteral (Risperdal Consta)
Thioridazine (generic)
Thiothixene (generic)
Trifluoperazine (generic)
Ziprasidone (Geodon)

Sedative Hypnotics

Dexmedetomidine (Precedex)
Diphenhydramine (Benadryl OTC)
Doxepin (Silenor)
Estazolam (ProSom, generic) [C-IV]
Eszopiclone (Lunesta)
Etomidate (Amidate)
Flurazepam (Dalmane) [C-IV]

Hydroxyzine (Atarax, Vistaril)
Midazolam (generic) [C-IV]
Pentobarbital (Nembutal, others)
Phenobarbital
Propofol (Diprivan, generic)
Ramelteon (Rozerem)
Secobarbital (Seconal)

Temazepam (Restoril, generic) [C-IV]
Triazolam (Halcion, generic)
Zaleplon (Sonata)
Zolpidem (Ambien IR, Ambien CR, Edluar, ZolpiMist, generic) [C-IV]

Stimulants

Armodafinil (Nuvigil)
Atomoxetine (Strattera)
Dexmethylphenidate (Focalin, Focalin XR)
Dextroamphetamine (Dexedrine, Procentra) [C-II]
Guanfacine (Intuniv)

Lisdexamfetamine (Vyvanse)
Methylphenidate, oral (Concerta, Metadate CD, Metadate SR, Methylin, Ritalin, Ritalin LA, Ritalin SR, Quillivant XR) [C-II]

Methylphenidate, transdermal (Daytrana)
Modafinil (Provigil, generic) [C-IV]

Miscellaneous CNS Agents

Clomipramine (Anafranil)
Clonidine, oral, extended-release (Kapvay)
Dalfampridine (Ampyra)
Fingolimod (Gilenya)
Gabapentin enacarbil (Horizant)

Interferon beta-1a (Avonex, Rebif)
Meclizine (Antivert) (Dramamine [OTC])
Natalizumab (Tysabri)
Nimodipine (Nimotop)
Rizatriptan (Maxalt, Maxalt-MLT, generic)

Sodium oxybate (Xyrem)
Teriflunomide (Aubagio)
Tetrabenazine (Xenazine)

DERMATOLOGIC AGENTS

Acitretin (Soriatane)
Acyclovir (Zovirax)
Adapalene (Differin)
Adapalene/benzoyl
  peroxide (Epiduo Gel)
Alefacept (Amevive)
Amphotericin B
  (Amphocin,
  Fungizone)
Anthralin (Dritho,
  Zithranol,
  Zithranol-RR)
Bacitracin, topical
  (Baciguent)
Bacitracin/polymyxin B,
  topical (Polysporin)
Bacitracin/neomycin/
  polymyxin B, topical
  (Neosporin ointment)
Bacitracin/neomycin/
  polymyxin B/
  hydrocortisone,
  topical (Cortisporin)
Botulinum toxin type A
  [abobotulinumtoxin A]
  (Dysport)
Botulinum toxin type A
  [onabotulinumtoxin
  A] (Botox, Botox
  Cosmetic)
Calcipotriene (Dovonex)
Calcitriol ointment
  (Vectical)
Capsaicin (Capsin,
  Zostrix, others)
Ciclopirox (Ciclodan,
  CNL8, Loprox,
  Pedipirox-4 nail kit,
  Penlac)

Ciprofloxacin (Cipro,
  Cipro XR, Proquin XR)
Clindamycin (Cleocin,
  Cleocin T, others)
Clindamycin/benzoyl
  peroxide (Benzaclin)
Clindamycin/tretinoin
  (Veltin Gel)
Clotrimazole/
  betamethasone
  (Lotrisone)
Dapsone, topical
  (Aczone)
Dibucaine (Nupercainal)
Diclofenac, topical
  (Solaraze)
Doxepin, topical
  (Zonalon, Prudoxin)
Econazole (Spectazole)
Erythromycin, topical
  (Akne-Mycin, Ery,
  Erythra-Derm,
  generic)
Erythromycin/benzoyl
  peroxide (Benzamycin)
Finasteride (Propecia)
Fluorouracil, topical
  [5-FU] (Efudex)
Gentamicin, topical
  (generic)
Imiquimod cream
  (Aldara, Zyclara)
Ingenol mebutate (Picato)
Isotretinoin
  (Amnesteem, Claravis,
  Myorisan, Sotret,
  Zentane, generic)
Ketoconazole
  (Nizoral, generic)

Ketoconazole, topical
  (Extina, Nizoral A-D
  Shampoo, Xolegel)
  [Shampoo OTC]
Kunecatechins
  [sinecatechins]
  (Veregen)
Lactic acid/ammonium
  hydroxide [Ammonium
  Lactate] (Lac-Hydrin)
Lindane (generic)
Metronidazole (Flagyl,
  Flagyl ER,
  MetroCream,
  MetroGel,
  MetroLotion)
Miconazole (Monistat
  1 combination pack,
  Monistat 3, Monistat 7)
  [OTC], (Monistat-
  Derm)
Miconazole/zinc oxide/
  petrolatum (Vusion)
Minocycline (Arestin,
  Dynacin, Minocin,
  Solodyn, generic)
Minoxidil, topical
  (Theroxidil, Rogaine)
  [OTC]
Mupirocin (Bactroban,
  Bactroban Nasal)
Naftifine (Naftin)
Nystatin (Mycostatin)
Oxiconazole (Oxistat)
Penciclovir (Denavir)
Permethrin (Elimite,
  Nix, generic [OTC])
Pimecrolimus (Elidel)

Podophyllin (Condylox, Condylox Gel 0.5%, Podocon-25)

Pramoxine (Anusol Ointment, ProctoFoam NS)

Pramoxine and hydrocortisone (Proctofoam-HC)

Selenium sulfide (Exsel Shampoo, Selsun Blue shampoo, Selsun shampoo)

Silver sulfadiazine (Silvadene, Thermazene, generic)

Steroids, topical (*See* Table 3, p 302)

Tacrolimus, ointment (Protopic)

Tazarotene (Avage, Fabior, Tazorac)

Terbinafine (Lamisil, Lamasil AT [OTC])

Tolnaftate (Tinactin, generic [OTC])

Tretinoin, topical [retinoic acid] (Avita, Retin-A, Retin-A Micro, Renova)

Ustekinumab (Stelara)

Vorinostat (Zolinza)

DIETARY SUPPLEMENTS

Calcium acetate (Calphron, Phos-Ex, PhosLo)

Calcium glubionate (Calcionate)

Calcium salts [chloride, gluconate, gluceptate]

Cholecalciferol [vitamin D_3] (Delta-D)

Cyanocobalamin [vitamin B_{12}] (Nascobal)

Ferric gluconate complex (Ferrlecit)

Ferrous gluconate (Fergon [OTC], others)

Ferrous sulfate

Ferumoxytol (Feraheme)

Fish oil (Lovaza, others [OTC])

Folic acid, injectable, oral (generic)

Iron dextran (Dexferrum, INFeD)

Iron sucrose (Venofer)

Magnesium oxide (Mag-Ox 400, others [OTC])

Magnesium sulfate (various)

Multivitamins, oral [OTC] (*See* Table 12, p 322)

Phytonadione [vitamin K_1] (Mephyton, generic)

Potassium supplements (*See* Table 6, p 314)

Pyridoxine [vitamin B_6] (generic)

Sodium bicarbonate [$NaHCO_3$] (generic)

Thiamine [vitamin B_1] (generic)

EAR (OTIC) AGENTS

Acetic acid/aluminum acetate, otic (Domeboro Otic)

Benzocaine/antipyrine (Auralgan)

Ciprofloxacin, otic (Cetraxal)

Ciprofloxacin/ dexamethasone, otic (Ciprodex)

Ciprofloxacin/ hydrocortisone, otic (Cipro HC Otic)

Neomycin/colistin/ hydrocortisone (Cortisporin-TC Otic Drops)

Neomycin/colistin/
hydrocortisone/
thonzonium
(Cortisporin-TC Otic
Suspension)

Ofloxacin otic (Floxin
Otic, Floxin Otic
Singles)
Sulfacetamide (Bleph-10,
Cetamide, Klaron,
generic)

Sulfacetamide/
prednisolone
(Blephamide)

ENDOCRINE SYSTEM AGENTS

Antidiabetic Agents

Acarbose (Precose)
Bromocriptine mesylate
(Cycloset)
Chlorpropamide
(Diabinese)
Glimepiride (Amaryl,
generic)
Glimepiride/pioglitazone
(Duetact)
Glipizide (Glucotrol,
Glucotrol XL, generic)
Glyburide (DiaBeta,
Glynase, generic)

Glyburide/metformin
(Glucovance, generic)
Insulins, injectable (See
Table 4, p 305)
Metformin (Fortmet,
Glucophage,
Glucophage XR,
Glumetza, Riomet,
generic)
Miglitol (Glyset)
Nateglinide (Starlix,
generic)

Pioglitazone (Actos,
generic)
Pioglitazone/metformin
(ACTOplus Met,
ACTOplus MET XR,
generic)
Repaglinide (Prandin)
Repaglinide/metformin
(PrandiMet)
Rosiglitazone (Avandia)
Tolazamide (generic)
Tolbutamide (generic)

DIPEPTIDYL PEPTIDASE-4 (DPP-4) INHIBITORS

Alogliptin (Nesina)
Alogliptin/metformin
(Kazano)
Alogliptin/pioglitazone
(Oseni)

Linagliptin (Tradjenta)
Saxagliptin (Onglyza)
Saxagliptin/metformin
(Kombiglyze XR)
Sitagliptin (Januvia)

Sitagliptin/metformin
(Janumet)
Sitagliptin/simvastatin
(Juvisync)

GLUCAGON-LIKE PEPTIDE-1 (GLP-1) RECEPTOR AGONISTS

Exenatide (Byetta)
Exenatide ER (Bydureon)

Liraglutide recombinant
(Victoza)

SODIUM-GLUCOSE CO-TRANSPORTER 2 (SGLT2) INHIBITORS

Canagliflozin (Invokana)

Hormone and Synthetic Substitutes

Calcitonin (Fortical, Miacalcin)

Calcitriol (Rocaltrol, Calcijex)

Cortisone, systemic and topical (*See* Table 2, p 301, and Table 3, p 302)

Desmopressin (DDAVP, Stimate)

Dexamethasone, systemic and topical (Decadron)

Fludrocortisone (Florinef, generic)

Fluoxymesterone (Androxy) [C-III]

Glucagon, recombinant (GlucaGen)

Hydrocortisone, topical/ systemic (Cortef, Solu-Cortef, generic)

Methylprednisolone (A-Methapred, Depo-Medrol, Medrol, Medrol Dosepak, Solu-Medrol, generic) (*See* Steroids, p 259, and Table 2, p 301)

Prednisolone (Flo-Pred, Omnipred, Orapred, Pediapred, generic) (*See* Steroids,

p 259, and Table 2, p 301)

Prednisone (generic) (*See* Steroids, p 259, and Table 2, p 301)

Testosterone (AndroGel 1%, AndroGel 1.62% Androderm, Axiron, Fortesta, Striant, Testim, Testopel)

Vasopressin [antidiuretic hormone, ADH] (Pitressin)

Hypercalcemia/Osteoporosis Agents

Alendronate (Fosamax, Fosamax Plus D)

Denosumab (Prolia, Xgeva)

Etidronate (Didronel)

Gallium nitrate (Ganite)

Ibandronate (Boniva, generic)

Pamidronate (generic)

Raloxifene (Evista)

Risedronate (Actonel, Actonel w/ Calcium, generic)

Risedronate, delayed-release (Atelvia)

Teriparatide (Forteo)

Zoledronic acid (Reclast, Zometa,generic)

Obesity

Lorcaserin (Belviq)

Orlistat (Xenical, Alli [OTC])

Phentermine (Adipex-P, Suprenza, generic)

Phentermine/topiramate (Qsymia) [C-IV]

Thyroid/Antithyroid

Levothyroxine (Synthroid, Levoxyl, others)

Liothyronine [T_3] (Cytomel, Triostat)

Methimazole (Tapazole, generic)

Potassium iodide (Lugol's Solution, Iosat, SSKI, Thyro-Block, ThyroSafe, ThyroShield) [OTC]

Propylthiouracil (generic)

Miscellaneous Endocrine Agents

Cinacalcet (Sensipar)
Demeclocycline (Declomycin)
Diazoxide (Proglycem)
Mifepristone (Korlym)

Pasireotide (Signifor)
Somatropin (Genotropin, Nutropin AQ, Omnitrope, Saizen, Serostim, Zorbtive)

Tesamorelin (Egrifta)

EYE (OPHTHALMIC) AGENTS

Glaucoma Agents

Acetazolamide (Diamox)
Apraclonidine (Iopidine)
Betaxolol, ophthalmic (Betoptic)
Brimonidine (Alphagan P)
Brimonidine/timolol (Combigan)
Brinzolamide (Azopt)

Carteolol, ophthalmic
Dipivefrin (Propine)
Dorzolamide (Trusopt)
Dorzolamide/timolol (Cosopt)
Echothiophate iodide, ophthalmic (Phospholine Iodide)

Latanoprost (Xalatan)
Levobunolol (AK-Beta, Betagan)
Tafluprost (Zioptan)
Timolol, ophthalmic (Betimol, Timoptic, Timoptic XE, generic)

Ophthalmic Antibiotics

Azithromycin, ophthalmic, 1% (AzaSite)
Bacitracin, ophthalmic (AK-Tracin Ophthalmic)
Bacitracin/neomycin/ polymyxin B (Neo-polycin, Neosporin Ophthalmic)
Bacitracin/neomycin/ polymyxin B/hydrocortisone (Neo-polycin HC Cortisporin Ophthalmic)
Bacitracin/polymyxin B, ophthalmic (AK-Poly-Bac Ophthalmic, Polysporin Ophthalmic)
Besifloxacin (Besivance)

Ciprofloxacin, ophthalmic (Ciloxan)
Erythromycin, ophthalmic (Ilotycin)
Gentamicin, ophthalmic (Garamycin, Genoptic, Gentak, generic)
Gentamicin/prednisolone, ophthalmic (Pred-G Ophthalmic)
Levofloxacin ophthalmic (Quixin, Iquix)
Moxifloxacin ophthalmic (Vigamox)
Neomycin/polymyxin B/hydrocortisone (Cortisporin Ophthalmic, Cortisporin Otic)

Neomycin/dexamethasone (AK-Neo-Dex Ophthalmic, NeoDecadron Ophthalmic)
Neomycin/polymyxin B/dexamethasone, ophthalmic (Maxitrol)
Neomycin/polymyxin B/prednisolone (Poly-Pred Ophthalmic)
Norfloxacin, ophthalmic (Chibroxin)
Ofloxacin, ophthalmic (Ocuflox)
Silver nitrate (generic)
Sulfacetamide, ophthalmic (Bleph-10, Cetamide, Sodium Sulamyd)

Sulfacetamide/
prednisolone,
ophthalmic
(Blephamide, others)

Tobramycin ophthalmic
(AKTob, Tobrex,
generic)
Tobramycin/
dexamethasone
ophthalmic (TobraDex)

Trifluridine, ophthalmic
(Viroptic)

Miscellaneous Ophthalmic Agents

Aflibercept (Eylea)
Alcaftadine, ophthalmic
(Lastacaft)
Artificial tears (Tears
Naturale [OTC])
Atropine (Isopto
Atropine, generic)
Bepotastine besilate
(Bepreve)
Cidofovir (Vistide)
Cromolyn sodium
(Opticrom)
Cyclopentolate (Cyclogyl,
Cyclate)
Cyclopentolate/
phenylephrine
(Cyclomydril)
Cyclosporine (Restasis)

Dexamethasone,
ophthalmic (AK-Dex
Ophthalmic, Decadron
Ophthalmic, Maxidex)
Diclofenac (Voltaren)
Emedastine (Emadine)
Epinastine (Elestat)
Ganciclovir, ophthalmic
gel (Zirgan)
Ketotifen (Alaway,
Claritin Eye, Zaditor,
Zyrtec Itchy Eye)
[OTC]
Ketorolac (Acular,
Acular LS, Acular PF)
Levocabastine (Livostin)
Lodoxamide (Alomide)
Loteprednol (Alrex,
Lotemax)

Naphazoline (Albalon,
Naphcon, generic)
Naphazoline/
pheniramine (Naphcon
A, Visine A, generic)
Nepafenac (Nevanac)
Olopatadine (Patanol,
Pataday)
Pemirolast (Alamast)
Phenylephrine (Neo-
Synephrine
Ophthalmic, AK-
Dilate, Zincfrin [OTC])
Ranibizumab (Lucentis)
Rimexolone (Vexol)
Scopolamine ophthalmic

GASTROINTESTINAL (GI) AGENTS

Antacids

Alginic acid/aluminum
hydroxide/magnesium
trisilicate (Gaviscon)
[OTC]
Aluminum hydroxide
(Amphojel,
AlternaGEL,
Dermagran) [OTC]

Aluminum hydroxide/
magnesium carbonate
(Gaviscon Extra
Strength Liquid)
[OTC]
Aluminum hydroxide/
magnesium hydroxide
(Maalox)

Aluminum hydroxide/
magnesium hydroxide/
simethicone (Mylanta,
Mylanta II, Maalox
Plus) [OTC]
Aluminum hydroxide/
magnesium trisilicate
(Gaviscon Regular
Strength) [OTC]

Calcium carbonate (Tums, Alka-Mints) [OTC]

Magaldrate (Riopan Plus) [OTC]

Simethicone (generic [OTC])

Antidiarrheals

Bismuth subsalicylate (Pepto-Bismol) [OTC]
Diphenoxylate/atropine (Lomotil, Lonox)
Lactobacillus (Lactinex Granules) [OTC]

Loperamide (Diamode, Imodium) [OTC]
Octreotide (Sandostatin, Sandostatin LAR, generic)

Paregoric [camphorated tincture of opium]
Rifaximin (Xifaxan, Xifaxan 550)

Antiemetics

Aprepitant (Emend)
Chlorpromazine (Thorazine)
Dimenhydrinate (Dramamine, others) [OTC]
Dolasetron (Anzemet)
Dronabinol (Marinol) [C-III]
Droperidol (Inapsine)
Fosaprepitant (Emend, Injection)

Granisetron (generic)
Meclizine (Antivert, Bonine, Dramamine [OTC])
Metoclopramide (Reglan, Clopra, Octamide)
Nabilone (Cesamet)
Ondansetron (Zofran, Zofran ODT)
Ondansetron, oral soluble film (Zuplenz)

Palonosetron (Aloxi)
Prochlorperazine (Compazine)
Promethazine (Promethegan, generic)
Scopolamine (Transderm Scop)
Trimethobenzamide (Tigan, generic)

Antiulcer Agents

Bismuth subcitrate/ metronidazole/ tetracycline (Pylera)
Cimetidine (Tagamet, Tagamet HB 200 [OTC])
Dexlansoprazole (Dexilant, Kapidex)
Esomeprazole (Nexium)
Famotidine (Fluxid Pepcid, Pepcid AC, generic, [OTC])
Lansoprazole (Prevacid, Prevacid 24HR [OTC])

Nizatidine (Axid, Axid AR [OTC], generic)
Omeprazole (Prilosec, Prilosec [OTC], generic)
Omeprazole, sodium bicarbonate (Zegerid, Zegerid [OTC])
Omeprazole, sodium bicarbonate, magnesium hydroxide (Zegerid w/ Magnesium Hydroxide)

Pantoprazole (Protonix, generic)
Rabeprazole (AcipHex)
Ranitidine (Zantac, Zantac EFFERDose [OTC], generic)
Sucralfate (Carafate, generic)

Cathartics/Laxatives

Bisacodyl (Dulcolax [OTC])

Citric acid/magnesium oxide/sodium picosulfate (Prepopik)

Docusate calcium (Surfak)

Docusate potassium (Dialose)

Docusate sodium (DOSS, Colace)

Glycerin suppository

Lactulose (Constulose, Generlac, Chronulac,

Cephulac, Enulose, others)

Magnesium citrate (Citroma, others) [OTC]

Magnesium hydroxide (Milk of Magnesia) [OTC]

Mineral oil [OTC]

Mineral oil enema (Fleet Mineral Oil) [OTC]

Polyethylene glycol-electrolyte solution

[PEG-ES] (GoLYTELY, CoLyte)

Polyethylene glycol [PEG] 3350 (MiraLAX) [OTC]

Psyllium (Konsyl, Metamucil, generic)

Sodium phosphate (OsmoPrep, Visicol)

Sorbitol (generic)

Enzymes

Pancrelipase (Creon, Pancreaze, Panakare Plus, Pertzye, Ultresa, Voikace, Zenpep, generic)

Miscellaneous GI Agents

Alosetron (Lotronex)

Alvimopan (Entereg)

Budesonide, oral (Entocort EC)

Balsalazide (Colazal)

Certolizumab pegol (Cimzia)

Crofelemer (Fulyzaq)

Dexpanthenol (Ilopan-Choline Oral, Ilopan)

Dibucaine (Nupercainal)

Dicyclomine (Bentyl)

Fidaxomicin (Dificid)

Hydrocortisone, rectal (Anusol-HC Suppository,

Cortifoam Rectal, Proctocort, others, generic)

Hyoscyamine (Anaspaz, Cystospaz, Levsin, others, generic)

Hyoscyamine/atropine/scopolamine/phenobarbital (Donnatal, others)

Infliximab (Remicade)

Linaclotide (Linzess)

Lubiprostone (Amitiza)

Mesalamine (Apriso, Asacol, Asacol HD, Canasa, Lialda,

Pentasa, Rowasa, generic)

Methylnaltrexone bromide (Relistor)

Metoclopramide (Reglan, Clopra, Octamide)

Mineral oil/pramoxine HCl/zinc oxide (Tucks Ointment) [OTC]

Misoprostol (Cytotec, generic)

Neomycin (Neo-Fradin, generic)

Olsalazine (Dipentum)

Oxandrolone (Oxandrin, generic) [C-III]
Pramoxine (Anusol Ointment, ProctoFoam NS, others)
Pramoxine/ hydrocortisone (Enzone, Proctofoam-HC)

Propantheline (Pro-Banthine, generic)
Starch, topical, rectal (Tucks Suppositories) [OTC]
Sulfasalazine (Azulfidine, Azulfidine EN, generic)

Teduglutide [rDNA origin] (Gattex)
Vasopressin [antidiuretic hormone (ADH)] (Pitressin)
Witch hazel (Tucks Pads, others [OTC])

HEMATOLOGIC AGENTS

Anticoagulants

Antithrombin, recombinant (ATryn)
Argatroban (generic)
Bivalirudin (Angiomax)
Dabigatran (Pradaxa)
Dalteparin (Fragmin)

Desirudin (Iprivask)
Enoxaparin (Lovenox)
Fondaparinux (Arixtra, generic)
Heparin (generic)
Lepirudin (Refludan)

Protamine (generic)
Warfarin (Coumadin, Jantoven, generic)

Antiplatelet Agents

Abciximab (ReoPro)
Aspirin (Bayer, Ecotrin, St. Joseph's) [OTC]
Cilostazol (Pletal)
Clopidogrel (Plavix)

Dipyridamole (Persantine)
Dipyridamole/aspirin (Aggrenox)
Eptifibatide (Integrilin)

Prasugrel (Effient)
Rivaroxaban (Xarelto)
Ticagrelor (Brilinta)
Ticlopidine (Ticlid)
Tirofiban (Aggrastat)

Antithrombotic Agents

Alteplase, recombinant [tPA] (Activase)
Aminocaproic acid (Amicar)

Anistreplase (Eminase)
Apixaban (Eliquis)
Dextran 40 (Gentran 40, Rheomacrodex)

Reteplase (Retavase)
Streptokinase (generic)
Tenecteplase (TNKase)

Hematinic Agents

Darbepoetin alfa (Aranesp)
Eltrombopag (Promacta)
Epoetin alfa [erythropoietin (EPO)] (Epogen, Procrit)

Filgrastim [G-CSF] (Neupogen)
Iron dextran (Dexferrum, INFeD)
Iron sucrose (Venofer)
Oprelvekin (Neumega)

Pegfilgrastim (Neulasta)
Plerixafor (Mozobil)
Romiplostim (Nplate)
Sargramostim [GM-CSF] (Leukine)

Volume Expanders

Albumin (Albuked, Albuminar 20, AlbuRx 25, Albutein, Buminate, Kedbumin, Plasbumin)

Dextran 40 (Gentran 40, Rheomacrodex)

Hetastarch (Hespan)

Plasma protein fraction (Plasmanate)

Miscellaneous Hematologic Agents

Antihemophilic factor VIII (Monoclate-P)

Antihemophilic factor [recombinant] (Advate, Hexilate FS, Kogenate FS, Recombinate, Xyntha)

Decitabine (Dacogen)

Deferiprone (Ferriprox)

Desmopressin (DDAVP, Stimate)

Lenalidomide (Revlimid)

Pentoxifylline (Trental, generic)

Prothrombin complex concentrate (human) (Kcentra)

Ruxolitinib (Jakafi)

IMMUNE SYSTEM AGENTS

Immunomodulators

Icatibant (Firazyr)

Interferon alfa (Roferon-A, Intron A)

Interferon alfacon-1 (Infergen)

Interferon beta-1a (Rebif)

Interferon beta-1b (Betaseron, Extavia)

Interferon gamma-1b (Actimmune)

Natalizumab (Tysabri)

Peginterferon alfa-2a [pegylated interferon] (Pegasys)

Peginterferon alfa-2b [pegylated interferon] (PegIntron)

Immunomodulators: Disease-Modifying Antirheumatic Drugs (DMARDs)

Abatacept (Orencia)

Adalimumab (Humira)

Anakinra (Kineret)

Certolizumab pegol (Cimzia)

Etanercept (Enbrel)

Golimumab (Simponi)

Infliximab (Remicade)

Tocilizumab (Actemra)

Tofacitinib (Xeljanz)

Immunosuppressive Agents

Azathioprine (Imuran)

Basiliximab (Simulect)

Belatacept (Nulojix)

Cyclosporine (Gengraf, Neoral, Sandimmune)

Daclizumab (Zenapax)

Everolimus (Zortress)

Lymphocyte immune globulin [antithymocyte globulin (ATG)] (Atgam)

Mycophenolate mofetil (CellCept, generic)

Mycophenolic acid (Myfortic, generic)

Sirolimus [rapamycin] (Rapamune)

Steroids, systemic (*See* Table 2, p 301)

Tacrolimus (Prograf, generic)

MUSCULOSKELETAL AGENTS

Antigout Agents

Allopurinol (Zyloprim, Lopurin, Aloprim)
Colchicine

Febuxostat (Uloric)
Pegloticase (Krystexxa)

Probenecid (Probalan, generic)

Muscle Relaxants

Baclofen (Lioresal Intrathecal, Gablofen)
Carisoprodol (Soma)
Chlorzoxazone (Parafon Forte DSC, others)
Cyclobenzaprine (Flexeril)

Cyclobenzaprine, extended-release (Amrix)
Dantrolene (Dantrium, Revonto)
Diazepam (Diastat, Valium)

Metaxalone (Skelaxin)
Methocarbamol (Robaxin, generic)
Orphenadrine (Norflex, generic)

Neuromuscular Blockers

Atracurium (Tracrium)
Botulinum toxin type A [incobotulinumtoxinA] (Xeomin)
Botulinum toxin type A [onabotulinumtoxinA] (Botox, Botox Cosmetic)

Botulinum toxin type B [rimabotulinumtoxinB] (Myobloc)
Pancuronium (generic)
Rocuronium (Zemuron, generic)

Succinylcholine (Anectine, Quelicin, generic)
Vecuronium (generic)

Miscellaneous Musculoskeletal Agents

Edrophonium (Enlon)
Leflunomide (Arava)
Methotrexate (Rheumatrex Dose Pack, Trexall, generic)

Sulfasalazine (Azulfidine, Azulfidine EN)

Tizanidine (Zanaflex, generic)

OB/GYN AGENTS

Contraceptives

Copper intrauterine device (IUD) (ParaGard T 380A)

Ethinyl estradiol/ norelgestromin (Ortho Evra)

Etonogestrel, implant (Implanon)

Etonogestrel/ethinyl estradiol, vaginal insert (NuvaRing)

Levonorgestrel intrauterine device (IUD) (Mirena)

Medroxyprogesterone (Provera,

Depo-Provera, Depo-Sub Q Provera, generic)

Oral contraceptives (*See* p 217, and Table 5, p 306)

Emergency Contraceptives

Levonorgestrel (Next Choice, Plan B One-Step, generic [OTC])

Ulipristal acetate (Ella)

Estrogen Supplementation

ESTROGEN ONLY

Estradiol, oral (Delestrogen, Estrace, Femtrace, others)

Estradiol, metered gel (Elestrin, Estrogel)

Estradiol, spray (Evamist)

Estradiol, transdermal (Alora, Climara, Estraderm, Vivelle Dot)

Estradiol, vaginal (Estring, Femring, Vagifem)

Estrogen, conjugated (Premarin)

Estrogen, conjugated-synthetic (Cenestin, Enjuvia)

Esterified estrogens (Menest)

COMBINATION ESTROGEN/PROGESTIN

Estradiol/levonorgestrel, transdermal (Climara Pro)

Estradiol/norethindrone (Activella, generic)

Estrogen, conjugated/ medroxyprogesterone (Prempro, Premphase)

Vaginal Preparations

Amino-Cerv pH 5.5 cream

Miconazole (Monistat 1 combination pack, Monistat 3, Monistat 7) [OTC], (Monistat-Derm)

Nystatin (Mycostatin)

Terconazole (Terazol 3, Terazol 7, generic)

Tioconazole (generic [OTC])

Miscellaneous OB/GYN Agents

Clomiphene (Clomid)
Dinoprostone (Cervidil
  Vaginal Insert, Prepidil
  Gel, Prostin E2)
Leuprolide (Lupron)
Magnesium sulfate
  (various)

Medroxyprogesterone
  (Provera, Depo-
  Provera, Depo-SubQ
  Provera)
Methylergonovine
  (Methergine)
Mifepristone [RU 486]
  (Mifeprex)

Nafarelin, metered spray
  (SYNAREL)
Oxytocin (Pitocin,
  generic)
Paroxetine (Brisdelle)
Terbutaline (generic)
Tranexamic acid
  (Lysteda, generic)

PAIN MEDICATIONS

Local/Topical (*See also* Local Anesthetics Table 1, p 300)

Benzocaine (Americaine,
  Lanacane, Hurricane,
  various [OTC])
Benzocaine/antipyrine
  (Auralgan)
Bupivacaine (Marcaine)
Capsaicin (Capsin,
  Zostrix, others) [OTC]
Cocaine
Dibucaine (Nupercainal)

Lidocaine, lidocaine/
  epinephrine
  (Anestacon Topical,
  Xylocaine, Xylocaine
  Viscous, Xylocaine
  MPF, others)
Lidocaine/prilocaine
  (EMLA, LMX)
Lidocaine/tetracaine,
  transdermal (Synera)

Mepivacaine
  (Carbocaine)
Procaine (Novocaine)
Pramoxine (Anusol
  Ointment, ProctoFoam
  NS, others)

Migraine Headache

Acetaminophen/butalbital,
  w/ and w/o caffeine
  (Fioricet, Margesic,
  Esgic, Dologic Plus,
  Bupap, Sedapap,
  Phrenilin)
Almotriptan (Axert)
Aspirin/butalbital/
  caffeine compound
  (Fiorinal)

Aspirin/butalbital/
  caffeine/codeine
  (Fiorinal w/ Codeine)
Eletriptan (Relpax)
Frovatriptan (Frova)
Naratriptan (Amerge,
  generic)
Sumatriptan (Alsuma,
  Imitrex, Imitrex
  Statdose, Imitrex
  Nasal Spray, generic)

Sumatriptan/naproxen
  sodium (Treximet)
Sumatriptan needleless
  system (Sumavel
  DosePro)
Zolmitriptan (Zomig,
  Zomig ZMT, Zomig
  Nasal)

Narcotic Analgesics

Acetaminophen/codeine
(Tylenol 2, 3, 4)
Alfentanil (Alfenta)
Buprenorphine
(Buprenex)
Buprenorphine/naloxone
(Suboxone)
Buprenorphine,
transdermal (Butrans)
Butorphanol (Stadol)
Codeine
Fentanyl (Sublimaze)
Fentanyl, transdermal
(Duragesic, generic)
[C-II]
Fentanyl, transmucosal
(Abstral, Actiq,
Fentora, Lazanda,
Onsolis, generic)
[C-II]
Hydrocodone/
acetaminophen (Lorcet,
Vicodin, Hycet, others)

Hydrocodone/ibuprofen
(Vicoprofen, generic)
[C-III]
Hydromorphone
(Dilaudid, Dilaudid
HP, generic) [C-II]
Hydromorphone,
extended-release
(Exalgo)
Levorphanol (Levo-
Dromoran)
Meperidine (Demerol,
Meperitab, generic)
[C-II]
Methadone (Dolophine,
Methadose, generic)
[C-II]
Morphine (Avinza XR,
Astramorph/PF,
Duramorph,
Infumorph, MS Contin,
Kadian SR, Oramorph
SR, Roxanol) [C-II]
Morphine/naltrexone
(Embeda)

Nalbuphine (generic)
Oxycodone (OxyContin,
Roxicodone, generic)
[C-II]
Oxycodone/
acetaminophen
(Percocet, Tylox)
Oxycodone/aspirin
(Percodan)
Oxycodone/ibuprofen
(Combunox)
Oxymorphone (Opana,
Opana ER)
Pentazocine (Talwin,
Talwin Compound,
Talwin NX) [C-IV]
Propoxyphene
(Darvon-N),
propoxyphene/
acetaminophen
(generic),
propoxyphene/aspirin
(generic) [C-IV]

Nonnarcotic Analgesics

Acetaminophen,
injection (Ofirmev)
Acetaminophen, oral
[N-acetyl-p-
aminophenol (APAP)]
(Acephen, Tylenol,
others, generic)
Acetaminophen/
butalbital/± caffeine
(Fioricet, Medigesic,
Repan, Sedapap-10,
Two-Dyne, Triapin,
Axocet, Phrenilin
Forte)

Aspirin (Bayer, Ecotrin,
St. Joseph's) [OTC]
Tramadol (Rybix ODT,
Ryzolt ER, Ultram,
Ultram ER, generic)
Tramadol/acetaminophen
(Ultracet)

Nonsteroidal Anti-inflammatory Drugs (NSAIDs)

Celecoxib (Celebrex)
Diclofenac, oral
  (Cataflam, Voltaren,
  Voltaren-XR)
Diclofenac, topical
  (Flector Patch,
  Pennsaid, Voltaren gel)
Diclofenac/misoprostol
  (Arthrotec)
Diflunisal (Dolobid)
Etodolac
Fenoprofen (Nalfon,
  generic)
Flurbiprofen (Ansaid,
  Ocufen, generic)

Ibuprofen, oral (Advil,
  Motrin, Motrin IB,
  Rufen, others, generic)
  [OTC]
Ibuprofen, parenteral
  (Caldolor)
Indomethacin (Indocin,
  generic)
Ketoprofen (Orudis,
  Oruvail)
Ketorolac (Toradol)
Ketorolac, nasal (Sprix)
Meloxicam (Mobic,
  generic)
Nabumetone (Relafen,
  generic)

Naproxen (Aleve [OTC],
  Anaprox, Anaprox
  DS, EC-Naprosyn,
  Naprelan, Naprosyn,
  generic)
Naproxen/esomeprazole
  (Vimovo)
Oxaprozin (Daypro,
  Daypro ALTA)
Piroxicam (Feldene,
  generic)
Sulindac (Clinoril,
  generic)
Tolmetin (generic)

Miscellaneous Pain Medications

Amitriptyline (Elavil)
Clonidine, epidural
  (Duraclon)
Imipramine (Tofranil)

Pregabalin (Lyrica,
  generic)
Tapentadol (Nucynta)

Tramadol (Ultram,
  Ultram ER)
Ziconotide (Prialt)

RESPIRATORY AGENTS

Antitussives, Decongestants, and Expectorants

Acetylcysteine
  (Acetadote, Mucomyst)
Benzonatate (Tessalon,
  Zonatuss)
Codeine
Dextromethorphan
  (Benylin DM, Delsym,
  Mediquell, PediaCare
  1, others) [OTC]
Guaifenesin (Robitussin,
  others, generic)
Guaifenesin/codeine
  (Robafen AC, others,
  generic)

Guaifenesin/
  dextromethorphan
  (many OTC bands)
Hydrocodone/
  homatropine
  (Hycodan, Hydromet,
  others, generic)
  [C-III]
Hydrocodone/
  pseudoephedrine
  (Detussin, Histussin-D,
  others, generic)
  [C-III]

Potassium iodide
  (Lugol's Solution,
  SSKI)
Pseudoephedrine (Many
  Mono and
  Combination Brands
  [OTC])

Bronchodilators

Albuterol (Proventil, Ventolin, Proair)

Albuterol/ipratropium (Combivent, DuoNeb)

Aminophylline (generic)

Arformoterol (Brovana)

Ephedrine (generic)

Epinephrine (Adrenalin, Sus-Phrine, EpiPen, EpiPen Jr, others)

Formoterol fumarate (Foradil, Performist)

Indacaterol (Arcapta Neohaler)

Isoproterenol (Isuprel)

Levalbuterol (Xopenex, Xopenex HFA)

Metaproterenol (Alupent, Metaprel)

Pirbuterol (Maxair, generic)

Salmeterol (Serevent, Serevent Diskus)

Terbutaline (Brethine, Bricanyl)

Theophylline (Theo24, Theochron, Theolair, generic)

Respiratory Inhalants

Acetylcysteine (Acetadote, Mucomyst)

Beclomethasone (QVAR)

Beclomethasone, nasal (Beconase AQ)

Budesonide (Rhinocort Aqua, Pulmicort)

Budesonide/formoterol (Symbicort)

Ciclesonide, inhaled (Alvesco)

Ciclesonide, nasal (Omnaris, Zettona)

Cromolyn sodium (Intal, NasalCrom, Opticrom, others)

Fluticasone furoate, nasal (Veramyst)

Fluticasone propionate, nasal (Flonase, generic)

Fluticasone propionate, inhaled (Flovent HFA, Flovent Diskus)

Fluticasone propionate/ salmeterol xinafoate (Advair Diskus, Advair HFA)

Formoterol fumarate (Foradil Aerolizer, Perforomist)

Ipratropium (Atrovent HFA, Atrovent Nasal, generic)

Mometasone/formoterol (Dulera)

Mometasone, inhaled (Asmanex Twisthaler)

Mometasone, nasal (Nasonex)

Olopatadine, nasal (Patanase)

Phenylephrine, nasal (Neo-Synephrine Nasal [OTC])

Roflumilast (Daliresp)

Tiotropium (Spiriva)

Tobramycin, inhalation (TOBI, TOBI Podhaler)

Triamcinolone (Azmacort)

Surfactants

Beractant (Survanta)

Calfactant (Infasurf)

Lucinactant (Surfaxin)

Miscellaneous Respiratory Agents

Alpha-1-protease inhibitor (Glassia, Prolastin C)

Aztreonam, inhaled

Dornase alfa (Pulmozyme, DNase)

Mannitol, inhalation (Aridol)

Montelukast (Singulair)

Omalizumab (Xolair)

Tadalafil (Adcirca)

Zafirlukast (Accolate, generic)

Zileuton (Zyflo, Zyflo CR)

UROGENITAL SYSTEM

Benign Prostatic Hyperplasia

Alfuzosin (Uroxatral)

Doxazosin (Cardura, Cardura XL)

Dutasteride (Avodart)

Dutasteride and tamsulosin (Jalyn)

Finasteride (Proscar, generic)

Silodosin (Rapaflo)

Tamsulosin (Flomax, generic)

Terazosin (Hytrin, generic)

Bladder Agents

Belladonna/opium, suppositories (B&O) (generic)

Bethanechol (Urecholine)

Butabarbital/ hyoscyamine/ phenazopyridine (Pyridium Plus)

Darifenacin (Enablex)

Fesoterodine (Toviaz)

Flavoxate (generic)

Hyoscyamine (Anaspaz, Cystospaz, Levsin)

Hyoscyamine, atropine, scopolamine/ phenobarbital (Donnatal, others, generic)

Methenamine hippurate (Hiprex), methenamine mandelate (Urex, Uroquid-Acid No. 2)

Mirabegron (Myrbetriq)

Oxybutynin (Ditropan, Ditropan XL, generic)

Oxybutynin transdermal system (Oxytrol)

Oxybutynin, topical (Gelnique)

Phenazopyridine (Pyridium, Azo-Standard, Urogesic, many others [OTC])

Solifenacin (VESIcare)

Tolterodine (Detrol, Detrol LA, generic)

Trospium (Sanctura, Sanctura XR, generic)

Erectile Dysfunction

Alprostadil, intracavernosal (Caverject, Edex)

Alprostadil, urethral suppository (Muse)

Avandafil (Stendra)

Sildenafil (Viagra, Revatio)

Tadalafil (Cialis)

Vardenafil (Levitra, Stayxn)

Yohimbine (Yocon, Yohimex)

Urolithiasis

Potassium citrate
(Urocit-K, generic)

Sodium citrate/citric acid
(Bicitra, Oracit)

Miscellaneous Urology Agents

Ammonium aluminum
sulfate (Alum [OTC])
BCG [Bacillus Calmette-
Guérin] (TheraCys,
Tice BCG)
Dimethyl sulfoxide
[DMSO] (Rimso-50)
Methenamine, phenyl
salicylate, methylene

blue, benzoic acid,
hyoscyamine (Prosed)
Neomycin/polymyxin
bladder irrigant
(Neosporin GU
Irrigant)
Nitrofurantoin
(Furadantin, Macrobid,
Macrodantin, generic)

Pentosan polysulfate
sodium (Elmiron)
Trimethoprim (Trimpex,
Proloprim)

VACCINES/SERUMS/TOXOIDS

Cytomegalovirus
immune globulin
[CMV-IG IV]
(CytoGam)
Diphtheria & tetanus
toxoids (Td) (Decavac,
Tenivac for > 7 y)
Diphtheria/tetanus
toxoids [DT] (generic
only, for < 7 y)
Diphtheria/tetanus
toxoids/acellular
pertussis, adsorbed
[DTaP; for < 7 y]
(Daptacel, Infanrix,
Tripedia)
Diphtheria/tetanus
toxoids/acellular
pertussis, adsorbed
[Tdap; for > 10–11 y]
(Boosters: Adacel,
Boostrix)

Diphtheria/tetanus
toxoids/acellular
pertussis, adsorbed/
inactivated poliovirus
vaccine [IPV]/
Haemophilus b
conjugate vaccine
combined (Pentacel)
Diphtheria/tetanus
toxoids/acellular
pertussis, adsorbed,
hepatitis B
[recombinant], and
inactivated poliovirus
vaccine [IPV]
combined (Pediarix)
Haemophilus b
conjugate vaccine
(ActHIB, HibTITER,
PedvaxHIB, others)
Hepatitis A [inactivated]
and hepatitis B

[recombinant] vaccine
(Twinrix)
Hepatitis A vaccine
(Havrix, Vaqta)
Hepatitis B immune
globulin (HyperHep B,
HepaGam B,
Nabi-HB, H-BIG)
Hepatitis B vaccine
(Engerix-B,
Recombivax HB)
Human papillomavirus
recombinant vaccine
(Cervarix [types 16,
18], Gardasil
[types 6, 11, 16, 18])
Immune globulin, IV
(Gamimune N,
Gammaplex, Gammar
IV, Sandoglobulin,
others)

Immune globulin,
subcutaneous
(Vivaglobin)

Influenza vaccine,
inactivated, trivalent
(IIV3) (Afluria,
Fluarix, Flucelvax,
FluLaval, Fluvirin,
Fluzone, Fluzone
High Dose, Fluzone
Intradermal)

Influenza vaccine,
inactivated,
quadrivalent (IIV4)
(Fluarix Quadrivalent,
Fluzone Quadrivalent)

Influenza vaccine, live-
attenuated,
quadrivalent (LAIV4)
(FluMist)

Influenza vaccine,
recombinant, trivalent
(RIV3) (FluBlok)

Measles/mumps/rubella
vaccine, live [MMR]
(M-M-R II)

Measles/mumps/rubella/
varicella virus
vaccine, live [MMRV]
(ProQuad)

Meningococcal
conjugate vaccine
[quadrivalent, MCV4]
(Menactra, Menveo)

Meningococcal groups C
and Y and
Haemophilus b
tetanus toxoid
conjugate vaccine
(Menhibrix)

Meningococcal
polysaccharide
vaccine [MPSV4]
(Menomune A/C/
Y/W-135)

Pneumococcal 13-valent
conjugate vaccine
(Prevnar 13)

Pneumococcal vaccine,
polyvalent
(Pneumovax-23)

Rotavirus vaccine, live,
oral, monovalent
(Rotarix)

Rotavirus vaccine, live,
oral, pentavalent
(RotaTeq)

Smallpox vaccine
(ACAM2000)

Tetanus immune globulin
(generic)

Tetanus toxoid (TT)
(generic)

Varicella immune
globulin (VarZIG)

Varicella virus vaccine
(Varivax)

Zoster vaccine, live
(Zostavax)

WOUND CARE

Becaplermin
(Regranex Gel)

MISCELLANEOUS THERAPEUTIC AGENTS

Acamprosate (Campral)

Alglucosidase alfa
(Lumizyme,
Myozyme)

C1 esterase inhibitor
[human] (Berinert,
Cinryze)

Cilostazol (Pletal)

Dextrose 50%/25%

Ecallantide (Kalbitor)

Eculizumab (Soliris)

Ivacaftor (Kalydeco)

Ketamine (Ketalar,
generic) [C-III]

Lanthanum carbonate
(Fosrenol)

Mecasermin (Increlex)

Megestrol acetate
(Megace, Megace-ES,
generic)

Methylene blue (Urolene
Blue, various)

Naltrexone (ReVia,
Vivitrol, generic)

Nicotine, gum (Nicorette, others)

Nicotine, nasal spray (Nicotrol NS)

Nicotine, transdermal (Habitrol, NicoDerm CQ [OTC], others)

Palifermin (Kepivance)

Potassium iodide (Lugol's Solution,

SSKI, Thyro-Block, ThyroSafe, ThyroShield) [OTC]

Sevelamer carbonate (Renvela)

Sevelamer hydrochloride (Renagel)

Sodium polystyrene sulfonate (Kayexalate, Kionex, generic)

Talc (Sterile Talc Powder)

Taliglucerase alfa (Elelyso)

Varenicline (Chantix)

NATURAL AND HERBAL AGENTS

Black cohosh

Chamomile

Cranberry (*Vaccinium macrocarpon*)

Dong quai (*Angelica polymorpha, sinensis*)

Echinacea (*Echinacea purpurea*)

Ephedra/ma huang

Evening primrose oil

Feverfew (*Tanacetum parthenium*)

Fish oil supplements (omega-3 polyunsaturated fatty acid)

Garlic (*Allium sativum*)

Ginger (*Zingiber officinale*)

Ginkgo biloba

Ginseng

Glucosamine sulfate (chitosamine) and chondroitin sulfate

Kava kava (kava kava root extract, *Piper methysticum*)

Melatonin

Milk thistle (*Silybum marianum*)

Red yeast rice

Resveratrol

Saw palmetto (*Serenoa repens*)

St. John's wort (*Hypericum perforatum*)

Valerian (*Valeriana officinalis*)

Yohimbine (*Pausinystalia yohimbe*) (Yocon, Yohimex)

GENERIC AND SELECTED BRAND DRUG DATA

Abacavir (Ziagen) **BOX:** Allergy (fever, rash, fatigue, GI, resp) reported; stop drug immediately & do not rechallenge; lactic acidosis & hepatomegaly/steatosis reported **Uses:** *HIV Infxn in combo w/ other antiretrovirals* **Acts:** NRTI **Dose:** *Adults.* 300 mg PO bid or 600 mg PO daily *Peds.* 8 mg/kg bid 16–20 mg/kg daily (stable CD$, undetect VRL) 300 mg bid max **W/P:** [C, –] CDC rec: HIV-infected mothers not breast-feed (transmission risk) **Disp:** Tabs 300 mg; soln 20 mg/mL **CI:** Mod–severe hepatic impair hypersens **SE:** See Box, ↑ LFTs, fat redistribution, N, V, HA, chills **Notes:** Many drug interactions; HLA-B*5701 ↑ risk for fatal hypersens Rxn, genetic screen before use

Abatacept (Orencia) **Uses:** *Mod–severe RAs, juvenile idiopathic arthritis* **Acts:** Selective costimulation modulator; ↓ T-cell activation **Dose:** *Adults.* Initial 500 mg (< 60 kg), 750 mg (60–100 kg); 1 g (> 100 kg) IV over 30 min; repeat at 2 and 4 wk, then q4wk; SQ regimen: after IV dose, 125 mg SQ w/in 24 h of Inf, then 125 SQ weekly *Peds 6–17 y.* 10 mg/kg (< 75 kg), 750 mg (75–100 kg), IV over 30 min; repeat at 2 and 4 wk then q4wk (> 100 kg, adult dose) **W/P:** [C; ?/–] w/ TNF blockers, anakinra; COPD; Hx predisposition to Infxn; w/ immunosuppressants **CI:** w/ Live vaccines w/in 3 mo of D/C abatacept **Disp:** IV soln 125 mg/mL **SE:** HA, URI, N, nasopharyngitis, Infxn, Inf Rxns/hypersens (dizziness, HA, HTN), COPD exacerbations, cough, dyspnea **Notes:** Screen for TB before use

Abciximab (ReoPro) **Uses:** *Prevent acute ischemic comps in PCI*, MI **Acts:** ↓ Plt aggregation (glycoprotein IIb/IIIa inhib) **Dose:** *ECC 2010.* ACS w/ immediate PCI: 0.25 mg/kg IV bolus 10–60 min before PCI, then 0.125 mcg/kg/min max 10 mcg/min IV for 12 h; w/ heparin. ACS w/ planned PCI w/in 24 h: 0.25 mg/kg IV bolus, then 10 mcg/min IV over 18–24 h concluding 1 h post-PCI; *PCI:* 0.25 mg/kg bolus 10–60 min pre-PTCA, then 0.125 mcg/kg/min (max = 10 mcg/min) cont Inf for 12 h **W/P:** [C, ?/–] **CI:** Active/recent (w/in 6 wk) internal hemorrhage, CVA w/in 2 y or CVA w/ sig neuro deficit, bleeding diathesis or PO anticoagulants w/in 7 d (unless PT < 1.2 × control), ↓ plt (< 100,000 cells/mcL), recent trauma or major surgery (w/in 6 wk), CNS tumor, AVM, aneurysm, severe uncontrolled HTN, vasculitis, dextran use w/ PTCA, murine protein allergy, w/ other glycoprotein IIb/IIIa inhib **Disp:** Inj 2 mg/mL **SE:** Back pain, ↓ BP, CP, allergic Rxns, bleeding, ↓ plt **Notes:** Use w/ heparin/ASA

Abiraterone (Zytiga) **Uses:** *Castrate-resistant metastatic PCa* **Acts:** CYP17 inhibitor; ↓ testosterone precursors **Dose:** 1000 mg PO qd w/ 5 mg prednisone bid; w/o food 2 h ac and 1 h pc; ↓ w/ hepatic impair **W/P:** [X, N/A] w/ Severe CHF, monitor for adrenocortical Insuff/excess, w/ CYP2D6 substrate/CYP3A4

35

inhib or inducers **CI:** PRG **Disp:** Tabs 250 mg **SE:** ↑ LFTs, jt swell, ↑ TG, ↓ K⁺, ↓ PO₄⁻³ edema, muscle pain, hot flush, D, UTI, cough,↑ BP, ↑ URI, urinary frequency, dyspepsia **Notes:** ✓ LFTs, K⁺; CYP17 inhib may ↑ mineralocorticoid SEs; prednisone ↓ ACTH limiting SEs

Acamprosate (Campral) **Uses:** *Maintain abstinence from EtOH* **Acts:** ↓ Glutamatergic transmission; ↓ NMDA receptors; related to GABA **Dose:** 666 mg PO tid; CrCl 30–50 mL/min: 333 mg PO tid **W/P:** [C; ?/–] **CI:** CrCl < 30 mL/min **Disp:** Tabs 333 mg EC **SE:** N/D, depression, anxiety, insomnia **Notes:** Does not eliminate EtOH withdrawal Sx; continue even if relapse occurs

Acarbose (Precose) **Uses:** *Type 2 DM* **Acts:** α-Glucosidase inhib; delays carbohydrate digestion to ↓ glucose **Dose:** 25–100 mg PO tid w/ 1st bite each meal; 50 mg tid (< 60 kg); 100 mg tid (> 60 kg); usual maint 50–100 mg PO tid **W/P:** [B, ?] w/ Scr > 2 mg/dL; can affect digoxin levels **CI:** IBD, colonic ulceration, partial intestinal obst; cirrhosis **Disp:** Tabs 25, 50, 100 mg **SE:** Abd pain, D, flatulence, ↑ LFTs, hypertens Rxn **Notes:** OK w/ sulfonylureas; ✓ LFTs q3ᵐᵒ for 1st y

Acebutolol (Sectral) **Uses:** *HTN, arrhythmias* chronic stable angina **Acts:** Blocks β-adrenergic receptors, β₁, & ISA **Dose:** *HTN:* 400–800 mg/d 2 ÷ doses *Arrhythmia:* 400–1200 mg/d 2 ÷ doses; ↓ 50% w/ CrCl < 50 mL/min, elderly; max 800 mg/d ↓ 75% w/ CrCl < 25 mL/min; max 400 mg/d **W/P:** [B, + M] Can exacerbate ischemic heart Dz, do not D/C abruptly **CI:** 2nd-/3rd-degree heart block, cardiac failure, cardiogenic shock **Disp:** Caps 200, 400 mg **SE:** Fatigue, HA, dizziness, ↓ HR

Acetaminophen [APAP, N-acetyl-p-Aminophenol] (Acephen, Ofirmev, IV [Rx], Tylenol, Other Generic) [OTC] **Uses:** *Mild–mod pain, HA, fever* **Acts:** Nonnarcotic analgesic; ↓ CNS synth of prostaglandins & hypothalamic heat-regulating center **Dose:** *Adults.* 650 mg PO or PR q4–6h or 1000 mg PO q6h; max 3 g/24 h *Peds < 12 y.* 10–15 mg/kg/dose PO or PR q4–6h; max 5 doses/24 h. Administer q6h if CrCl 10–50 mL/min & q8h if CrCl < 10 mL/min **W/P:** [C, +] w/ Hepatic/renal impair in elderly & w/ EtOH use (> 3 drinks/d) w/ > 4 g/dL; EtOH liver Dz, G6PD deficiency; w/ warfarin **CI:** Hypersens **Disp:** Tabs melt away/dissolving 80, 160 mg; tabs: 325, 500, 650 mg; chew tabs 80, 160 mg; gel caps 500 mg liq 100 mg/mL, 160 mg/5 mL, 325 mg/5 mL, 500 mg/15 mL, 80 mg/0.8 mL; *Acephen* supp 80, 120, 125, 325, 650 mL **SE:** hepatotoxic; OD hepatotoxic at 10 g; 15 g can be lethal; Rx w/ N-acetylcysteine **Notes:** No anti-inflammatory or plt-inhibiting action; avoid EtOH risk of liver injury primarily occurs when pts take multiple products containing acetaminophen at one time and exceed the current max dose of 3000 mg within a 24-h period; FDA has requested that all APAP-containing meds be max of 325 mg to limit tox, and change OTC liquids to uniform conc 160 mg/5 mL

Acetaminophen, Injection (Ofirmev) **Uses:** *Mild–mod pain, fever* **Acts:** Nonnarcotic analgesic; CNS synth of prostaglandins & hypothalamic heat-regulating center **Dose:** *Adults & Peds > 50 kg.* 1000 mg q6h or 650 mg q4h IV;

4000 mg max/d. **< 50 kg:** 15 mg/kg q6h or 12.5 mg/kg q4h, 75 mg/kg/d max. **Peds ≥ 2–12 y:** 15 mg/kg q6h or 12.5 mg/kg q4h IV, 75 mg/kg/d max. Min. interval of 4 h **W/P:** [C, +] Excess dose can cause hepatic injury; caution w/ liver Dz, alcoholism, malnutrition, hypovolemia, CrCl < 30 g/min **CI:** Hypersens to components, severe/active liver Dz **Disp:** IV 1000 mg (10 mg/mL) **SE:** N/V, HA, insomnia (adults); N/V, constipation, pruritus, agitation, atelectasis (peds) **Notes:** Min. dosing interval 4 h; infuse over 15 min. No anti-inflammatory or plt-inhibiting action

Acetaminophen + Butalbital ± Caffeine (Fioricet, Margesic, Esgic, Repan, Sedapap, Dolgic Plus, Bupap, Phrenilin Forte) [C-III]

Uses: *Tension HA*, mild pain **Acts:** Nonnarcotic analgesic w/ barbiturate **Dose:** 1–2 tabs or caps PO q4–6h PRN; ↓ in renal/hepatic impair; 3 g/24 h APAP max **W/P:** [C, ?/–] Alcoholic liver Dz, G6PD deficiency **CI:** Hypersens **Disp:** Caps *Dolgic Plus:* ↑ butalbital 50 mg, caffeine 40 mg, APAP 750 mg; Caps *Margesic, Esgic:* butalbital 50 mg, caffeine 40 mg, APAP 325 mg; Caps *Phrenilin Forte:* butalbital 50 mg + APAP 650 mg; Caps: *Esgic-Plus, Zebutal:* butalbital 50 mg, caffeine 40 mg, APAP 500 mg; liq *Dolgic LQ:* butalbital 50 mg, caffeine 40 mg, APAP 325 mg/15 mL. Tabs: *Medigesic, Fioricet, Repan:* butalbital 50 mg, caffeine 40 mg, APAP 325 mg; *Phrenilin:* butalbital 50 mg + APAP 325 mg, *Sedapap:* butalbital 50 mg + APAP 650 mg **SE:** Drowsiness, dizziness, "hangover" effect, N/V **Notes:** Butalbital habit forming; avoid EtOH; see Acetaminophen note p 36

Acetaminophen + Codeine (Tylenol No. 2, 3, and 4) [C-III, C-V]

Uses: *Mild–mod pain (No. 2–3); mod–severe pain (No. 4)* **Acts:** Combined APAP & narcotic analgesic **Dose:** *Adults.* 1–2 tabs q4–6h PRN or 30–60 mg/ codeine q4–6h based on codeine content (max dose APAP = 4 g/d). *Peds.* APAP 10–15 mg/kg/dose; codeine 0.5–1 mg/kg dose q4–6h (max: 3–6 y, 5 mL/dose; 7–12 y, 10 mL/dose) max 2.6 g/d if < 12 y; ↓ in renal/hepatic impair **W/P:** [C, ?] Alcoholic liver Dz; G6PD deficiency **CI:** Hypersens **Disp:** Tabs 300 mg APAP + codeine (No. 2 = 15 mg, No. 3 = 30 mg, No. 4 = 60 mg); susp (C-V) APAP 120 mg + codeine 12 mg/5 mL **SE:** Drowsiness, dizziness, N/V **Notes:** See Acetaminophen note p 36

Acetazolamide (Diamox)

Uses: *Diuresis, drug and CHF edema, glaucoma, prevent high-altitude sickness, refractory epilepsy*, metabolic alkalosis, resp stimulant in COPD **Acts:** Carbonic anhydrase inhib; ↓ renal excretion of hydrogen & ↑ renal excretion of Na^+, K^+, HCO_3^-, & H_2O **Dose:** *Adults.* Diuretic: 250–375 mg IV or PO q24h *Glaucoma:* 250–1000 mg PO q24h in ÷ doses *Epilepsy:* 8–30 mg/kg/d PO in ÷ doses *Altitude sickness:* 500–1000 mg/d ÷ dose q8–12h or SR q12–24h start 24 h before & 48–72 h after highest ascent *Metabolic alkalosis:* 500 mg IV × 1 *Resp stimulant:* 25 mg bid *Peds. Epilepsy:* 8–30 mg/kg/24 h PO in ÷ doses; max 1 g/d *Diuretic:* 5 mg/kg/24 h PO or IV *Alkalinization of urine:* 5 mg/kg/dose PO bid-tid *Glaucoma:* 8–30 mg/kg/24 h PO in 3 ÷ doses; max 1 g/d; ↓ dose w/ CrCl 10–50 mL/min; avoid if CrCl < 10 mL/min **W/P:** [C, +/–]

CI: Renal/hepatic/adrenal failure, sulfa allergy, hyperchloremic acidosis **Disp:** Tabs 125, 250 mg; ER caps 500 mg; Inj 500 mg/vial, powder for recons **SE:** Malaise, metallic taste, drowsiness, photosens, hyperglycemia **Notes:** Follow Na$^+$ & K$^+$; watch for metabolic acidosis; ✓ CBC & plts; SR forms not for epilepsy

Acetic Acid & Aluminum Acetate (Otic Domeboro) Uses: *Otitis externa* Acts: Anti-infective **Dose:** 4–6 gtt in ear(s) q2–3h **W/P:** [C, ?] **CI:** Perforated tympanic membranes **Disp:** 2% otic soln **SE:** Local irritation

Acetylcysteine (Acetadote, Mucomyst) Uses: *Mucolytic, antidote to APAP hepatotox/OD* adjuvant Rx chronic bronchopulmonary Dzs & CF* prevent contrast-induced renal dysfunction **Acts:** Splits mucoprotein disulfide linkages; restores glutathione in APAP OD to protect liver **Dose:** *Adults & Peds.* Nebulizer: 3–5 mL of 20% soln diluted w/ equal vol of H$_2$O or NS tid-qid *Antidote:* PO or NG: 140 mg/kg load, then 70 mg/kg q4h × 17 doses (dilute 1:3 in carbonated beverage or OJ), repeat if emesis w/in 1 h of dosing *Acetadote:* 150 mg/kg IV over 60 min, then 50 mg/kg over 4 h, then 100 mg/kg over 16 h *Prevent renal dysfunction:* 600–1200 mg PO bid × 2 d **W/P:** [B, ?] **Disp:** Soln, inhaled and oral 10%, 20%; Acetadote IV soln 20% **SE:** Bronchospasm (inhaled), N/V, drowsiness, anaphylactoid Rxns w/ IV **Notes:** Activated charcoal adsorbs PO acetylcysteine for APAP ingestion; start Rx for APAP OD w/in 6–8 h

Acitretin (Soriatane) BOX: Not to be used by females who are PRG or who intend to become PRG during/for 3 y following drug D/C; no EtOH during/2 mo following D/C; no blood donation for 3 y following D/C; hepatotoxic Uses: *Severe psoriasis*; other keratinization Dz (lichen planus, etc) Acts: Retinoid-like activity **Dose:** 25–50 mg/d PO, w/ main meal; **W/P:** [X, ?/–] Renal/hepatic impair; in women of reproductive potential **CI:** See Box; ↑ serum lipids; w/ MTX or tetracyclines **Disp:** Caps 10, 17.5, 25 mg **SE:** Hyperesthesia, cheilitis, skin peeling, alopecia, pruritus, rash, arthralgia, GI upset, photosens, thrombocytosis, ↑ triglycerides, ↑ Na$^+$, K$^+$, PO$_4$$^{-2}$ **Notes:** ✓ LFTs/lytes/lipids; response takes up to 2–3 mo; informed consent & FDA guide w/ each Rx required

Aclidinium Bromide (Tudorza Pressair) Uses: *Bronchospasm w/ COPD* Acts: LA anticholinergic, blocks ACH receptors **Dose:** 400 mcg/inhal, 1 inhal bid **W/P:** [C, ?] w/ Atropine hypersens, NAG, BPH, or MG; avoid w/ milk allergy **CI:** None **Disp:** Inhal powder, 30/60 doses **SE:** HA, D, nasopharyngitis, cough **Notes:** Not for acute exacerbation; lactose in powder, avoid w/ milk allergy; OK w/ renal impair

Acyclovir (Zovirax) Uses: *Herpes simplex* (HSV) (genital/mucocutaneous, encephalitis, keratitis), *Varicella zoster, Herpes zoster* (shingles) **Acts:** Interferes w/ viral DNA synth **Dose:** *Adults.* Dose on IBW if obese (> 125% IBW) PO: *Initial genital HSV:* 200 mg PO q4h while awake (5 caps/d) × 10 d or 400 mg PO tid × 7–10 d *Chronic HSV suppression:* 400 mg PO bid *Intermittent HSV Rx:* As initial, except Rx × 5 d, or 800 mg PO bid, at prodrome *Topical: Initial herpes genitalis:* Apply q3h (6×/d) for 7 d *HSV encephalitis:* 10 mg/kg IV q8h × 10 d

Herpes zoster: 800 mg PO 5×/d for 7–10 d *IV:* 10 mg/kg/dose IV q8h × 7 d *Peds.*
Genital HSV: 3 mo–12 y: 40–80 mg/kg/d ÷ 3–4 doses (max 1 g); ≥ *12 y:* 200 mg
5×/d or 400 mg 3 × /d × 5–10 d; IV: 5 mg/kg/dose q8h × 5–7 d *HSV/encephalitis:*
3 mo–12 y: 60 mg/kg/d IV ÷ q8h × 14–21 d > *12 y:* 30 mg/kg/d IV ÷ q8h × 14–21 d
Chickenpox: ≥2 *y:* 20 mg/kg/dose qid × 5 d *Shingles:* < *12 y:* 30 mg/kg/d PO
or 1500 mg/m²/d IV ÷ q8h × 7–10 d; ↓ w/ CrCl < 50 mL/min **W/P:** [B, +] **CI:**
Component hypersens **Disp:** Caps 200 mg; tabs 400, 800 mg; susp 200 mg/5 mL;
Inj 500 & 1000 mg/vial; Inj soln, 50 mg/mL oint 5% and cream 5% **SE:** Dizziness,
lethargy, malaise, confusion, rash, IV site inflammation; transient ↑ Cr/BUN
Notes: PO better than topical for herpes genitalis

Adalimumab (Humira) **BOX:** Cases of TB have been observed; ✓ TB skin
test prior to use; hep B reactivation possible, invasive fungal, and other opportunistic
Infxns reported; lymphoma/other CA possible in children/adolescents **Uses:** *Mod-
severe RA w/ an inadequate response to one or more DMARDs, psoriatic arthritis
(PA), juvenile idiopathic arthritis (JIA), plaque psoriasis, ankylosing spondylitis (AS),
Crohn Dz, ulcerative colitis* **Acts:** TNF-α inhib **Dose:** *RA, PA, AS:* 40 mg SQ q other
wk; may ↑ 40 mg qwk if not on MTX. JIA 15–30 kg 20 mg q other wk *Crohn Dz/
ulcerative colitis:* 160 mg d 1, 80 mg 2 wk later, then 2 wk later start maint 40 mg q
other wk **W/P:** [B, ?/–] See Box; do not use w/ live vaccines **CI:** None **Disp:** Prefilled
0.4 mL (20 mg) & 0.8 mL (40 mg) syringe **SE:** Inj site Rxns, HA, rash, ↑ CHF,
anaphylaxis, pancytopenia (aplastic anemia) demyelinating Dz, new onset psoriasis
Notes: Refrigerate prefilled syringe, rotate Inj sites, OK w/ other DMARDs

Adapalene (Differin) **Uses:** *Acne vulgaris* **Acts:** Retinoid-like, modulates
cell differentiation/keratinization/inflammation **Dose:** *Adults & Peds > 12 y.* Apply
1×/d to clean/dry skin QHS **W/P:** [C, ?/–] products w/ sulfur/resorcinol/salicylic
acid ↑ irritation **CI:** Component hypersens **Disp:** Top lotion, gel, cream 0.1%; gel
0.3% **SE:** Skin redness, dryness, burning, stinging, scaling, itching, sunburn
Notes: Avoid exposure to sunlight/sunlamps; wear sunscreen

Adapalene & Benzoyl Peroxide (Epiduo) **Uses:** *Acne vulgaris*
Acts: Retinoid-like, modulates cell differentiation, keratinization, and inflamma-
tion w/ antibacterial **Dose:** *Adults & Peds > 12 y.* Apply 1 × daily to clean/dry skin
W/P: [C, ?/–] Bleaching effects, photosensitivity **CI:** Component hypersens **Disp:**
Topical gel: adapalene 0.1% and benzoyl peroxide 2.5% (45g) **SE:** Local irritation,
dryness **Notes:** Vit A may ↑ SE

Adefovir (Hepsera) **BOX:** Acute exacerbations of hep B seen after D/C Rx
(monitor LFTs); nephrotoxic w/ underlying renal impair w/ chronic use (monitor
renal Fxn); HIV resistance/untreated may emerge; lactic acidosis & severe
hepatomegaly w/ steatosis reported **Uses:** *Chronic active hep B* **Acts:** Nucleotide
analog **Dose:** CrCl > 50 mL/min: 10 mg PO daily; CrCl 20–49 mL/min: 10 mg PO
q48h; CrCl 10–19 mL/min: 10 mg PO q72h; HD: 10 mg PO q7d postdialysis
W/P: [C, ?/–] **Disp:** Tabs 10 mg **SE:** Asthenia, HA, D, hematuria Abd pain; see
Box **Notes:** ✓ HIV status before use

Adenosine (Adenocard, Adenoscan) Uses: *Adenocard* *PSVT*; including w/ WPW; *Adenoscan* (pharmacologic stress testing) Acts: Class IV antiarrhythmic; slows AV node conduction Dose: *Stress test.* 140 mcg/kg/min × 6 min cont Inf *Adults. ECC 2010.* 6-mg rapid IV push, then 20-mL NS bolus. Elevate extremity; repeat 12 mg in 1–2 min PRN *Peds. ECC 2010. Symptomatic SVT*: 0.1 mg/kg rapid IV/IO push (max dose 6 mg); can follow w/ 0.2 mg/kg rapid IV/IO push (max dose 12 mg); follow each dose w/ ≥ 5 mL NS flush W/P: [C, ?] Hx bronchospasm CI: 2nd-/3rd-degree AV block or SSS (w/o pacemaker); Afib/flutter w/ WPW, V tachycardia, recent MI or CNS bleed, asthma Disp: Inj 3 mg/mL SE: Facial flushing, HA, dyspnea, chest pressure, ↓ BP, pro-arrhythmic Notes: Doses > 12 mg not OK; can cause momentary asystole w/ use; caffeine, theophylline antagonize effects

Aflibercept (Eylea) Uses: *Neovascular age-related macular degeneration* Acts: Binds VGEF-A & placental growth factor; ↓ neovascularization & vascular permeability Dose: *Adults.* 2 mg (0.05 mL) intravitreal Inj q4wk × 3 mo, then q8wk W/P: [C, ?] may cause endophthalmitis or retinal detachment CI: Ocular or periocular Infxn, active intraocular inflammation, hypersens Disp: Inj 40 mg/mL/vial SE: Blurred vision, eye pain, conjunctival hemorrhage, cataract, ↑ IOP, vitreous detachment, floaters, arterial thrombosis Notes: For ophthalmic intravitreal Inj only

Albumin (Albuked, Albuminar 20, AlbuRx 25, Albutein, Buminate, Kedbumin, Plasbumin) Uses: *Plasma vol expansion for shock (eg, burns, hemorrhage),* others based on specific product label: ovarian hyperstimulation synd, CABG support, hypoalbuminemia Acts: ↑ intravascular oncotic pressure Dose: *Adults.* Initial 25 g IV; then based on response; 250 g/48 h max Peds. 0.5–1 g/kg/dose; max 6 g/kg/d W/P: [C, ?] Severe anemia; cardiac, renal, or hepatic Insuff d/t protein load & hypervolemia avoid 25% albumin in preterm infants CI: CHF, severe anemia Disp: Soln 5%, vials 20%, 25% SE: Chills, fever, CHF, tachycardia, ↑↓ BP, hypervolemia Notes: Contains 130–160 mEq Na⁺/L; may cause pulm edema; max Inf rates: 25% vial: 2–3 mL/min; 5% soln: 5–10 mL/min

Albuterol (Proventil, Ventolin, ProAir) Uses: *Asthma, COPD, prevent exercise-induced bronchospasm* Acts: β-Adrenergic sympathomimetic bronchodilator; relaxes bronchial smooth muscle Dose: *Adults. Inhaler:* 2 Inh q4–6h PRN; q4–6h *PO:* 2–4 mg PO tid-qid *Nebulizer:* 1.25–5 mg (0.25–1 mL of 0.5% soln in 2–3 mL of NS) q4–8h PRN *Prevent exercise-induced asthma:* 2 puffs 5–30 min prior to activity *Peds. Inhaler:* 2 Inh q4–6h *PO:* 0.1–0.2 mg/kg/dose PO; max 2–4 mg PO tid *Nebulizer:* 0.63–5 mg in 2–3 mL of NS q4–8h PRN W/P: [C, ?] Disp: Tabs 2, 4 mg; XR tabs 4, 8 mg; syrup 2 mg/5 mL; 90 mcg/dose metered-dose inhaler; soln for nebulizer 0.083, 0.5% SE: Palpitations, tachycardia, nervousness, GI upset

Albuterol & Ipratropium (Combivent, DuoNeb) Uses: *COPD* Acts: Combo of β-adrenergic bronchodilator & quaternary anticholinergic Dose: 2 Inh qid;

nebulizer 3 mL q6h; max 3 mL q4h **W/P:** [C, ?] **CI:** Peanut/soybean allergy **Disp:** Metered-dose inhaler, 18 mcg ipratropium & 90 mcg albuterol/puff (contains ozone-depleting CFCs; will be gradually removed from US market); nebulization soln (DuoNeb) ipratropium 0.5 mg & albuterol 2.5 mg/3 mL **SE:** Palpitations, tachycardia, nervousness, GI upset, dizziness, blurred vision

Alcaftadine (Lastacaft) Uses: *Allergic conjunctivitis* **Acts:** Histamine H_1-receptor antag **Dose:** 1 gtt in eye(s) daily **W/P:** [B, ?] **Disp:** Ophth soln 0.25% **SE:** Eye irritation Notes: Remove contacts before use

Aldesleukin [IL-2] (Proleukin) BOX: Restrict to pts w/ nl cardiac/pulmonary Fxns as defined by formal testing. Caution w/ Hx of cardiac/pulmonary Dz. Administer in hospital setting w/ physician experienced w/ anticancer agents. Assoc w/ capillary leak syndrome (CLS) characterized by ↓ BP and organ perfusion w/ potential for cardiac/respiratory tox, GI bleed/infarction, renal insufficiency, edema, and mental status changes. Increased risk of sepsis and bacterial endocarditis. Treat bacterial Infxn before use. Pts w/ central lines are at ↑ risk for Infxn. Prophylaxis w/ oxacillin, nafcillin, ciprofloxacin, or vancomycin may reduce staphylococcal Infxn. Hold w/ mod–severe severe lethargy or somnolence; continued use may result in coma Uses: *Met RCC & melanoma* **Acts:** Acts via IL-2 receptor; many immunomodulatory effects **Dose:** 600,000 Int units/kg q8h × max 14 doses d 1–5 and d 15–19 of 28-d cycle (FDA-dose/schedule for RCC); other schedules (eg, "high dose" 720,000 Int units/kg IV q8h up to 12 doses, repeat 10–15 d later) **W/P:** [C, ?/–] **CI:** Organ allografts; abnormal thallium stress test or PFT **Disp:** Powder for recons 22×10^6 Int units, when reconstituted 18 mill Int units/mL = 1.1 mg/mL **SE:** Flu-like synd (malaise, fever, chills), N/V/D, ↑ bili; capillary leak synd; ↓ BP, tachycardia, pulm & periph edema, fluid retention, & Wt gain; renal & mild hematologic tox (↓ Hgb, plt, WBC), eosinophilia; cardiac tox (ischemia, atrial arrhythmias); neurotox (CNS depression, somnolence, delirium, rare coma); pruritic rashes, urticaria, & erythroderma common

Alefacept (Amevive) Uses: *Mod-severe chronic plaque psoriasis* **Acts:** Binds CD2, ↓ T-lymphocyte activation **Dose:** 7.5 mg IV or 15 mg IM once/wk × 12 wk; may repeat course 12 wk later if CD4 OK **W/P:** [B, ?/–] PRG registry; associated w/ serious Infxn; ✓ CD4 before each dose; w/ hold if < 250; D/C if < 250 × 1 mo **CI:** HIV **Disp:** 15-mg powder vial **SE:** Pharyngitis, myalgia, Inj site Rxn, malignancy, Infxn, ↑ LFT (monitor for liver damage) **Notes:** Immunizations up to date before use

Alemtuzumab (Campath relaunch as Lemtrada) BOX: Serious, including fatal, cytopenias, Inf Rxns, and Infxns can occur; limit dose to 30 mg (single) & 90 mg (weekly), higher doses ↑ risk of pancytopenia; ↓ dose gradually & monitor during Inf, D/C for Grade 3 or 4 Inf Rxns; give prophylaxis for PCP & herpes virus Infxns Uses: *B-cell CLL* **Acts:** CD52-directed cytolytic Ab **Dose:** *Adults.* 3 mg d 1, then ↑ dose to 30 mg/d IV 3×/wk for 12 wk (see label for escalation strategy); infuse over 2 h; premedicate w/ oral antihistamine & APAP **W/P:**

[C, ?/–] Do not give live vaccines; D/C for autoimmune/severe hematologic Rxns **Disp:** Inj 30 mq/mL (1 mL) **SE:** Cytopenias, Infxns, Inf Rxns, ↓/↑ BP, Inj site Rxn N/V/D, insomnia, anxiety **Notes:** ✓ CBC & plt weekly & CD4 counts after Rx until > 200 cells/μL

Alendronate (Fosamax, Fosamax Plus D) Uses: *Rx & prevent osteoporosis male & postmenopausal female, Rx steroid-induced osteoporosis, Paget Dz* **Acts:** ↓ Nl & abnormal bone resorption, ↓ osteoclast action **Dose:** *Osteoporosis:* Rx: 10 mg/d PO or 70 mg qwk; Fosamax plus D 1 tab qwk *Steroid-induced osteoporosis:* Rx: 5 mg/d PO, 10 mg/d postmenopausal not on estrogen *Prevention:* 5 mg/d PO or 35 mg qwk *Paget Dz:* 40 mg/d PO × 6 mo **W/P:** [C, ?] Not OK if CrCl < 35 mL/min, w/ NSAID use **CI:** Esophageal anomalies, inability to sit/stand upright for 30 min, ↓ Ca²⁺ **Disp:** Tabs 5, 10, 35, 40, 70 mg, *Fosamax plus D:* Alendronate 70 mg w/ cholecalciferol (vit D₃) 2800 or 5600 Int units **SE:** Abd pain, acid regurgitation, constipation, D/N, dyspepsia, musculoskeletal pain, jaw osteonecrosis (w/ dental procedures, chemo) **Notes:** Take 1st thing in AM w/ H₂O (8 oz) > 30 min before 1st food/beverage of day; do not lie down for 30 min after. Use Ca²⁺ & vit D supl w/ regular tab; may ↑ atypical subtrochanteric femur fractures

Alfentanil (Alfenta) [C-II] Uses: *Adjunct in maint of anesthesia; analgesia* **Acts:** Short-acting narcotic analgesic **Dose:** *Adults & Peds > 12 y.* 3–75 mcg/kg (IBW) IV Inf; total depends on duration of procedure **W/P:** [C, –] ↑ ICP, resp depression **Disp:** Inj 500 mcg/mL **SE:** ↓ HR, ↓ BP arrhythmias, peripheral vasodilation, ↑ ICP, drowsiness, resp depression, N/V/constipation, ADH release

Alfuzosin (Uroxatral) Uses: *Symptomatic BPH* **Acts:** α-Blocker **Dose:** 10 mg PO daily immediately after the same meal **W/P:** [B, ?/–]w/ any Hx ↓ BP; use w/ PDE5 inhibitors may ↓ BP; may ↑ QTc interval; IFIS during cataract surgery **CI:** CYP3A4 inhib; mod–severe hepatic impair; protease inhibitors for HIV **Disp:** Tabs 10 mg ER **SE:** Postural ↓ BP, dizziness, HA, fatigue **Notes:** Do not cut or crush

Alginic Acid + Aluminum Hydroxide & Magnesium Trisilicate (Gaviscon) [OTC] Uses: *Heartburn* **Acts:** Protective layer blocks gastric acid **Dose:** Chew 2–4 tabs or 15–30 mL PO qid followed by H₂O **W/P:** [C, ?] Avoid w/ renal impair or Na⁺-restricted diet **Disp:** Chew tabs, susp **SE:** D, constipation

Alglucosidase Alfa (Lumizyme, Myozyme) ↓ CV/resp Fxn Uses: *Rx Pompe DZ* **Acts:** Recombinant acid α-glucosidase; degrades glycogen in lysosomes **Dose:** *Peds 1 mo–3.5 y.* 20 mg/kg IV q2wk over 4 h (see PI) **W/P:** [B, ?/–] Illness at time of Inf may ↑ Inf Rxns **Disp:** Powder 50 mg/vial limited distribution **SE:** Hypersens, fever, rash, D, V, gastroenteritis, pneumonia, URI, cough, resp distress/failure, Infxns, cardiac arrhythmia, ↑/↓ HR, flushing, anemia, pain, constipation

Aliskiren (Tekturna) Uses: *HTN* **Acts:** 1st direct renin

inhib **Dose:** 150–300 mg/d PO **W/P:** [D, ?/–]; Avoid w/ CrCl < 30 mL/min; ketoconazole and other CYP3A4 inhib may ↑ aliskiren levels **CI:** Anuria, sulfur sensitivity **Disp:** Tabs 150, 300 mg **SE:** D, Abd pain, dyspepsia, GERD, cough, ↑ K+,
angioedema, ↓ BP, dizziness, ↑ BUN, ↑ SCr

Aliskiren & Amlodipine (Tekamlo) **BOX:** May cause fetal injury & death;
D/C immediately when PRG detected **Uses:** *HTN* **Acts:** Renin inhib w/ dihydro-
pyridine CCB **Dose:** *Adult.* 150/5 mg PO 1×/d; max 300/10 mg/d); max effect in
2 wk **W/P:** [D, ?/–] do not use w/ cyclosporine/itraconazole avoid CrCl < 30 mL/min
Disp: Tabs (aliskiren mg/amlodipine mg) 150/5, 150/10, 300/5, 300/10 **SE:** ↓ BP, ↑
K+, angioedema, peripheral edema, D, dizziness, angina, MI, ↑ SCr, ↑ BUN

Aliskiren, Amlodipine, Hydrochlorothiazide (Amturnide) **BOX:**
May cause fetal injury & death; D/C immediately when PRG detected **Uses:**
HTN **Acts:** Renin inhib, dihydropyridine CCB, & thiazide diuretic **Dose:** *Adult.*
Titrate q2wk PRN to 300/10/25 mg PO max/d **W/P:** [D, ?/–] Avoid w/ CrCl < 30
mL/min; do not use w/ cyclosporine/itraconazole; ↓ BP in salt/volume depleted
pts; HCTZ may exacerbate/activate SLE; D/C if myopia or NAG **CI:** Anuria, sulfonamide allergy **Disp:** Tabs (aliskiren mg/amlodipine mg/HCTZ mg) 150/5/12.5,
300/5/12.5, 300/5/25, 300/10/12.5, 300/10/25 **SE:** ↓ BP, ↑ K+, hyperuricemia,
angioedema, peripheral edema, D, HA, dizziness, angina, MI, nasopharyngitis

Aliskiren/Hydrochlorothiazide (Tekturna HCT) **BOX:** May cause
injury and death to a developing fetus; D/C immediately when PRG detected **Uses:**
HTN **Acts:** Renin inhib w/ thiazide diuretic **Dose:** 150 mg/12.5 mg PO q day;
may ↑ after 2–4 wk up to *max* 300 mg/25 mg **W/P:** [D, –] Avoid w/ CrCl ≤ 30 mL/
min; avoid w/ CYP3A4 inhib (Li, ketoconazole, etc) may ↑ aliskiren levels; ↓ BP in
salt/volume depleted pts sulfonamide allergy HCTZ may exacerbate/activate SLE
Disp: Tabs (aliskiren mg/HCTZ mg) 150/12.5, 150/25, 300/12.5, 300/25 **SE:** Dizziness, influenza, D, cough, vertigo, asthenia, arthralgia, angioedema, ↑ BUN

Allopurinol (Zyloprim, Aloprim) **Uses:** *Gout, hyperuricemia of malignancy, uric acid urolithiasis* **Acts:** Xanthine oxidase inhib; ↓ uric acid production **Dose:** *Adults. PO:* Initial 100 mg/d; usual 300 mg/d; max 800 mg/d; ÷ dose
if > 300 mg/d *IV:* 200–400 mg/m²/d (max 600 mg/24 h); (after meal w/ plenty of
fluid) *Peds.* Only for hyperuricemia of malignancy if < 10 y: 10 mg/kg/d PO
(max 800 mg) or 50–100 mg/m² q8h (max 300 mg/m²/d); 200–400 mg/m²/d IV
(max 600 mg) ↓ in renal impair **W/P:** [C, M] **Disp:** Tabs 100, 300 mg, Inj
500 mg/30 mL (Aloprim) **SE:** Rash, N/V, renal impair, angioedema **Notes:** Aggra-
vates acute gout; begin after acute attack resolves; IV dose of 6 mg/mL final conc
as single daily Inf or ÷ 6-, 8-, or 12-h intervals

Almotriptan (Axert) **Uses:** *Rx acute migraine* **Acts:** Vascular serotonin
receptor agonist **Dose:** *Adults. PO:* 6.25–12.5 mg PO, repeat in 2 h PRN; 2 dose/24 h
max PO dose; w/ hepatic/renal impair, w/ potent CYP3A4 6.25–mg single dose (max
12.5 mg/d) **W/P:** [C, ?/–] **CI:** Angina, ischemic heart Dz, coronary artery vasospasm, hemiplegic or basilar migraine, uncontrolled HTN, ergot use, w/ sulfonamide

allergy MAOI use w/in 14 d **Disp:** Tabs 6.25, 12.5 **SE:** N, somnolence, paresthesias, HA, dry mouth, weakness, numbness, coronary vasospasm, HTN

Alogliptin (Nesina) **Uses:** *Monotherapy type 2 DM* **Acts:** DDP-4 inhib, ↑ insulin synth/release **Dose:** 25 mg/d PO; if CrCl 30–60 mL/min 12.5 mg/d; CrCl < 30 mL/min 6.25 mg/d **W/P:** [B, M] 0.2% pancreatitis risk, hepatic failure, hypersens Rxn **CI:** Hypersens **Disp:** Tabs 6.25, 12.5, 25 mg **SE:** Hypoglycemia, HA, nasopharyngitis, URI

Alogliptin/Metformin (Kazano) **BOX:** Lactic acidosis w/ metformin accumulation; ↑ risk w/ sepsis, vol depletion, CHF, renal/hepatic impair, excess alcohol; w/ lactic acidosis suspected D/C and hospitalize **Uses:** *Combo type 2 DM* **Acts:** DDP-4 inhib; ↑ insulin synth/release w/ biguanide; ↓ hepatic glucose prod & absorption; ↑ insulin sens **Dose:** Max daily 25 mg alogliptin, 2000 mg metformin **W/P:** [B, M] may cause lactic acidosis, pancreatitis, hepatic failure, hypersens Rxn, vit B_{12} def **CI:** hx of hypersens, renal impair (♀ SCr ≥ 1.4 mg/dL or ♂ ≥ 1.5 mg/dL), metabolic acidosis **Disp:** Tabs (alogliptin mg/metformin mg): 12.5/500, 12.5/1000 **SE:** ↓ glucose, HA, nasopharyngitis, D, ↑ BP, back pain, URI **Notes:** Warn against excessive EtOH intake, may ↑ metformin lactate effect; temp D/C w/ surgery or w/ iodinated contrast studies

Alogliptin/Pioglitazone (Oseni) **BOX:** May cause/worsen CHF **Uses:** *Combo type 2 DM* **Acts:** DDP-4 inhibitor, ↑ insulin synth/release w/ thiazolidinedione; ↑ insulin sens **Dose:** 25 mg alogliptin/15 mg pioglitazone or 25 mg/30 mg/d; NYHA Class I/II, start 25 mg/15 mg **W/P:** [C, –] **CI:** CHF NYHA Class III/IV, hx of hypersens **Disp:** Tabs (alogliptin mg/pioglitazone mg): 25/15, 25/30, 25/45, 12.5/15, 12.5/30, 12.5/45 **SE:** Back pain, nasopharyngitis, URI **Notes:** 25 mg/15 mg max w/ strong CYP2C8 inhib; may ↑ bladder CA risk (~↑ 3/10,000)

Alosetron (Lotronex) **BOX:** Serious GI SEs, some fatal, including ischemic colitis reported. Prescribed only through participation in the prescribing program **Uses:** *Severe D/predominant IBS in women who fail conventional Rx* **Acts:** Selective 5-HT₃ receptor antagonist **Dose:** *Adults.* 0.5 mg PO bid; ↑ to 1 mg bid max after 4 wk; D/C after 8 wk not controlled **W/P:** [B, ?/–] **CI:** Hx chronic/severe constipation, GI obst, strictures, toxic megacolon, GI perforation, adhesions, ischemic/UC, Crohn Dz, diverticulitis, thrombophlebitis, hypercoagulability **Disp:** Tabs 0.5, 1 mg **SE:** Constipation, Abd pain, N, fatigue, HA **Notes:** D/C immediately if constipation or Sxs of ischemic colitis develop; informed consent prior to use

Alpha-1-Protease Inhibitor (Glassia, Prolastin C) **Uses:** *α₁-Antitrypsin deficiency* **Acts:** Replace human α₁-protease inhib **Dose:** 60 mg/kg IV once/wk **W/P:** [C, ?] **CI:** Selective IgA deficiencies w/ IgA antibodies **Disp:** Inj 500, 1000 mg powder; 1000 mg soln vial for Inj **SE:** HA, CP, edema, MS discomfort, fever, dizziness, flu-like Sxs, allergic Rxns, ↑ AST/ALT

Alprazolam (Xanax, Niravam) [C-IV] **Uses:** *Anxiety & panic disorders*, anxiety w/ depression* **Acts:** Benzodiazepine; antianxiety agent **Dose:** *Anxiety:* Initial, 0.25–0.5 mg tid; ↑ to 4 mg/d max ÷ doses *Panic:* Initial, 0.5 mg tid; may gradually ↑ to response; ↓ in elderly, debilitated, & hepatic impair **W/P:** [D, –] **CI:** NAG, concomitant itra-/ketoconazole **Disp:** Tabs 0.25, 0.5, 1, 2 mg; Xanax XR 0.5, 1, 2, 3 mg; Niravam (ODTs) 0.25, 0.5, 1, 2 mg; soln 1 mg/mL **SE:** Drowsiness, fatigue, irritability, memory impair, sexual dysfunction, paradoxical Rxns **Notes:** Avoid abrupt D/C after prolonged use

Alprostadil [Prostaglandin E₁] (Prostin VR) **BOX:** Apnea in up to 12% of neonates especially < 2 kg at birth **Uses:** *Conditions where ductus arteriosus flow must be maintained*, sustain pulm/systemic circulation until OR (eg, pulm atresia/stenosis, transposition) **Acts:** Vasodilator (ductus arteriosus very sensitive), plt inhib **Dose:** 0.05–0.1 mcg/kg/min IV; ↓ to response **ECC 2010:** Maintain ductus patency: 0.01–0.4 mcg/kg/min **W/P:** [X, –] **CI:** Neonatal resp distress synd **Disp:** Inj 500 mcg/mL **SE:** Cutaneous vasodilation, Sz-like activity, jitteriness, ↑ temp, ↓ K⁺, thrombocytopenia, ↓ BP; may cause apnea **Notes:** Keep intubation kit at bedside

Alprostadil, Intracavernosal (Caverject, Edex) **Uses:** *ED* **Acts:** Relaxes smooth muscles, dilates cavernosal arteries, ↑ lacunar spaces w/ blood entrapment **Dose:** 2.5–60 mcg intracavernosal; titrate in office **W/P:** [X,] **CI:** ↑ risk of priapism (eg, sickle cell); penile deformities/implants; men in whom sexual activity inadvisable **Disp:** *Caverject:* 5-, 10-, 20-, 40-mcg powder for Inj vials ± diluent syringes 10-, 20-, 40-mcg amp *Caverject Impulse:* Self-contained syringe (29 gauge) 10 & 20 mcg *Edex:* 10-, 20-, 40-mcg cartridges **SE:** Local pain w/ Inj **Notes:** Counsel about priapism, penile fibrosis, & hematoma risks, titrate dose in office

Alprostadil, Urethral Suppository (Muse) **Uses:** *ED* **Acts:** Urethral absorption; vasodilator, relaxes smooth muscle of corpus cavernosa **Dose:** 125–250 mcg PRN to achieve erection (max 2 systems/24 h) duration 30–60 min **W/P:** [X, –] **CI:** ↑ Priapism risk (especially sickle cell, myeloma, leukemia) penile deformities/implants; men in whom sex inadvisable **Disp:** 125, 250, 500, 1000 mcg w/ transurethral system **SE:** ↓ BP, dizziness, syncope, penile/testicular pain, urethral burning/bleeding, priapism **Notes:** Titrate dose in office

Alteplase, Recombinant [tPA] (Activase) **Uses:** *AMI, PE, acute ischemic stroke, & CV cath occlusion* **Acts:** Thrombolytic; binds fibrin in thrombus, initiates fibrinolysis **Dose:** **ECC 2010:** STEMI: 15-mg bolus; then 0.75 mg/kg over 30 min (50 mg max); then 0.50 mg/kg over next 60 min (35 mg max; max total dose 100 mg) Acute ischemic stroke: 0.9 mg/kg IV (max 90 mg) over 60 min; give 10% of total dose over 1 min; remaining 90% over 1 h (or 3-h Inf) *PE:* 100 mg over 2 h (submassive PE: can administer 10-mg bolus, then 90 mg over 2 h) *Cath occlusion:* 10–29 kg 1 mg/mL; ≥ 30 kg 2 mg/L **W/P:** [C, ?] **CI:** Active internal bleeding; uncontrolled HTN (SBP > 185 mm Hg, DBP > 110 mm Hg); recent (w/in 3 mo) CVA, GI bleed, trauma; intracranial or intraspinal surgery or Dzs (AVM/aneurysm/subarachnoid hemorrhage/neoplasm), prolonged cardiac massage; suspected aortic dissection, w/ anticoagulants or INR > 1.7, heparin w/in 48 h, plts < 100,000, Sz at the time of stroke, significant closed head/facial trauma **Disp:** Powder for Inj 2, 50, 100 mg **SE:** Bleeding, bruising (eg, venipuncture sites), ↓ BP **Notes:** Give heparin to prevent reocclusion; in AMI, doses of > 150 mg associated w/ intracranial bleeding

Altretamine (Hexalen) **BOX:** BM suppression, neurotox common should be administered by experienced chemo MD **Uses:** *Palliative Rx persistent or recurrent ovarian CA* **Acts:** Unknown; ? cytotoxic/alkylating agent; ↓ nucleotide incorporation **Dose:** 260 mg/m²/d in 4 ÷ doses for 14–21 d of a 28-d Rx cycle; after meals and hs **W/P:** [D, ?/–] **CI:** Preexisting BM depression or neurologic tox **Disp:** Gel caps 50 mg **SE:** N/V/D, cramps; neurotox (neuropathy, CNS depression); myelosuppression, anemia, ↓ PLT, ↓ WBC **Notes:** ✓ CBC, routine neurologic exams

Aluminum Hydroxide (Amphojel, AlternaGEL, Dermagran) [OTC] **Uses:** *Heartburn, upset or sour stomach, or acid indigestion*; supl to Rx of ↑PO₄²⁻; *minor cuts, burns (Dermagran)* **Acts:** Neutralizes gastric acid; binds PO_4^{2-} **Dose:** *Adults.* 10 30 mL or 300 1200 mg PO q4 6h *Peds.* 5 15 mL PO q4–6h or 50–150 mg/kg/24 h PO ÷ q4–6h (hyperphosphatemia) **W/P:** [C, ?] **Disp:** Tabs 300, 600 mg; susp 320, 600 mg/5 mL; oint 0.275% (*Dermagran*) **SE:** Constipation **Notes:** OK w/ renal failure; topical ointment for cuts/burns

Aluminum Hydroxide + Alginic Acid + Magnesium Carbonate (Gaviscon Extra Strength, Liquid) [OTC] **Uses:** *Heartburn, acid indigestion* **Acts:** Neutralizes gastric acid **Dose:** *Adults.* 15–30 mL PO pc & hs; 2–4 chew tabs up to qid. **W/P:** [C, ?] ↑ Mg²⁺, avoid w/in renal impair **Disp:** Liq w/ AlOH 95 mg/Mg carbonate 358 mg/15 mL; Extra Strength liq AlOH 254 mg/Mg carbonate 237 mg/15 mL; chew tabs AlOH 160 mg/Mg carbonate 105 mg **SE:** Constipation, ↓ Notes: Qid doses best pc & hs; may ↓ absorption of some drugs, take 2–3 h apart to ↓ effect

Aluminum Hydroxide + Magnesium Hydroxide (Maalox, Mylanta Ultimate Strength) [OTC] **Uses:** *Hyperacidity* (peptic ulcer, hiatal hernia, etc) **Acts:** Neutralizes gastric acid **Dose:** *Adults.* 10–20 mL or 1–2 tabs PO qid or PRN **W/P:** [C, ?] **Disp:** Chew tabs, susp **SE:** May ↑ Mg²⁺ w/ renal Insuff, constipation, ↓ Notes: Doses qid best pc & hs

Aluminum Hydroxide + Magnesium Hydroxide & Simethicone (Mylanta Regular Strength, Maalox Advanced) [OTC] **Uses:** *Hyperacidity w/ bloating* **Acts:** Neutralizes gastric acid & defoaming **Dose:** *Adults.* 10–20 mL or 1–2 tabs PO qid or PRN, avoid in renal impair **W/P:** [C, ?] **Disp:** Tabs, susp, liq **SE:** ↑ Mg²⁺ in renal Insuff, ↓, constipation **Notes:** Mylanta II contains twice Al & Mg hydroxide of Mylanta; may affect absorption of some drugs

Aluminum Hydroxide + Magnesium Trisilicate (Gaviscon, Regular Strength) [OTC] **Uses:** *Relief of heartburn, upset or sour stomach, or acid indigestion* **Acts:** Neutralizes gastric acid **Dose:** Chew 1–2 tabs qid; avoid in renal impair **W/P:** [C, ?] **CI:** Mg²⁺, sensitivity **Disp:** AlOH 80 mg/Mg trisilicate 20 mg/tab **SE:** ↑ Mg²⁺ in renal Insuff, constipation, ↓ **Notes:** May affect absorption of some drugs

Alvimopan (Entereg) BOX: For short-term hospital use only (max 15 doses) Uses: *↓ Time to GI recovery w/ bowel resection and primary anastomosis* Acts: Opioid (μ) receptor antagonist; selectively binds GI receptors, antagonizes effects of opioids on GI motility/secretion Dose: 12 mg 30 min–5 h preop PO, then 12 mg bid up to 7 d; max 15 doses W/P: [B, ?/–] Not rec in complete bowel obstruction surgery, hepatic/renal impair CI: Therapeutic opioids > 7 consecutive days prior Disp: Caps 12 mg SE: ↓ K+, dyspepsia, urinary retention, anemia, back pain Notes: Hospitals must be registered to use

Amantadine (Symmetrel) Uses: *Rx/prophylaxis influenza A (no longer recommended d/t resistance), Parkinsonism, & drug-induced EPS* Acts: Prevents infectious viral nucleic acid release into host cell; releases dopamine and blocks reuptake of dopamine in presynaptic nerves Dose: *Adults. Influenza A:* 200 mg/d PO or 100 mg PO bid w/in 48 h of Sx *EPS:* 100 mg PO bid (up to 300 mg/d ÷ doses) *Parkinsonism:* 100 mg PO daily-bid (up to 400 mg/d) *Peds 1–9 y.* 4.4–8.8 mg/kg/24 h to 150 mg/24 h max ÷ doses daily-bid *10–12 y.* 100–200 mg/d in 2 ÷ doses; ↓ in renal impair W/P: [C, ?/–] Disp: Caps 100 mg; tabs 100 mg; soln 50 mg/5 mL SE: Orthostatic ↓ BP, edema, insomnia, depression, irritability, hallucinations, dream abnormalities, N/D, dry mouth Notes: Not for influenza use in US d/t resistance including H1N1

Ambrisentan (Letairis) BOX: CI in PRG; ✓ monthly PRG tests; limited access program Uses: *Pulm arterial HTN* Acts: Endothelin receptor antagonist Dose: *Adults.* 5 mg PO/d, max 10 mg/d; not OK w/ hepatic impair W/P: [X, –] w/ Cyclosporine, strong CYP3A or 2C19 inhib, inducers of P-glycoprotein, CYPs and UGTs CI: PRG Disp: Tabs 5, 10 mg SE: Edema, ↓ Hct/Hgb nasal congestion, sinusitis, dyspnea, flushing, constipation, HA, palpitations, hepatotoxic Notes: Available only through the Letairis Education and Access Program (LEAP); D/C AST/ALT > 5× ULN or bili > 2× ULN or S/Sx of liver dysfunction; childbearing females must use 2 methods of contraception

Amifostine (Ethyol) Uses: *Xerostomia prophylaxis during RT (head, neck, etc) where parotid is in radiation field; ↓ renal tox w/ repeated cisplatin* Acts: Prodrug, dephosphorylated to active thiol metabolite, free radical scavenger binds cisplatin metabolites Dose: Chemo prevent: 910 mg/m²/d 15-min IV Inf 30 min pre-chemo; *Xerostomia Px:* 200 mg/m² over 2 min IV/d 15 min pre-rad W/P: [C, ?/–] Disp: 500-mg vials powder, reconstitute in NS SE: Transient ↓ BP (> 60%), N/V, flushing w/ hot or cold chills, dizziness, ↓ Ca²⁺, somnolence, sneezing, serious skin Infxn Notes: Does not ↓ effectiveness of cyclophosphamide + cisplatin chemotherapy

Amikacin (Amikin) BOX: May cause nephrotoxicity, neuromuscular blockade, & respiratory paralysis Uses: *Serious gram(–) bacterial Infxns* & mycobacteria Acts: Aminoglycoside; ↓ protein synth Spectrum: Good gram(–) bacterial coverage: *Pseudomonas* & *Mycobacterium* sp Dose: *Adults & Peds. Conventional:* 5–7.5 mg/kg/dose q8h; once daily; 15–20 mg/kg q24h; ↑ interval w/ renal impair

Neonates < 1200 g, 0–4 wk: 7.5 mg/kg/dose q18h–24h *Age < 7 d, 1200–2000 g:* 7.5 mg/kg/dose q12h *> 2000 g:* 7.5–10 mg/kg/dose q12h *Age > 7 d, 1200–2000 g:* 7.5–10 mg/kg/dose q8–12h *> 2000 g:* 7.5–10 mg/kg/dose q8h **W/P:** [O, +/–] Avoid w/ diuretics **Disp:** Inj 50 & 250 mg/mL **SE:** Renal impairment, oto **Notes:** May be effective in gram(–) resistance to gentamicin & tobramycin; follow Cr; Levels: *Peak:* 30 min after Inf *Trough* < 0.5 h before next dose *Therapeutic: Peak* 20–30 mcg/mL, *Trough:* < 8 mcg/mL; *Toxic peak* > 35 mcg/mL; *half-life:* 2 h

Amiloride (Midamor)   **BOX:** ↑ K⁺ esp renal Dz DM, elderly **Uses:** *HTN, CHF, & thiazide or loop diuretic induced ↓ K⁺* **Acts:** K⁺-sparing diuretic; interferes w/ K⁺/Na⁺ exchange in distal tubule & collecting duct **Dose:** *Adults.* 5–10 mg PO daily (max 20 mg/d) *Peds.* 0.4–0.625 mg/kg/d; ↓ w/ renal impair **W/P:** [B, ?] avoid CrCl < 10 mL/min **CI:** ↑ K⁺, acute or chronic renal Dz, diabetic neuropathy, w/ other K⁺-sparing diuretics **Disp:** Tabs 5 mg **SE:** ↑ K⁺; HA, dizziness, dehydration, impotence **Notes:** ✓ K⁺

Aminocaproic Acid (Amicar)   **Uses:** *Excessive bleeding from systemic hyperfibrinolysis & urinary fibrinolysis* **Acts:** ↓ Fibrinolysis; inhibits TPA, inhibits conversion of plasminogen to plasmin **Dose:** *Adults.* 4–5 g IV or PO (1st h) then 1 g/h IV or 1.25 g/h PO × 8 h or until bleeding controlled; 30 g/d max *Peds.* 100 mg/kg IV (1st h) then 1 g/m²/h; max 18 g/m²/d; ↓ w/ renal Insuff **W/P:** [C, ?] Not for upper urinary tract bleeding **CI:** DIC **Disp:** Tabs 500 mg, syrup 1.25 g/5 mL; Inj 250 mg/mL **SE:** ↓ BP, ↓ HR, dizziness, HA, fatigue, rash, GI disturbance, skeletal muscle weakness, ↓ plt Fxn **Notes:** Administer × 8 h or until bleeding controlled

Aminoglutethimide (Cytadren)   **Uses:** *Cushing synd*, adrenocortical carcinoma, breast CA & PCa* **Acts:** ↓ Adrenal steroidogenesis & conversion of androgens to estrogens; ↓w/ aromatase inhib **Dose:** Initial 250 mg PO 4× d, titrate q1–2wk max 2 g/d; w/ hydrocortisone 20–40 mg/d; ↓ w/ renal Insuff **W/P:** [D, ?] **Disp:** Tabs 250 mg **SE:** Adrenal Insuff ("medical adrenalectomy"), hypothyroidism, masculinization,* rash, myalgia, fever, drowsiness, lethargy, anorexia **Notes:** Give q6h to ↓ N

Aminophylline (Generic)   **Uses:** *Asthma, COPD*, & bronchospasm **Acts:** Relaxes smooth muscle (bronchi, pulm vessels); stimulates diaphragm **Dose:** *Adults. Acute asthma:* Load 5.7 mg/kg IV, then 0.38–0.51 mg/kg/h (900 mg/d max) *Chronic asthma:* 380 mg/d PO ÷ q6–8h; maint ↑ 760 mg/d *Peds.* Load 5.7 mg/kg/dose IV; *1 ≤ 9 y:* 1.01 mg/kg/h; *9 ≤ 12 y:* 0.89 mg/kg/h; w/ hepatic Insuff & w/ some drugs (macrolide & quinolone antib, cimetidine, propranolol) **W/P:** [C, +] Uncontrolled arrhythmias, HTN, Sz disorder, hyperthyroidism, peptic ulcers **Disp:** Tabs 100, 200 mg; PR tabs 100, 200 mg, soln 105 mg/5 mL, Inj 25 mg/mL **SE:** N/V, irritability, tachycardia, ventricular arrhythmias, Szs **Notes:** Individualize dosage *Level:* 10–20 mcg/mL, toxic > 20 mcg/mL; aminophylline 85% theophylline; erratic rectal absorption

Amiodarone (Cordarone, Nexterone, Pacerone) BOX: Liver tox, exacerbation of arrhythmias and lung damage reported **Uses:** *Recurrent VF or unstable VT*, supraventricular arrhythmias, AF **Acts:** Class III antiarrhythmic inhibits alpha/beta adrenergic system (Table 9, p 318) **Dose:** *Adults. Ventricular arrhythmias:* IV: 15 mg/min × 10 min, then 1 mg/min × 6 h, maint 0.5-mg/min cont Inf or *PO:* Load: 800–1600 mg/d PO × 1–3 wk Maint: 600–800 mg/d PO for 1 mo, then 200–400 mg/d *Supraventricular arrhythmias: IV:* 300 mg IV over 1 h, then 20 mg/kg for 24 h, then 600 mg PO daily for 1 wk, maint 100–400 mg daily or *PO:* Load 600–800 mg/d PO for 1–4 wk *Maint:* Slow ↓ to 100–400 mg daily *ECC 2010. VF/VT cardiac arrest refractory to CPR, shock and pressor:* 300 mg IV/IO push; can give additional 150 mg IV/IO once; *Life-threatening arrhythmias:* Max dose: 2.2 g IV/24 h; rapid Inf: 150 mg IV over first 10 min (15 mg/min); can repeat 150 mg IV q10min PRN; slow Inf: 360 mg IV over 60 min (1 mg/min); maint: 540 mg IV over 18 h (0.5 mg/min) *Peds.* 10–15 mg/kg/24 h ÷ q12h PO for 7–10 d, then 5 mg/kg/24 h ÷ q12h or daily (infants require ↑ loading) *ECC 2010. Pulseless VT/Refractory VF:* 5 mg/kg IV/IO bolus, repeat PRN to 15 mg/kg (2.2 g in adolescents)/24 h; max single dose 300 mg; *Perfusing SVT/Ventricular arrhythmias:* 5 mg/kg IV/IO load over 20–60 min; repeat PRN to 15 mg/kg (2.2 g in adolescents)/24h **W/P:** [D, –] May require ↓ digoxin/warfarin dose, ↓ w/ liver Insuff; many drug interactions **CI:** Sinus node dysfunction, 2nd-/3rd-degree AV block, sinus brady (w/o pacemaker), iodine sensitivity **Disp:** Tabs 100, 200, 400 mg; Inj 50 mg/mL; Premixed Inf 150, 360 mg **SE:** Pulm fibrosis, exacerbation of arrhythmias, ↑ QT interval; CHF, hypo-/hyperthyroidism, ↑ LFTs, liver failure, ↓ BP/↓ HR (Inf related) dizziness, HA, corneal microdeposits, optic neuropathy/neuritis, peripheral neuropathy, photosens; blue skin **Notes:** IV conc > 2.0 mg/mL central line only Levels: *Trough:* just before next dose *Therapeutic:* 0.5–2.5 mcg/mL *Toxic:* > 2.5 mcg/mL *Half-life:* 40–55 d (↓ peds)

Amitriptyline (Elavil) BOX: Antidepressants may ↑ suicide risk; consider risks/benefits of use. Monitor pts closely **Uses:** *Depression (not bipolar depression)* peripheral neuropathy, chronic pain, tension HAs, migraine HA prophylaxis PTSD* **Acts:** TCA; ↓ reuptake of serotonin & norepinephrine by presynaptic neurons **Dose:** *Adults. Initial:* 25–150 mg PO hs; may ↑ to 300 mg hs *Peds.* Not OK < 12 y unless for chronic pain *Initial:* 0.1 mg/kg PO hs, ↑ over 2–3 wk to 0.5–2 mg/kg PO hs; taper to D/C **W/P:** CV Dz, Szs [D,+/–] NAG, hepatic impair **CI:** w/ MAOIs or w/in 14 d of use, during AMI recovery **Disp:** Tabs 10, 25, 50, 75, 100, 150 mg; Inj 10 mg/mL **SE:** Strong anticholinergic SEs; OD may be fatal; urine retention, sedation, ECG changes BM suppression, orthostatic ↓ BP, photosens **Notes:** Levels: *Therapeutic:* 100–250 mg/mL *Toxic:* > 500 mg/mL; levels may not correlate w/ effect

Amlodipine (Norvasc) Uses: *HTN, stable or unstable angina* **Acts:** CCB; relaxes coronary vascular smooth muscle **Dose:** 2.5–10 mg/d PO; ↓ w/ hepatic impair **W/P:** [C, ?] **Disp:** Tabs 2.5, 5, 10 mg **SE:** Edema, HA, palpitations, flushing, dizziness **Notes:** Take w/o regard to meals

Amlodipine/Atorvastatin (Caduet) Uses: *HTN, chronic stable/vasospastic angina, control cholesterol & triglycerides* Acts: CCB & HMG-CoA reductase inhib Dose: Amlodipine 2.5–10 mg w/ atorvastatin 10–80 mg PO daily W/P: [X, –] CI: Active liver Dz, ↑ LFTs Disp: Tabs amlodipine/atorvastatin: 2.5/10, 2.5/20, 2.5/40, 5/10, 5/20, 5/40, 5/80, 10/10, 10/20, 10/40, 10/80 SE: Edema, HA, palpitations, flushing, myopathy, arthralgia, myalgia, GI upset, liver failure Notes: ✓ LFTs; instruct pt to report muscle pain/weakness

Amlodipine/Olmesartan (Azor) BOX: Use of renin-angiotensin agents in PRG can cause injury and death to fetus, D/C immediately when PRG detected Uses: *Hypertension* Acts: CCB w/ angiotensin II receptor blocker Dose: *Adults.* Initial 5 mg/20 mg, max 10 mg/40 mg q day W/P: [D, –] w/ K⁺ supl or K⁺-sparing diuretics, renal impair, RAS, severe CAD, AS CI: PRG Disp: Tabs amlodipine/olmesartan 5 mg/20 mg, 10/20, 5/40, 10/40 SE: Edema, vertigo, dizziness, ↓ BP

Amlodipine/Valsartan (HA Exforge) BOX: Use of renin-angiotensin agents in PRG can cause fetal injury and death, D/C immediately when PRG detected Uses: *HTN* Acts: CCB w/ angiotensin II receptor blocker Dose: *Adults.* Initial 5 mg/160 mg, may ↑ after 1–2 wk, max 10 mg/320 mg q day, start elderly at 1/2 initial dose W/P: [D /–] w/ K⁺ supl or K⁺-sparing diuretics, renal impair, RAS, severe CAD SE: Edema, vertigo, nasopharyngitis, URI, dizziness, ↓ BP

Amlodipine/Valsartan/HCTZ (Exforge HCT) BOX: Use of renin-angiotensin agents in PRG can cause fetal injury and death, D/C immediately when PRG detected Uses: *Hypertension (not initial Rx)* Acts: CCB, angiotensin II receptor blocker, & thiazide diuretic Dose: 5–10/160–320/12.5–25 mg 1 tab 1 × d may ↑ dose after 2 wk; max dose 10/320/25 mg W/P: [D, –] w/ Severe hepatic or renal impair CI: Anuria, sulfonamide allergy Disp: Tabs amlodipine/valsartan/HCTZ: 5/160/12.5, 10/160/12.5, 5/160/25, 10/160/25, 10/320/25 mg SE: edema, dizziness, HA, fatigue, ↑/↓ K⁺ ↑ BUN, ↑ SCr, nasopharyngitis, dyspepsia, N, back pain, muscle spasm, ↓ BP

Ammonium Aluminum Sulfate [Alum] [OTC] Uses: *Hemorrhagic cystitis when saline bladder irrigation fails* Acts: Astringent Dose: 1–2% soln w/ constant NS bladder irrigation W/P: [+/–] Disp: Powder for recons SE: Encephalopathy possible; ✓ aluminum levels, especially w/ renal Insuff; can precipitate & occlude catheters Notes: Safe w/o anesthesia & w/ vesicoureteral reflux

Amoxicillin (Amoxil, Moxatag) Uses: *Ear, nose, & throat, lower resp, skin, urinary tract Infxns from susceptible gram(+) bacteria* endocarditis prophylaxis, H. pylori eradication w/ other agents (gastric ulcers) Acts: β-Lactam antibiotic; ↓ cell wall synth Spectrum: Gram(+) (Streptococcus sp, Enterococcus sp); some gram(–) (H. influenzae, E. coli, N. gonorrhoeae, H. pylori, & P. mirabilis) Dose: *Adults.* 250–500 mg PO tid or 500–875 mg bid ER 775 mg 1 × d Peds. 25–100 mg/kg/24 h PO ÷ q8h, ↓ in renal impair W/P: [B, +] Disp: Caps 250, 500 mg;

chew tabs 125, 200, 250, 400 mg, susp 50, 125, 200, 250 mg/mL & 400 mg/5 mL; tabs 500, 875 mg; tab ER 775 mg **SE:** D; rash **Notes:** Cross hypersens w/ PCN; many *E. coli* strains resistant; chew tabs contain phenylalanine

Amoxicillin & Clavulanic Acid (Augmentin, Augmentin 600 ES, Augmentin XR) Uses: *Ear, lower resp, sinus, urinary tract, skin Infxns caused by β-lactamase–producing *H. influenzae*, *S. aureus*, & *E. coli** **Acts:** β-Lactam antibiotic w/ β-lactamase inhib *Spectrum:* Gram(+) same as amoxicillin alone, MSSA; gram(−) as w/ amoxicillin alone, β-lactamase–producing *H. influenzae*, *Klebsiella* sp, *M. catarrhalis* **Dose:** *Adults.* 250–500 mg PO q8h or 875 mg q12h; XR 2000 mg PO q12h *Peds.* 20–40 mg/kg/d as amoxicillin PO ÷ q8h or 45–90 mg/kg/d ÷ q12h; ↓ in renal impair; take w/ food **W/P:** [B, enters breast milk] **Disp:** Supplied (as amoxicillin/clavulanic): Tabs 250/125, 500/125, 875/125 mg; chew tabs 125/31.25, 200/28.5, 250/62.5, 400/57 mg; susp 125/31.25, 250/62.5, 200/28.5, 400/57 mg/5 mL; susp ES 600/42.9 mg/5 mL; XR tab 1000/62.5 mg **SE:** Abd discomfort, N/V/D, allergic Rxn, vaginitis **Notes:** Do not substitute two 250-mg tabs for one 500-mg tab (possible OD of clavulanic acid); max clavulanic acid 125 mg/dose

Amphotericin B (Fungizone) Uses: *Severe, systemic fungal Infxns; oral & cutaneous candidiasis* **Acts:** Binds ergosterol in the fungal membrane to alter permeability **Dose:** *Adults & Peds.* 0.25–1.5 mg/kg/24 h IV over 2–6 h (25–50 mg/d or q other day). Total varies w/ indication ↑ PR, N/V **W/P:** [B, ?] **Disp:** Powder (Inj) 50 mg/vial **SE:** ↓ K⁺/Mg²⁺ from renal wasting; anaphylaxis, HA, fever, chills, nephrotox, ↓ BP, anemia, rigors **Notes:** ✓ Cr/LFTs/K⁺/Mg²⁺; ↓ in renal impair; pretreatment w/ APAP & diphenhydramine ± hydrocortisone, ↓ SE

Amphotericin B Cholesteryl (Amphotec) Uses: *Aspergillosis if intolerant/refractory to conventional amphotericin B*, systemic candidiasis* **Acts:** Binds ergosterol in fungal membrane, alters permeability **Dose:** *Adults & Peds.* 3–4 mg/kg/d; 1 mg/kg/h Inf, 7.5 mg/kg/d max; ↓ w/ renal Insuff **W/P:** [B, ?] **Disp:** Powder for Inj 50, 100 mg/vial **SE:** Anaphylaxis; fever, chills, HA, ↓ PLT, N/V, ↑ HR, ↓ K⁺, ↓ Mg²⁺, nephrotox, ↓ BP, infusion Rxns, anemia **Notes:** Do not use in-line filter; ✓ LFTs/lytes

Amphotericin B Lipid Complex (Abelcet) Uses: *Refractory invasive fungal Infxn in pts intolerant to conventional amphotericin B* **Acts:** Binds ergosterol in fungal membrane, alters permeability **Dose:** *Adults & Peds.* 2.5–5 mg/kg/d IV × 1 daily **W/P:** [B, ?] **Disp:** Inj 5 mg/mL **SE:** Anaphylaxis; fever, chills, HA, ↓ K⁺, ↑ SCr ↓ Mg²⁺, nephrotox, ↓ BP, anemia **Notes:** Filter w/ 5-micron needle; do not mix in electrolyte containing solns; if Inf > 2 h, manually mix bag

Amphotericin B Liposomal (AmBisome) Uses: *Refractory invasive fungal Infxn w/ intolerance to conventional amphotericin B; cryptococcal meningitis in HIV; empiric for febrile neutropenia; visceral leishmaniasis* **Acts:** Binds ergosterol in fungal membrane, alters membrane permeability **Dose:** *Adults & Peds.* 3–6 mg/kg/d, Inf 60–120 min; varies by indication; ↓ in renal Insuff **W/P:**

[B, ?] **Disp:** Powder Inj 50 mg **SE:** Anaphylaxis, fever, chills, HA, ↓ K+, ↓ Mg2+ peripheral edema, insomnia, rash, ↑ LFTs, nephrotox, ↓ BP, anemia **Notes:** Do not use < 1-micron filter

Ampicillin **Uses:** *Resp, GU, or GI tract Infxns, meningitis d/t gram(−) & (+) bacteria; SBE prophylaxis* **Acts:** β-Lactam antibiotic; ↓ cell wall synth *Spectrum:* Gram(+) (*Streptococcus* sp, *Staphylococcus* sp, *Listeria*); gram(−) (*Klebsiella* sp, *E. coli, H. influenzae, P. mirabilis, Shigella* sp, *Salmonella* sp) **Dose: Adults.** 1000 mg–2 g IM or IV q4–6h or 250–500 mg PO q6h; varies by indication *Peds Neonates < 7 d.* 50–100 mg/kg/24 h ÷ q8h *Term infants.* 75–150 mg/kg/24 h ÷ q6–8h IV or PO *Children > 1 mo.* 200 mg/kg/24 h ÷ q6h IM or IV; 50–100 mg/kg/24 h ÷ q6h PO up to 250 mg/dose *Meningitis:* 200–400 mg/kg/24 h; ↓ w/ renal impair; take on empty stomach **W/P:** [B, M] Cross-hypersens w/ PCN **Disp:** Caps 250, 500 mg; susp, 125 mg/5 mL, 250 mg/5 mL; powder (Inj) 125, 250, 500 mg, 1, 2, 10 g/vial **SE:** D, rash, allergic Rxn **Notes:** Many *E. coli* resistant

Ampicillin-Sulbactam (Unasyn) **Uses:** *Gynecologic, intra-Abd, skin Infxns d/t β-lactamase–producing S. aureus, Enterococcus, H. influenzae, P. mirabilis, & Bacteroides* sp* **Acts:** β-Lactam antibiotic & β-lactamase inhib *Spectrum:* Gram(+) & (−) as for amp alone; also *Enterobacter, Acinetobacter, Bacteroides* **Dose: Adults.** 1.5–3 g IM or IV q6h *Peds.* 100–400 mg ampicillin/kg/d (150–300 mg Unasyn) q6h; ↓ w/ renal Insuff **W/P:** [B, M] **Disp:** Powder for Inj 1.5, 3 g/vial, 15 g bulk package **SE:** Allergic Rxns, rash, D, Inj site pain **Notes:** A 2:1 ratio ampicillin:sulbactam

Anakinra (Kineret) **Uses:** *Reduce S/Sxs of mod–severe active RA, failed 1 or more DMARDs* **Acts:** Human IL-1 receptor antagonist **Dose:** 100 mg SQ daily; w/ CrCl < 30 mL/min, q other day **W/P:** [B, ?] Only > 1% y avoid in active Inf **CI:** *E. coli*-derived protein allergy **Disp:** 100-mg prefilled syringes; 100 mg (0.67 mL/vial) **SE:** ↓ WBC especially w/ TNF-blockers, Inj site Rxn (may last up to 28 d), Infxn, N/D, Abd pain, flu-like sx, HA **Notes:** ✓ immunization up to date prior to starting Rx

Anastrozole (Arimidex) **Uses:** *Breast CA: postmenopausal w/ metastatic breast CA, adjuvant Rx postmenopausal early hormone-receptor(+) breast CA* **Acts:** Selective nonsteroidal aromatase inhib, ↓ circulatory estradiol **Dose:** 1 mg/d **W/P:** [X, ?/–] **CI:** PRG **Disp:** Tabs 1 mg **SE:** May ↑ cholesterol; N/V/D, HTN, flushing, ↑ bone/tumor pain, HA, somnolence, mood disturbance, depression, rash, fatigue, weakness **Notes:** No effect on adrenal steroids or aldosterone

Anidulafungin (Eraxis) **Uses:** *Candidemia, esophageal candidiasis, other Candida Infxn (peritonitis, intra-Abd abscess)* **Acts:** Echinocandin; ↓ cell wall synth *Spectrum: C. albicans, C. glabrata, C. parapsilosis, C. tropicalis* **Dose:** Candidemia, others: 200 mg IV × 1, then 100 mg IV daily [Tx ≥ 14 d after last (+)culture]; Esophageal candidiasis: 100 mg IV × 1, then 50 mg IV daily (Tx > 14 d and 7 d after resolution of Sx); 1.1 mg/min max Inf rate **W/P:** [B, ?/–] **CI:** Echinocandin hypersens **Disp:** Powder 50, 100 mg/vial **SE:** Histamine-mediated Inf Rxns (urticaria, flushing, ↓ BP, dyspnea, etc), fever, N/V/D, ↓ K⁺, HA, ↑ LFTs, hep, worsening hepatic failure **Notes:** ↓ Inf rate to < 1.1 mg/min w/ Inf Rxns

Anthralin (Dritho, Zithranol, Zithranol-RR) Uses: *Psoriasis* **Acts:** Keratolytic **Dose:** Apply daily **W/P:** [C, ?] **CI:** Acutely inflamed psoriatic eruptions, erythroderma **Disp:** Cream, 0.5, 1, 1.2%; shampoo **SE:** Irritation; hair/fingernails/skin discoloration, erythema

Antihemophilic Factor [AHF, Factor VIII] (Monoclate) Uses: *Classic hemophilia A* **Acts:** Provides factor VIII needed to convert prothrombin to thrombin **Dose:** *Adults & Peds.* 1 AHF unit/kg ↑ factor VIII level by 2 Int unit/dL; units required = (Wt in kg) × (desired factor VIII ↑ as % nl) × (0.5); minor hemorrhage = 20–40% nl; mod hemorrhage/minor surgery = 30–50% nl; major surgery, life-threatening hemorrhage = 80–100% nl **W/P:** [C, ?] **Disp:** ✓ each vial for units contained, powder for recons **SE:** Rash, fever, HA, chills, N/V **Notes:** Determine % nl factor VIII before dosing

Antihemophilic Factor (Recombinant) (Advate, Helixate FS, Kogenate FS, Recombinate, Xyntha) Uses: *Control/prevent bleeding & surgical prophylaxis in hemophilia A* **Acts:** ↑ Levels of factor VIII **Dose:** *Adults.* Required units = body Wt (kg) × desired factor VIII rise (Int units/dL or % of nl) × 0.5 (Int units/kg per Int units/dL); frequency/duration determined by type of bleed (see PI) **W/P:** [C, ?/–] Severe hypersens Rxn possible **CI:** None **Disp:** ✓ each vial for units contained, powder for recons **SE:** HA, fever, N/V/D, weakness, allergic Rxn **Notes:** Monitor for the development of factor VIII neutralizing antibodies

Antithrombin, Recombinant (Atryn) Uses: *Prevent periop/peripartum thromboembolic events w/ hereditary antithrombin (AT) deficiency* **Acts:** Inhibits thrombin and factor Xa **Dose:** *Adults.* Based on pre-Rx AT level, BW (kg) and drug monitoring; see package. Goal AT levels 0.8–1.2 Int units/mL **W/P:** [C, +/–] Hypersensitivity Rxns; ↑ effect of heparin/LMWH **CI:** Hypersens to goat/goat milk proteins **Disp:** Powder 1750 Int units/vial **SE:** Bleeding, infusion site Rxn **Notes:** ✓aPTT and anti-factor Xa; monitor for bleeding or thrombosis

Antithymocyte Globulin (See Lymphocyte Immune Globulin, p 181)

Apixaban (Eliquis) BOX: ↑ Risk of spinal/epidural hematoma w/ paralysis & ↑ thrombotic events w/ D/C in afib pts; monitor closely **Uses:** *Prevent CVA/TE in nonvalvular afib* **Acts:** Factor Xa inhib **Dose:** 5 mg bid; 2.5 mg w/2 of the following: ≥ 80 y, Wt ≤ 60 kg, SCr ≥ 1.5; 2.5 mg w/ strong dual inhib of CYP3A4 and P-glycoprotein; if on 2.5 mg do **NOT** use w/ strong dual inhib of CYP3A4 and P-glycoprotein **W/P:** [B, –] Do not use w/ prosthetic valves **CI:** Pathological bleeding & apixaban hypersens **Disp:** Tabs 2.5, 5 mg **SE:** Bleeding **Notes:** If missed dose, do **NOT** double next dose; no antidote to reverse; anticoagulant effect can last 24 h after dose

Apomorphine (Apokyn) Uses: *Acute, intermittent hypomobility ("off") episodes of Parkinson Dz* **Acts:** Dopamine agonist **Dose:** *Adults.* 0.2 mL SQ supervised test dose; if BP OK, initial 0.2 mL (2 mg) SQ during "off" periods; only 1 dose per "off" period; titrate dose; 0.6 mL (6 mg) max single doses; use w/ anti-emetic; ↓ in renal impair **W/P:** [C, ?] Avoid EtOH; antihypertensives, vasodilators, cardio-/cerebrovascular Dz, hepatic impair **CI:** IV administration 5-HT₃ antagonists, sulfite allergy **Disp:** Inj 10 mg/mL, 3-mL pen cartridges **SE:** Emesis, syncope, ↑ QT, orthostatic ↓ BP, somnolence, ischemia, Inj site Rxn, edema, N/V, hallucination abuse potential, dyskinesia, fibrotic conditions, priapism, CP/angina, yawning, rhinorrhea **Notes:** Daytime somnolence may limit activities; trimethobenzamide 300 mg tid PO or other non–5-HT₃ antagonist antiemetic given 3 d prior to & up to 2 mo following initiation

Apraclonidine (Iopidine) Uses: *Control, postop intraocular HTN* **Acts:** α₂-Adrenergic agonist **Dose:** 1–2 gtt of 0.5% tid; 1 gtt of 1% before and after surgical procedure **W/P:** [C, ?] **CI:** w/in 14 d of or w/ MAOI **Disp:** 0.5, 1% soln **SE:** Ocular irritation, lethargy, xerostomia, blurred vision

Aprepitant (Emend, Oral) Uses: *Prevents N/V associated w/ emetogenic CA chemotherapy (eg, cisplatin) (use in combo w/ other antiemetics)*, postop N/V* **Acts:** Substance P/neurokinin 1 (NK₁) receptor antagonist **Dose:** 125 mg PO day 1, 1 h before chemotherapy, then 80 mg PO qam days 2 & 3; postop N/V: 40 mg w/in 3 h of induction **W/P:** [B, ?/–]; substrate & mod CYP3A4 inhib; CYP2C9 inducer (Table 10, p 319); ↓ Effect OCP and warfarin **CI:** Use w/ pimozide or cisapride **Disp:** Caps 40, 80, 125 mg **SE:** Fatigue, asthenia, hiccups **Notes:** See also fosaprepitant (Emend, Injection)

Arformoterol (Brovana) **BOX:** Long-acting β₂-adrenergic agonists may increase the risk of asthma-related death. Use only for pts not adequately controlled on other asthma-controller meds; safety + efficacy in asthma not established Uses: *Maint in COPD* **Acts:** Selective LA β₂-adrenergic agonist **Dose:** *Adults.* 15 mcg bid nebulization **W/P:** [C, ?] **CI:** Hypersens **Disp:** Soln 15 mcg/2 mL **SE:** Pain, back pain, CP, D, sinusitis, nervousness, palpitations, allergic Rxn, peripheral edema, rash, leg **Notes:** Not for acute bronchospasm. Refrigerate, use immediately after opening

Argatroban (Generic) Uses: *Prevent/Tx thrombosis in HIT, PCI in pts w/ HIT risk* **Acts:** Anticoagulant, direct thrombin inhib **Dose:** 2 mcg/kg/min IV; adjust until aPTT 1.5–3 × baseline not to exceed 100 s; 10 mcg/kg/min max; ↓ w/ hepatic impair **W/P:** [B, ?] Avoid PO anticoagulants, ↑ bleeding risk; avoid use w/ thrombolytics in critically ill pts **CI:** Overt major bleed **Disp:** Inj 100 mg/mL; Premixed Inf* 50, 125 mg **SE:** AF, cardiac arrest, cerebrovascular disorder, ↓ BP, VT, N/V/D, sepsis, cough, renal tox, ↓ Hgb **Notes:** Steady state in 1–3 h; ✓ aPTT w/ Inf start and after each dose change

Aripiprazole (Abilify, Abilify Discmelt) **BOX:** Increased mortality in elderly w/ dementia-related psychosis; ↑ suicidal thinking in children, adolescents, and young adults w/ MDD Uses: *Schizophrenia adults and peds 13–17 y, mania or mixed episodes associated w/ bipolar disorder, MDD in adults, agitation w/ schizophrenia* **Acts:** Dopamine & serotonin antagonist **Dose:** *Adults. Schizophrenia:* 10–15 mg PO/d

Acute agitation: 9.75 mg/1.3 mL IM *Bipolar:* 15 mg/d, *MDD adjunct* w/ other antidepressants initial 2 mg/d. *Peds. Schizophrenia: 13–17 y:* Start 2 mg/d, usual 10 mg/d; max 30 mg/d for all adult and peds uses; ↓ dose w/ CYP3A4/CYP2D6 inhib (Table 10, p 319); ↑ dose w/ CYP3A4 inducer W/P: [C, –] w/ Low WBC, CV Dz **Disp:** Tabs 2, 5, 10, 15, 20, 30 mg; Discmelt (disintegrating tabs 10, 15 mg), soln 1 mg/mL, Inj 7.5 mg/mL **SE:** Neuroleptic malignant synd, tardive dyskinesia, orthostatic ↓ BP, cognitive & motor impair, ↑ glucose, leukopenia, neutropenia, and agranulocytosis **Notes:** Discmelt contains phenylalanine; monitor CBC

Armodafinil (Nuvigil) Uses: *Narcolepsy, SWSD, and OSAHS* Acts: ?; binds dopamine receptor, ↓ dopamine reuptake Dose: *Adults. OSAHS/narcolepsy:* 150 or 250 mg PO daily in A.M. *SWSD:* 150 mg PO q day 1 h prior to start of shift; ↓ w/ hepatic impair; monitor for interactions w/ substrates CYP3A4/5, CYP7C19 W/P: [C, ?] CI: Hypersens to modafinil/armodafinil Disp: Tabs 50, 150, 250 mg SE: HA, N, dizziness, insomnia, xerostomia, rash including SJS, angioedema, anaphylactoid Rxns, multiorgan hypersens Rxns

Artemether & Lumefantrine (Coartem) Uses: *Acute, uncomplicated malaria (*P. falciparum*)* Acts: Antiprotozoal/Antimalarial Dose: *Adults > 16 y, 25–< 35 kg:* 3 tabs hour 0 & 8 day 1, then 3 tabs bid day 2 & 3 (18 tabs/course) *≥ 35 kg:* 4 tabs hour 0 & 8 day 1, then 4 tabs bid day 2 & 3 (24 tabs/course) *Peds 2 mo–< 16 y. 5–< 15 kg:* 1 tab at hour 0 & 8 day 1, then 1 tab bid day 2 & 3 (6 tabs/course) *15–< 25 kg:* 2 tabs hour 0 & 8 day 1, then 2 tabs bid day 2 & 3 (12 tabs/course) *25–< 35 kg:* 3 tabs at hour 0 & 8 day 1, then 3 tabs bid on day 2 & 3 (18 tabs/course) *≥ 35 kg:* See Adult dose W/P: [C, ?] ↑ QT, hepatic/renal impair, CYP3A4 inhib/substrate/inducers, CYP2D6 substrates CI: Component hypersens Disp: Tabs artemether 20 mg/lumefantrine 120 mg SE: Palp, HA, dizziness, chills, sleep disturb, fatigue, anorexia, N/V/D, Abd pain, weakness, arthralgia, myalgia, cough, splenomegaly, fever, anemia, hepatomegaly, ↑ AST, ↑ QT Notes: Not rec w/ other agents that ↑ QT

Artificial Tears (Tears Naturale) [OTC] Uses: *Dry eyes* Acts: Ocular lubricant Dose: 1–2 gtt PRN Disp: OTC soln SE: Mild stinging, temp blurred vision

Asenapine Maleate (Saphris) BOX: ↑Mortality in elderly w/ dementia-related psychosis Uses: *Schizophrenia; manic/mixed bipolar disorder* Acts: Dopamine/serotonin antagonist Dose: *Adults. Schizophrenia:* 5 mg twice daily; max 20 mg/d *Bipolar disorder:* 5–10 mg twice daily W/P: [C, ?/–] Disp: SL tabs 5, 10 mg SE: Dizziness, insomnia, ↑ TG, edema, ↑/↓ BP, somnolence, akathisia, oral hypoesthesia, EPS, ↑ weight, ↑ glucose, ↑ QT interval, hyperprolactinemia, ↓ WBC, neuroleptic malignant syndrome, severe allergic Rxns Notes: Do not swallow/crush/chew tab; avoid eating/drinking 10 min after dose

L-Asparaginase (Elspar) Uses: *ALL* (in combo w/ other agents) Acts: Protein synth inhib Dose: Unit/m²/dose based on protocol W/P: [C, ?] CI: Active/ Hx pancreatitis; Hx of allergic Rxn, thrombosis or hemorrhagic event w/ prior Rx w/ asparaginase Disp: Powder (Inj) 10,000 units/vial SE: Allergy 15–35%

(urticaria to anaphylaxis); fever, chills, N/V, anorexia, coma, azotemia, Abd cramps, depression, agitation, Sz, pancreatitis, ↑ glucose or LFTs, coagulopathy **Notes:** Test dose OK, ✓ glucose, coagulation studies, LFTs

Aspirin (Bayer, Ecotrin, St. Joseph's) [OTC] Uses: *CABG, PTCA, carotid endarterectomy, ischemic stroke, TIA, ACS/MI, arthritis, pain, HA, fever, inflammation* **Acts:** Prostaglandin inhib by COX-2 inhib **Dose: Adults.** *Pain, fever:* 325–650 mg q4–6h PO or PR (4 g/d max) *Plt inhib:* 81–325 mg PO daily; *Prevent MI:* 81 (preferred)–325 mg PO daily; *ECC 2010. ACS:* 160–325 mg nonenteric coated PO ASAP (chewing preferred at ACS onset) **Peds.** *Antipyretic:* 10–15 mg/kg/dose PO or PR q4–6h; *Kawasaki Dz:* 80–100 mg/kg/d ÷ q6h, 3–5 mg/kg/d after fever resolves for at least 48 h or total 14 d; for all uses 4 g/d max; avoid w/ CrCl < 10 mL/min, severe liver Dz **W/P:** [C, M] linked to Reye synd; avoid w/ viral illness in peds < 16 y **CI:** Allergy to ASA, chickenpox/ flu Sxs, synd of nasal polyps, angioedema, & bronchospasm to NSAIDs, bleeding disorder **Disp:** Tabs 325, 500 mg; chew tabs 81 mg; EC tabs 81, 162, 325, 500 mg; effervescent tabs 500 mg; supp 300, 600 mg; caplets 81, 375, 500 mg **SE:** GI upset, erosion, & bleeding **Notes:** D/C 1 wk preop; avoid/limit EtOH; Salicylate levels: *Therapeutic:* 100–250 mcg/mL *Toxic:* > 300 mcg/mL

Aspirin, Butalbital & Caffeine Compound (Fiorinal) [C-III] Uses: *Tension HA*, pain **Acts:** Barbiturate w/ analgesic **Dose:** 1–2 PO q4h PRN, max 6 tabs/d; dose in renal/hepatic Dz **W/P:** [C (D w/ prolonged use or high doses at term)] **CI:** ASA allergy, GI ulceration, bleeding disorder, porphyria, synd of nasal polyps, angioedema, & bronchospasm to NSAIDs **Disp:** Caps/tabs ASA 325 mg/ butalbital 50 mg/caffeine 40 mg **SE:** Drowsiness, dizziness, GI upset, ulceration, bleeding, light-headedness heartburn, confusion, HA **Notes:** Butalbital habit-forming; D/C 1 wk prior to surgery, avoid or limit EtOH

Aspirin + Butalbital, Caffeine, & Codeine (Fiorinal + Codeine) [C-III] Uses: *Complex tension HA* **Acts:** Sedative and narcotic analgesic **Dose:** 1–2 tabs/caps PO q4h max 6/d **W/P:** [C, –] **CI:** Allergy to ASA and codeine; synd of nasal polyps, angioedema, & bronchospasm to NSAIDs; bleeding diathesis, peptic ulcer or sig GI lesions, porphyria **Disp:** Caps contain 325 mg ASA, 40 mg caffeine, 50 mg butalbital, 30 mg codeine **SE:** Drowsiness, dizziness, GI upset, ulceration, bleeding **Notes:** D/C 1 wk prior to surgery, avoid/limit EtOH

Atazanavir (Reyataz) Uses: *HIV-1 Infxn* **Acts:** Protease inhib **Dose:** Antiretroviral naïve 300 mg PO daily w/ ritonavir 100 mg or 400 mg PO daily; experienced pts 300 mg w/ ritonavir 100 mg; when given w/ efavirenz 600 mg, administer atazanavir 400 mg + ritonavir 100 mg once/d; separate doses from didanosine; ↓ w/ hepatic impair **W/P:** CDC rec: HIV-infected mothers not breast-feed [B, –]; ↑ levels of statins sildenafil, antiarrhythmics, warfarin, cyclosporine, TCAs; w/ St. John's wort, PPIs H₂-receptor antagonists; do not use w/ salmeterol, colchicine (w/renal/hepatic failure); adjust dose w/ bosentan, tadalafil for PAH **CI:** w/ Midazolam, triazolam, ergots, pimozide, simvastatin, lovastatin, cisapride, etravirine, indinavir, irinotecan, rifampin, alpha 1-adrenoreceptor antagonist (alfuzosin), PDE5 inhibitor sildenafil **Disp:** Caps 100, 150, 200, 300 mg **SE:** HA, N/V/D, Bilirubin, rash, Abd pain, DM, photosens, ↑ PR interval **Notes:** Administer w/ food; may have less-adverse effect on cholesterol; if given w/ H₂ blocker, separate by 10 h H₂; if given w/ proton pump inhib, separate by 12 h; concurrent use not OK in experienced pts

Atenolol (Tenormin) **BOX:** Avoid abrupt withdrawl (esp CAD pts), gradual taper to ↓, acute ↑ HR, HTN +/− ischemia **Uses:** *HTN, angina, post-MI* **Acts:** selective β-adrenergic receptor blocker **Dose:** *HTN & angina:* 25–100 mg/d PO *ECC 2010. AMI:* 5 mg IV over 5 min; in 10 min, 5 mg slow IV; if tolerated in 10 min, start 50 mg PO, titrate; ↓ in renal impair **W/P:** [D, M] DM, bronchospasm; abrupt D/C can exacerbate angina & ↑ MI risk **CI:** ↓ HR, cardiogenic shock, cardiac failure, 2nd /3rd-degree AV block, sinus node dysfunction, pulm edema **Disp:** Tabs 25, 50, 100 mg **SE:** ↓ HR, ↓ BP, 2nd/3rd-degree AV block, dizziness, fatigue

Atenolol & Chlorthalidone (Tenoretic) **Uses:** *HTN* **Acts:** β-Adrenergic blockade w/ diuretic **Dose:** 50–100 mg/d PO based on atenolol; ↓ dose w/ CrCl < 35 mL/min **W/P:** [D, ?/] DM, bronchospasm **CI:** See atenolol; anuria, sulfonamide, cross-sensitivity **Disp:** Atenolol 50 mg/chlorthalidone 25 mg, atenolol 100 mg/chlorthalidone 25 mg **SE:** ↓ HR, ↓ BP, 2nd/3rd-degree AV block, dizziness, fatigue, ↓ K⁺, photosens

Atomoxetine (Strattera) **BOX:** ↑ Frequency of suicidal thinking; monitor closely especially in peds pts. **Uses:** *ADHD* **Acts:** Selective norepinephrine reuptake inhib **Dose:** *Adults & Peds > 70 kg.* 40 mg PO/d, after 3 d minimum, ↑ to 80–100 mg ÷ daily-bid *Peds < 70 kg.* 0.5 mg/kg × 3 d, then ↑ 1.2 mg/kg daily or bid (max 1.4 mg/kg or 100 mg); ↓ dose w/ hepatic Insuff or in combo w/ CYP2D6 inhib (Table 10, p 319) **W/P:** [C, ?/–] Known structural cardiac anomalies, cardiac Hx hepatoxicity **CI:** NAG, w/in 2 wk of D/C an MAOI **Disp:** Caps 10, 18, 25, 40, 60, 80, 100 mg **SE:** HA, insomnia, dry mouth, Abd pain, N/V, anorexia ↑ BP, tachycardia, Wt loss, somnolence, sexual dysfunction, jaundice, ↑ LFTs **Notes:** AHA rec: All children receiving stimulants for ADHD receive CV assessment before Rx initiated; D/C immediately w/ jaundice

Atorvastatin (Lipitor) **Uses:** dyslipidemia, primary prevention CV Dz **Acts:** HMG-CoA reductase inhib **Dose:** Initial 10–20 mg/d, may ↑ to 80 mg/d **W/P:** [X, –] **CI:** Active liver Dz, unexplained ↑ LFTs **Disp:** Tabs 10, 20, 40, 80 mg **SE:** Myopathy, HA, arthralgia, myalgia, GI upset, CP, edema, insomnia dizziness, liver failure **Notes:** Monitor LFTs, instruct pt to report unusual muscle pain or weakness

Atovaquone (Mepron) **Uses:** *Rx & prevention PCP*; *Toxoplasma gondii* encephalitis, babesiosis (w/ azithromycin) **Acts:** ↓ Nucleic acid & ATP synth **Dose:** *Rx:* 750 mg PO bid for 21 d *Prevention:* 1500 mg PO once/d (w/ meals) **W/P:** [C, ?] **Disp:** Susp 750 mg/5 mL **SE:** Fever, HA, anxiety, insomnia, rash, N/V, cough, pruritus, weakness

Atovaquone/Proguanil (Malarone) Uses: *Prevention or Rx *P. falciparum* malaria* Acts: Antimalarial Dose: *Adults. Prevention:* 1 tab PO 1–2 d before, during, & 7 d after leaving endemic region *Rx:* 4 tabs PO single dose daily × 3 d *Peds.* See PI W/P: [C, ?/–] CI: Prophylactic use when CrCl < 30 mL/min Disp: Tabs atovaquone 250 mg/proguanil 100 mg; peds 62.5/25 mg SE: HA, fever, myalgia, Abd pain dizziness, weakness N/V, ↑ LFTs

Atracurium (Tracrium) Uses: *Anesthesia adjunct to facilitate ET intubation, facilitate ventilation in ICU pts* Acts: Nondepolarizing neuromuscular blocker Dose: *Adults & Peds > 2 y.* 0.4–0.5 mg/kg IV bolus, then 0.08–0.1 mg/kg q20–45min PRN; ICU: 0.4–0.5 mg/kg/min titrated W/P: [C, ?] Disp: Inj 10 mg/mL SE: Flushing Notes: Pt must be intubated & on controlled ventilation; use adequate amounts of sedation & analgesia

Atropine, Ophthalmic (Isopto Atropine, Generic) Uses: *Mydriasis, cycloplegia, uveitis* Acts: Antimuscarinic; cycloplegic, dilates pupils Dose: *Adults. Refraction:* 1–2 gtt 1 h before *Uveitis:* 1–2 gtt daily-qid CI: NAG, adhesions between iris and lens Disp: 1% ophthal soln, 1% oint SE: Local irritation, burning, blurred vision, light sensitivity Notes: Compress lacrimal sac 2–3 min after instillation; effects can last 1–2 wk

Atropine, Systemic (AtroPen Auto-Injector) Uses: *Preanesthetic; symptomatic ↓ HR & asystole, AV block, organophosphate (insecticide) and acetylcholinesterase (nerve gas) inhib antidote; cycloplegic* Acts: Antimuscarinic; blocks acetylcholine at parasympathetic sites, cycloplegic Dose: *Adults. ECC 2010. Asystole or PEA:* Routine use for asystole or PEA no longer recommended; *Bradycardia:*0.5 mg IV q3–5min as needed; max 3 mg or 0.04 mg/kg *Preanesthetic:* 0.4–0.6 mg IM/IV *Poisoning:* 1–2 mg IV bolus, repeat q3–5min PRN to reverse effects *Peds. ECC 2010. Symptomatic bradycardia:* 0.02 mg/kg IV/IO (min dose 0.1 mg, max single dose 0.5 mg); repeat PRN X1; max total dose 1 mg or 0.04 mg/kg child, 3 mg adolescent W/P: B/[C, +] CI: NAG, adhesions between iris and lens, pyloric stenosis, prostatic hypertrophy Disp: Inj 0.05, 0.1, 0.4, 1 mg/mL *AtroPen Auto-injector:* 0.25, 0.5, 1, 2 mg/dose SE: Flushing, mydriasis, tachycardia, dry mouth & nose, blurred vision, urinary retention, constipation, psychosis Notes: SLUDGE are Sx of organophosphate poisoning; *Auto-injector* limited distribution; see ophthal forms below

Atropine/Pralidoxime (DuoDote) Uses: *Nerve agent (tabun, sarin, others), or organophosphate insecticide poisoning* Acts: Atropine blocks effects of excess acetylcholine; pralidoxime reactivates acetylcholinesterase inactivated by poisoning Dose: 1 Inj midlateral thigh; 10–15 min for effect; w/ severe Sx, give 2 additional Inj; if alert/oriented no more doses W/P: [C, ?] Disp: Auto-injector 2.1 mg atropine/600 mg pralidoxime SE: Dry mouth, blurred vision, dry eyes, photophobia, confusion, HA, tachycardia, ↑ BP, flushing, urinary retention, constipation, Abd pain N, V, emesis Notes: See "SLUDGE" under Atropine, Systemic; limited distribution; for use by personnel w/ appropriate training; wear protective garments; do not rely solely on medication; evacuation and decontamination ASAP

Avanafil (Stendra) Uses: *ED* Acts: ↓ Phosphodiesterase type 5 (PDE5) (responsible for cGMP breakdown); ↑ cGMP activity to relax smooth muscles to ↑ flow to corpus cavernosum Dose: (men only) 100 mg PO 30 min before sex activity, no more than 1X/d; ↑/↓ dose 50–200 mg based on effect; do not use w/ strong CYP3A4 inhib; use 50 mg w/ mod CYP3A4 inhib; w/ or w/o food W/P: [C, ?] Priapism risk; hypotension w/ BP meds or substantial alcohol; seek immediate attention w/ hearing loss or acute vision loss (may be NAION); w/ CYP3A4 inhib (eg, ketoconazole, ritonavir, erythromycin) ↑ effects; do not use w/ severe renal/ hepatic impair CI: w/ Nitrates or if sex not advised Disp: Tabs 50, 100, 200 mg SE: HA, flushing, nasal congestion, nasopharyngitis back pain Notes: More rapid onset than sildenafil (15–30 min)

Axitinib (Inlyta) Uses: *Advanced RCC* Acts: TKI inhibitor Dose: Adults. 5 mg PO q12h; if tolerated > 2 wk, ↑ to 7 mg q12h, then 10 mg q12h; w/ or w/o food; swallow whole; ↓ dose by ½ w/ moderate hepatic impair; avoid w/ or ↓ dose by ½ if used w/ strong CYP3A4/5 inhib W/P: [D, ?] w/ brain mets, recent GI bleed Disp: Tabs 1, 5 mg SE: N/V/D/C, HTN, fatigue, asthenia, ↓ appetite, ↓ Wt, LFTs, hand-foot synd, venous/arterial thrombosis; hemorrhage, ↓ thyroid, GI perf/ fistula, proteinuria, hypertensive crisis, impaired wound healing, reversible posterior leukoencephalopathy synd Notes: Hold 24 h prior to surgery

Azathioprine (Imuran, Azasan) BOX: May ↑ neoplasia w/ chronic use; mutagenic and hematologic tox possible Uses: *Adjunct to prevent renal transplant rejection, RA*, SLE, Crohn Dz, UC Acts: Immunosuppressive; antagonizes purine metabolism Dose: Adults. Crohn and UC: Start 50 mg/d, ↑ 25 mg q1–2wk, target dose 2–3 mg/kg/d Adults & Peds. Renal transplant: 3–5 mg/kg/d IV/PO single daily dose, then 1–3 mg/kg/d maint; RA: 1 mg/kg/d once daily or ÷ bid × 6–8 wk, ↑ 0.5 mg/kg/d q4wk to 2.5 mg/kg/d; w/ renal Insuff W/P: [D, ?/–] CI: PRG Disp: Tabs 50, 75, 100 mg; powder for Inj 100 mg SE: GI intolerance, fever, chills, leukopenia, ↑ LFTs, bilirubin, ↑ risk Infxns, thrombocytopenia Notes: Handle Inj w/ cytotoxic precautions; interaction w/ allopurinol; do not administer live vaccines on drug; ✓ CBC and LFTs; dose per local transplant protocol, usually start 1–3 d pretransplant

Azelastine (Astelin, Astepro, Optivar) Uses: *Allergic rhinitis (rhinorrhea, sneezing, nasal pruritus), vasomotor rhinitis; allergic conjunctivitis* Acts: Histamine H₁-receptor antagonist Dose: Adults & Peds > 12 y. Nasal: 1–2 sprays/ nostril bid Ophth: 1 gtt in each affected eye bid Peds 5–11 y. 1 spray/nostril 1× d W/P: [C, ?/–] CI: Component sensitivity Disp: Nasal 137 mcg/spray; ophthal soln 0.05% SE: Somnolence, bitter taste, HA, colds Sx (rhinitis, cough)

Azilsartan (Edarbi) BOX: Use in 2nd/3rd trimester can cause fetal injury and death; D/C when PRG detected Uses: *HTN* Acts: ARB Dose: Adults. 80 mg PO 1 × d; consider 40 mg PO 1 × d if on high dose diuretic W/P: [D, ?] correct vol/ salt depletion before Disp: Tabs 40, 80 mg SE: D, ↓ BP, N, asthenia, fatigue, dizziness, cough

Azilsartan & Chlorthalidone (Edarbyclor) BOX: Use in 2nd/3rd trimester can cause fetal injury and death; D/C when PRG detected Uses: *HTN* Acts: ARB w/ thiazide diuretic Dose: *Adults.* 40/12.5 mg–40/25 mg PO 1 × d W/P: [D, ?] Correct vol/salt depletion prior to use; use w/ lithium, NSAIDs CI: Anuria Disp: Tabs (azilsartan/chlorthalidone) 40/12.5, 40/25 mg SE: N/D, ↓ BP, asthenia, fatigue, dizziness, cough, ↓ K⁺, hyperuricemia, photosens, ↑ glucose

Azithromycin (Zithromax) Uses: *Community-acquired pneumonia, pharyngitis, otitis media, skin Infxns, nongonococcal (chlamydial) urethritis, chancroid & PID; Rx & prevention of MAC in HIV* Acts: Macrolide antibiotic; bacteriostatic; ↓ protein synth Spectrum: *Chlamydia, H. ducreyi, H. influenzae, Legionella, M. catarrhalis, M. pneumoniae, M. hominis, N. gonorrhoeae, S. aureus, S. aglactiae, S. pneumoniae, S. pyogenes* Dose: *Adults.* Resp tract Infxns: PO: Caps 500 mg day 1, then 250 mg/d PO × 4 d Sinusitis: 500 mg/d PO × 3 d IV: 500 mg × 2 d, then 500 mg PO × 7–10 d Nongonococcal urethritis: 1 g PO × 1 Gonorrhea, uncomplicated: 2 g PO × 1 Prevent MAC: 1200 mg PO once/wk Peds. Otitis media: 10 mg/kg PO day 1, then 5 mg/kg/d days 2–5 Pharyngitis (≥ 2 y): 12 mg/kg/d PO × 5 d; take susp on empty stomach; tabs OK w/ or w/o food; ↓ w/ CrCl < 10 mL/mg W/P: [B, +] May ↑ QTc w/ arrhythmias Disp: Tabs 250, 500, 600 mg; Z-Pack (5-d, 250 mg); Tri-Pack (500-mg tabs × 3); susp 2 g; single-dose packet (Zmax) ER susp (2 g); susp 100, 200 mg/5 mL; Inj powder 500 mg; 2.5 mL SE: GI upset, metallic taste

Azithromycin Ophthalmic 1% (AzaSite) Uses: *Bacterial conjunctivitis* Acts: Bacteriostatic Dose: *Adults & Peds ≥ 1 y.* 1 gtt bid, q8–12 h × 2 d, then 1 gtt q day × 5 d W/P: [↑ B, ?] CI: None Disp: 1% in 2.5-mL bottle SE: Irritation, burning, stinging, contact dermatitis, corneal erosion, dry eye, dysgeusia, nasal congestion, sinusitis, ocular discharge, keratitis

Aztreonam (Azactam) Uses: *Aerobic gram(–) UTIs, lower resp, intra-Abd, skin, gynecologic Infxns & septicemia* Acts: Monobactam: ↓ Cell wall synth Spectrum: Gram(–) (*Pseudomonas, E. coli, Klebsiella, H. influenzae, Serratia, Proteus, Enterobacter, Citrobacter*) Dose: *Adults.* 1–2 g IV/IM q6–12 h UTI: 500 mg–1 g IV q8–12h Meningitis: 2 g IV q6–8h Peds. 90–120 mg/kg/d ÷ q6–8h ↓ in renal impair W/P: [B, +] Disp: Inj (soln), 1 g, 2 g/50 mL Inj powder for recons 1 g, 2 g SE: N/V/D, rash, pain at Inj site Notes: No gram(+) or anaerobic activity; OK in PCN-allergic pts

Aztreonam, Inhaled (Cayston) Uses: *Improve respiratory Sx in CF pts w/ P. aeruginosa* Acts: Monobactam: ↓ cell wall synth Dose: *Adults & Peds ≥ 7 y.* One dose 3×/d × 28 d (space doses q4h) W/P: [B, +] w/ Beta-lactam allergy CI: Allergy to aztreonam Disp: Lyophilized SE: Allergic Rxn, bronchospasm, cough, nasal congestion, wheezing, pharyngolaryngeal pain, V, Abd pain, chest discomfort, pyrexia, rash Notes: Use immediately after reconstitution, use only w/ Altera Nebulizer System; bronchodilator prior to use

Bacitracin & Polymyxin B, Ophthalmic (AK-Poly-Bac Ophthalmic, Polysporin Ophthalmic); Bacitracin, Neomycin, & Polymyxin B,

Ophthalmic (Neo-Polycin Neosporin Ophthalmic); Bacitracin, Neomycin, Polymyxin B, & Hydrocortisone, Ophthalmic (Neo-Polycin HC Cortisporin Ophthalmic) Uses: *Steroid-responsive inflammatory ocular conditions* Acts: Topical antibiotic w/ anti-inflammatory Dose: Apply q3–4h into conjunctival sac W/P: [C, ?] CI: Viral, mycobacterial, fungal eye Infxn Disp: See Bacitracin, topical equivalents, next listing

Bacitracin, Topical (Baciguent); Bacitracin & Polymyxin B, Topical (Polysporin); Bacitracin, Neomycin, & Polymyxin B, Topical (Neosporin); Bacitracin, Neomycin, Polymyxin B, & Hydrocortisone, Topical (Cortisporin) Uses: Prevent/Rx of *minor skin Infxns* Acts: Topical antibiotic w/ added components (anti-inflammatory & analgesic) Dose: Apply sparingly bid-qid W/P: [C, ?] Not for deep wounds, puncture, or animal bites Disp: Bacitracin 500 units/g oint; bacitracin 500 units/polymyxin B sulfate 10,000 units/g oint & powder; bacitracin 400 units/neomycin 3.5 mg/polymyxin B 5000 units/g oint; bacitracin 400 units/neomycin 3.5 mg/polymyxin B 5000 units/hydrocortisone 10 mg/g oint; Bacitracin 500 units/neomycin 3.5 mg/polymyxin B 5000 units/lidocaine 40 mg/g oint Notes: Ophthal, systemic, & irrigation forms available, and generally used d/t potential tox

Baclofen (Lioresal Intrathecal, Gablofen) BOX: Abrupt discontinuation especially IT use can lead to organ failure, rhabdomyolysis, and death Uses: *Spasticity d/t severe chronic disorders (eg, MS, amyotrophic lateral sclerosis, or spinal cord lesions)*, trigeminal neuralgia, intractable hiccups Acts: Centrally acting skeletal muscle relaxant; ↓ transmission of monosynaptic & polysynaptic cord reflexes Dose: *Adults.* Initial, 5 mg PO tid; ↑ q3d to effect; max 80 mg/d *IT.* Via implantable pump (see PI) *Peds 2–7 y.* 20–30 mg ÷ q8h (max 60 mg) > *8 y:* Max 120 mg/d *IT:* Via implantable pump (see PI); ↓ in renal impair; take w/ food or milk W/P: [C, +] Epilepsy, neuropsychological disturbances; Disp: Tabs 10, 20 mg; IT Inj 50, 500, 1000, 2000 mcg/mL SE: Dizziness, drowsiness, insomnia, rash, fatigue, ataxia, weakness, ↓ BP

Balsalazide (Colazal) Uses: *Ulcerative colitis* Acts: 5-ASA derivative, anti-inflammatory Dose: 2.25 g (3 caps) tid × 8–12 wk W/P: [B, ?/–] Severe renal failure CI: Mesalamine or salicylate hypersens Disp: Caps 750 mg SE: Dizziness, HA, N, Abd pain, agranulocytosis, renal impair, allergic Rxns Notes: Daily dose of 6.75 g = 2.4 g mesalamine, UC exacerbation upon initiation of Rx

Basiliximab (Simulect) BOX: Use only under the supervision of a physician experienced in immunosuppression Rx in an appropriate facility Uses: *Prevent acute transplant rejection* Acts: IL-2 receptor antagonists Dose: *Adults & Peds > 35 kg.* 20 mg IV 2 h before transplant, then 20 mg IV 4 d posttransplant *Peds < 35 kg.* 10 mg 2 h prior to transplant; same dose IV 4 d posttransplant W/P: [B, ?/–] CI: Hypersens to murine proteins Disp: Inj powder 10, 20 mg SE: Edema, ↓ BP, HTN, HA, dizziness, fever, pain, Infxn, GI effects, electrolyte disturba Notes: A murine/human MoAb

BCG [Bacillus Calmette-Guérin] (TheraCys, Tice BCG) BOX: Contains live, attenuated mycobacteria; transmission risk; handle as biohazard; nosocomial & disseminated Infxns reported in immunosuppressed; Uses: *Bladder CA (superficial)*, TB prophylaxis: Routine US adult BCG immunization not recommended. Children who are PPD(−) and continually exposed to untreated/ineffectively treated adults or whose TB strain is INH/rifampin resistant. Healthcare workers in high-risk environments Acts: Attenuated live BCG culture, immunomodulator Dose: Bladder CA, 1 vial prepared & instilled in bladder for 2 h. Repeat once/wk × 6 wk; then 1 Tx at 3, 6, 12, 18, & 24 mo after W/P: [C, ?] Asthma w/ TB immunization CI: Immunosuppression, PRG, steroid use, febrile illness, UTI, gross hematuria, w/ traumatic catheterization Disp: Powder 81 mg (TheraCys), 50 mg (Tice BCG) SE: Intravesical: Hematuria, urinary frequency, dysuria, bacterial UTI, rare BCG sepsis malaise, fever, chills, pain, N/V, anorexia, anemia Notes: PPD is not CI in BCG vaccinated persons; intravesical use, dispose/void in toilet w/ chlorine bleach

Becaplermin (Regranex Gel) BOX: Increased mortality d/t malignancy reported; use w/ caution in known malignancy Uses: Local wound care adjunct w/ *diabetic foot ulcers* Acts: Recombinant PDGF, enhances granulation tissue Dose: Adults. Based on lesion: Calculate the length of gel, measure the greatest length of ulcer by the greatest width; tube size and measured result determine the formula used in the calculation. Recalculate q1–2wk based on change in lesion size. 15-g tube: [length × width] × 0.6 = length of gel (in inches) or for 2-g tube: [length × width] × 1.3 = length of gel (in inches) Peds. See PI W/P: [C, ?] CI: Neoplasmatic site Disp: 0.01% gel in 2-, 15-g tubes SE: Rash Notes: Use w/ good wound care; wound must be vascularized; reassess after 10 wk if ulcer not ↓ by 30% or not healed by 20 wk

Beclomethasone (QVAR) Uses: Chronic *asthma* Acts: Inhaled corticosteroid Dose: Adults & Peds 5–11 y. 40–160 mcg 1–4 Inhs bid; initial 40–80 mcg Inh bid if on bronchodilators alone; 40–160 mcg bid w/ other inhaled steroids; 320 mcg bid max; taper to lowest effective dose bid; rinse mouth/throat after W/P: [C, ?] CI: Acute asthma Disp: PO metered-dose inhaler; 40, 80 mcg/Inh SE: HA, cough, hoarseness, oral candidiasis Notes: Not effective for acute asthma; effect in 1–2 d or as long as 2 wk; rinse mouth after use

Beclomethasone Nasal (Beconase AQ) Uses: *Allergic rhinitis, nasal polyps* Acts: Inhaled steroid Dose: Adults & Peds. Aqueous inhaler: 1–2 sprays/nostril bid W/P: [C, ?] Disp: Nasal metered-dose inhaler 42 mcg/spray SE: Local irritation, burning, epistaxis Notes: Effect in days to 2 wk

Bedaquiline Fumarate (Sirturo) BOX: ↑ QT can occur and may be additive w/ other QT-prolonging drugs; ↑ risk of death vs placebo, only use when an active TB regimen cannot be provided Uses: *Tx of MDR TB* Acts: diarylquinoline antimycobacterial Dose: 400 mg/d × 2 wk, then 200 mg 3 ×/wk wk W/P: [B, –] ↑ QT, ✓ ECG freq; D/C if ventricular arrhythmias or QTc

> 500 ms; hepatic Rxn, ✓ LFTs, D/C w/ AST/ALT > 8× ULN, T bili > 2× ULN or LFTs persist > 2 wk; w/ renal failure **CI**: w/ drugs that ↑ QTc **Disp**: Tabs 100 mg **SE**: HA, N, arthralgias, hemoptysis, CP **Notes**: Frequent ✓ ECG; ✓ LFTs; avoid use of potent CYP3A4 inducers; avoid w/in < 14 d use of CYP3A4 inhib

Belatacept (Nulojix) **BOX**: May ↑ risk of posttransplant lymphoproliferative disorder (PTLD) mostly CNS; ↑ risk of Infxn; for use by physicians experienced in immunosuppressive therapy; ↑ risk of malignancies; not for liver transplant **Uses**: *Prevention rejection in EBV positive kidney transplant recipients* **Acts**: T-cell costimulation blocker **Dose**: Day 1 (transplant day, preop) & day 5 10 mg/kg; end of wk 2, wk 4, wk 8, wk 12 after transplant 10 mg/kg; Maint: End of wk 16 after transplant wk 4 5 mg/kg **W/P**: [C, –] w/ CYP3A4 inhib/inducers, other anticoagulants or plt inhib **CI**: EBV seronegative or unknown EBV status **Disp**: 250 mg Inj **SE**: anemia, N/V/D, UTI, edema, constipation, ↑ BP, pyrexia, graft dysfunction, cough, HA, ↑/↓ K⁺, ↓ WBC **Notes**: REMS; use in combo w/ basiliximab, mycophenolate mofetil (MMF), & steroids; PML w/ excess belatacept dosing

Belimumab (Benlysta) **Uses**: *SLE* **Acts**: B-lymphocyte inhib **Dose**: *Adults*. 10 mg/kg IV q2wk × 3 doses, then q4wk; Inf over 1 h; premed against Inf & hypersens Rxns **W/P**: [C, ?/–] h/o active or chronic Infxn; possible ↑ mortality **CI**: Live vaccines, hypersens **Disp**: Inj powder 120, 400 mg/vial **SE**: N/D, bronchitis, nasopharyngitis, pharyngitis, insomnia, extremity pain, pyrexia, depression, migraine, serious/fatal, hypersens, anaphylaxis **Notes**: Not for severe active lupus nephritis or CNS lupus or w/ other biologics or IV cyclophosphamide

Belladonna & Opium Suppositories (Generic) [C-II] **Uses**: *Mod–severe pain associated w/ bladder spasms* **Acts**: Antispasmodic, analgesic **Dose**: 1 supp PR 1–2/d (up to 4 doses/d) **W/P**: [C, ?] **CI**: Glaucoma, resp depression, severe renal or hepatic dz, convulsive disorder, acute alcoholism **Disp**: 30 mg opium/16.2 mg belladonna extract; 60 mg opium/16.2 mg belladonna extract **SE**: Anticholinergic (eg, sedation, urinary retention, constipation)

Benazepril (Lotensin) **BOX**: PRG abrupt stop **Uses**: *HTN* **Acts**: ACE inhib **Dose**: 10–80 mg/d PO **W/P**: [D, –] **CI**: Angioedema **Disp**: Tabs 5, 10, 20, 40 mg **SE**: Symptomatic ↓ BP w/ diuretics; dizziness, HA, ↑ K⁺, nonproductive cough, ↑ SCr

Bendamustine (Treanda) **Uses**: *CLL B-cell NHL* **Acts**: Mechlorethamine derivative; alkylating agent **Dose**: *Adults*. 100 mg/m² IV over 30 min on days 1 & 2 of 28-d cycle, up to 6 cycles (w/ tox see PI for dose changes); NHL: 120 mg/m² IV over 30 min d 1 & 2 of 21-d tx cycle up to 8 cycles; do not use w/ CrCl < 40 mL/min, severe hepatic impair **W/P**: [D, ?/–] Do not use w/ CrCl < 40 mL/min, severe hepatic impair **CI**: Hypersens to bendamustine or mannitol **Disp**: Inj powder, 25 mg, 100 mg **SE**: Pyrexia, N/V, dry mouth, fatigue, cough, stomatitis, rash, myelosuppression, Infxn, Inf Rxns & anaphylaxis, tumor lysis synd, skin Rxns, extravasation **Notes**: Consider use of allopurinol to prevent tumor lysis synd

Benzocaine (Americaine, Hurricane Lanacane, Various [OTC]) **Uses**: *Topical anesthetic, lubricant on ET tubes, catheters, etc; pain relief in external otitis, cerumen removal, skin conditions, sunburn, insect bites, mouth and gum irritation, hemorrhoids* **Acts:** Topical local anesthetic **Dose:** *Adults & Peds > 1 y. Anesthetic lubricant:* Apply evenly to tube/instrument; other uses per manufacturer instructions **W/P:** [C, –] Do not use on broken skin; see provider if condition does not respond; avoid in infants and those w/ pulmonary Dzs **Disp:** Many site-specific OTC forms creams, gels, liquids, sprays, 2–20% **SE:** Itching, irritation, burning, edema, erythema, pruritus, rash, stinging, tenderness, urticaria; methemoglobinemia (infants or in COPD) **Notes:** Use minimum amount to obtain effect; methemoglobinemia S/Sxs: HA, lightheadedness, SOB, anxiety, fatigue, pale, gray or blue colored skin, and tachycardia

Benzocaine & Antipyrine (Auralgan) **Uses:** *Analgesia in severe otitis media* **Acts:** Anesthetic w/ local decongestant **Dose:** Fill ear & insert a moist cotton plug; repeat 1–2 h PRN **W/P:** [C, ?] **CI:** w/ Perforated eardrum **Disp:** Soln 5.4% antipyrine, 1.4% benzocaine **SE:** Local irritation, methemoglobinemia, ear discharge

Benzonatate (Tessalon, Zonatuss) **Uses:** Symptomatic relief of *nonproductive cough* **Acts:** Anesthetizes the stretch receptors in the resp passages **Dose:** *Adults & Peds > 10 y.* 100 mg PO tid (max 600 mg/d) **W/P:** [C, ?] **Disp:** Caps 100, 150, 200 mg **SE:** Sedation, dizziness, GI upset **Notes:** Do not chew or puncture the caps; deaths reported in peds < 10 y w/ ingestion

Benztropine (Cogentin) **Uses:** *Parkinsonism & drug-induced extrapyramidal disorders* **Acts:** Anticholinergic & antihistaminic effects **Dose:** *Adults. Parkinsonism:* initial 0.5–1 mg PO/IM/IV qhs, ↑ q 5–6 d PRN by 0.5 mg, usual dose 1–2 mg/d, 6 mg/d max. *Extrapyramidal:* 1–4 mg PO/IV/IM q day-bid. *Peds > 3 y.* 0.02–0.05 mg/kg/dose 1–2/d **W/P:** [C, ?] w/ Urinary Sxs, NAG, hot environments, CNS or mental disorders, other phenothiazines or TCA **CI:** < 3 y pyloric/duodenal obstruction, myasthenia gravis **Disp:** Tabs 0.5, 1, 2 mg; Inj 1 mg/mL **SE:** Anticholinergic (tachycardia, ileus, N/V, etc), anhidrosis, heat stroke

Benzyl Alcohol (Ulesfia) **Uses:** *Head lice* **Acts:** Pediculicide **Dose:** Apply volume for hair length to dry hair; saturate the scalp; leave on 10 min; rinse w/ water; repeat in 7 d; *Hair length 0–2 in:* 4–6 oz; *2–4 in:* 6–8 oz; *4–8 in:* 8–12 oz; *8–16 in:* 12–24 oz; *16–22 in:* 24–32 oz; *> 22 in:* 32–48 oz **W/P:** [B, ?] Avoid eyes **CI:** none **Disp:** 5% lotion 4-, 8-oz bottles **SE:** Pruritus, erythema, irritation (local, eyes) **Notes:** Use fine-tooth/nit comb to remove nits and dead lice; no ovocidal activity

Bepotastine Besilate (Bepreve) **Uses:** *Allergic conjunctivitis* **Acts:** H₁-receptor antagonist **Dose:** *Adults.* 1 gtt into affected eye(s) twice daily **W/P:** [C, ?/–] Do not use while wearing contacts **Disp:** Soln 1.5% **SE:** Mild taste, eye irritation, HA, nasopharyngitis

Beractant (Survanta) **Uses:** *Prevention & Rx RDS in premature infants* **Acts:** Replaces pulm surfactant **Dose:** 100 mg/kg via ET tube; repeat q6h PRN; max 4 doses **Disp:** Susp 25 mg of phospholipid/mL **SE:** Transient ↓ HR, desaturation, apnea

Besifloxacin (Besivance) Uses: *Bacterial conjunctivitis* Acts: Inhibits DNA gyrase & topoisomerase IV. Dose: *Adults & Peds > 1 y.* 1 gtt into eye(s) tid 4–12 h apart × 7 d W/P: [C, ?] Remove contacts during Tx CI: None Disp: 0.6% susp SE: HA, redness, blurred vision, irritation

Betaxolol (Kerlone) Uses: *HTN* Acts: Competitively blocks β-adrenergic receptors, β$_1$ W/P: [C, ?/–] CI: Sinus ↓ HR, AV conduction abnormalities, uncompensated cardiac failure Dose: 5–20 mg/d Disp: Tabs 10, 20 mg SE: Dizziness, HA, ↓ HR, edema, CHF, fatigue, lethargy

Betaxolol, Ophthalmic (Betoptic) Uses: Open-angle glaucoma Acts: Competitively blocks β$_1$-adrenergic receptors, Dose: 1–2 gtt bid W/P: [C, ?/–] Disp: Soln 0.5%; susp 0.25% SE: Local irritation, photophobia

Bethanechol (Urecholine) Uses: *Acute postop/postpartum nonobstructive urinary retention; neurogenic bladder w/ retention* Acts: Stimulates cholinergic smooth muscle in bladder & GI tract Dose: *Adults.* Initial 5–10 mg PO, then repeat qh until response or 50 mg, typical 10–50 mg tid-qid, 200 mg/d max tid-qid; 2.5–5 mg SQ tid-qid & PRN. *Peds.* 0.3–0.6 mg/kg/24 h PO ÷ tid-qid; take on empty stomach W/P: [C, –] CI: BOO, PUD, epilepsy, hyperthyroidism, ↓ HR, COPD, AV conduction defects, Parkinsonism, ↓ BP, vasomotor instability Disp: Tabs 5, 10, 25, 50 mg SE: Abd cramps, D, salivation, ↓ BP

Bevacizumab (Avastin) BOX: Associated w/ GI perforation, wound dehiscence, & fatal hemoptysis Uses: *Met colorectal CA w/5 FU, NSCLC w/ paclitaxel and carboplatin; glioblastoma; metastatic RCC w/ IFN-alpha* Acts: Vascular endothelial GF inhibitor Dose: *Adults.* Colon: 5 mg/kg or 10 mg/kg IV q14d; *NSCLC:* 15 mg/kg q21d; 1st dose over 90 min; 2nd over 60 min, 3rd over 30 min if tolerated; *RCC:* 10 mg/kg IV q2wk w/ IFN-α IV W/P: [C, –] Do not use w/in 28 d of surgery if time for separation of drug & anticipated surgical procedures is unknown; D/C w/ serious adverse effects CI: None Disp: 100 mg/4 mL 400 mg/16 mL vials SE: Wound dehiscence, GI perforation, tracheoesophageal fistula, arterial thrombosis, hemoptysis, hemorrhage, HTN, proteinuria, CHF, Inf Rxns, D, leukopenia Notes: Monitor for ↑ BP & proteinuria

Bicalutamide (Casodex) Uses: *Advanced PCa w/ GnRH agonists (eg, leuprolide, goserelin)* Acts: Nonsteroidal antiandrogen Dose: 50 mg/d W/P: [X, ?] CI: Women Disp: Caps 50 mg SE: Hot flashes, ↓ loss of libido, impotence, edema, pain, D/N/V, gynecomastia, ↑ LFTs

Bicarbonate (See Sodium Bicarbonate, p 256)

Bisacodyl (Dulcolax) [OTC] Uses: *Constipation; preop bowel prep* Acts: Stimulates peristalsis Dose: *Adults.* 5–15 mg PO or 10 mg PR PRN. *Peds < 2 y.* 5 mg PR PRN. *> 2 y:* 5 mg PO or 10 mg PR PRN (do not chew tabs or give w/in 1 h of antacids or milk) W/P: [C, ?] CI: Abd pain or obstruction; N/V Disp: EC tabs 5, 10 mg supp 10 mg, enema soln 10 mg/30 mL SE: Abd cramps, proctitis, & inflammation w/ supps

Bismuth Subcitrate/Metronidazole/Tetracycline (Pylera) Uses: *H. pylori Infxn w/ omeprazole* Acts: Eradicates H. pylori, see agents Dose: 3 caps qid w/ omeprazole 20 mg bid for × 10 d W/P: [D, −] CI: PRG, peds < 8 y (tetracycline during tooth development causes teeth discoloration), w/ renal/hepatic impair, component hypersens Disp: Caps w/ 140-mg bismuth subcitrate potassium, 125-mg metronidazole, & 125-mg tetracycline hydrochloride SE: Stool abnormality, N, anorexia, D, dyspepsia, Abd pain, HA, flu-like synd, taste perversion, vaginitis, dizziness; see SE for each component Notes: Metronidazole carcinogenic in animals

Bismuth Subsalicylate (Pepto-Bismol) [OTC] Uses: Indigestion, N, & *D*; combo for Rx of *H. pylori Infxn* Acts: Antisecretory & anti-inflammatory Dose: **Adults.** 2 tabs or 30 mL PO PRN (max 8 doses/24 h). **Peds.** (For all max 8 doses/24 h). **3–6 y:** 1/3 tab or 5 mL PO PRN. **6–9 y:** 2/3 tab or 10 mL PO PRN. **9–12 y:** 1 tab or 15 mL PO PRN W/P: [C, D (3rd tri), −] Avoid w/ renal failure; Hx severe GI bleed; influenza or chickenpox (↑ risk of Reye synd) CI: h/o severe GI bleeding or coagulopathy, ASA allergy Disp: Chew tabs, caplets 262 mg; liq 262, 525 mg/15 mL; susp 262 mg/15 mL SE: May turn tongue & stools black

Bisoprolol (Zebeta) Uses: *HTN* Acts: Competitively blocks β₁-adrenergic receptors Dose: 2.5–10 mg/d (max dose 20 mg/d); ↓ w/ renal impair W/P: [C, ?/−] CI: Sinus bradycardia, AV conduction abnormalities, uncompensated cardiac failure Disp: Tabs 5, 10 mg SE: Fatigue, lethargy, HA, ↓ HR, edema, CHF Notes: Not dialyzed

Bivalirudin (Angiomax) Uses: *Anticoagulant w/ ASA in unstable angina undergoing PTCA, PCI, or in pts undergoing PCI w/ or at risk for HIT/HITTS* Acts: Anticoagulant, thrombin inhib Dose: 0.75 mg/kg IV bolus, then 1.75 mg/kg/h for duration of procedure and up to 4 h postprocedure; ✓ ACT 5 min after bolus, may repeat 0.3 mg/kg bolus if necessary (give w/ aspirin ASA 300–325 mg/d; start pre-PTCA) W/P: [B, ?] CI: Major bleeding Disp: Powder 250 mg for Inj SE: ↓ BP, bleeding, back pain, N, HA

Bleomycin Sulfate (Generic) BOX: Idiopathic Rxn (↓ BP, fever, chills, wheezing) in lymphoma pts; pulm fibrosis; should be administered by chemo-experienced physician Uses: *Testis CA; Hodgkin Dz & NHLs; cutaneous lymphomas; & squamous cell CA (head & neck, larynx, cervix, skin, penis); malignant pleural effusion sclerosing agent* Acts: Induces DNA breakage (scission) Dose: (per protocols); ↓ w/ renal impair W/P: [D, ?] CI: w/ Hypersens, idiosyncratic Rxn Disp: Powder (Inj) 15, 30 units Disp: Hyperpigmentation & allergy (rash to anaphylaxis); fever in 50%; lung tox (idiosyncratic & dose related); pneumonitis w/ fibrosis; Raynaud phenomenon, N/V Notes: Test dose 1 unit, especially in lymphoma pts; lung tox w/ total dose > 400 units or single dose > 30 units; avoid high FiO₂ in general anesthesia to ↓ tox

Boceprevir (Victrelis) Uses: *Chronic hep C, genotype 1, w/ compensated liver Dz, including naive to Tx or failed Tx w/ peginterferon and ribavirin* Acts:

Hep C antiviral **Dose:** *Adults.* After 4 wk of peginterferon and ribavirin, then 800 mg tid w/ food for 44 wk w/ peginterferon and ribavirin; must be used w/ peginterferon and ribavirin **W/P:** [B, X w/ peginterferon and ribavirin, –] (X because must be used w/ peginterferon and ribavirin, class B by itself) **CI:** All CIs to peginterferon and ribavirin; men if PRG female partner; drugs highly dependent on CYP3A4/5 including alfuzosin, sildenafil, tadalafil, lovastatin, simvastatin, ergotamines, cisapride, triazolam, midazolam, rifampin, St. John's wort, phenytoin, carbamazepine, phenobarbital, drosperinone strong inhib CYP3A4/5 **Disp:** Caps 200 mg **SE:** Anemia, ↓ WBCs, neutrophils, fatigue, insomnia, HA, anorexia, N/V/D, dysgeusia, alopecia **Notes:** (NS3/4A protease inhib); ✓ HCV-RNA levels wk 4, 8, 12, 24, end of Tx; ✓ WBC w/ diff at wk 4, 8, 12

Bortezomib (Velcade) Uses: *Rx multiple myeloma or mantel cell lymphoma w/ one failed previous Rx* **Acts:** Proteasome inhib **Dose:** Per protocol or PI, ↓ dose w/ hematologic tox, neuropathy **W/P:** [D, ?/–] w/ Drugs CYP450 metabolized (Table 10, p 319) **Disp:** 3.5 mg vial Inj powder **SE:** Asthenia, GI upset, anorexia, dyspnea, HA, orthostatic ↓ BP, edema, insomnia, dizziness, rash, pyrexia, arthralgia, neuropathy

Bosutinib Monohydrate (Bosulif) Uses: *Ph+ CML intol/resist to prior therapy* **Acts:** TKI **Dose:** 500 mg/d, ↑ dose to 600 mg/d by wk 8 w/ incomplete reponse, or by wk 12 w/ cytogenetic incomplete response and no grade 3/greater adverse Rxn; w/ hepatic impair 200 mg/d **W/P:** [D, –] GI toxicity; ↓ BM, ✓ CBC/LFTs q mo; fluid retention; hold/↓ dose or D/C w/ toxicity **CI:** Hypersens **Disp:** Tabs 100, 500 mg **SE:** N, V, D, Abd pain, fever, rash, fatigue, anemia, ↓ plts **Notes:** Avoid w/ mod/strong CYP3A inhib & inducers; avoid use of PPIs

Botulinum Toxin Type A [abobotulinumtoxinA] (Dysport) BOX: Effects may spread beyond Tx area leading to swallowing and breathing difficulties (may be fatal); Sxs may occur hours to weeks after Inj Uses: *Cervical dystonia (adults), glabellar lines (cosmetic)* **Acts:** Neurotoxin, ↓ ACH release from nerve endings, ↓ neuromuscular transmission **Dose:** *Cervical dystonia:* 500 units IM ÷ dose units into muscles; retreat no less than 12–16 wk PRN dose range 250–100 units based on response. *Glabellar lines:* 50 units ÷ in 10 units/Inj into muscles, do not administer at intervals < q3mo repeat no less than q3mo **W/P:** [C, ?] Sedentary pt to resume activity slowly after Inj; aminoglycosides and nondepolarizing muscle blockers may ↑↑ effects; do not exceed dosing **CI:** Hypersens to components (cow milk), Infxn at Inj site **Disp:** 300, 500 units, Inj **SE:** Anaphylaxis, erythema multiforme, dysphagia, dyspnea, syncope, HA, NAG, Inj site pain **Notes:** Botulinum toxin products not interchangeable

Botulinum Toxin Type A [incobotulinumtoxinA] (Xeomin) BOX: Effects may spread beyond Tx area leading to swallowing and breathing difficulties (may be fatal); Sxs may occur hours to weeks after Inj Uses: *Cervical dystonia (adults), glabellar lines* **Acts:** Neurotoxin, ↓ ACH release from nerve endings, ↓ neuromuscular transmission **Dose:** *Cervical dystonia:* 120 units IM ÷ dose into muscles; *Glabellar lines:* 4 units into each of the 5 sites (total = 20 units) do not administer at intervals < q3mo **W/P:** [C, ?] Sedentary pt to resume activity slowly after Inj; aminoglycosides and nondepolarizing muscle blockers may ↑↑ effects; do not exceed dosing **CI:** Hypersens to components (cow milk), infect at Inj site **Disp:** 50, 100 units, Inj **SE:** Dysphagia, neck/musculoskeletal pain, muscle weakness, Inj site pain **Notes:** Botulinum toxin products not interchangeable

Botulinum Toxin Type A [onabotulinumtoxinA] (Botox, Botox Cosmetic) **BOX:** Effects may spread beyond Tx area leading to swallowing/breathing difficulties (may be fatal); Sxs may occur hours to weeks after Inj **Uses:** *Glabellar lines (cosmetic) < 65 y, blepharospasm, cervical dystonia, axillary hyperhidrosis, strabismus, chronic migraine, upper limb spasticity, incontinence in OAB due to neurologic Dz* **Acts:** Neurotoxin, ↓ ACH release from nerve endings; denervates sweat glands/muscles **Dose:** *Adults. Glabellar lines (cosmetic):* 0.1 mL IM × 5 sites q3–4mo; *Blepharospasm:* 1.25–2.5 units IM/site q3mo; max 200 units/30 d total; *Cervical dystonia:* 198–300 units IM ÷ < 100 units into muscle; *Hyperhidrosis:* 50 units intradermal/each axilla; *Strabismus:* 1.25–2.5 units IM/site q3mo; inject eye muscles w/ EMG guidance; *Chronic migraine:* 155 units total, 0.1 mL (5 unit) Inj ÷ into 7 head/neck muscles; *Upper limb spasticity:* Dose based on Hx use EMG guidance **W/P:** [C, ?] w/ Neurologic Dz; do not exceed rec doses; sedentary pt to resume activity slowly after Inj; aminoglycosides and nondepolarizing muscle blockers may ↑↑ effects; Do not exceed dosing **CI:** Hypersens to components, Infxn at Inj site **Disp:** Inj powder, single-use vial (dilute w/ NS); (*Botox cosmetic*) 50, 100 units; (*Botox*) 100, 200 unit vials; store 2–8°C **SE:** Anaphylaxis, erythema multiforme, dysphagia, dyspnea, syncope, HA, NAG, Inj site pain **Notes:** Botulinum toxin products not interchangeable; do not exceed total dose of 360 units q12–16wk

Botulinum Toxin Type B [rimabotulinumtoxinB] (Myobloc) **BOX:** Effects may spread beyond Tx area leading to swallowing and breathing difficulties (may be fatal); Sxs may occur hours to weeks after Inj **Uses:** *Cervical dystonia (adults)* **Acts:** Neurotoxin, ↓ ACH release from nerve endings, ↓ neuromuscular transmission **Dose:** *Cervical dystonia:* 2500–5000 units IM ÷ dose units into muscles; lower dose if naïve **W/P:** [C, ?] Sedentary pt to resume activity slowly after Inj; aminoglycosides and nondepolarizing muscle blockers may ↑↑ effects; do not exceed dosing **CI:** Hypersens to components, Infxn at Inj site **Disp:** Inj 5000 units/mL **SE:** Anaphylaxis, erythema multiforme, dysphagia, dyspnea, syncope, HA, NAG, Inj site pain **Notes:** Effect 12–16 wk w/ 5000–10,000 units; botulinum toxin products not interchangeable

Brentuximab Vedotin (Adcetris) **BOX:** JC virus Infxn leading to PML and death may occur **Uses:** *Hodgkin lymphoma, systemic anaplastic large cell lymphoma* **Acts:** CD30-directed antibody-drug conjugate **Dose:** *Adult.* 1.8 mg/kg IV over 30 min q 3 wk; max 16 cycles; pts > 100 kg, dose based on Wt of 100 kg; ↓ dose w/ periph neuropathy & neutropenia (see label) **W/P:** [D, ?/–] w/ Strong

CYP3A4 inhib/inducers **CI:** w/ Bleomycin **Disp:** Inj (powder) 50 mg/vial **SE:** Periph neuropathy, ↓ WBC/Hgb/plt, N/V/D, HA, dizziness, pain, arthralgia, myalgia, insomnia, anxiety, alopecia, night sweats, URI, fatigue, pyrexia, rash, cough, dyspnea, Inf Rxns, tumor lysis synd, PML, SJS, pulmonary tox

Brimonidine (Alphagan P) Uses: *Open-angle glaucoma, ocular HTN* **Acts:** α₂-Adrenergic agonist **Dose:** 1 gtt in eye(s) tid (wait 15 min to insert contacts) **W/P:** [B, ?] **CI:** MAOI Rx **Disp:** 0.15, 0.1, 0.2%, soln **SE:** Local irritation, HA, fatigue

Brimonidine/Timolol (Combigan) Uses: *↓ IOP in glaucoma or ocular HTN* **Acts:** Selective α₂-adrenergic agonist & nonselective β-adrenergic antagonist **Dose:** *Adults & Peds ≥ 2 y.* 1 gtt bid **W/P:** [C, −] **CI:** Asthma, severe COPD, sinus brady, 2nd-/3rd-degree AV block, CHF cardiac failure, cardiogenic shock, component hypersens **Disp:** Soln: (2 mg/mL brimonidine, 5 mg/mL timolol) 5, 10, 15 mL **SE:** Allergic conjunctivitis, conjunctival folliculosis, conjunctival hyperemia, eye pruritus, ocular burning & stinging **Notes:** Instill other ophthal products 5 min apart

Brinzolamide (Azopt) Uses: *Open-angle glaucoma, ocular HTN* **Acts:** Carbonic anhydrase inhib **Dose:** 1 gtt in eye(s) tid **W/P:** [C, ?/−] **CI:** Sulfonamide allergy **Disp:** 1% susp **SE:** Blurred vision, dry eye, blepharitis, taste disturbance, HA

Bromocriptine (Parlodel) Uses: *Parkinson Dz, hyperprolactinemia, acromegaly, pituitary tumors* **Acts:** Agonist to striatal dopamine receptors; ↓ prolactin secretion **Dose:** Initial, 1.25 mg PO bid; titrate to effect, w/ food **W/P:** [B, −] **CI:** uncontrolled HTN, PRG, severe CAD or CVS Dz **Disp:** Tabs 2.5 mg; caps 5 mg **SE:** ↓ BP, Raynaud phenomenon, dizziness, N, GI upset, hallucinations

Bromocriptine Mesylate (Cycloset) Uses: *Improve glycemic control in adults w/ type 2 DM* **Acts:** Dopamine receptor agonist; ? DM mechanism **Dose:** *Initial:* 0.8 mg PO daily, ↑ weekly by 1 tab; usual dose 1.6–4.8 mg 1×/d; w/in 2 h after waking w/ food **W/P:** [B, −] May cause orthostatic ↓ BP, psychotic disorders; not for type 1 DM or DKA; w/ strong inducers/inhib of CYP3A4, avoid w/ dopamine antagonists/receptor agonists **CI:** Hypersens to ergots drugs, w/ syncopal migraine, nursing mothers **Disp:** Tabs 0.8 mg **SE:** N/V, fatigue, HA, dizziness, somnolence

Budesonide (Rhinocort Aqua, Pulmicort) Uses: *Allergic & nonallergic rhinitis, asthma* **Acts:** Steroid **Dose:** *Adults. Rhinocort Aqua:* 1 spray each nostril/d *Pulmicort Flexhaler:* 1–2 Inh bid *Peds. Rhinocort Aqua intranasal:* 1 spray each nostril/d; *Pulmicort flexhaler* 1–2 Inh bid; *Respules:* 0.25–0.5 mg daily or bid (rinse mouth after PO use) **W/P:** [B, ?/−] **CI:** w/ Acute asthma **Disp:** *Flexhaler:* 90, 180 mcg/Inh; *Respules:* 0.25, 0.5,1 mg/2 mL; *Rhinocort Aqua:* 32 mcg/spray **SE:** HA, N, cough, hoarseness, *Candida* Infxn, epistaxis

Budesonide, Oral (Entocort EC) Uses: *Mild–mod Crohn Dz* **Acts:** Steroid, anti-inflammatory **Dose:** *Adults.* Initial: 9 mg PO q A.M. to 8 wk max: maint 6 mg PO q A.M. taper by 3 mo; avoid grapefruit juice **CI:** Hypersens **W/P:** [C, ?/−]

DM, glaucoma, cataracts, HTN, CHF **Disp:** Caps 3 mg ER **SE:** HA, N, ↑ Wt, mood change, *Candida* Infxn, epistaxis **Notes:** Do not cut/crush/chew; taper on D/C

Budesonide/Formoterol (Symbicort) **BOX:** Long-acting β₂-adrenergic agonists may ↑ risk of asthma-related death. Use only for pts not adequately controlled on other meds **Uses:** *Rx of asthma, main in COPD (chronic bronchitis and emphysema)* **Acts:** Steroid w/ LA β₂-adrenergic agonist **Dose:** *Adults & Peds > 12 y.* 2 Inh bid (use lowest effective dose), 640/18 mcg/d max **W/P:** [C, ?/–] **CI:** Status asthmaticus/acute asthma **Disp:** Inh (budesonide/formoterol): 80/4.5 mcg, 160/4.5 mcg **SE:** HA, GI discomfort, nasopharyngitis, palpitations, tremor, nervousness, URI, paradoxical bronchospasm, hypokalemia, cataracts, glaucoma **Notes:** Not for acute bronchospasm; not for transferring pt from chronic systemic steroids; rinse & spit w/ water after each dose

Bumetanide (Bumex) **BOX:** Potent diuretic, may result in profound fluid & electrolyte loss **Uses:** *Edema from CHF, hepatic cirrhosis, & renal Dz* **Acts:** Loop diuretic; ↓ reabsorption of Na⁺ & Cl⁻, in ascending loop of Henle & the distal tubule **Dose:** *Adults.* 0.5–2 mg/d PO; 0.5–1 mg IV/IM q8–24h (max 10 mg/d). *Peds.* 0.015–0.1 mg/kg PO q6–24h (max 10 mg/d) **W/P:** [C, ?/–] **CI:** Anuria, hepatic coma, severe electrolyte depletion **Disp:** Tabs 0.5, 1, 2 mg; Inj 0.25 mg/mL **SE:** ↓ K⁺, ↓ Na⁺, ↑ Cr, ↑ uric acid, dizziness, ototox **Notes:** Monitor fluid & lytes

Bupivacaine (Marcaine) **BOX:** Avoid 0.75% for OB anethesia d/t reports of cardiac arrest and death **Uses:** *Local, regional, & spinal anesthesia, obstetrical procedures* local & regional analgesia **Acts:** Local anesthetic **Dose:** *Adults & Peds.* Dose dependent on procedure (tissue vascularity, depth of anesthesia, etc) (Table 1, p 300) **W/P:** [C, –] Severe bleeding, ↓ BP, shock & arrhythmias, local Infxns at site, septicemia **CI:** Obstetrical paracervical block anesthesia **Disp:** Inj 0.25, 0.5, 0.75% **SE:** ↓ BP, ↑ HR, dizziness, anxiety

Buprenorphine (Buprenex) [C-III] **Uses:** *Mod–severe pain* **Acts:** Opiate agonist-antagonist **Dose:** 0.3–0.6 mg IM or slow IV push q6h PRN **W/P:** [C, –] **Disp:** 0.3 mg/mL **SE:** Sedation, ↓ BP, resp depression **Notes:** Withdrawal if opioid-dependent

Buprenorphine & Naloxone (Suboxone) [C-III] **Uses:** *Maint opioid withdrawal* **Acts:** Opioid agonist-antagonist + opioid antagonist **Dose:** Usual: 4–24 mg/d SL; ↑/↓ by 2/0.5 mg or 4/1 mg to effect of S/Sxs **W/P:** [C, +/–] **CI:** Hypersens **Disp:** SL film buprenorphine/naloxone: 2/0.5, 8/2 mg **SE:** Oral hypoparesthesia, HA, V, pain, constipation, diaphoresis **Notes:** Not for analgesia

Buprenorphine, Transdermal (Butrans) [C-III] **BOX:** Limit use to severe around-the-clock chronic pain; assess for opioid abuse/addiction before use; 20 mcg/h max due to ↑ QTc; avoid heat on patch, may result in OD **Uses:** *Mod–severe chronic pain requiring around-the-clock opioid analgesic* **Acts:** Opiate agonist-antagonist **Dose:** Wear patch ×7/d; if opioid naïve, start 5 mcg/h; see label for conversion from opioid; wait 72 h before Δ dose; wait 3 wk before using same application site **W/P:** [C, –] **CI:** Resp depression, severe asthma, ileus, component hypersens, short-term opioid need, postop/mild/intermittent pain **Disp:** Transdermal patch 5, 10, 20 mcg/h **SE:** N/V, HA, site Rxns pruritus, dizziness, constipation, somnolence, dry mouth **Notes:** Taper on D/C

Bupropion (Aplenzin XR, Wellbutrin, Wellbutrin SR, Wellbutrin XL, Zyban)
BOX: All pts being treated w/ bupropion for smoking cessation Tx should be observed for neuropsychiatric S/Sxs (hostility, agitation, depressed mood, and suicide-related events; most during/after *Zyban*; Sxs may persist following D/C; closely monitor for worsening depression or emergence of suicidality, increased suicidal behavior in young adults **Uses:** *Depression, smoking cessation adjunct*, ADHD, not for peds use **Acts:** Weak inhib of neuronal uptake of serotonin & norepinephrine; ↓ neuronal dopamine reuptake **Dose:** *Depression:* 100–450 mg/d ÷ bid-tid; SR 150–200 mg bid; XL 150–450 mg daily. *Smoking cessation (Zyban, Wellbutrin XR):* 150 mg/d × 3 d, then 150 mg bid × 8–12 wk, last dose before 6 P.M.; ↓ dose w/ renal/hepatic impair **W/P:** [C, ?/–] **CI:** Sz disorder, Hx anorexia nervosa or bulimia, MAOI w/in 14 d; abrupt D/C of EtOH or sedatives; inhibitors/inducers of CYP2B6 (Table 10, p 319) **Disp:** Tabs 75, 100 mg; SR tabs 100, 150, 200 mg; XL tabs 150, 300 mg; Zyban tabs 150 mg; Aplenzin XR tabs: 175, 348, 522 mg **SE:** Xerostomia, dizziness, Szs, agitation, insomnia, HA, tachycardia, ↓ Wt **Notes:** Avoid EtOH & other CNS depressants, SR & XR do not cut/chew/crush, may ↑ adverse events including Szs

Buspirone
Uses: *Generalized anxiety disorder* **Acts:** Antianxiety; antagonizes CNS serotonin and dopamine receptors **Dose:** Initial: 7.5 mg PO bid; ↑ by 5 mg q2–3d to effect; usual 20–30 mg/d; max 60 mg/d **CI:** Hypersens **W/P:** [B, ?/–] Avoid w/ severe hepatic/renal Insuff w/ MAOI **Disp:** Tabs 5, 7.5, 10, 15, 30 mg **SE:** Drowsiness, dizziness, HA, N, EPS, serotonin synd, hostility, depression **Notes:** No abuse potential or physical/psychological dependence

Busulfan (Myleran, Busulfex)
BOX: Can cause severe bone marrow suppression, should be administered by an experienced physician **Uses:** *CML*, preparative regimens for allogeneic & ABMT in high doses **Acts:** Alkylating agent **Dose:** (per protocol) Oral 1.8 mg/kg/d; Inj 60 mg/10 mL **SE:** Bone marrow suppression, ↑ BP, pulm fibrosis, N (w/ high dose), gynecomastia, adrenal Insuff, skin hyperpigmentation, ↑ HR, rash, weakness, Sz

Butabarbital, Hyoscyamine Hydrobromide, Phenazopyridine (Pyridium Plus)
Uses: *Relieve urinary tract pain w/ UTI, procedures, trauma* **Acts:** Phenazopyridine (topical anesthetic), hyoscyamine (parasympatholytic, ↓ spasm), & butabarbital (sedative) **Dose:** 1 PO qid, pc & hs; w/ antibiotic for UTI, 2 d max **W/P:** [D, ?] **Disp:** Tab butabarbital/hyoscyamine/phenazopyridine, 15 mg/0.3 mg/150 mg **SE:** HA, rash, itching, GI distress, methemoglobinemia, hemolytic anemia, anaphylactoid-like Rxns, dry mouth, dizziness, drowsiness, blurred vision **Notes:** Colors urine orange, may tint skin, sclera; stains clothing/contacts

Butorphanol (Stadol) [C-IV] Uses: **Anesthesia adjunct, pain & migraine HA** Acts: Opiate agonist-antagonist w/ central analgesic actions Dose: 0.5–4 mg IM or IV q3–4h PRN. *Migraine:* 1 spray in 1 nostril, repeat × 1 60–90 min, then q3–4h; ↓ in renal impair W/P: [C, +] Disp: Inj 1, 2 mg/mL; nasal 1 mg/spray (10 mg/mL) SE: Drowsiness, dizziness, nasal congestion Notes: May induce withdrawal in opioid dependency

C1 Esterase Inhibitor [Human] (Berinert, Cinryze) Uses: **Berinert:* Rx acute Abd or facial attacks of HAE*, **Cinryze:* Prophylaxis of HAE** Acts: ↓ complement system by ↓ factor XIIa and kallikrein activation Dose: *Adults & Adolescents. Berinert:* 20 units/kg IV × 1; *Cinryze:* 1000 units IV q3–4d W/P: [C, ?/–] Hypersens Rxns, monitor for thrombotic events, may contain infectious agents CI: Hypersens Rxns to C1 esterase inhibitor preparations Disp: 500 units/vial SE: HA, Abd pain, N/V/D, muscle spasms, pain, subsequent HAE attack, anaphylaxis, thromboembolism

Cabazitaxel (Jevtana) BOX: Neutropenic deaths reported; ✓ CBCs, CI w/ ANC ≤ 1500 cells/mm³; severe hypersens (rash/erythema, ↓ BP, bronchospasm) may occur, D/C drug & Tx; CI w/ Hx of hypersens to cabazitaxel or others formulated w/ polysorbate 80 Uses: **Hormone refractory metastatic PCa after taxotere** Acts: Microtubule inhib Dose: 25 mg/m² IV Inf (over 1 h) q3wk w/ prednisone 10 mg PO daily; premed w/ antihistamine, corticosteroid, H₂ antagonist; do not use w/ bili ≥ ULN, AST/ALT ≥ 1.5 × ULN W/P: [D, ?/–] w/ CYP3A inhib/inducers CI: See Box Disp: 40 mg/mL Inj SE: ↓ WBC, ↓ Hgb, ↓ plt, sepsis, N/V/D, constipation, Abd/back/jt pain, dysgeusia, fatigue, hematuria, neuropathy, anorexia, cough, dyspnea, alopecia, pyrexia, hypersens Rxn, renal failure Notes: Monitor closely pts > 65 y

Cabozantinib (Cometriq) BOX: GI perf/fistulas, severe and sometimes fatal hemorrhage (3%) including GI bleed/hemoptysis Uses: **Metastatic medullary thyroid CA** Acts: Multi TKI Dose: 140 mg/d, do NOT eat 2 h ac or 1 h pc W/P: [D, –] D/C w/ arterial thromboembolic events; dehiscence; ↑ BP, ONJ; palmar-plantar erythrodysesthesia synd; proteinuria; reversible posterior leukoencephalopathy CI: w/ Severe bleed Disp: Caps 20, 80 mg SE: N, V, Abd pain, constipation, stomatitis, oral pain, dysgeusia, fatigue, ↓ Wt, anorexia, ↑ BP, ↑ AST/ALT, ↑ alk phos, ↑ bili, ↓ Ca, ↓ PO₄, ↓ plts, ↓ lymphocytes, ↓ neutrophils Notes: A CYP3A4 subs, w/ strong CYP3A4 induc ↓ cabozantinib exposure, w/ strong CYP3A4 inhib ↑ cabozantinib exposure; ✓ for hemorrhage

Calcipotriene (Dovonex) Uses: **Plaque psoriasis** Acts: Synthetic vitamin D₃ analog Dose: Apply bid W/P: [C, ?] CI: ↑ Ca²⁺; vit D tox; do not apply to face Disp: Cream; foam oint; soln 0.005% SE: Skin irritation, dermatitis

Calcitonin (Fortical, Miacalcin) Uses: *Miacalcin:* *Paget Dz, emergent Rx hypercalcemia, postmenopausal osteoporosis*; *Fortical:* *Postmenopausal osteoporosis** Acts: Polypeptide hormone (salmon derived), inhibits osteoclasts Dose: *Paget Dz:* 100 units/d IM/SQ initial, 50 units/d or 50–100 units q1–3d maint. *Hypercalcemia:* 4 units/kg IM/SQ q12h; ↑ to 8 units/kg q12h, max q6h. *Osteoporosis:* 100 units/q other day IM/SQ; intranasal 200 units = 1 nasal spray/d **W/P:** [C, ?] **Disp:** *Fortical, Miacalcin* nasal spray 200 Int units/activation; Inj, *Miacalcin* 200 units/mL (2 mL) **SE:** Facial flushing, N, Inj site edema, nasal irritation, polyuria, may ↑ granular casts in urine **Notes:** For nasal spray alternate nostrils daily; ensure adequate calcium and vit D intake; *Fortical* is rDNA derived from salmon

Calcitriol (Rocaltrol, Calcijex) **Uses:** *Predialysis reduction of ↑ PTH levels to treat bone Dz; ↑ Ca²⁺ on dialysis* **Acts:** 1,25-Dihydroxycholecalci-ferol (vit D analog);↑ Ca²⁺ and phosphorus absorption; ↑ bone mineralization **Dose:** *Adults. Renal failure:* 0.25 mcg/d PO, ↑ 0.25 mcg/d q4–8wk PRN; 0.5–4 mcg 3×/wk IV, ↑ PRN *Hypoparathyroidism.* 0.5–2 mcg/d. *Peds. Renal failure:* 15 ng/kg/d, ↑ PRN; maint 30–60 ng/kg/d. *Hypoparathyroidism:* < *5 y:* 0.25–0.75 mcg/d. > *6 y:* 0.5–2 mcg/d **W/P:** [C, ?] ↑ Mg²⁺ possible w/ antacids **CI:** ↑ Ca²⁺; vit D tox **Disp:** Inj 1 mcg/mL (in 1 mL); caps 0.25, 0.5 mcg; soln 1 mcg/mL **SE:** ↑ Ca²⁺ possible **Notes:** ✓ To keep Ca²⁺ WNL; use nonaluminum phosphate binders and low-phosphate diet to control serum phosphate

Calcitriol, Ointment (Vectical) **Uses:** *Mild–moderate plaque psoriasis* **Acts:** Vitamin D₃ analog **Dose:** *Adults.* Apply to area BID; max 200 g/wk **W/P:** [C, ?/–] Avoid excess sunlight **CI:** None **Disp:** Oint 3 mcg/g (5-, 100-g tube) **SE:** Hypercalcemia, hypercalciuria, nephrolithiasis, worsening psoriasis, pruritus, skin discomfort

Calcium Acetate (PhosLo) **Uses:** *ESRD-associated hyperphosphatemia* **Acts:** Ca²⁺ supl w/o aluminum to ↓ PO₄²⁻ absorption **Dose:** 2–4 tabs PO w/ meals usual 2001–2668 mg PO w/ meals **W/P:** [C, +] **CI:** ↑ Ca²⁺ renal calculi **Disp:** Gel-Cap 667 mg **SE:** Can ↑ Ca²⁺, hypophosphatemia, constipation **Notes:** Monitor Ca²⁺

Calcium Carbonate (Tums, Alka-Mints) [OTC] **Uses:** *Hyperacidity-associated w/ peptic ulcer Dz, hiatal hernia, etc* **Acts:** Neutralizes gastric acid **Dose:** 500 mg–2 g PO PRN, 7 g/d max; ↓ w/ impair renal **W/P:** [C, ?] **CI:** ↑ CA, ↓ phos, renal calculi, suspected digoxin tox **Disp:** Chew tabs 350, 420, 500, 550, 750, 850 mg; susp **SE:** ↑ Ca²⁺, ↓ PO₄⁻, constipation

Calcium Glubionate (Calcionate) [OTC] **Uses:** *Rx & prevent calcium deficiency* **Acts:** Ca²⁺ supl **Dose:** *Adults.* 1000–1200 mg/d ÷ doses. *Peds.* 200–1300 mg/d **W/P:** [C, ?] **Disp:** OTC syrup 1.8 g/5 mL = elemental Ca 115 mg/5 mL **SE:** ↑ Ca²⁺, ↓ PO₄⁻, constipation

Calcium (Chloride, Gluconate, Gluceptate) **Uses:** *Ca²⁺ replacement*, VF, Ca²⁺ blocker tox (CCB), *severe ↑ Mg²⁺ tetany*, *hyperphosphatemia in ESRD* **Acts:** Ca²⁺ supl/replacement **Dose:** *Adults. Replacement:* 1–2 g/d PO. *Tetany:* 1 g CaCl over 10–30 min; repeat in 6 h PRN; *ECC 2010. Hyperkalemia/ hypermagnesemia/CCB OD:* 500–1000 mg (5–10 mL of 10% soln) IV; repeat PRN; comparable dose of 10% calcium gluconate is 15–30 mL *Peds. Tetany:* 10 mg/kg CaCl over 5–10 min; repeat in 6–8 h or use Inf (200 mg/kg/d max).

ECC 2010. Hypocalcemia/hyperkalemia/hypermagnesemia/CCB OD: Calcium chloride or gluconate 20 mg/kg (0.2 mL/kg) slow IV/IO, repeat PRN; central venous route preferred *Adults & Peds.* ↓ Ca²⁺ d/t citrated blood Inf: 0.45 mEq Ca/100 mL citrated blood Inf (↓ in renal impair) **W/P:** [C, ?] **CI:** ↑ Ca²⁺, suspected digoxin tox **Disp:** CaCl Inj 10% = 100 mg/mL = Ca 27.2 mg/mL = 10-mL amp; Ca gluconate Inj 10% = 100 mg/mL = Ca 9 mg/mL; tabs 500 mg = 45-mg Ca, 650 mg = 58.5-mg Ca, 975 mg = 87.75-mg Ca, 1 g = 90-mg Ca; Ca gluceptate Inj 220 mg/mL = 18-mg/mL Ca **SE:** ↓ HR, cardiac arrhythmias, ↑ Ca²⁺, constipation **Notes:** CaCl 270 mg (13.6 mEq) elemental Ca/g & calcium gluconate 90 mg (4.5 mEq) Ca/g. RDA for Ca intake: *Peds < 6 mo.* 200 mg/d; *6 mo–1 y:* 260 mg/d; *1–3 y:* 700 mg/d; *4–8 y:* 1000 mg/d; *10–18 y:* 1300 mg/d. *Adults.* 1000 mg/d; > *50 y:* 1200 mg/d

Calfactant (Infasurf) Uses: *Prevention & Rx of RSD in infants* Acts: Exogenous pulm surfactant Dose: 3 mL/kg instilled into lungs. Can repeat 3 total doses given 12 h apart **W/P:** [?, ?] **Disp:** Intratracheal susp 35 mg/mL **SE:** Monitor for cyanosis, airway obst, ↓ HR during administration

Canagliflozin (Invokana) Uses: *Type 2 DM* Acts: Sodium-glucose co-transporter 2 (SGLT2) inhib Dose: *Adults.* Start 100 mg/d; ↑ to 300 mg PRN w/ GFR > 60 mL/min **W/P:** [C, –] ↓ BP from ↓ vol from glucosuria; ↑ K⁺; ↑ Cr, √renal Fxn; genital mycotic infections; hypoglycemia lower risk than insulin & sulfonylureas; hypersens **CI:** Hypersens reaction, severe renal impairment (GFR < 45 mL/min) **Disp:** Tabs 100, 300 **SE:** UTI, genital mycotic infections (3–15%) less likely to occur in circumcised males, polyuria, ↑ K⁺, ↑ PO₄⁻³, ↑ Mg²⁺, ↑ creat, ↑ LDL-chol **Notes:** First in class w/ FDA approval; may ↑ CV morbidity in first 30 d of Tx; CrCl 45–60 mL/min 100 mg/d max, do NOT use w/ CrCl < 45 mL/min; Wt loss likely; do not use w/ severe liver Dz; ↑ adverse events in geriatric pop; metabolized by UDP-glucuronosyltransferase 1A9 & 2B4, concomitant rifampin, phenytoin, or ritonavir use reduces exposure, may need to ↑ dose; may need to ↓ digoxin dose

Candesartan (Atacand) BOX: w/ PRG D/C immediately Uses: *HTN, CHF* Acts: Angiotensin II receptor antagonist Dose: 4–32 mg/d (usual 16 mg/d) **W/P:** [C(1st tri), D (2nd tri), ?/–] w/ renal Dz **CI:** Component hypersens **Disp:** Tabs 4, 8, 16, 32 mg **SE:** Dizziness, HA, flushing, angioedema, ↑ K⁺, ↑ SCr

Capsaicin (Capsin, Zostrix, Others) [OTC] Uses: Pain d/t *postherpetic neuralgia*, *arthritis, diabetic neuropathy*,*minor pain of muscles & joints* Acts: Topical analgesic Dose: Apply tid-qid **W/P:** [B, ?] **Disp:** OTC creams; gel; lotions; roll-ons **SE:** Local irritation, neurotox, cough **Notes:** Wk to onset of action

Captopril (Capoten, Others) Uses: *HTN, CHF, MI*, LVD, diabetic nephropathy Acts: ACE inhib Dose: *Adults. HTN:* Initial, 25 mg PO bid-tid; ↑ to maint q1–2wk by 25-mg increments/dose (max 450 mg/d) *CHF:* Initial, 6.25–12.5 mg PO tid; titrate PRN *LVD:* 50 mg PO tid. *DN:* 25 mg PO tid. *Peds* infants 0.15–0.3 mg/kg/dose PO ÷ 1–4 doses *Children:* Initial, 0.3–0.5 mg/kg/dose PO; ↑ to

6 mg/kg/d max in 2–4 ÷ doses; 1 h ac; ↓ dose renal impairment **W/P:** [D, –] **CI:** Hx angioedema **Disp:** Tabs 12.5, 25, 50, 100 mg **SE:** Rash, proteinuria, cough, ↑ K⁺

Carbamazepine (Tegretol XR, Carbatrol, Epitol, Equetro) BOX:

Aplastic anemia & agranulocytosis have been reported w/ carbamazepine; pts w/ Asian ancestry should be tested to determine potential for skin Rxns **Uses:** *Epilepsy, trigeminal neuralgia, acute mania w/ bipolar disorder (Equetro)* EtOH withdrawal **Acts:** Anticonvulsant **Dose:** *Adults. Initial:* 200 mg PO bid or 100 mg 4 ×/d as susp; ↑ by 200 mg/d; usual 800–1200 mg/d ÷ doses. *Acute Mania (Equetro):* 400 mg/d, ÷ bid, adjust by 200 mg/d to response 1600 mg/d max. *Peds < 6 y.* 10–20 mg/kg ÷ bid-tid or qid (susp) *6–12 y: Initial:* 200 mg/d bid (tab) or qid (susp), ↑ 100 mg/d, usual: 400–800 mg/d, max 1000 mg/d; ↓ in renal impair; take w/ food **W/P:** [D, M] **CI:** w/in 14 d, w/ nefazodone, MAOI use, Hx BM suppression **Disp:** Tabs 200 mg; chew tabs 100 mg, XR tabs 100, 200,400 mg; *Equetro* Caps ER 100, 200, 300 mg; susp 100 mg/5 mL **SE:** Drowsiness, dizziness, blurred vision, N/V, rash, SJS/toxic epidermal necrolysis (TEN), ↓ Na⁺, leukopenia, agranulocytosis **Notes:** Monitor CBC & levels: *Trough:* Trough before next dose; *Therapeutic: Peak:* 8–12 mcg/mL (monotherapy), 4–8 mcg/mL (polytherapy); *Toxic Trough:* > 15 mcg/mL; *Half-life:* 15–20 h; generic products not interchangeable, many drug interactions, administer susp in 3–4 ÷ doses daily; skin tox (SJS/TEN) ↑ w/ HLA-B*1502 allele

Carbidopa/Levodopa (Sinemet, Parcopa) **Uses:** *Parkinson Dz*

Acts: ↑ CNS dopamine levels **Dose:** 25/100 mg tid, ↑ as needed (max 200/2000 mg/d) **W/P:** [C, ?] **CI:** NAG, suspicious skin lesion (may activate melanoma), melanoma, MAOI use (w/in 14 d) **Disp:** Tabs (mg carbidopa/mg levodopa) 10/100, 25/100, 25/250; tabs SR (mg carbidopa/mg levodopa) 25/100, 50/200; ODT 10/100, 25/100, 25/250 **SE:** Psych disturbances, orthostatic ↓ BP, dyskinesias, cardiac arrhythmias

Carboplatin (Paraplatin) BOX: Administration only by physician experi-

enced in CA chemotherapy; ↓ PLT, anemia, ↑ Infxn; BM suppression possible; anaphylaxis and V may occur **Uses:** *Ovarian*, lung, head & neck, testicular, urothelial, & brain CA, NHL & allogeneic & ABMT in high doses **Acts:** DNA cross-linker; forms DNA-platinum adducts **Dose:** Per protocols based on target (Calvert formula: mg = AUC × [25 + calculated GFR]); adjust based on plt count, CrCl, & BSA (Egorin formula); up to 1500 mg/m² used in ABMT setting (per protocols) **W/P:** [D, ?] severe hepatic tox **CI:** Severe BM suppression, excessive bleeding **Disp:** Inj 50-, 150-, 450-, 650-mg vial (10 mg/mL) **SE:** Pain, ↓ Na⁺/Mg²⁺/Ca²⁺/K⁺, anaphylaxis, ↓ BM, N/V/D, nephrotox, hematuria, neurotox, ↑ LFTs **Notes:** Physiologic dosing based on Calvert or Egorin formula allows ↑ doses w/ ↓ tox

Carfilzomib (Kyprolis) **Uses:** *Multiple myeloma w/ > 2 prior therapies

and prog w/in 60 d* **Acts:** Proteasome inhib **Dose:** 20 mg/m²/d, if tolerated ↑ to 27 mg/m²/d; IV over 2–10 min; cycle = 2 consecutive d/wk × 3 wk, then 12-d rest; hydrate before and after admin, premedicate w/ dexamethasone first cycle, dose escalation or if infusion reactions **W/P:** [D, –] CHF, cardiac ischemia; pulm HTN, dyspnea; tumor lysis synd; ↓ plts, ✓ plts; hepatic toxicity, ✓ LFTs **CI:** None **Disp:** Vial, 60 mg powder **SE:** N, D, fever, fatigue, dyspnea, ARF, anemia, ↓ plts, ↓ lymphocytes, ↑ LFTs, peripheral neuropathy

Carisoprodol (Soma) **Uses:** *Acute (limit 2–3 wk) painful musculoskeletal conditions* **Acts:** Centrally acting muscle relaxant **Dose:** 250–350 mg PO tid-qid **W/P:** [C, M] Tolerance may result; w/ renal/hepatic impair, w/ CYP219 poor metabolizers **CI:** Allergy to meprobamate; acute intermittent porphyria **Disp:** Tabs 250, 350 mg **SE:** CNS depression, drowsiness, dizziness, HA, tachycardia, weakness, rare Sz **Notes:** Avoid EtOH & other CNS depressants; avoid abrupt D/C; available in combo w/ ASA or codeine.

Carmustine [BCNU] (BiCNU, Gliadel) **BOX:** BM suppression, dose-related pulm tox possible; administer under direct supervision of experienced physician **Uses:** *Primary or adjunct brain tumors, multiple myeloma, Hodgkin and non-Hodgkin lymphomas*, induction for autologous stem cell or BMT (off label) surgery & RT adjunct high-grade glioma and recurrent glioblastoma *(Gliadel implant)* **Acts:** Alkylating agent; nitrosourea forms DNA cross-links to inhibit DNA **Dose:** 150–200 mg/m² q6–8wk single or ÷ dose daily Inj over 2 d; 20–65 mg/m² q4–6wk; 300–600 mg/m² in BMT (per protocols); up to 8 implants in CNS op site; ↓ w/ hepatic and renal impair **W/P:** [D, ?/–] ↓ WBC, RBC, plt counts, renal/ hepatic impair **CI:** ↓ BM, PRG **Disp:** Inj 100 mg/vial; *Gliadel* wafer 7.7 mg **SE:** Inf Rxn, ↓ BP, N/V, ↓ WBC & plt, phlebitis, facial flushing, hepatic/renal dysfunction, pulm fibrosis (may occur years after), optic neuroretinitis; heme tox may persist 4–6 wk after dose **Notes:** Do not give course more frequently than q6wk (cumulative tox); ✓ baseline PFTs, monitor pulm status

Carteolol Ophthalmic (Generic) **Uses:** *↑ IOP pressure, chronic open-angle glaucoma* **Acts:** Blocks β-adrenergic receptors (β₁, β₂), mild ISA **Dose:** Ophthal 1 gtt in eye(s) bid **W/P:** [C, ?/–] Cardiac failure, asthma **CI:** Sinus brady-cardia; heart block > 1st degree; bronchospasm **Disp:** Ophthal soln 1% **SE:** Conjunctival hyperemia, anisocoria, keratitis, eye pain **Notes:** Oral forms no longer available in US

Carvedilol (Coreg, Coreg CR) **Uses:** *HTN, mild–severe CHF, LVD post-MI* **Acts:** Blocks adrenergic receptors, β₁, β₂, α₁ **Dose:** *HTN:* 6.25–12.5 mg bid or CR 20–80 mg PO daily. *CHF:* 3.125–50 mg bid; w/ food to minimize orthostatic ↓ BP **W/P:** [C, ?/–] asthma, DM **CI:** Decompensated CHF, 2nd-/3rd-degree heart block, SSS, severe ↓ HR w/o pacemaker, acute asthma, severe hepatic impair **Disp:** Tabs 3.125, 6.25, 12.5, 25 mg; CR tabs 10, 20, 40, 80 mg **SE:** Dizziness, fatigue, hyperglycemia, may mask/potentiate hypoglycemia, ↓ HR, edema, hypercholesterolemia **Notes:** Do not D/C abruptly; ↑ digoxin levels

Caspofungin (Cancidas) **Uses:** *Invasive aspergillosis refractory/intolerant to standard Rx, candidemia & other candida Inf*, empiric Rx in febrile neutropenia w/ presumed fungal Infxn **Acts:** Echinocandin; ↓ fungal cell wall synth; highest activity in regions of active cell growth **Dose:** 70 mg IV load day 1, 50 mg/d IV;

slow Inf over 1 h; ↓ in hepatic impair **W/P:** [C, ?/–] Do not use w/ cyclosporine **CI:** Allergy to any component **Disp:** Inj 50, 70 mg powder for recons **SE:** Fever, HA, N/V, thrombophlebitis at site, ↑ LFTs ↓ BP, edema, ↑ HR, rash, ↓ K, D, Inf Rxn **Notes:** Monitor during Inf; limited experience beyond 2 wk of Rx

Cefaclor (Ceclor, Raniclor) **Uses:** *Bacterial Infxns of the upper & lower resp tract, skin, bone, urinary tract* **Acts:** 2nd-gen cephalosporin; ↓ cell wall synth. *Spectrum:* More gram(–) activity than 1st-gen cephalosporins; effective against gram(+) (*Streptococcus* sp, *S. aureus*); gram(–) against *H. influenzae, E. coli, Klebsiella, Proteus* **Dose:** *Adults.* 250–500 mg PO > q8h. *Peds.* 20–40 mg/kg/d PO ÷ 8–12 h; ↓ renal impair **W/P:** [B, M] **CI:** Cephalosporin/PCN allergy **Disp:** Caps 250, 500 mg; tabs ER 500 mg; susp 125, 250, 375 mg/5 mL **SE:** N/D, rash, eosinophilia, ↑ LFTs, HA, rhinitis, vaginitis

Cefadroxil (Duricef) **Uses:** *Infxns skin, bone, upper & lower resp tract, urinary tract* **Acts:** 1st-gen cephalosporin; ↓ cell wall synth. *Spectrum:* Good gram(+) (group A β-hemolytic *Streptococcus, Staphylococcus*); gram(–) (*E. coli, Proteus, Klebsiella*) **Dose:** *Adults.* 1–2 g/d PO, 2 ÷ doses *Peds.* 30 mg/kg/d ÷ bid; ↓ in renal impair **W/P:** [B, M] **CI:** Cephalosporin/PCN allergy **Disp:** Caps 500 mg; tabs 1 g; susp, 250, 500 mg/5 mL **SE:** N/V/D, rash, eosinophilia, ↑ LFTs

Cefazolin (Ancef, Kefzol) **Uses:** *Infxns of skin, bone, upper & lower resp tract, urinary tract* **Acts:** 1st-gen cephalosporin; β-lactam ↓ cell wall synth. *Spectrum:* Good gram(+) bacilli & cocci (*Streptococcus, Staphylococcus* [except *Enterococcus*]); some gram(–) (*E. coli, Proteus, Klebsiella*) **Dose:** *Adults.* 1–2 g IV q8h *Peds.* 25–100 mg/kg/d IV ÷ q6–8h; ↓ in renal impair **W/P:** [B, M] **CI:** Cephalosporin/PCN allergy **Disp:** Inj **SE:** D, rash, eosinophilia, ↑ LFTs, Inj site pain **Notes:** Widely used for surgical prophylaxis

Cefdinir (Omnicef) **Uses:** *Infxns of the resp tract, skin, and skin structure* **Acts:** 3rd-gen cephalosporin; ↓ cell wall synth *Spectrum:* Many gram(+) & (–) organisms; more active than cefaclor & cephalexin against *Streptococcus, Staphylococcus*; some anaerobes **Dose:** *Adults.* 300 mg PO bid or 600 mg PO qd. *Peds.* 7 mg/kg PO bid or 14 mg/kg PO qd; ↓ in renal impair **W/P:** [B, M] w/ PCN-sensitive pts **CI:** Hypersens to cephalosporins **Disp:** Caps 300 mg; susp 125, 250 mg/5 mL **SE:** Anaphylaxis, D, rare pseudomembranous colitis, HA

Cefditoren (Spectracef) **Uses:** *Acute exacerbations of chronic bronchitis, pharyngitis, tonsillitis; skin Infxns* **Acts:** 3rd-gen cephalosporin; ↓ cell wall synth. *Spectrum:* Good gram(+) (*Streptococcus & Staphylococcus*); gram(–) (*H. influenzae & M. catarrhalis*) **Dose:** *Adults & Peds > 12 y.* Skin also *pharyngitis, tonsillitis:* 200 mg PO bid × 10 d. *Chronic bronchitis:* 400 mg PO bid × 10 d; avoid antacids w/in 2 h; take w/ meals; ↓ in renal impair **W/P:** [B, ?] Renal/hepatic impair **CI:** Cephalosporin/PCN allergy, milk protein, or carnitine deficiency **Disp:** Tabs 200, 400 mg **SE:** HA, N/V/D, colitis, nephrotox, hepatic dysfunction, SJS, toxic epidermal necrolysis, allergic Rxns **Notes:** Causes renal excretion of carnitine; tabs contain milk protein

Cefepime (Maxipime) Uses: *Comp/uncomp UTI, pneumonia, empiric febrile neutropenia, skin/soft-tissue Infxns, comp intra-Abd Infxns* Acts: 4th-gen cephalosporin; ↓ cell wall synth. *Spectrum:* Gram(+) *S. pneumoniae, S. aureus*, gram(−) *K. pneumoniae, E. coli, P. aeruginosa, & Enterobacter* sp Dose: *Adults.* 1–2 g IV q8–12h. *Peds.* 50 mg/kg q8h for febrile neutropenia; 50 mg/kg bid for skin/soft-tissue Infxns; ↓ in renal impair W/P: [B, +]; Sz risk w/ CrCl < 60 mL/min; adjust dose w/ renal Insuff CI: Cephalosporin/PCN allergy Disp: Inj 500 mg, 1, 2 g SE: Rash, pruritus, N/V/D, fever, HA, (+) Coombs test w/o hemolysis Notes: Can give IM or IV; concern over ↑ death rates not confirmed by FDA

Cefixime (Suprax) Uses: *Resp tract, skin, bone, & urinary tract Infxns* Acts: 3rd-gen cephalosporin; ↓ cell wall synth. *Spectrum: S. pneumoniae, S. pyogenes, H. influenzae, & enterobacteria* Dose: *Adults.* 400 mg PO ÷ daily-bid. *Peds.* 8 mg/kg/d PO ÷ daily-bid; ↓ w/ renal impair W/P: [B, ?] CI: Cephalosporin/PCN allergy Disp: Tabs 400 mg, 100, 200 mg chew tab, susp 100, 200 mg/5 mL SE: N/V/D, flatulence, & Abd pain Notes: ✓Renal & hepatic Fxn; use susp for otitis media

Cefotaxime (Claforan) Uses: *Infxns of lower resp tract, skin, bone & jt, urinary tract, meningitis, sepsis, PID, GC* Acts: 3rd-gen cephalosporin; ↓ cell wall synth. *Spectrum:* Most gram(−) (not *Pseudomonas*), some gram(+) cocci *S. pneumoniae, S. aureus* (penicillinase/nonpenicillinase producing), *H. influenzae* (including ampicillin-resistant), not *Enterococcus*; many PCN-resistant pneumococci Dose: *Adults. Uncomplicated Infxn:* 1 g IV/IM q12h; *Mod–severe Infxn:* 1–2 g IV/IM q 8–12 h; *Severe/septicemia:* 2 g IV/IM q4–8h; *GC urethritis, cervicitis, rectal in female:* 0.5 g IM × 1; rectal GC men 1 g IM × 1; *Peds.* 50–200 mg/kg/d IV ÷ q6–8h; ↓ w/ renal/hepatic impair W/P: [B, +] Arrhythmia w/ rapid Inj; w/ colitis CI: Cephalosporin/PCN allergy Disp: Powder for Inj 500 mg, 1, 2, 10 g, premixed Inf 20 mg/mL, 40 mg/mL SE: D, rash, pruritus, colitis, eosinophilia, ↑ transaminases

Cefotetan Uses: *Infxns of the upper & lower resp tract, skin, bone, urinary tract, Abd, & gynecologic system* Acts: 2nd-gen cephalosporin; ↓ cell wall synth *Spectrum:* Less active against gram(+) anaerobes including *B. fragilis*; gram(−), including *E. coli, Klebsiella, & Proteus* Dose: *Adults.* 1–3 g IV q12h. *Peds.* 20–40 mg/kg/dose IV ÷ q12h (6 g/d max) ↓ w/ renal impair W/P: [B, +] May ↑ bleeding risk; w/ Hx of PCN allergies, w/ renal-nephrotoxic drugs CI: Cephalosporin/PCN allergy Disp: Powder for Inj 1, 2, 10 g SE: D, rash, eosinophilia, ↑ transaminases, hypoprothrombinemia, & bleeding (d/t MTT side chain) Notes: May interfere w/ warfarin

Cefoxitin (Mefoxin) Uses: *Infxns of the upper & lower resp tract, skin, bone, urinary tract, Abd, & gynecologic system* Acts: 2nd-gen cephalosporin; ↓ cell wall synth. *Spectrum:* Good gram(−) against enteric bacilli (i.e., *E. coli, Klebsiella, & Proteus*); anaerobic: *B. fragilis* Dose: *Adults.* 1–2 g IV q6–8h. *Peds.* 80–160 mg/kg/d ÷ q4–6h (12 g/d max); ↓ w/ renal impair W/P: [B, M] CI: Cephalosporin/PCN allergy Disp: Powder for Inj 1, 2, 10 g SE: D, rash, eosinophilia, ↑ transaminases

Cefpodoxime (Vantin) Uses: *Rx resp, skin, & urinary tract Infxns* Acts: 3rd-gen cephalosporin; ↓ cell wall synth. Spectrum: *S. pneumoniae* or non-β-lactamase–producing *H. influenzae*; acute uncomplicated *N. gonorrhoeae*; some uncomplicated gram(–) (*E. coli, Klebsiella, Proteus*) Dose: *Adults.* 100–400 mg PO q12h. *Peds.* 10 mg/kg/d PO ÷ bid; ↓ in renal impair, w/ food W/P: [B, M] CI: Cephalosporin/PCN allergy Disp: Tabs 100, 200 mg; susp 50, 100 mg/5 mL SE: D, rash, HA, eosinophilia, ↑ transaminases Notes: Drug interactions w/ agents that ↑ gastric pH

Cefprozil (Cefzil) Uses: *Rx resp tract, skin, & urinary tract Infxns* Acts: 2nd-gen cephalosporin; ↓ cell wall synth. Spectrum: Active against MSSA, Streptococcus, & gram(–) bacilli (*E. coli, Klebsiella, P. mirabilis, H. influenzae, Moraxella*) Dose: *Adults.* 250–500 mg PO daily-bid. *Peds.* 7.5–15 mg/kg/d PO ÷ bid; ↓ in renal impair W/P: [B, M] CI: Cephalosporin/PCN allergy Disp: Tabs 250, 500 mg; susp 125, 250 mg/5 mL SE: D, dizziness, rash, eosinophilia, ↑ transaminases Notes: Use higher doses for otitis & pneumonia

Ceftaroline (Teflaro) Uses: *Tx skin/skin structure Infxn & CAP* Acts: Unclassified ("5th gen") cephalosporin; ↓ cell wall synthesis; Spectrum: Gram(+) Staph aureus (MSSA/MRSA), Strep pyogenes, Strep agalactiae, Strep pneumo—niae; Gram(–) *E. coli, K. pneumoniae, K. oxytoca, H. influenzae* Dose: *Adults.* 600 mg IV q12h, CrCl 30–50 mL/min: 400 mg IV q12h; CrCl 15–29 mL/min: 300 mg IV q12h; CrCl < 15 mL/min: 200 mg IV q12h; Inf over 1 h W/P: [B, ?/–] monitor for *C. difficile*-associated D CI: Cephalsporin sensitivity Disp: Inj 600 mg SE: Hypersens Rxn, D/N, rash, constipation, ↓ K+, phlebitis, ↑ LFTs

Ceftazidime (Fortaz, Tazicef) Uses: *Rx resp tract, skin, bone, urinary tract Infxns, meningitis, & septicemia* Acts: 3rd-gen cephalosporin; ↓ cell wall synth. Spectrum: *P. aeruginosa* sp, good gram(–) activity Dose: *Adults.* 500–2 g IV/IM q8–12h. *Peds.* 30–50 mg/kg/dose IV q8h 6g/d max; ↓ renal impair W/P: [B, +] PCN sensitivity CI: Cephalosporin/PCN allergy Disp: Powder for Inj 500 mg, 1, 2, 6 g SE: D, rash, eosinophilia, ↑ transaminases Notes: Use only for proven or strongly suspected Infxn to ↓ development of drug resistance

Ceftibuten (Cedax) Uses: *Rx resp tract, skin, urinary tract Infxns, & otitis media* Acts: 3rd-gen cephalosporin; ↓ cell wall synth. Spectrum: *H. influenzae* & *M. catarrhalis*; weak against *S. pneumoniae* Dose: *Adults.* 400 mg/d PO. *Peds.* 9 mg/kg/d PO; ↓ in renal impair; take on empty stomach (susp) W/P: [B, +/–] CI: Cephalosporin/PCN allergy Disp: Caps 400 mg; susp 90 mg/5 mL SE: D, rash, eosinophilia, ↑ transaminases

Ceftriaxone (Rocephin) BOX: Avoid in hyperbilirubinemic neonates or co-infusion w/ calcium-containing products Uses: *Resp tract (pneumonia), skin, bone, Abd & urinary tract Infxns, meningitis, septicemia, GC, PID, perioperative* Acts: 3rd-gen cephalosporin; ↓ cell wall synth. Spectrum: Mod gram(+); excellent β-lactamase producers Dose: *Adults.* 1–2 g IV/IM q12–24h. *Peds.* 50–100 mg/kg/d IV/IM ÷ q12–24h W/P: [B, +] CI: Cephalosporin allergy; hyperbilirubinemic neonates **Disp:** Powder for Inj 250 mg, 500 mg, 1, 2, 10 g; premixed 20, 40 mg/mL **SE:** D, rash, ↑ WBC, thrombocytosis, eosinophilia, ↑ LFTs

Cefuroxime (Ceftin [PO], Zinacef [Parenteral]) **Uses:** *Upper & lower resp tract, skin, bone, urinary tract, Abd, gynecologic Infxns* **Acts:** 2nd-gen cephalosporin; ↓ cell wall synth *Spectrum:* Staphylococci, group B streptococci, *H. influenzae, E. coli, Enterobacter, Salmonella, & Klebsiella* **Dose:** *Adults.* 750 mg–1.5 g IV q8h or 250–500 mg PO bid *Peds.* 75–150 mg/kg/d IV ÷ q8h or 20–30 mg/kg/d PO ÷ bid; ↓ w/ renal impair; take PO w/ food **W/P:** [B, +] **CI:** Cephalosporin/PCN allergy **Disp:** Tabs 250, 500 mg; susp 125, 250 mg/5 mL; powder for Inj 750 mg, 1.5, 7.5 g **SE:** D, rash, eosinophilia, ↑ LFTs **Notes:** Cefuroxime film-coated tabs & susp not bioequivalent; do not substitute on a mg/mg basis; IV crosses blood–brain barrier

Celecoxib (Celebrex) **BOX:** ↑ Risk of serious CV thrombotic events, MI, & stroke; can be fatal; ↑ risk of serious GI adverse events including bleeding, ulceration, & perforation of the stomach or intestines; can be fatal **Uses:** *OA, RA, ankylosing spondylitis, acute pain, primary dysmenorrhea, preventive in FAP* **Acts:** NSAID; ↓ COX-2 pathway **Dose:** 100–200 mg/d or bid; *FAP:* 400 mg PO bid; ↓ w/ hepatic impair; take w/ food/milk **W/P:** [C/D (3rd tri), ?] w/ Renal impair **CI:** Sulfonamide allergy, perioperative CABG **Disp:** Caps 50, 100, 200, 400 mg **SE:** See Box; GI upset, HTN, edema, renal failure, HA **Notes:** Watch for Sxs of GI bleed; no effect on plt/bleeding time; can affect drugs metabolized by P-450 pathway

Centruroides (Scorpion) Immune F(ab′)₂ (Anascorp) **Uses:** *Antivenom for scorpion envenomation w/ symptoms* **Acts:** IgG, bind/neutralize *Centruroides sculpturatus* toxin **Dose:** *Adult/Peds.* 3 vials, recons w/ 5 mL NS, combine all 3, dilute to 50 mL, Inf IV over 10 min; 1 vial q 30–60 min PRN Sx **W/P:** [C, M] hypersens, especially w/ Hx equine protein Rxn **CI:** None **Disp:** Vial **SE:** Fever, N, V, pruritus, rash, myalgias, serum sickness **Notes:** Use only w/ important symptoms (loss of muscle control, abn eye movements, slurred speech, resp distress, salivation, vomiting); may contain infectious agents

Cephalexin (Keflex, Generic) **Uses:** *Skin, bone, upper/lower resp tract (streptococcal pharyngitis), otitis media, uncomp cystitis Infxns* **Acts:** 1st-gen cephalosporin; ↓ cell wall synth. *Spectrum: Streptococcus* (including β-hemolytic), *Staphylococcus, E. coli, Proteus, & Klebsiella* **Dose:** *Adults & Peds > 15 y.* 250–1000 mg PO qid; *Peds < 15 y.* 25–100 mg/kg/d PO ÷ bid-qid; ↓ in renal impair; w/ or w/o food **W/P:** [B, +] **CI:** Cephalosporin/ PCN allergy **Disp:** Caps 250, 500 mg; susp, 125, 250 mg; susp 125, 250 mg/5 mL **SE:** D, rash, eosinophilia, gastritis, dyspepsia, ↑ LFTs, *C. difficile* colitis, vaginitis

Certolizumab Pegol (Cimzia) **BOX:** Serious Infxns (bacterial, fungal, TB, opportunistic) possible. D/C w/ severe Infxn/sepsis, test and monitor for TB w/ Tx; lymphoma/other CA possible in children/adolescents **Uses:** *Crohn Dz w/ inadequate response to conventional Tx; mod–severe RA* **Acts:** TNF-α blocker **Dose:** *Crohn: Initial:* 400 mg SQ, repeat 2 & 4 wk after; *Maint:* 400 mg SQ q4wk. *RA:*

Initial: 400 mg SQ, repeat 2 & 4 wk after; *Maint:* 200 mg SQ q other wk or 400 mg SQ q4wk. **W/P:** [B, ?] Infxn, TB, autoimmune Dz, demyelinating CNS Dz, hep B reactivation **CI:** None **Disp:** Inj, powder for reconstitution 200 mg; Inj, soln: 200 mg/mL (1 mL) **SE:** HA, N, URI, serious Infxns, TB, opportunistic Infxns, malignancies, demyelinating Dz, CHF, pancytopenia, lupus-like synd, new-onset psoriasis **Notes:** 400 mg dose 2 Inj of 200 mg each. Monitor for Infxn. Do not give live/attenuated vaccines during Rx; avoid use w/ anakinra

Cetirizine (Zyrtec, Zyrtec D) [OTC] Uses: *Allergic rhinitis & other allergic Sxs including urticaria* **Acts:** Nonsedating antihistamine; *Zyrtec D* contains decongestant **Dose:** *Adults & Children > 6 y:* 5–10 mg/d; *Zyrtec D* 5/120 mg PO bid whole **Peds 6–11 mo.** 2.5 mg daily. *12 mo–5 y:* 2.5 mg daily-bid; ↓ to q day in renal/hepatic impair **W/P:** [C, ?/–] w/ HTN, BPH, rare CNS stimulation, DM, heart Dz **CI:** Allergy to cetirizine, hydroxyzine **Disp:** Tabs 5, 10 mg; chew tabs 5, 10 mg; syrup 5 mg/5 mL; *Zyrtec D:* Tabs 5/120 mg (cetirizine/pseudoephedrine) **SE:** HA, drowsiness, xerostomia **Notes:** Can cause sedation; swallow ER tabs whole

Cetuximab (Erbitux) BOX: Severe Inf Rxns including rapid onset of airway obst (bronchospasm, stridor, hoarseness), urticaria, & ↓ BP; permanent D/C required; ↑ risk sudden death and cardiopulmonary arrest Uses: *EGFR + metastatic colorectal CA w/ or w/o irinotecan, unresectable head/neck small cell carcinoma w/ RT; monotherapy in metastatic head/neck CA* **Acts:** Human/mouse recombinant MoAb; binds EGFR, ↓ tumor cell growth **Dose:** Per protocol; load 400 mg/m² IV over 2 h; 250 mg/m² given over 1 h weekly **W/P:** [C, –] **Disp:** Inj 100 mg/50 mL **SE:** Aceneform rash, asthenia/malaise, N/V/D, Abd pain, alopecia, Inf Rxn, derm tox, interstitial lung Dz, fever, sepsis, dehydration, kidney failure, PE **Notes:** Assess tumor for EGFR before Rx; pretreatment w/ diphenhydramine; w/ mild SE ↓ rate by 50%; limit sun exposure

Charcoal, Activated (Actidose-Aqua, CharcoCaps, EZ Char, Kerr Insta-Char, Requa Activated Charcoal) Uses: *Emergency poisoning by most drugs & chemicals (see CI)* **Acts:** Adsorbent detoxicant **Dose:** Give w/ 70% sorbitol (2 mL/kg); repeated use of sorbitol not OK **Adults.** *Acute intoxication:* 25–100 g/dose. *GI dialysis:* 20–50 g q6h for 1–2 d. **Peds 1–12 y.** *Acute intoxication:* 1–2 g/kg/dose. *GI dialysis:* 5–10 g/dose q4–8h **W/P:** [C, ?] May cause V (hazardous w/ petroleum & caustic ingestions); do not mix w/ dairy **CI:** Not effective for cyanide, mineral acids, caustic alkalis, organic solvents, iron, EtOH, methanol poisoning, Li; do not use sorbitol in pts w/ fructose intolerance, intestinal obst, nonintact GI tracts **Disp:** Powder, liq, caps, tabs **SE:** Some liq dosage forms in sorbitol base (a cathartic); V/D, black stools, constipation **Notes:** Charcoal w/ sorbitol not OK in children < 1 y; monitor for ↓ K⁺ & Mg²⁺; protect airway in lethargic/comatose pts

Chlorambucil (Leukeran) BOX: Myelosuppressive, carcinogenic, teratogenic, associated w/ infertility Uses: *CLL, Hodgkin Dz*, Waldenström macroglobulinemia **Acts:** Alkylating agent (nitrogen mustard) **Dose:** (per protocol) 0.1–0.2 mg/kg/d for 3–6 wk or 0.4 mg/kg/dose q2wk; ↓ w/ renal impair **W/P:** [D, ?] Sz disorder & BM suppression; affects human fertility **CI:** Previous resistance; alkylating agent allergy; w/ live vaccines **Disp:** Tabs 2 mg **SE:** ↓ BM, CNS stimulation, N/V, drug fever, rash, secondary leukemias, alveolar dysplasia, pulm fibrosis, hepatotoxic **Notes:** Monitor LFTs, CBC, plts, serum uric acid; ↓ dose if pt has received radiation

Chlordiazepoxide (Librium, Mitran, Libritabs) [C-IV]   **Uses:** *Anxiety, tension, EtOH withdrawal*, & preop apprehension **Acts:** Benzodiazepine; antianxiety agent **Dose:** *Adults. Mild anxiety:* 5–10 mg PO tid-qid or PRN. *Severe anxiety:* 25–50 mg PO q6–8h or PRN **Peds > 6 y.** 5 mg PO q6–8h; ↓ in renal impair, elderly **W/P:** [D, ?] Resp depression, CNS impair, Hx of drug dependence; avoid in hepatic impair **CI:** Preexisting CNS depression, NAG **Disp:** Caps 5, 10, 25 mg **SE:** Drowsiness, CP, rash, fatigue, memory impair, xerostomia, Wt gain **Notes:** Erratic IM absorption

Chlorothiazide (Diuril)   **Uses:** *HTN, edema* **Acts:** Thiazide diuretic **Dose:** *Adults.* 500 mg–1 g PO daily-bid; 500–1000 mg/d IV (for edema only). *Peds > 6 mo.* 10–20 mg/kg/24 h PO ÷ bid; 4 mg/kg + daily bio IV; OK w/ food **W/P:** [C, +] **CI:** Sensitivity to thiazides/sulfonamides, anuria **Disp:** Tabs 250, 500 mg; susp 250 mg/5 mL; Inj 500 mg/vial **SE:** ↓ K+, Na+, dizziness, hyperglycemia, hyperuricemia, hyperlipidemia, photosens **Notes:** Do not use IM/SQ; take early in the day to avoid nocturia; use sunblock; monitor lytes

Chlorpheniramine (Chlor-Trimeton, Others) [OTC]   **BOX:** OTC meds w/ chlorpheniramine should not be used in peds < 2 y **Uses:** *Allergic rhinitis*, common cold **Acts:** Antihistamine **Dose:** *Adults.* 4 mg PO q4–6h or 8–12 mg PO bid of SR 24 mg/d max *Peds.* 0.35 mg/kg/24 h PO ÷ q4–6h or 0.2 mg/kg/24 h SR **W/P:** [C, ?/–] BOO; NAG; hepatic Insuff **CI:** Allergy Disp: Tabs 4 mg; SR tabs 12 mg **SE:** Anticholinergic SE & sedation common, postural ↓ BP, QT changes, extrapyramidal Rxns, photosens **Notes:** Do not cut/crush/chew ER forms; deaths in pts < 2 y associated w/ cough and cold meds [MMWR 2007;56(01):1–4]

Chlorpromazine (Thorazine)   **Uses:** *Psychotic disorders, N/V*, apprehension, intractable hiccups **Acts:** Phenothiazine antipsychotic; antiemetic **Dose:** *Adults. Psychosis:* 30–800 mg/d in 1–4 ÷ doses, start low dose, ↑ PRN; typical 200–600 mg/d; 1–2 g/d may be needed in some cases. *Severe Sxs:* 25 mg IM/IV initial; may repeat in 1–4 h; then 25–50 mg PO or PR tid. *Hiccups:* 25–50 mg PO tid-qid. *Children > 6 mo: Psychosis & N/V:* 0.5–1 mg/kg/dose PO q4–6h or IM/IV q6–8h; **W/P:** [C, ?/–] Safety in children < 6 mo not established; Szs, avoid w/ hepatic impair, BM suppression **CI:** Sensitivity w/ phenothiazines; NAG **Disp:** Tabs 10, 25, 50, 100, 200 mg; Inj 25 mg/mL **SE:** Extrapyramidal SE & sedation; α-adrenergic blocking properties; ↓ BP; ↑ QT interval **Notes:** Do not D/C abruptly

Chlorpropamide (Diabinese)   **Uses:** *Type 2 DM* **Acts:** Sulfonylurea; ↑ pancreatic insulin release; ↑ peripheral insulin sensitivity; ↓ hepatic glucose output **Dose:** 100–500 mg/d; w/ food, ↓ hepatic impair **W/P:** [C, ?/–] CrCl

< 50 mL/min; ↓ in hepatic impair **CI:** Cross-sensitivity w/ sulfonamides **Disp:** Tabs 100, 250 mg **SE:** HA, dizziness, rash, photosens, hypoglycemia, SIADH **Notes:** Avoid EtOH (disulfiram-like Rxn)

Chlorthalidone **Uses:** *HTN* **Acts:** Thiazide diuretic **Dose:** *Adults.* 25–100 mg PO daily. **Peds.** (Not approved) 0.3–2 mg/kg/dose PO 3×/wk or 1–2 mg/kg/d PO; ↓ in renal impair; OK w/ food, milk **W/P:** [B, +] **CI:** Cross-sensitivity w/ thiazides or sulfonamides; anuria **Disp:** Tabs 25, 50, 100 mg **SE:** ↓ K+, dizziness, photosens, ↑ glucose, hyperuricemia, sexual dysfunction

Chlorzoxazone (Parafon Forte DSC, Others) **Uses:** *Adjunct to rest & physical therapy Rx to relieve discomfort associated w/ acute, painful musculoskeletal conditions* **Acts:** Centrally acting skeletal muscle relaxant **Dose:** *Adults.* 500–750 mg PO tid–qid. **Peds.** 20 mg/kg/d in 3–4 ÷ doses W/P: [C, ?] Avoid EtOH & CNS depressants **CI:** Severe liver Dz **Disp:** Tabs 250, 500, 750 mg **SE:** Drowsiness, tachycardia, dizziness, hepatotox, angioedema

Cholecalciferol [Vitamin D₃] (Delta D) **Uses:** Dietary supl to Rx vit D deficiency **Acts:** ↑ intestinal Ca²⁺ absorption **Dose:** 400–1000 Int units/d PO **W/P:** [A (D doses above the RDA), +] **CI:** ↑ Ca²⁺, hypervitaminosis, allergy **Disp:** Tabs 400, 1000 Int units **SE:** Vit D tox (renal failure, HTN, psychosis) **Notes:** 1 mg cholecalciferol = 40,000 Int units vit D activity

Cholestyramine (Questran, Questran Light, Prevalite) **Uses:** *Hypercholesterolemia; hyperlipidemia; pruritus associated w/ partial biliary obst; D associated w/ excess fecal bile acids* pseudomembranous colitis, dig tox, hyperoxaluria **Acts:** Binds intestinal bile acids, forms insoluble complexes **Dose:** *Adults.* Titrate: 4 g/d-bid ↑ to max 24 g/d ÷ 1–6 doses/d. **Peds.** 240 mg/kg/d in 2–3 ÷ doses max 8 g/d **W/P:** [C, ?] Constipation, phenylketonuria, may interfere w/ other drug absorption; consider supl w/ fat-soluble vits **CI:** Complete biliary or bowel obst; w/ mycophenolate hyperlipoproteinemia types III, IV, V **Disp:** (*Questran*) 4 g cholestyramine resin/9 g powder; (*Prevalite*) w/ aspartame: 4 g resin/5.5 g powder; (*Questran Light*) 4 g resin/5 g powder **SE:** Constipation, Abd pain, bloating, HA, rash, vit K deficiency **Notes:** OD may cause GI obst; mix 4 g in 2–6 oz of noncarbonated beverage; take other meds 1–2 h before or 6 h after; ✓ lipids

Ciclesonide, Inhalation (Alvesco) **Uses:** *Asthma maint* **Acts:** Inhaled steroid **Dose:** *Adults & Peds > 12 y. On bronchodilators alone:* 80 mcg bid (320 mcg/d max). *Inhaled corticosteroids:* 80 mcg bid (640 mcg/d max). *On oral corticosteroids:* 320 mcg bid, (640 mcg/d max) **W/P:** [C, ?] **CI:** Status asthmaticus or other acute episodes of asthma, hypersens **Disp:** Inh 80, 160 mcg/actuation 60 doses **SE:** HA, nasopharyngitis, sinusitis, pharyngolaryngeal pain, URI, arthralgia, nasal congestion **Notes:** Oral *Candida* risk, rinse mouth and spit after, taper systemic steroids slowly when transferring to ciclesonide, monitor growth in pediatric pts, counsel on use of device, clean mouthpiece weekly

Ciclesonide, Nasal (Omnaris, Zettona) **Uses:** Allergic rhinitis **Acts:** Nasal corticosteroid **Dose:** *Adults/Peds > 12 y. Omnaris* 2 sprays, *Zettona* 1 spray each nostril 1 ×/d; **W/P:** [C, ?/–] w/ ketoconazole; monitor peds for growth ↓ **CI:** Component allergy **Disp:** Intranasal spray, *Omnaris* 50 mcg/spray (120 doses); *Zettona* 37 mcg/spray (60 doses) **SE:** Adrenal suppression, delayed nasal wound healing, URI, HA, ear pain, epistaxis ↑ risk viral Dz (eg, chickenpox), delayed growth in children

Ciclopirox (Ciclodan, CNL8, Loprox, Pedipirox-4 Nail Kit, Penlac)

Uses: *Tinea pedis, tinea cruris, tinea corporis, cutaneous candidiasis, tinea versicolor, tinea rubrum* **Acts:** Antifungal antibiotic; cellular depletion of essential substrates &/or ions **Dose:** *Adults & Peds > 10 y.* Massage into affected area bid. *Onychomycosis:* Apply to nails daily, w/ removal q7d **W/P:** [B, ?] **CI:** Component sensitivity **Disp:** Cream 0.77%, gel 0.77%, topical susp 0.77%, shampoo 1%, nail lacquer 8% **SE:** Pruritus, local irritation, burning **Notes:** D/C w/ irritation; avoid dressings; gel best for athlete's foot

Cidofovir (Vistide)

BOX: Renal impair is the major tox. Neutropenia possible, ✓ CBC before dose. Follow administration instructions. Possible carcinogenic, teratogenic **Uses:** *CMV retinitis w/ HIV* **Acts:** Selective inhib viral DNA synth **Dose:** *Rx:* 5 mg/kg IV over 1 h once/wk × 2 wk w/ probenecid. *Maint:* 5 mg/kg IV once/2 wk w/ probenecid (2 g PO 3 h prior to cidofovir, then 1 g PO at 2 h & 8 h after cidofovir); ↓ w/ renal impair **W/P:** [C, –] SCr > 1.5 mg/dL or CrCl < 55 mL/min or urine protein ≥ 100 mg/dL; w/ other nephrotoxic drugs **CI:** Probenecid/sulfa allergy **Disp:** Inj 75 mg/mL **SE:** Renal tox, chills, fever, HA, N/V/D, ↓ plt, ↓ WBC **Notes:** Hydrate w/ NS prior to each Inf

Cilostazol (Pletal)

BOX: PDE III inhib have ↓ survival w/ class III/IV heart failure **Uses:** *↓ Sxs of intermittent claudication* **Acts:** Phosphodiesterase III inhib; ↑ cAMP in plts & blood vessels, vasodilation & inhibit plt aggregation **Dose:** 100 mg PO bid, 1/2 h before or 2 h after breakfast & dinner **W/P:** [C, ?] ↓ dose w/ drugs that inhibit CYP3A4 & CYP2C19 (Table 10, p 319) **CI:** CHF, hemostatic disorders, active bleeding **Disp:** Tabs 50, 100 mg **SE:** HA, palpitation, D

Cimetidine (Tagamet, Tagamet HB 200 [OTC])

Uses: *Duodenal ulcer; ulcer prophylaxis in hypersecretory states (eg, trauma, burns); & GERD* **Acts:** H₂-receptor antagonist **Dose:** *Adults.* *Active ulcer:* 2400 mg/d IV cont Inf or 300 mg IV q6h; 400 mg PO bid or 800 mg hs. *Maint:* 400 mg PO hs. *GERD:* 300–600 mg PO q6h; maint 800 mg PO hs *Peds Infants.* 10–20 mg/kg/24 h PO or IV ÷ q6–12h. *Children:* 20–40 mg/kg/24 h PO or IV ÷ q6h; ↓ w/ renal Insuff & in elderly **W/P:** [B, +] Many drug interactions (P-450 system); do not use w/ clopidogrel (↓ effect) **CI:** Component sensitivity **Disp:** Tabs 200 (OTC), 300, 400, 800 mg; liq 300 mg/5 mL; Inj 300 mg/2 mL **SE:** Dizziness, HA, agitation, ↓ plt, gynecomastia **Notes:** 1 h before or 2 h after antacids; avoid EtOH

Cinacalcet (Sensipar)

Uses: *Secondary hyperparathyroidism in CRF; ↑ Ca²⁺ in parathyroid carcinoma* **Acts:** ↓ PTH by ↑ calcium-sensing receptor sensitivity **Dose:** *Secondary hyperparathyroidism:* 30 mg PO daily. *Parathyroid*

carcinoma: 30 mg PO bid; titrate q2–4wk based on calcium & PTH levels; swallow whole; take w/ food **W/P:** [C, ?/–] w/ Szs, adjust w/ CYP3A4 inhib (Table 10, p 319) **Disp:** Tabs 30, 60, 90 mg **SE:** N/V/D, myalgia, dizziness, ↓ Ca²⁺ **Notes:** Monitor Ca²⁺, PO₄⁻, PTH

Ciprofloxacin (Cipro, Cipro XR) BOX: ↑ risk of tendonitis and tendon rupture; ↑ risk w/ age > 60, transplant pts may worsen MG Sxs **Uses:** *Rx lower resp tract, sinuses, skin & skin structure, bone/joints, complex intra-Abd Infxn (w/ metronidazole), typhoid, infectious D, uncomp GC, inhal anthrax UT Infxns, including prostatitis* **Acts:** Quinolone antibiotic; ↓ DNA gyrase. *Spectrum:* Broad gram(+) & (–) aerobics; little *Streptococcus*; good *Pseudomonas, E. coli, B. fragilis, P. mirabilis, K. pneumoniae, C. jejuni,* or *Shigella* **Dose:** *Adults.* 250–750 mg PO q12h; XR 500–1000 mg PO q24h; or 200–400 mg IV q12h; ↓ in renal impair **W/P:** [C, ?/–] Children < 18 y; avoid in MG **CI:** Component sensitivity; w/ tizanidine **Disp:** Tabs 100, 250, 500, 750 mg; tabs XR 500, 1000 mg; susp 5 g/100 mL, 10 g/100 mL; Inj 200, 400 mg; premixed piggyback 200, 400 mg/100 mL **SE:** Restlessness, N/V/D, rash, ruptured tendons, ↑ LFTs, peripheral neuropathy risk **Notes:** Avoid antacids; reduce/restrict caffeine intake; interactions w/ theophylline, caffeine, sucralfate, warfarin, antacids, most tendon problems in Achilles, rare shoulder and hand

Ciprofloxacin, Ophthalmic (Ciloxan) Uses: *Rx & prevention of ocular Infxns (conjunctivitis, blepharitis, corneal abrasions)* **Acts:** Quinolone antibiotic; ↓ DNA gyrase **Dose:** 1–2 gtt in eye(s) q2h while awake for 2 d, then 1–2 gtt q1h while awake for 5 d, oint 1/2-in ribbon in eye tid × 2 d, then bid × 5 d **W/P:** [C, ?/–] **CI:** Component sensitivity **Disp:** Soln 3.5 mg/mL; oint 0.3%, 3.5 g **SE:** Local irritation

Ciprofloxacin, Otic (Cetraxal) Uses: *Otitis externa* **Acts:** Quinolone antibiotic; ↓ DNA gyrase. *Spectrum: P. aeruginosa, S. aureus* **Dose:** *Adults & Peds > 1 y.* 0.25 mL in ear(s) q 12 h × 7 d **W/P:** [C, ?/–] **CI:** Component sensitivity **Disp:** Soln 0.2% **SE:** Hypersens Rxn, ear pruritus/pain, HA, fungal superinfection

Ciprofloxacin & Dexamethasone, Otic (Ciprodex Otic) Uses: *Otitis externa, otitis media peds* **Acts:** Quinolone antibiotic; ↓ DNA gyrase; w/ steroid **Dose:** *Adults.* 4 gtt in ear(s) bid × 7 d. *Peds > 6 mo.* 4 gtt in ear(s) bid for 7 d **W/P:** [C, ?/–] **CI:** Viral ear Infxns **Disp:** Susp ciprofloxacin 0.3% & dexamethasone 1% **SE:** Ear discomfort **Notes:** OK w/ tympanostomy tubes

Ciprofloxacin & Hydrocortisone, Otic (Cipro HC Otic) Uses: *Otitis externa* **Acts:** Quinolone antibiotic; ↓ DNA gyrase; w/ steroid **Dose:** *Adults & Peds > 1 y.* 3 gtt in ear(s) bid × 7 d **W/P:** [C, ?/–] **CI:** Perforated tympanic membrane, viral Infxns of the external canal **Disp:** Susp ciprofloxacin 0.2% & hydrocortisone 1% **SE:** HA, pruritus

Cisplatin (Platinol, Platinol AQ) BOX: Anaphylactic-like Rxn, ototox, cumulative renal tox; doses > 100 mg/m² q3–4wk rarely used, do not confuse w/ carboplatin **Uses:** *Testicular, bladder, ovarian*, SCLC, NSCLC, breast, head &

neck, & penile CAs; osteosarcoma; peds brain tumors **Acts:** DNA-binding; denatures double helix; intrastrand cross-linking **Dose:** 10–20 mg/m²/d for 5 d q3wk; 50–120 mg/m² q3–4wk (per protocols); ↓ w/ renal impair **W/P:** [D, –] Cumulative renal tox may be severe; ↓ BM, hearing impair, preexisting renal Insuff **CI:** w/ Anthrax or live vaccines, platinum-containing compound allergy; w/ cidofovir **Disp:** Inj 1 mg/mL **SE:** Allergic Rxns, N/V, nephrotox (↑ w/ administration of other nephrotoxic drugs; minimize by NS Inf & mannitol diuresis), high-frequency hearing loss in 30%, peripheral "stocking glove"-type neuropathy, cardiotox (ST, T-wave changes), ↓ Mg²⁺, mild ↓ BM, hepatotox; renal impair dose-related & cumulative **Notes:** Give taxanes before platinum derivatives; ✓ Mg²⁺, lytes before & w/in 48 h after cisplatin

Citalopram (Celexa) **BOX:** Closely monitor for worsening depression or emergence of suicidality, particularly in pts < 24 y; not for peds **Uses:** *Depression* **Acts:** SSRI **Dose:** Initial 20 mg/d, may ↑ to 40 mg/d max dose; ↓ 20 mg/d max > 60 y, w/ cimetidine, or hepatic/renal Insuff **W/P:** [C, +/–] Hx of mania, Szs & pts at risk for suicide, ↑ risk serotonin synd (p 321) w/ triptans, linezolid, lithium, tramadol, St. John's wort; use w/ other SSRIs, SNRIs, or tryptophan not rec **CI:** MAOI or w/in 14 d of MAOI use **Disp:** Tabs 10, 20, 40 mg; soln 10 mg/5 mL **SE:** Somnolence, insomnia, anxiety, xerostomia, N, diaphoresis, sexual dysfunction; may ↑ Qt interval and cause arrhythmias; ↓ Na⁺/SIADH

Citric Acid/Magnesium Oxide/Sodium Picosulfate (Prepopik) **Uses:** *Colonoscopy colon prep* **Acts:** Stimulant/osmotic laxative **Dose:** Powder recons w/ 5-oz cold water; *"Split Dose":* 1st dose night before and 2nd dose morning of procedure; OR *"Day Before":* 1st dose afternoon/early eve day before and 2nd dose later evening; clear liquids after dose **W/P:** [B, ?] Fluid/electrolyte abnormalities, arrhythmias, seizures; ↑ risk in renal Insuff or w/ nephrotox drugs; mucosal ulcerations; aspiration risk **CI:** CrCl < 30 mL/min; GI perf/obstr/ileus/ gastric retention/toxic colitis/megacolon **Disp:** Packets, 16.1 g powder (10 mg sodium picosulfate, 3.5 g mag oxide, 12 g anhyd citric acid) w/ dosing cup **SE:** N, V, D, HA, Abd pain, cramping, bloating **Notes:** Meds taken 1 h w/in dose might not be absorbed

Cladribine (Leustatin) **BOX:** Dose-dependent reversible myelosuppression; neurotox, nephrotox, administer by physician w/ experience in chemotherapy regimens **Uses:** *HCL, CLL, NHLs, progressive MS* **Acts:** Induces DNA strand breakage; interferes w/ DNA repair/synth; purine nucleoside analog **Dose:** 0.09–0.1 mg/kg/d cont IV Inf for 1–7 d (per protocols); ↓ w/ renal impair **W/P:** [D, ?/–] Causes neutropenia & Infxn **CI:** Component sensitivity **Disp:** Inj 1 mg/mL **SE:** ↓ BM, T lymphocyte ↓ may be prolonged (26–34 wk), fever in 46%, tumor lysis synd, Infxns (especially lung & IV sites), rash (50%), HA, fatigue, N/V **Notes:** Consider prophylactic allopurinol; monitor CBC

Clarithromycin (Biaxin, Biaxin XL) **Uses:** *Upper/lower resp tract, skin/ skin structure Infxns, H. pylori Infxns, & Infxns caused by nontuberculosis (atypical) Mycobacterium; prevention of MAC Infxns in HIV Infxn* **Acts:** Macrolide antibiotic, ↓ protein synth. *Spectrum:* H. influenzae, M. catarrhalis, S. pneumoniae, M. pneumoniae, & H. pylori **Dose:** *Adults.* 250–500 mg PO bid or 1000 mg (2 × 500 mg XL tab)/d. *Mycobacterium:* 500 mg PO bid. *Peds > 6 mo.* 7.5 mg/kg/dose PO bid; ↓ w/ renal impair **W/P:** [C, ?] Antibiotic-associated colitis; rare ↑ QT & ventricular arrhythmias; not rec w/ PDE5 inhib **CI:** Macrolide allergy; w/ Hx jaundice w/ Biaxin; w/ cisapride, pimozide, astemizole, terfenadine, ergotamines; w/ colchicine & renal impair; w/ statins; w/ ↑ QT or ventricular arrhythmias **Disp:** Tabs 250, 500 mg; susp 125, 250 mg/5 mL; 500 mg XL tab **SE:** ↑ QT interval, causes metallic taste, N/D, Abd pain, HA, rash **Notes:** Multiple drug interactions, ↑ theophylline & carbamazepine levels; do not refrigerate susp

Clemastine Fumarate (Tavist, Dayhist, Antihist-1) [OTC] Uses: *Allergic rhinitis & Sxs of urticaria* **Acts:** Antihistamine **Dose:** *Adults & Peds > 12 y.* 1.34 mg bid–2.68 mg tid; max 8.04 mg/d, 6–12 y: 0.67–1.34 mg bid (max 4.02/d), < 6 y: 0.335–0.67 mg/d ÷ into 2–3 doses (max 1.34 mg/d), **W/P:** [B, M] BOO; Do not take w/ MAOI **CI:** NAG **Disp:** Tabs 1.34, 2.68 mg; syrup 0.67 mg/5 mL **SE:** Drowsiness, dyscoordination, epigastric distress, urinary retention **Notes:** Avoid EtOH

Clevidipine (Cleviprex) Uses: *HTN when PO not available/desirable* **Acts:** Dihydropyridine CCB, potent arterial vasodilator **Dose:** 1–2 mg/h IV then maint 4–6 mg/h; max 21 mg/h **W/P:** [C, ?] ↓ BP, syncope, rebound HTN, reflex tachycardia, CHF **CI:** Hypersens: component or formulation (soy, egg products); impaired lipid metabolism; severe aortic stenosis **Disp:** Inj 0.5 mg/mL (50 mL, 100 mL) **SE:** AF, fever, insomnia, N/V, HA, renal impair

Clindamycin (Cleocin, Cleocin-T, Others) BOX: Pseudomembranous colitis may range from mild to lifethreatening Uses: *Rx aerobic & anaerobic Infxns; topical for severe acne & Vag Infxns* **Acts:** Bacteriostatic; interferes w/ protein synth. *Spectrum:* Streptococci (eg, staphylococci, staphylococci, & gram(+) & (-) anaerobes; no activity against gram(-) aerobes **Dose:** *Adults.* PO: 150–450 mg PO q6–8h. *IV:* 300–600 mg IV q6h or 900 mg IV q8h. *Vag cream:* 1 applicator hs × 7 d. *Vag supp:* Insert 1 qhs × 3 d *Topical:* Apply 1% gel, lotion, or soln bid. *Peds Neonates.* (Avoid use; contains benzyl alcohol) 10–15 mg/kg/24 h ÷ q8–12h. *Children > 1 mo:* 10–30 mg/kg/24 h ÷ q6–8h, to a max of 1.8 g/d PO or 4.8 g/d IV. *Topical:* Apply 1%, gel, lotion, or soln bid; ↓ in severe hepatic impair **W/P:** [B, +] Can cause fatal colitis **CI:** Hx pseudomembranous colitis **Disp:** Caps 75, 150, 300 mg; susp 75 mg/5 mL; Inj 300 mg/2 mL; Vag cream 2%, topical soln 1%, gel 1%, lotion 1%, Vag supp 100 mg **SE:** D may be *C. difficile* pseudomembranous colitis, rash, ↑ LFTs **Notes:** D/C drug w/ D, evaluate for *C. difficile*

Clindamycin/Benzoyl Peroxide (Benzaclin) Uses: *Topical for acne vulgaris* **Acts:** Bacteriostatic antibiotic w/ keratolytic **Dose:** Apply bid (A.M. & P.M.) **W/P:** [C, ?] Pseudomembranous colitis reported **CI:** Component sensitivity, Hx UC/antib-assoc colitis **Disp:** Gel 10 mg (clindamycin [1%] and benzoyl peroxide [5%]) **SE:** Dry skin, pruritus, peeling, erythema, sunburn, allergic Rxns **Notes:** May bleach hair/fabrics; not approved in peds

Clindamycin/Tretinoin (Veltin Gel, Ziana) Uses: *Acne vulgaris* Acts: Lincosamide abx (↓ protein synthesis) w/ a retinoid; *Spectrum:* P. acnes Dose: *Adults (> 12 y).* Apply pea-size amount to area qd W/P: [C, ?/–] do not use w/ erythromycin products CI: Hx regional enteritis/UC/abx-assoc colitis Disp: Top Gel (clindamycin 1.2%/tretinoin 0.025%) SE: Dryness, irritation, erythema, pruritis, exfoliation, dermatitis, sunburn Notes: Avoid eyes, lips, mucous membranes

Clobazam (Onfi)[C IV] Uses: *Szs assoc w/ Lennox-Gastaut synd* Acts: Potentiates GABA neurotransmission; binds to benzodiazepine GABA$_A$ receptor Dose: *Adults & Peds ≥ 2y.* ≤ *30 kg:* 5 mg PO/d, titrate weekly 20 mg/d max; > *30 kg:* 10 mg daily, titrate weekly 40 mg/d max; divide dose bid if > 5 mg/d; may crush & mix w/ applesauce; ↓ dose in geriatric pts, CYP2C19 poor metabolizers, & mild–mod hepatic impair; ↓ dose weekly by 5–10 mg/d w/ D/C W/P: [C, ±] physical/psychological dependence & suicidal ideation/behavior; withdrawal Sxs w/ rapid dose ↓; alcohol ↑ clobazam levels by 50%; adjust w/ CYP2C19 inhib, ↓ dose of drugs metabolized by CYP2D6; may ↓ contraceptive effect Disp: Tabs 5, 10, 20 mg; susp 2.5 mg/mL SE: Somnolence, sedation, cough, V, constipation, drooling, UTI, aggression, dysarthria, fatigue, insomnia, ataxia, pyrexia, lethargy, ↑/↓ appetite

Clofarabine (Clolar) Uses: Rx relapsed/refractory ALL after at least 2 regimens in children 1–21 y Acts: Antimetabolite; ↓ ribonucleotide reductase w/ false nucleotide base-inhibiting DNA synth Dose: 52 mg/m² IV over 2 h daily × 5 d (repeat q2–6wk); per protocol; ↓ w/ renal impair W/P: [D, –] Disp: Inj 20 mg/20 mL SE: N/V/D, anemia, leukopenia, thrombocytopenia, neutropenia, Infxn, ↑ AST/ALT Notes: Monitor for tumor lysis synd & SIRS/capillary leak synd; hydrate well

Clomiphene (Clomid, Serophene) Uses: *Tx ovulatory dysfunction in women desiring PRG* Acts: Nonsteroidal ovulatory stimulant; estrogen antagonist Dose: 50 mg × 5 d; if no ovulation ↑ to 100 mg × 5 d @ 30 d later; ovulation usually 5–10 d postcourse, time coitus w/ expected ovulation time W/P: [X, ?/–] r/o PRG & ovarian enlargement CI: Hypersens, uterine bleed, PRG, ovarian cysts (not due to polycystic ovary synd), liver Dz, thyroid/adrenal dysfunction Disp: Tabs 50 mg SE: Ovarian enlargement, vasomotor flushes

Clomipramine (Anafranil) BOX: <mark>Closely monitor for suicidal ideation or unusual behavior changes</mark> Uses: *OCD*, depression, chronic pain, panic attacks Acts: TCA; ↑ synaptic serotonin & norepinephrine Dose: *Adults.* Initial 25 mg/d PO in ÷ doses; ↑ over few wk 250 mg/d max QHS. *Peds > 10 y.* Initial 25 mg/d PO in ÷ doses; ↑ over few wk 200 mg/d or 3 mg/kg/d max given hs W/P: [C, +/–] CI: w/ MAOI, linezolid, IV methylene blue (risk serotonin synd), TCA allergy, during AMI recovery Disp: Caps 25, 50, 75 mg SE: Anticholinergic (xerostomia, urinary retention, constipation), somnolence

Clonazepam (Klonopin) [C-IV] Uses: *Lennox-Gastaut synd, akinetic & myoclonic Szs, absence Szs, panic attacks*, RLS, neuralgia, parkinsonian dysarthria, bipolar disorder **Acts:** Benzodiazepine; anticonvulsant **Dose:** *Adults.* 1.5 mg/d PO in 3 ÷ doses; ↑ by 0.5–1 mg/d q3d PRN up to 20 mg/d. *Peds.* 0.01–0.03 mg/kg/24 h PO ÷ tid; ↑ to 0.1–0.2 mg/kg/24 h ÷ tid; 0.2 mg/kg/d max; avoid abrupt D/C **W/P:** [D, M] Elderly pts, resp Dz, CNS depression, severe hepatic impair, NAG **CI:** Severe liver Dz, acute NAG **Disp:** Tabs 0.5, 1, 2 mg, oral disintegrating tabs 0.125, 0.25, 0.5, 1, 2 mg **SE:** CNS (drowsiness, dizziness, ataxia, memory impair) **Notes:** Can cause retrograde amnesia; a CYP3A4 substrate

Clonidine, Epidural (Duraclon) **BOX:** Dilute 500 mcg/mL before use; not rec for OB, postpartum or periop pain management due to ↓ BP/HR **Uses:** *w/ Opiates for severe pain in cancer patients uncontrolled by opiates alone* **Acts:** Centrally acting analgesic **Dose:** 30 mcg/h by epidural Inf **W/P:** [C, ?/M] May ↓ HR/resp **CI:** See Box; clonidine sens, Inj site Infxn, anticoagulants, bleed diathesis, use above C4 dermatome **Disp:** 500 mcg/mL; dilute to 100 mcg/mL w/ NS (preservative free) **SE:** ↓ BP, dry mouth, N/V, somnolence, dizziness, confusion, sweating, confusion, hallucinations, tinnitus **Notes:** Avoid abrupt D/C; may cause nervousness, rebound ↑ BP

Clonidine, Oral (Catapres) **Uses:** *HTN*; opioid, EtOH, & tobacco withdrawal, ADHD **Acts:** Centrally α-adrenergic stimulant **Dose:** *Adults.* 0.1 mg PO tid, ↑ by 0.1 mg/d q wk (max 2.4 mg/d). *Peds.* 5–10 mcg/kg/d ÷ q8–12h (max 0.9 mg/d); ↓ in renal impair **W/P:** [C, +/–] Avoid w/ β-blocker, elderly, severe CV Dz, renal impair; use w/ agents that affect sinus node may cause severe ↓ HR **CI:** Component sensitivity **Disp:** Tabs 0.1, 0.2, 0.3 mg **SE:** drowsiness, orthostatic ↓ BP, xerostomia, constipation, ↓ HR, dizziness **Notes:** More effective for HTN if combined w/ diuretics; withdraw slowly, rebound HTN w/ abrupt D/C of doses > 0.2 mg bid; ADHD use in peds needs CV assessment before starting epidural clonidine (Duraclon) used for chronic CA pain

Clonidine, Oral, Extended-Release (Kapvay) **Uses:** *ADHD alone or as adjunct* **Acts:** Central α-adrenergic stimulant **Dose:** *Adults, Peds > 6 y.* initial 0.1 mg qhs, then adjust weekly to bid; split dose based on table; do not crush/chew; do not substitute other products as mg dosing differs; > 0.4 mg/d not rec

Kapvay Total Daily Dose	Morning Dose	Bedtime Dose
0.1 mg	N/A	0.1 mg
0.2 mg	0.1 mg	0.1 mg
0.3 mg	0.1 mg	0.2 mg
0.4 mg	0.2 mg	0.2 mg

W/P: [C, +/−] May cause severe ↓ HR and ↓ BP; w/ BP meds **CI:** Component sensitivity **Disp:** Tabs ER 0.1, 0.2 mg **SE:** Somnolence, fatigue, URI, irritability, sore throat, insomnia, nightmares, emotional disorder, constipation, congestion, ↑ temperature, dry mouth, ear pain **Notes:** On D/C, ↓ no more than 0.1 mg q3–7d

Clonidine, Transdermal (Catapres TTS) **Uses:** *HTN* **Acts:** Centrally acting α-adrenergic stimulant **Dose:** 1 patch q7d to hairless area (upper arm/torso); titrate to effect; ↓ w/ severe renal impair; **W/P:** [C, +/−] Avoid w/ β-blocker, withdraw slowly, in elderly, severe CV Dz and w/ renal impair; use w/agents that affect sinus node may cause severe ↓ HR **CI:** Component sensitivity **Disp:** TTS-1, TTS-2, TTS-3 (delivers 0.1, 0.2, 0.3 mg, respectively, of clonidine/d for 1 wk) **SE:** Drowsiness, orthostatic ↓ BP, xerostomia, constipation, ↓ HR **Notes:** Do not D/C abruptly (rebound HTN); doses > 2 TTS-3 usually not associated w/ ↑ efficacy; steady state in 2–3 d

Clopidogrel (Plavix, Generic) **Uses:** *Reduce atherosclerotic events*, administer ASAP in ECC setting w/ high-risk ST depression or T-wave inversion **Acts:** ↓ Plt aggregation **Dose:** 75 mg/d; *ECC 2010.* ACS: 300–600 mg PO loading dose, then 75 mg/d PO; full effects take several days **W/P:** [B, ?] Active bleeding; risk of bleeding from trauma & other; TTP; liver Dz; other CYP2C19 (eg, fluconazole); OK w/ ranitidine, famotidine **CI:** Coagulation disorders, active/ intracranial bleeding; CABG planned w/in 5–7 d **Disp:** Tabs 75, 300 mg **SE:** ↑ bleeding time, GI intolerance, HA, dizziness, rash, thrombocytopenia, ↓ WBC **Notes:** Plt aggregation to baseline ~ 5 d after D/C, plt transfusion to reverse acutely; clinical response highly variable

Clorazepate (Tranxene) [C-IV] **Uses:** *Acute anxiety disorders, acute EtOH withdrawal Sxs, adjunctive therapy Rx partial Szs* **Acts:** Benzodiazepine; antianxiety agent **Dose:** *Adults.* 15–60 mg/d PO single or ÷ doses. *Elderly & debilitated pts:* Initial 7.5–15 mg/d in ÷ doses. *EtOH withdrawal:* Day 1: Initial 30 mg; then 30–60 mg ÷ doses; Day 2: 45–90 mg ÷ doses; Day 3: 22.5–45 mg ÷ doses; Day 4: 15–30 mg ÷ doses. After day 4: 15–30 mg ÷ doses, then 7.5–15 mg/d ÷ doses *Peds.* 3.75–7.5 mg/dose bid to 60 mg/d max ÷ bid-tid **W/P:** [D, ?/−] Elderly; Hx depression **CI:** NAG; Not OK < 9 y of age **Disp:** Tabs 3.75, 7.5, 15 mg **SE:** CNS depressant effects (drowsiness, dizziness, ataxia, memory impair), ↓ BP **Notes:** Monitor pts w/ renal/hepatic impair (drug may accumulate); avoid abrupt D/C; may cause dependence

Clotrimazole (Lotrimin, Mycelex, Others) [OTC] **Uses:** *Candidiasis & tinea Infxns* **Acts:** Antifungal; alters cell wall permeability. *Spectrum:* Oropharyngeal candidiasis, dermatophytoses, superficial mycoses, cutaneous candidiasis, & vulvovaginal candidiasis **Dose:** *PO: Prophylaxis:* 1 troche dissolved in mouth tid *Rx:* 1 troche dissolved in mouth 5×/d for 14 d. *Vag 1% cream:* 1 applicator-full hs for 7 d. *2% cream:* 1 applicator-full hs for 3 d *Tabs:* 100 mg vaginally hs for 7 or 200 mg (2 tabs) vaginally hs for 3 d or 500-mg tabs vaginally hs once. *Topical:*

Apply bid 10–14 d **W/P:** [B (C if PO), ?] Not for systemic fungal Infxn; safety in children < 3 y not established **CI:** Component allergy **Disp:** 1% cream; soln; troche 10 mg; vag cream 1%, 2% **SE:** *Topical:* Local irritation; *PO:* N/V, ↑ LFTs **Notes:** PO prophylaxis immunosuppressed pts

Clotrimazole & Betamethasone (Lotrisone) Uses: *Fungal skin Infxns* **Acts:** Imidazole antifungal & anti-inflammatory. *Spectrum:* Tinea pedis, cruris, & corporis **Dose:** *Children ≥ 17 y.* Apply & massage into area bid for 2–4 wk **W/P:** [C, ?] Varicella Infxn **CI:** Children < 12 y **Disp:** Cream 1/0.05% 15, 45 g; lotion 1/0.05% 30 mL **SE:** Local irritation, rash **Notes:** Not for diaper dermatitis or under occlusive dressings

Clozapine (Clozaril, FazaClo, Versacloz) BOX: Myocarditis, agranulocytosis, Szs, & orthostatic ↓ BP associated w/ clozapine; ↑ mortality in elderly w/ dementia-related psychosis **Uses:** *Refractory severe schizophrenia*; childhood psychosis; obsessive-compulsive disorder (OCD); bipolar disorder **Acts:** "Atypical" TCA **Dose:** 12.5 mg daily or bid initial; ↑ to 300–450 mg/d over 2 wk; maintain lowest dose possible; do not D/C abruptly **W/P:** [B, +/–] Monitor for psychosis & cholinergic rebound **CI:** Uncontrolled epilepsy; comatose state; WBC < 3500 cells/mm³ and ANC < 2000 cells/mm³ before Rx or < 3000 cells/mm³ during Rx, Eos > 4000/mm³ **Disp:** Orally disintegrating tabs (ODTs) 12.5, 25, 100, 150, 200 mg; tabs 25, 100 mg; susp 50 mg/mL **SE:** Sialorrhea, tachycardia, drowsiness, ↑ Wt, constipation, incontinence, rash, Szs, CNS stimulation, hyperglycemia **Notes:** Avoid activities where sudden loss of consciousness could cause harm; benign temperature ↑ may occur during the 1st 3 wk of Rx, weekly CBC mandatory 1st 6 mo, then q other wk

Cocaine [C-II] Uses: *Topical anesthetic for mucous membranes* **Acts:** Narcotic analgesic, local vasoconstrictor **Dose:** Lowest topical amount that provides relief; 3 mg/kg max **W/P:** [C, ?] PRG, ocular anesthesia **Disp:** Topical soln & viscous preparations 4–10%; powder **SE:** CNS stimulation, nervousness, loss of taste/smell, chronic rhinitis, CV tox, abuse potential **Notes:** Use only on PO, laryngeal, & nasal mucosa; do not use on extensive areas of broken skin

Codeine [C-II] Uses: *Mild–mod pain; symptomatic relief of cough* **Acts:** Narcotic analgesic; ↓ cough reflex **Dose:** *Adults. Analgesic:* 15–60 mg PO or IM q4h PRN; 360 mg max/24 h. *Antitussive:* 10–20 mg PO q4h PRN; max 120 mg/d. *Peds. Analgesic:* 0.5–1 mg/kg/dose PO or q4–6h PRN. *Antitussive:* 1–1.5 mg/kg/24 h PO ÷ q4h; max 30 mg/24 h; ↓ in renal/hepatic impair **W/P:** [C (D if prolonged use or high dose at term), +] CNS depression, Hx drug abuse, severe hepatic impair **CI:** Component sensitivity **Disp:** Tabs 15, 30, 60 mg; soln 30 mg/5 mL; Inj 15, 30 mg **SE:** Drowsiness, constipation, ↓ BP **Notes:** Usually combined w/ APAP for pain or w/ agents (eg, terpin hydrate) as an antitussive; 120 mg IM = 10 mg IM morphine

Colchicine (Colcrys) Uses: *Acute gouty arthritis & prevention of recurrences; familial Mediterranean fever*; primary biliary cirrhosis **Acts:** ↓ migration of leukocytes; ↓ leukocyte lactic acid production **Dose:** *Acute gout*: 1.2 mg load, 0.6 mg 1 h later, then prophylactic 0.6 mg/qd-bid *FMF: Adult* 1.2–2.4 mg/d *Peds > 4 y see label* **W/P:** [C, +] w/ P-glycoprotein or CYP3A4 inhib in pt w/ renal or hepatic impair, ↓ dose or avoid in elderly or w/ indinavir **CI:** Serious renal, GI, hepatic, or cardiac disorders; blood dyscrasias **Disp:** Tabs 0.6 mg **SE:** N/V/D, Abd pain, BM suppression, hepatotox

Colesevelam (Welchol) Uses: *↓ LDL & total cholesterol alone or in combo w/ an HMG-CoA reductase inhib, improve glycemic control in type 2 DM* **Acts:** Bile acid sequestrant **Dose:** 3 tabs PO bid or 6 tabs daily w/ meals **W/P:** [B, ?] Severe GI motility disorders; in pts w/ triglycerides > 300 mg/dL (may ↑ levels); use not established in peds **CI:** Bowel obst, serum triglycerides > 500; Hx hypertriglyceridemia-pancreatitis **Disp:** Tabs 625 mg; oral susp 1.875, 3.75 g **SE:** Constipation, dyspepsia, myalgia, weakness **Notes:** May ↓ absorption of fat-soluble vits

Colestipol (Colestid) Uses: *Adjunct to ↓ serum cholesterol in primary hypercholesterolemia, relieve pruritus associated w/ ↑ bile acids* **Acts:** Binds intestinal bile acids to form insoluble complex **Dose:** *Granules:* 5–30 g/d ÷ 2–4 doses; tabs: 2–16 g/d ÷ daily-bid **W/P:** [C, ?] Avoid w/ high triglycerides, GI dysfunction **CI:** Bowel obst **Disp:** Tabs 1 g; granules 5 g/pack or scoop **SE:** Constipation, Abd pain, bloating, HA, GI irritation & bleeding **Notes:** Do not use dry powder; mix w/ beverages, cereals, etc; may ↓ absorption of other meds and fat-soluble vits

Conivaptan HCL (Vaprisol) Uses: *Euvolemic & hypervolemic hyponatremia* **Acts:** Dual arginine vasopressin V_{1A}/V_2 receptor antagonist **Dose:** 20 mg IV × 1 over 30 min, then 20 mg cont IV Inf over 24 h; 20 mg/d cont IV Inf for 1–3 more d; may ↑ to 40 mg/d if Na^+ not responding; 4 d max use; use large vein, change site q24h **W/P:** [C, ?/–] Rapid ↑ Na^+ (> 12 mEq/L/24 h) may cause osmotic demyelination synd; impaired renal/hepatic Fxn; may ↑ digoxin levels; CYP3A4 inhib (Table 10, p 319) **CI:** Hypovolemic hyponatremia; w/ CYP3A4 inhib; anuria **Disp:** Inj 20 mg/100 mL **SE:** Inf site Rxns, HA, N/V/D, constipation, ↓ K^+, orthostatic ↓ BP, thirst, dry mouth, pyrexia, pollakiuria, polyuria, Infxn **Notes:** Monitor Na^+, vol and neurologic status; D/C w/ very rapid ↑ Na^+; mix only w/ 5% dextrose

Copper IUD Contraceptive (ParaGard T 380A) Uses: *Contraception, long-term (up to 10 y)* **Acts:** ?, interfere w/ sperm survival/transport **Dose:** Insert any time during menstrual cycle; replace at 10 y max **W/P:** [C, ?] Remove w/ intrauterine PRG, increased risk of comps w/ PRG and device in place **CI:** Acute PID or in high-risk behavior, postpartum endometritis, cervicitis **Disp:** 309 mg IUD **SE:** PRG, ectopic PRG, pelvic Infxn w/ or w/o immunocompromised, embedment, perforation, expulsion, Wilson Dz, fainting w/ insert, Vag bleeding, expulsion **Notes:** Counsel pt does not protect against STD/HIV; see PI for detailed instructions; 99% effective

Cortisone, Systemic and Topical See Steroids pp 259 & 260, and Tables 2 & 3 pp 301 & 302

Crizotinib (Xalkori) Uses: *Locally advanced/metastatic NSCLC w/ anaplastic lymphoma kinase (ALK)-positive* **Acts:** TKI **Dose:** *Adult.* 250 mg PO bid; swallow whole; see label for tox adjustments **W/P:** [D, ?/–] w/ Hepatic impair & CrCl < 30 mL/min; may cause ↑ QT (monitor); ↓ dose w/ CYP3A substrates; avoid w/ strong CYP3A inducers/inhib & CYP3A substrates w/ narrow therapeutic index **Disp:** Caps 200, 250 mg **SE:** N/V/D, constipation, Abd pain, stomatitis, edema, vision disorder, hepatotox, pneumonitis, pneumonia, PE, neutropenia, thrombocytopenia, lymphopenia, HA, dizziness, fatigue, cough, dyspnea, URI, fever, arthralgia, ↓ appetite, rash, neuropathy **Notes:** ✓ CBC & LFTs monthly

Crofelemer (Fulyzaq) Uses: *Noninfectious diarrhea w/ HIV on anti-retrovirals* **Acts:** Inhibits cAMP-stimulated CF transmembrane conductance regulator Cl⁻ channel and Ca activated Cl⁻ channels of intestinal epithelial cells, controls Cl⁻ and fluid secretion **Dose:** 125 mg bid **W/P:** [C, –] **CI:** None **Disp:** Tab 125 mg DR **SE:** Flatulence, cough, bronchitis, URI, ↑ bili **Notes:** r/o infectious D before; do not crush/chew tabs; minimal absorb, drug interact unlikely

Cromolyn Sodium (Intal, NasalCrom, Opticrom, Others) Uses: *Adjunct to the Rx of asthma; prevent exercise-induced asthma; allergic rhinitis; ophthal allergic manifestations; food allergy, systemic mastocytosis, IBD* **Acts:** Antiasthmatic; mast cell stabilizer **Dose:** *Adults & Children > 12 y.* **Inh:** 20 mg (as powder in caps) inhaled qid *PO:* 200 mg qid 15–20 min ac, up to 400 mg qid. *Nasal instillation.* Spray once in each nostril 2–6×/d. *Ophthal:* 1–2 gtt in each eye 4–6 × d. *Peds. Inh:* 2 puffs qid of metered-dose inhaler. *PO: Infants < 2 y:* (not OK) 20 mg/kg/d in 4 ÷ doses. *2–12 y:* 100 mg qid ac **W/P:** [B, ?] w/ Renal/hepatic impair **CI:** Acute asthmatic attacks **Disp:** PO conc 100 mg/5 mL; soln for nebulizer 20 mg/2 mL; nasal soln 40 mg/mL; ophthal soln 4% **SE:** Unpleasant taste, hoarseness, coughing **Notes:** No benefit in acute Rx; 2–4 wk for maximal effect in perennial allergic disorders

Cyanocobalamin [Vitamin B₁₂] (Nascobal) Uses: *Pernicious anemia & other vit B₁₂ deficiency states; ↑ requirements d/t PRG; thyrotoxicosis; liver or kidney Dz* **Acts:** Dietary vit B₁₂ supl **Dose:** *Adults.* 30 mcg/d × 5–10 d intranasal: 500 mcg once/wk for pts in remission, 100 mcg IM or SQ daily for 5–10 d, then 100 mcg IM 2×/wk for 1 mo, then 100 mcg IM monthly. *Peds.* Use 0.2 mcg/kg × 2 d test dose; if OK 30–50 mcg/d for 2 or more wk (total 1000 mcg) then maint: 100 mcg/mo. **W/P:** [A (C if dose exceeds RDA), +] **CI:** Allergy to cobalt; hereditary optic nerve atrophy; Leber Dz **Disp:** Tabs 50, 100, 250, 500, 1000, 2500, 5000 mcg; Inj 1000 mcg/mL; intranasal (Nascobal) gel 500 mcg/0.1 mL **SE:** Itching, D, HA, anxiety **Notes:** PO absorption erratic; OK for use w/ hyperalimentation

Cyclobenzaprine (Flexeril) Uses: *Relief of muscle spasm* **Acts:** Centrally acting skeletal muscle relaxant; reduces tonic somatic motor activity **Dose:** 5–10 mg PO bid-qid (2–3 wk max) **W/P:** [B, ?] Shares the toxic potential of the TCAs; urinary hesitancy, NAG **CI:** Do not use concomitantly or w/in 14 d of MAOIs;

hyperthyroidism; heart failure; arrhythmias **Disp:** Tabs 5, 10 mg **SE:** Sedation & anticholinergic effects **Notes:** May inhibit mental alertness or physical coordination

Cyclobenzaprine, Extended-Release (Amrix) **Uses:** *Muscle spasm* **Acts:** ? Centrally acting long-term muscle relaxant **Dose:** 15–30 mg PO daily 2–3 wk; 30 mg/d max **W/P:** [B, ?/–] w/ Urinary retention, NAG, w/ EtOH/CNS depressant **CI:** MAOI w/in 14 d, elderly, arrhythmias, heart block, CHF, MI recovery phase, ↑ thyroid **Disp:** Caps ER 15, 30 mg **SE:** Dry mouth, drowsiness, dizziness, HA, N, blurred vision, dysgeusia **Notes:** Avoid abrupt D/C w/ long-term use

Cyclopentolate, Ophthalmic (Cyclogyl, Cylate) **Uses:** *Cycloplegia, mydriasis* **Acts:** Cycloplegic mydriatic, anticholinergic inhibits iris sphincter and ciliary body **Dose:** *Adults.* 1 gtt in eye 40–50 min preprocedure, may repeat × 1 in 5–10 min *Peds.* As adult, children 0.5%; infants use 0.5% **W/P:** [C (may cause late-term fetal anoxia/↓ HR), +/–], w/ premature infants, HTN, Down synd, elderly, CI: NAG **Disp:** Ophthal soln 0.5, 1, 2% **SE:** Tearing, HA, irritation, eye pain, photophobia, arrhythmia, tremor, ↑ IOP, confusion **Notes:** Compress lacrimal sac for several min after dose; heavily pigmented irises may require ↑ strength; peak 25–75 min, cycloplegia 6–24 h, mydriasis up to 24 h; 2% soln may result in psychotic Rxns and behavioral disturbances in peds

Cyclopentolate With Phenylephrine (Cyclomydril) **Uses:** *Mydriasis greater than cyclopentolate alone* **Acts:** Cycloplegic mydriatic, α-adrenergic agonist w/ anticholinergic to inhibit iris sphincter **Dose:** 1 gtt in eye q 5–10 min (max 3 doses) 40–50 min preprocedure **W/P:** [C (may cause late-term fetal anoxia/↓ HR), +/–] HTN, w/ elderly w/ CAD **CI:** NAG **Disp:** Ophthal soln cyclopentolate 0.2%/phenylephrine 1% (2, 5 mL) **SE:** Tearing, HA, irritation, eye pain, photophobia, arrhythmia, tremor **Notes:** Compress lacrimal sac for several min after dose; heavily pigmented irises may require ↑ strength; peak 25–75 min, cycloplegia 6–24 h, mydriasis up to 24 h

Cyclophosphamide (Cytoxan, Neosar) **Uses:** *Hodgkin Dz & NHLs; multiple myeloma; small cell lung, breast, & ovarian CAs; mycosis fungoides; neuroblastoma; retinoblastoma; acute leukemias; allogeneic & ABMT in high doses; severe rheumatologic disorders (SLE, JRA, Wegner granulomatosis)* **Acts:** Alkylating agent **Dose:** *Adults.* (per protocol) 500–1500 mg/m^2 daily; single dose at 2- to 4-wk intervals; 1.8 g/m^2–160 mg/kg (or at 12 g/m^2 in 75-kg individual) in the BMT setting (per protocols). *Peds. SLE:* 500 mg–1g/m^2 q mo. *JRA:* 10 mg/kg q 2 wk; ↓ w/ renal impair **W/P:** [D, –] w/ BM suppression, hepatic Insuff **CI:** Component sensitivity **Disp:** Tabs 25, 50 mg; Inj 500 mg, 1 g, 2 g **SE:** ↓ BM; hemorrhagic cystitis, SIADH, alopecia, anorexia; N/V; hepatotox; rare interstitial pneumonitis; irreversible testicular atrophy possible; cardiotox rare; 2nd malignancies (bladder, ALL), risk 3.5% at 8 y, 10.7% at 12 y **Notes:** Hemorrhagic cystitis prophylaxis: cont bladder irrigation & MESNA uroprotection; encourage hydration, long-term bladder CA screening

Cyclosporine (Gengraf, Neoral, Sandimmune) BOX: ↑ risk neoplasm, ↑ risk skin malignancies, ↑ risk HTN and nephrotox Uses: *Organ rejection in kidney, liver, heart, & BMT w/ steroids; RA; psoriasis* Acts: Immunosuppressant; reversible inhibition of immunocompetent lymphocytes Dose: *Adults & Peds. PO:* 15 mg/kg/12h pretransplant; after 2 wk, taper by 5 mg/wk to 5–10 mg/kg/d. *IV:* If NPO, give 1/3 PO dose IV; ↓ in renal/hepatic impair W/P: [C, –] Dose-related risk of nephrotox/hepatotox/serious fatal Infxns; live, attenuated vaccines may be less effective; may induce fatal malignancy; many drug interactions; ↑ risk of Infxns after D/C CI: Renal impair; uncontrolled HTN; w/ lovastatin, simvastatin Disp: Caps 25, 100 mg; PO soln 100 mg/mL; Inj 50 mg/mL SE: May ↑ BUN & Cr & mimic transplant rejection; HTN; HA; hirsutism Notes: Administer in glass container; *Neoral & Sandimmune* not interchangeable; monitor BP, Cr, CBC, LFTs, interaction w/ St. John's wort; Levels: *Trough:* Just before next dose: *Therapeutic:* Variable 150–300 ng/mL RIA

Cyclosporine, Ophthalmic (Restasis) Uses: *↑ Tear production suppressed d/t ocular inflammation* Acts: Immune modulator, anti-inflammatory Dose: 1 gtt bid each eye 12 h apart; OK w/ artificial tears, allow 15 min between W/P: [C, –] CI: Ocular Infxn, component allergy Disp: Single-use vial 0.05% SE: Ocular burning/hyperemia Notes: Mix vial well

Cyproheptadine (Periactin) Uses: *Allergic Rxns; itching* Acts: Phenothiazine antihistamine; serotonin antagonist Dose: *Adults.* 4–20 mg PO ÷ q8h; max 0.5 mg/kg/d. *Peds 2–6 y.* 2 mg bid-tid (max 12 mg/24 h). *7–14 y:* 4 mg bid-tid; ↓ in hepatic impair W/P: [B, ?] Elderly, CV Dz, asthma, thyroid Dz, BPH CI: Neonates or < 2 y; NAG; BOO; acute asthma; GI obst; w/ MAOI Disp: Tabs 4 mg; syrup 2 mg/5 mL SE: Anticholinergic, drowsiness Notes: May stimulate appetite

Cytarabine [ARA-C] (Cytosar-U) BOX: Administration by experienced physician in properly equipped facility; potent myelosuppressive agent Uses: *Acute leukemias, CML, NHL; IT for leukemic meningitis or prophylaxis* Acts: Antimetabolite; interferes w/ DNA synth Dose: 100–150 mg/m²/d for 5–10 d (low dose); 3 g/m² q12h for 6–12 doses (high dose); 1 mg/kg 1–2/wk (SQ maint); 5–75 mg/m² up to 3/wk IT (per protocols); ↓ in renal/hepatic impair W/P: [D, ?] In elderly, w/ marked BM suppression, ↓ dosage by ↓ the number of days of administration CI: Component sensitivity Disp: Inj 100, 500 mg, 1, 2 g, also 20, 100 mg/mL SE: ↓ BM, N/V/D, stomatitis, flu-like synd, rash on palms/soles, hepatic/cerebellar dysfunction w/ high doses, noncardiogenic pulm edema, neuropathy, fever Notes: Little use in solid tumors; high-dose tox limited by corticosteroid ophthal soln

Cytarabine Liposome (DepoCyt) BOX: Can cause chemical arachnoiditis (N/V/HA, fever) ↓ severity w/ dexamethasone. Administer by experienced physician in properly equipped facility Uses: *Lymphomatous meningitis* Acts: Antimetabolite; interferes w/ DNA synth Dose: 50 mg IT q14d for 5 doses, then 50 mg IT q28d × 4 doses; use dexamethasone prophylaxis W/P: [D, ?] May cause neurotox; blockage to CSF flow may ↑ the risk of neurotox; use in peds not established **CI:** Active meningeal Infxn **Disp:** IT Inj 50 mg/5 mL **SE:** Neck pain/rigidity, HA, confusion, somnolence, fever, back pain, N/V, edema, neutropenia, ↓ plt, anemia **Notes:** Cytarabine liposomes are similar in microscopic appearance to WBCs; caution in interpreting CSF studies

Cytomegalovirus Immune Globulin [CMV-IG IV] (CytoGam) **Uses:** *Prophylaxis/attenuation CMV Dz w/ transplantation* **Acts:** IgG antibodies to CMV **Dose:** 150 mg/kg/dose w/in 72 h of transplant and wk 2, 4, 6, 8: 100–150 mg/kg/dose wk 12, 16 posttransplant; 50–100 mg/kg/dose **W/P:** [C, ?] Anaphylactic Rxns; renal dysfunction **CI:** Allergy to immunoglobulins; IgA deficiency **Disp:** Inj 50 mg/mL **SE:** Flushing, N/V, muscle cramps, wheezing, HA, fever, non-cardiogenic pulm edema, renal Insuff, aseptic meningitis **Notes:** IV only in separate line; do not shake

Dabigatran (Pradaxa) **BOX:** Pradaxa D/C w/o adequate anticoagulation ↑ stroke risk **Uses:** *↓ Risk stroke/systemic embolism w/ nonvalvular afib* **Acts:** Thrombin inhibitor **Dose:** CrCl > 30 mL/min: 150 mg PO bid; CrCl 15–30 mL/min: 75 mg PO bid; do not chew/break/open caps **W/P:** [C, ?/–] Avoid w/ P-glycoprotein inducers (i.e., rifampin) **CI:** Active bleeding, prosthetic valve **Disp:** Caps 75, 150 mg **SE:** Bleeding, gastritis, dyspepsia **Notes:** See label to convert between anticoagulants; caps sensitive to humidity (30-d after opening bottle); routine coags not needed; ↑ PTT/INR/TT; w/ nl TT, no drug activity; ½ life 12–17 h

Dacarbazine (DTIC) **BOX:** Causes hematopoietic depression, hepatic necrosis, may be carcinogenic, teratogenic **Uses:** *Melanoma, Hodgkin Dz, sarcoma* **Acts:** Alkylating agent; antimetabolite as a purine precursor; ↓ protein synth, RNA, & especially DNA **Dose:** 2–4.5 mg/kg/d for 10 consecutive d or 250 mg/m²/d for 5 d (per protocols); ↓ in renal impair **W/P:** [C, –] In BM suppression; renal/hepatic impair **CI:** Component sensitivity **Disp:** Inj 100, 200 mg **SE:** ↓ BM, N/V, hepatotox, flu-like synd, ↓ BP, photosensa, alopecia, facial flushing, facial paresthesias, urticaria, phlebitis at Inj site **Notes:** Avoid extrav, ✓ CBC, plt

Daclizumab (Zenapax) **BOX:** Administer under skilled supervision in properly equipped facility **Uses:** *Prevent acute organ rejection* **Acts:** IL-2 receptor antagonist **Dose:** 1 mg/kg/dose IV; 1st dose pretransplant, then 1 mg/kg q14d × 4 doses **W/P:** [C, ?] **CI:** Component sensitivity **Disp:** Inj 5 mg/mL **SE:** Hyperglycemia, edema, HTN, ↓ BP, constipation, HA, dizziness, anxiety, nephrotox, pulm edema, pain, anaphylaxis/hypersens **Notes:** Administer w/in 4 h of prep

Dactinomycin (Cosmegen) **BOX:** Administer under skilled supervision in properly equipped facility; powder and soln toxic, corrosive, mutagenic, carcinogenic, and teratogenic; avoid exposure and use precautions **Uses:** *Choriocarcinoma, Wilms tumor, Kaposi and Ewing sarcomas, rhabdomyosarcoma, uterine and testicular CA* **Acts:** DNA-intercalating agent **Dose:** *Adults:* 15 mcg/kg/d for 5 d q3–6 wk or 400–600 mcg/m² for 5d q3–6 wk **Peds.** Sarcoma (per protocols); ↓ in renal impair **W/P:** [D, ?] **CI:** Concurrent/recent chickenpox or herpes zoster; infants < 6 mo **Disp:** Inj 0.5 mg **SE:** Myelo-/immunosuppression, severe N/V/D, alopecia, acne, hyperpigmentation, radiation recall phenomenon, tissue damage w/ extrav, hepatotox **Notes:** Classified as antibiotic but not used as antimicrobial

Dalfampridine (Ampyra) Uses: *Improve walking w/ MS* **Acts:** K^+ channel blocker **Dose:** 10 mg PO q12h max dose/d 20 mg **W/P:** [C, ?/–] Not w/ other 4-aminopyridines **CI:** Hx Sz; w/ CrCl ≤ 50 mL/min **Disp:** Tab ER 10 mg **SE:** HA, N, constipation, dyspepsia, dizziness, insomnia, UTI, nasopharyngitis, back pain, pharyngolaryngeal pain, asthenia, balance disorder, MS relapse, paresthesia, Sz **Notes:** Do not cut/chew/crush/dissolve tab

Dalteparin (Fragmin) **BOX:** ↑ Risk of spinal/epidural hematoma w/ LP Uses: *Unstable angina, non–Q-wave MI, prevent & Rx DVT following surgery (hip, Abd), pt w/ restricted mobility, extended therapy Rx for PE DVT in CA pt* **Acts:** LMW heparin **Dose:** *Angina/MI:* 120 units/kg (max 10,000 units) SQ q12h w/ ASA. *DVT prophylaxis:* 2500–5000 units SQ 1–2 h preop, then daily for 5–10 d. *Systemic anticoagulation:* 200 units/kg/d SQ or 100 units/kg bid SQ. *CA:* 200 Int units/kg (max 18,000 Int units) SQ q24h × 30 d, mo 2–6 150 Int units/kg SQ q24h (max 18,000 Int units) **W/P:** [B, ?] In renal/hepatic impair, active hemorrhage, cerebrovascular Dz, cerebral aneurysm, severe HTN **CI:** HIT; pork product allergy; w/ mifepristone **Disp:** Inj multiple ranging from 2500 units (16 mg/0.2 mL) to 25,000 units/mL (3.8 mL) prefilled vials **SE:** Bleeding, pain at site, ↓ plt **Notes:** Predictable effects eliminates lab monitoring; not for IM/IV use

Dantrolene (Dantrium, Revonto) **BOX:** Hepatotox reported; D/C after 45 d if no benefit observed Uses: *Rx spasticity d/t upper motor neuron disorders (eg, spinal cord injuries, stroke, CP, MS); malignant hyperthermia* **Acts:** Skeletal muscle relaxant **Dose:** *Adults. Spasticity:* 25 mg PO daily; ↑ 25 mg to effect to 100 mg PO q8h (400 mg/d max). *Peds.* 0.5 mg/kg/dose/d; ↑ by 0.5 mg/kg dose tid to 2 mg/kg/dose tid (max 400 mg/d) *Adults & Peds. Malignant hyperthermia: Rx:* Cont rapid IV, start 1 mg/kg until Sxs subside or 10 mg/kg is reached. *Postcrisis follow-up:* 4–8 mg/kg/d in 3–4 ÷ doses for 1–3 d to prevent recurrence **W/P:** [C, ?] Impaired cardiac/pulm/hepatic Fxn **CI:** Active hepatic Dz; where spasticity needed to maintain posture or balance **Disp:** Caps 25, 50, 100 mg; powder for Inj 20 mg/vial **SE:** Hepatotox, ↑ LFTs, drowsiness, dizziness, rash, muscle weakness, D/N/V, pleural effusion w/ pericarditis, blurred vision, hep, photosens **Notes:** Monitor LFTs; avoid sunlight/ EtOH/CNS depressants

Dapsone, Oral Uses: *Rx & prevent PCP; toxoplasmosis prophylaxis; leprosy* **Acts:** Unknown; bactericidal **Dose:** *Adults. PCP prophylaxis* 50–100 mg/d PO; Rx PCP 100 mg/d PO w/ TMP 15–20 mg/kg/d for 21 d. *Peds. PCP prophylaxis alternated dose:* (> 1 mo) 4 mg/kg/dose once/wk (max 200 mg); Rx *PCP:* 1–2 mg/kg/24 h PO daily; max 100 mg/d **W/P:** [C, +] G6PD deficiency; severe anemia **CI:** Component sensitivity **Disp:** Tabs 25, 100 mg **SE:** Hemolysis, methemoglobinemia, agranulocytosis, rash, cholestatic jaundice

Notes: Absorption ↑ by an acidic environment; for leprosy, combine w/ rifampin & other agents

Dapsone, Topical (Aczone) Uses: *Topical for acne vulgaris* **Acts:** Unknown; bactericidal **Dose:** Apply pea-size amount and rub into areas bid; wash hands after **W/P:** [C, +] G6PD deficiency; severe anemia **CI:** Component sensitivity **Disp:** 5% gel **SE:** Skin oiliness/peeling, dryness erythema **Notes:** Not for oral, ophthal, or intravag use; check G6PD levels before use; follow CBC if G6PD deficient

Daptomycin (Cubicin) Uses: *Complicated skin/skin structure Infxns d/t gram(+) organisms* *S. aureus*, bacteremia, MRSA endocarditis **Acts:** Cyclic lipopeptide; rapid membrane depolarization & bacterial death. *Spectrum: S. aureus* (including MRSA), *S. pyogenes, S. agalactiae, S. dysgalactiae* subsp *Equisimilis*, & *E. faecalis* (vancomycin-susceptible strains only) **Dose:** *Skin:* 4 mg/kg IV daily × 7–14 d (over 2 min); *Bacteremia & Endocarditis:* 6 mg/kg q24h; ↓ w/ CrCl < 30 mL/min or dialysis: q48h **W/P:** [B, ?] w/ HMG-CoA inhib **Disp:** Inj 500 mg/10 mL **SE:** Anemia, constipation, N/V/D, HA, rash, site Rxn, muscle pain/weakness, edema, cellulitis, hypo-/hyperglycemia, ↑ alkaline phosphatase, cough, back pain, Abd pain, ↓ K⁺, anxiety, CP, sore throat, cardiac failure, confusion, *Candida* Infxns **Notes:** ✓ CPK baseline & weekly; consider D/C HMG-CoA reductase inhib to ↓ myopathy risk; not for Rx PNA

Darbepoetin Alfa (Aranesp) BOX: Associated w/ ↑ CV, thromboembolic events and/or mortality; D/C if Hgb > 12 g/dL; may increase tumor progression and death in CA pts **Uses:** *Anemia associated w/ CRF*, anemia in nonmyeloid malignancy w/ concurrent chemotherapy **Acts:** ↑ Erythropoiesis, recombinant erythropoietin variant **Dose:** 0.45 mcg/kg single IV or SQ qwk; titrate, do not exceed target Hgb of 12 g/dL; use lowest doses possible, see PI to convert from *Epogen* **W/P:** [C, ?] May ↑ risk of CV &/or neurologic SE in renal failure; HTN; w/ Hx Szs **CI:** Uncontrolled HTN, component allergy **Disp:** 25, 40, 60, 100, 200, 300 mcg/mL, 150 mcg/0.75 mL in polysorbate or albumin excipient **SE:** May ↑ cardiac risk, CP, hypo-/hypertension, N/V/D, myalgia, arthralgia, dizziness, anemia, fatigue, fever, ↑ risk Infxn **Notes:** Longer half-life than *Epogen*; weekly CBC until stable

Darifenacin (Enablex) Uses: *OAB* Urinary antispasmodic **Acts:** Muscarinic receptor antagonist **Dose:** 7.5 mg/d PO; 15 mg/d max (7.5 mg/d w/ mod hepatic impair or w/ CYP3A4 inhib); w/ drugs metabolized by CYP2D (Table 10, p 319); swallow whole **W/P:** [C, ?/–] w/ Hepatic impair **CI:** Urinary/gastric retention, uncontrolled NAG, paralytic ileus **Disp:** Tabs ER 7.5, 15 mg **SE:** Xerostomia/ eyes, constipation, dyspepsia, Abd pain, retention, abnormal vision, dizziness, asthenia

Darunavir (Prezista) Uses: *Rx HIV w/ resistance to multiple protease inhib* **Acts:** HIV-1 protease inhib **Dose:** *Adults.* Rx-naïve and w/o darunavir resistance substitutions: 800 mg w/ ritonavir 100 mg qd. Rx experienced w/ 1 darunavir resistance: 600 mg w/ ritonavir 100 mg BID w/ food. *Peds 6–18 y and*

> **20 kg.** Dose based on body weight (see label); do not exceed the Rx experienced adult dose. Do not use qd dosing in peds; w/ food **W/P:** [C, ?/–] Hx sulfa allergy, CYP3A4 substrate, changes levels of many meds (↑ amiodarone, ↑ dihydropyridine, ↑ HMG-CoA reductase inhib [statins], ↓ SSRIs, ↓ methadone); do not use w/ salmeterol, colchicine (w/ renal impair; do not use w/ severe hepatic impair); adjust dose w/ bosentan, tadalafil for PAH **CI:** w/ Astemizole, rifampin, St. John's Wort, terfenadine, ergotamines, lovastatin, simvastatin, methylergonovine, pimozide, midazolam, triazolam, alpha 1-adrenoreceptor antagonist (alfuzosin), PDE5 inhibitors (eg, sildenafil) **Supplied:** Tabs 75, 150, 400, 600 mg **SE:** ↑ glucose, cholesterol, triglycerides, central redistribution of fat (metabolic synd), N, ↓ neutrophils, ↑ amylase

Dasatinib (Sprycel) Uses: CML, Ph + ALL Acts: Multi-TKI Dose: 100–140 mg PO day; adjust w/ CYP3A4 inhib/inducers (Table 10, p 319) **W/P:** [D, ?/–] **CI:** None **Disp:** Tabs 20, 50, 70, 80, 100, 140 mg **SE:** ↓ BM, edema, fluid retention, pleural effusions, N/V/D, Abd pain, bleeding, fever, ↑ QT **Notes:** Replace K+, Mg2+ before Rx

Daunorubicin (Cerubidine) BOX: Cardiac Fxn should be monitored d/t potential risk for cardiac tox & CHF, renal/hepatic dysfunction Uses: *Acute leukemias* Acts: DNA-intercalating agent; ↓ topoisomerase II, generates oxygen free radicals **Dose:** 45–60 mg/m^2/d for 3 consecutive d; 25 mg/m^2/wk (per protocols); ↓ w/ renal/hepatic impair **W/P:** [D, ?] **CI:** Component sens **Disp:** Inj 20, 50 mg **SE:** ↓ BM, mucositis, N/V, orange urine, alopecia, radiation recall phenomenon, hepatotox (↑ bili), tissue necrosis w/ extrav, cardiotox (1–2% CHF w/ 550 mg/m^2 cumulative dose) **Notes:** Prevent cardiotox w/ dexrazoxane (w/ > 300 mg/m^2 daunorubicin cum dose); IV use only; allopurinol prior to ↓ hyperuricemia

Decitabine (Dacogen) Uses: *MDS* Acts: Inhibits DNA methyltransferase **Dose:** 15 mg/m^2 cont Inf over 3 h; repeat q8h × 3 d; repeat cycle q6wk, min 4 cycles; delay Tx and ↓ dose if inadequate hematologic recovery at 6 wk (see PI); delay Tx w/ Cr > 2 mg/dL or bili > 2× ULN **W/P:** [D, ?/–]; avoid PRG; males should not father a child during or 2 mo after; renal/hepatic impair **Disp:** Powder 50 mg/vial **SE:** ↓ WBC, ↓ HgB, ↓ plt, febrile neutropenia, edema, petechiae, N/V/D, constipation, stomatitis, dyspepsia, cough, fever, fatigue, ↑ LFTs/bili, hyperglycemia, Infxn, HA **Notes:** ✓ CBC & plt before cycle and PRN; premedicate w/ antiemetic

Deferasirox (Exjade) BOX: May cause renal and hepatic tox/failure, GI bleed; follow labs Uses: *Chronic iron overload d/t transfusion in pts > 2 y* Acts: Oral iron chelator **Dose:** 20 mg/kg PO/d; adjust by 5–10 mg/kg q3–6mo based on monthly ferritin; 40 mg/kg/d max; on empty stomach 30 min ac; hold dose w/ ferritin < 500 mcg/L; dissolve in water/orange/apple juice (< 1 g/3.5 oz; > 1 g in 7 oz) drink immediately; resuspend residue and swallow; do not chew, do not swallow whole tabs or take w/ Al-containing antacids **W/P:** [B, ?/–] Elderly, renal impair, heme disorders; ↑ MDS in pt 60 y **Disp:** Tabs for oral susp 125, 250, 500 mg **SE:** N/V/D, Abd pain, skin rash, HA, fever, cough, ↑ Cr & LFTs, Infxn, hearing loss, dizziness, cataracts, retinal disorders, ↑ IOP **Notes:** ARF, cytopenias possible; ✓ Cr weekly 1st mo then q mo, ✓ CBC, urine protein, LFTs; do not use w/ other iron-chelator therapies; dose to nearest whole tab; initial auditory/ophthal testing and q12mo

Deferiprone (Ferriprox)   **BOX:** May cause neutropenia & agranulocytosis w/ Infxn & death. Monitor baseline ANC & weekly. D/C if Infxn develops. Advise pts to report any Sx of Infxn. **Uses:** *Transfusion iron overload in thalassemia synds* **Acts:** Iron chelator **Dose:** 25 mg/kg PO 3 × d (75 mg/kg/d); 33 mg/kg PO 3 × d (99 mg/kg/d) max round dose to nearest 1/2 tab **W/P:** [D, −] D/C w/ ANC < 1.5 × 10⁹/L **CI:** Hypersens **Disp:** Tabs (scored) 500 mg **SE:** N/V, Abd pain, chromaturia, arthralgia, ↑ ALT, neutropenia, agranulocytosis, ↑ QT, HA **Notes:** Separate by 4 h antacids & mineral supplements w/ polyvalent cations; ✓ plasma zinc

Degarelix (Firmagon)   **Uses:** *Advanced PCa* **Acts:** Reversible LHRH antagonist, ↓ LH and testosterone w/o flare seen w/ LHRH agonists (transient ↑ in testosterone) **Dose:** Initial 240 mg SQ in two 120 mg doses (40 mg/mL); maint 80 mg SQ (20 mg/mL) q28d **W/P:** [Not for women] **CI:** Women **Supplied:** Inj vial 120 mg (initial); 80 mg (maint) **SE:** Inj site Rxns, hot flashes, ↑ Wt, ↑ serum GGT **Notes:** Requires 2 Inj initial (volume); 44% testosterone castrate (< 50 ng/dL) at day 1, 96% day 3

Delavirdine (Rescriptor)   **Uses:** *HIV Infxn* **Acts:** Nonnucleoside RT inhib **Dose:** 400 mg PO tid **W/P:** [C, ?] CDC rec: HIV-infected mothers not breast-feed (transmission risk); w/ renal/hepatic impair **CI:** w/ Drugs dependent on CYP3A (Table 10, p 319) **Disp:** Tabs 100, 200 mg **SE:** Fat redistribution, immune reconstitution synd, HA, fatigue, rash, ↑ transaminases, N/V/D **Notes:** Avoid antacids; ↓ cytochrome P-450 enzymes; numerous drug interactions; monitor LFTs

Demeclocycline (Declomycin)   **Uses:** *SIADH* **Acts:** Antibiotic, antagonizes ADH action on renal tubules **Dose:** 600–1200 mg/d PO on empty stomach; ↓ in renal failure; avoid antacids **W/P:** [D, ?/−] Avoid in hepatic/renal impair & children **CI:** Tetracycline allergy **Disp:** Tabs 150, 300 mg **SE:** D, Abd cramps, photosens, DI **Notes:** Avoid sunlight, numerous drug interactions; not for peds < 8 y

Denosumab (Prolia, Xgeva)   **Uses:** *Tx osteoporosis postmenopausal women* ↑ BMD in men on ADT (*Prolia*); prevent skeletal events w/ bone mets from solid tumors (*Xgeva*) **Acts:** RANK ligand (RANKL) inhibitor (human IgG2 MoAb); inhibits osteoclasts **Dose:** *Prolia:* 60 mg SQ q6mo; *Xgeva:* 120 mg SQ q4wk; in upper arm, thigh, Abd **W/P:** [X (Xgeva), D (Prolia), ?/−] **CI:** Hypocalcemia **Disp:** Inj *Prolia* 60 mg/mL; *Xgeva* 70 mg/mL **SE:** ↓ Ca²⁺, hypophosphatemia, serious Infxns, dermatitis, rashes, eczema, jaw osteonecrosis, pancreatitis, pain (musculoskeletal, back), fatigue, asthenia, dyspnea, N, Abd pain, flatulence, hypercholesterolemia, anemia, cystitis **Notes:** Give w/ calcium 1000 mg & vit D 400 Int units/d

Desipramine (Norpramin)   **BOX:** Closely monitor for worsening depression or emergence of suicidality **Uses:** *Endogenous depression*, chronic pain, peripheral neuropathy **Acts:** TCA; ↑ synaptic serotonin or norepinephrine in CNS **Dose:** *Adults.* 100–200 mg/d single or ÷ dose; usually single hs dose (max 300 mg/d); ↓ dose in elderly *Peds 6–12 y.* 1–3 mg/kg/d ÷ dose, 5 mg/kg/d max **W/P:** [C, ?/–] w/ CV Dz, Sz disorder, hypothyroidism, elderly, liver impair **CI:** MAOIs w/in 14 d; during AMI recovery phase w/ linezolid or IV methylene blue (↑ risk serotonin synd) **Disp:** Tabs 10, 25, 50, 75, 100, 150 mg **SE:** Anticholinergic (blurred vision, urinary retention, xerostomia); orthostatic ↓ BP; ↑ QT, arrhythmias **Notes:** Numerous drug interactions; blue-green urine; avoid sunlight

Desirudin (Iprivask) **BOX:** Recent/planned epidural/spinal anesthesia, ↑ epidural/spinal hematoma risk w/ paralysis; consider risk vs benefit before neuraxial intervention **Uses:** *DVT Px in hip replacement* **Acts:** Thrombin inhibitor **Dose:** *Adults.* 15 mg SQ q12h, initial 5–15 min prior to surgery; CrCl 31–60 mL/min: 5 mg SQ q12h; CrCl < 31 mL/min: 1.7 mg SQ q12h; ✓ aPTT & SCr daily for dosage mod **W/P:** [C, ?/–] **CI:** Active bleeding, irreversible coags, hypersens to hirudins **Disp:** Inj 15 mg **SE:** Hemorrhage, N/V, Inj site mass, wound secretion, anemia, thrombophlebitis, ↓ BP, dizziness, anaphylactic Rxn, fever

Desloratadine (Clarinex) **Uses:** *Seasonal & perennial allergic rhinitis; chronic idiopathic urticaria* **Acts:** Active metabolite of Claritin, H₁-antihistamine, blocks inflammatory mediators **Dose:** *Adults & Peds > 12 y.* 5 mg PO daily; 5 mg PO q other day w/ hepatic/renal impair **W/P:** [C, ?/–] RediTabs contain phenylalanine **Disp:** Tabs 5 mg; *RediTabs* (rapid dissolving) 2.5, 5 mg, syrup 0.5 mg/mL **SE:** Allergy, anaphylaxis, somnolence, HA, dizziness, fatigue, pharyngitis, xerostomia, N, dyspepsia, myalgia

Desmopressin (DDAVP, Stimate) **BOX:** Not for hemophilia B or w/ factor VIII antibody; not for hemophilia A w/ factor VIII levels < 5% **Uses:** *DI; bleeding d/t uremia, hemophilia A, & type I von Willebrand Dz (parenteral), nocturnal enuresis* **Acts:** Synthetic analog of vasopressin (human ADH); ↑ factor VIII **Dose:** *DI: Intranasal: Adults.* 0.1–0.4 mL (10–40 mcg/d in 1–3 ÷ doses). *Peds 3 mo–12 y.* 0.05–0.3 mL/d (5 mcg/d) in 1 or 2 doses. *Parenteral: Adults.* 0.5–1 mL (2–4 mcg/d in 2 ÷ doses); converting from nasal to parenteral, use 1/10 nasal dose. *PO: Adults.* 0.05 mg bid; ↑ to max of 1.2 mg. *Hemophilia A & von Willebrand Dz (type I): Adults & Peds > 10 kg.* 0.3 mcg/kg in 50 mL NS, Inf over 15–30 min *Peds < 10 kg.* As above w/ dilution to 10 mL w/ NS. *Nocturnal enuresis: Peds > 6 y.* 20 mcg intranasally hs **W/P:** [B, M] Avoid overhydration **CI:** Hemophilia B; CrCl < 50 mL/min, severe classic von Willebrand Dz; pts w/ factor VIII antibodies; hyponatremia **Disp:** Tabs 0.1, 0.2 mg; Inj 4 mcg/mL; nasal spray 0.1 mg/mL (10 mcg)/spray 1.5 mg/mL (150 mcg)/spray) **SE:** Facial flushing, HA, dizziness, vulval pain, nasal congestion, pain at Inj site, ↓ Na⁺, H₂O intoxication **Notes:** In very young & old pts, ↓ fluid intake to avoid H₂O intoxication & ↓ Na⁺; ↓ urine output, ↑ urine osm, ↓ plasma osm

Desvenlafaxine (Pristiq) **BOX:** Monitor for worsening or emergence of suicidality, particularly in peds, adolescent, and young adult pts **Uses:** *MDD* **Acts:**

Selective serotonin and norepinephrine reuptake inhib **Dose:** 50 mg PO daily, ↓ w/ renal impair **W/P:** [C, ±/M] **CI:** Hypersens, MAOI w/in 14 d of stopping MAOI **Disp:** Tabs 50, 100 mg **SE:** N, dizziness, insomnia, hyperhidrosis, constipation, somnolence, decreased appetite, anxiety, and specific male sexual Fxn disorders **Notes:** Tabs should be taken whole, allow 7 d after stopping before starting an MAOI

Dexamethasone, Ophthalmic (AK-Dex Ophthalmic, Decadron Ophthalmic, Maxidex) Uses: *Inflammatory or allergic conjunctivitis* **Acts:** Anti-inflammatory corticosteroid **Dose:** Instill 1–2 gtt tid-qid **W/P:** [C, ?/–] **CI:** Active untreated bacterial, viral, & fungal eye Infxns **Disp:** Susp & soln 0.1% **SE:** Long-term use associated w/ cataracts

Dexamethasone, Systemic, Topical (Decadron)   See Steriods, Systemic p 259 and Steroids, Topical p 260. *Peds. ECC 2010. Croup:* 0.6 mg/kg IV/IM/ PO once; max dose 16 mg; *Asthma:* 0.6 mg/kg IV/IM/PO q24h; max dose 16 mg

Dexlansoprazole (Dexilant, Kapidex) Uses: *Heal and maint of erosive esophagitis (EE), GERD* PUD **Acts:** PPI, delayed release **Dose:** EE: 60 mg qd up to 8 wk; maint healed EE: 30 mg qd up to 6 mo; GERD 30 mg/QD × 4 wk; ↓ w/ hepatic impair **W/P:** [B, +/–] do not use w/ clopidogrel/atazanavir or drugs w/ pH based absorption (eg, ampicillin, iron salts, ketoconazole); may alter warfarin and tacrolimus levels **CI:** Component hypersensitivity **Disp:** Caps 30, 60 mg **SE:** N/V/D, flatulence, Abd pain, URI **Notes:** w/ or w/o food; take whole or sprinkle on tsp applesauce; clinical response does not r/o gastric malignancy; see also lansoprazole; ? ↑ risk of fractures w/ all PPI; risk of hypomagnesemia w/ long-term use, monitor

Dexmedetomidine (Precedex) Uses: *Sedation in intubated & nonintubated pts* **Acts:** Sedative; selective α_2-agonist **Dose:** *Adults. ICU Sedation:* 1 mcg/kg IV over 10 min then 0.2–0.7 mcg/kg/h; *Procedural sedation:* 0.5–1 mcg/ kg IV over 10 min then 0.2–1 mcg/kg/h; in elderly, liver Dz **W/P:** [C, ?/–] **CI:** None **Disp:** Inj 200 mcg/2 mL **SE:** Hypotension, bradycardia **Notes:** Tachyphylaxis & tolerance assoc w/ exposure > 24 h

Dexmethylphenidate (Focalin, Focalin XR)[C-II] **BOX:** Caution w/ Hx drug dependence/alcoholism. Chronic abuse may lead to tolerance, psychological dependence & abnormal behavior; monitor closely during withdrawal Uses: *ADHD* **Acts:** CNS stimulant, blocks reuptake of norepinephrine & DA **Dose:** *Adults. Focalin:* 2.5 mg PO twice daily, ↑ by 2.5–5 mg weekly; max 20 mg/d *Focalin XR:* 10 mg PO daily, ↑ 10 mg weekly; max 40 mg/d *Peds ≥ 6 y. Focalin:* 2.5 mg PO bid, ↑ 2.5–5 mg weekly; max 20 mg/d *Focalin XR:* 5 mg PO daily, ↑ 5 mg weekly; max 30 mg/d; if already on methylphenidate, start w/ half of current total daily dose **W/P:** [C, ?/–] Avoid w/ known cardiac abnorml; may ↓ metabolism of warfarin/anticonvulsants/antidepressants **CI:** Agitation, anxiety, tension, glaucoma, Hx motor tic, fam Hx/dx Tourette's w/in 14 d of MAOI; hypersens to methylphenidate **Disp:** Tabs 2.5, 5, 10 mg; caps ER 5, 10, 15, 20, 25, 30, 35, 40 mg **Acts:** HA, anxiety, dyspepsia, ↓ appetite, Wt loss, dry mouth, visual disturbances, ↑ HR, HTN, MI, stroke, sudden death, Szs, growth suppression, aggression, mania, psychosis **Notes:** ✓CBC w/ prolonged use; swallow ER caps whole or sprinkle contents on applesauce (do not crush/chew)

Dexpanthenol (Ilopan-Choline [Oral], Ilopan) **Uses:** *Minimize paralytic ileus, Rx postop distention* **Acts:** Cholinergic agent **Dose:** *Adults.* Relief of gas: 2–3 tabs PO tid. *Prevent postop ileus:* 250–500 mg IM stat, repeat in 2 h, then q6h PRN. *Ileus:* 500 mg IM stat, repeat in 2 h, then q6h, PRN **W/P:** [C, ?] **CI:** Hemophilia, mechanical bowel obst **Disp:** Inj 250 mg/mL; cream 2% (Panthoderm Cream [OTC]) **SE:** GI cramps

Dexrazoxane (Zinecard, Totect) **Uses:** *Prevent anthracycline-induced (eg, doxorubicin) cardiomyopathy (Zinecard), extrav of anthracycline chemotherapy (Totect)* **Acts:** Chelates heavy metals; binds intracellular iron & prevents anthracycline-induced free radicals **Dose:** *Systemic for cardiomyopathy (Zinecard):* 10:1 ratio dexrazoxane: doxorubicin 30 min before each dose, 5:1 ratio w/ CrCl < 40 mL/min *Extrav (Totect):* IV Inf over 1–2 h q day × 3 d, w/in 6 h of extrav. *Day 1:* 1000 mg/m² (max 2000 mg); *Day 2:* 1000 mg/m² (max 2000 mg); *Day 3:* 500 mg/m² (max: 1000 mg); w/ CrCl < 40 mL /min, ↓ dose by 50% **W/P:** [D, –] **CI:** Component sensitivity **Disp:** Inj powder 250, 500 mg (10 mg/mL) **SE:** ↓ BM, fever, Infxn, stomatitis, alopecia, N/V/D; ↑ LFTs, Inj site pain

Dextran 40 (Gentran 40, Rheomacrodex) **Uses:** *Shock, prophylaxis of DVT & thromboembolism, adjunct in peripheral vascular surgery* **Acts:** Expands plasma vol; ↓ blood viscosity **Dose:** *Shock:* 10 mL/kg IV Inf rapidly; 20 mL/ kg max 1st 24 h; beyond 24 h 10 mL/kg max; D/C after 5 d. *Prophylaxis of DVT & thromboembolism:* 10 mL/kg IV day of surgery, then 500 mL/d IV for 2–3 d, then 500 mL IV q2–3d based on risk for up to 2 wk **W/P:** [C, ?] Inf Rxns; w/ corticosteroids **CI:** Major hemostatic defects; cardiac decompensation; renal Dz w/ severe oliguria/anuria **Disp:** 10% dextran 40 in 0.9% NaCl or 5% dextrose **SE:** Allergy/ anaphylactoid Rxn (observe during 1st min of Inf), arthralgia, cutaneous Rxns, ↓ BP, fever **Notes:** Monitor Cr & lytes; keep well hydrated

Dextroamphetamine (Dexedrine, Procentra) [C-II] **BOX:** Amphetamines have a high potential for abuse. Long-term use may lead to dependence. Serious CV events, including death, w/ preexisting cardiac cond. **Uses:** *ADHD, narcolepsy* **Acts:** CNS stimulant; ↑ DA & norepinephrine release **Dose:** *ADHD ≥ 6 y:* 5 mg daily-bid, ↑ by 5 mg/d weekly PRN, max 60 mg/d ÷ bid-tid; *Peds 3–5 y.* 2.5 mg PO daily, ↑ 2.5 mg/d weekly PRN to response; *Peds < 3 y.* Not recommended; *Narcolepsy 6–12 y: 5 mg daily,* ↑ by 5 mg/d weekly PRN max 60 mg/d ÷ bid-tid; ≥ *12 y:* 10-60 mg/d ÷ bid-tid; ER caps once daily **W/P:** [C, +/–] Hx drug abuse; separate 14 d from MAOIs **CI:** Advanced arteriosclerosis, CVD, mod–severe HTN, hyperthyroidism, glaucoma **Disp:** Tabs 5, 10 mg; ER capsules 5, 10, 15 mg; soln 5 mg/5 mL **SE:** HTN, ↓ appetite, insomnia **Notes:** May open ER capsules, do not crush beads

Dextromethorphan (Benylin DM, Delsym, Mediquell, PediaCare 1, Others) [OTC] **Uses:** *Control nonproductive cough* **Acts:** Suppresses medullary cough center **Dose:** *Adults.* 10–30 mg PO q4h PRN (max 120 mg/24 h). *Peds 4–6 y.* 2.5–7.5 mg q4–8h (max 30 mg/24 h). *7–12 y:* 5–10 mg q4–8h (max 60 mg/24 h) **W/P:** [C, ?/–] Not for persistent or chronic cough **CI:** < 2 y **Disp:** Caps 30 mg; lozenges 2.5, 5, 7.5, 15 mg; syrup 15 mg/15 mL, 10 mg/5 mL; liq 10 mg/15 mL, 3.5, 7.5, 15 mg/5 mL; sustained-action liq 30 mg/5 mL **SE:** GI disturbances **Notes:** Found in combo OTC products w/ guaifenesin; deaths reported in pts < 2 y; no longer OTC for < 4 y; abuse potential; efficacy in children debated; do not use w/in 14 d of D/C MAOI

Dextrose 50%/25% **Uses:** Hypoglycemia, insulin OD **Acts:** Sugar source in the form of D-glucose **Dose:** *Adults.* One 50-mL amp of 50% soln IV *Peds. ECC 2010.* Hypoglycemia. 0.5–1 g/kg (25% max IV/IO conc); 50% Dextrose (0.5 g/mL): 1–2 mL/kg; 25% Dextrose (0.25 g/mL): 2–5 mL/kg; 10% Dextrose (0.1 g/mL): 5–10 mL/kg; 5% Dextrose (0.95 g/mL): 10–20 mL/kg if volume tolerated **W/P:** [C, M] w/ Suspected intracranial bleeding can ↑ ICP **CI:** None if used w/ documented hypoglycemia **Disp:** Inj forms **SE:** Burning at IV site, local tissue necrosis w/ extravasation; neurologic Sxs (Wernicke encephalopathy) if pt thiamine deficient **Notes:** If pt well enough to protect airway, use oral glucose first; do not routinely use in altered mental status w/o low glucose, can worsen outcome in stroke; lower concentrations dextrose used in IV fluids

Diazepam (Valium, Diastat) [C-IV] **Uses:** *Anxiety, EtOH withdrawal, muscle spasm, status epilepticus, panic disorders, amnesia, preop sedation* **Acts:** Benzodiazepine **Dose:** *Adults. Status epilepticus:* 5–10 mg q5–10min to 30 mg max in 8-h period. *Anxiety, muscle spasm:* 2–10 mg PO bid-qid or IM/IV q3–4h PRN. *Preop:* 5–10 mg PO or IM 20–30 min or IV just prior to procedure. *EtOH withdrawal:* 10 mg q3–4h × 24 h, then 5 mg PO q3–4h PRN or 5–10 mg IV q10–15min for CIWA withdrawal score ≥ 8, 100 mg/h max; titrate to agitation; avoid excessive sedation; may lead to aspiration or resp arrest. *Peds. Status epilepticus:* < *5 y:* 0.05–0.3 mg/kg/dose IV q15–30min up to a max of 5 mg. > *5 y:* to max of 10 mg. *Sedation, muscle relaxation:* 0.04–0.3 mg/kg/dose q2–4h IM or IV to max of 0.6 mg/kg in 8 h, or 0.12–0.8 mg/kg/24 h PO ÷ tid-qid; ↓ w/ hepatic impair **W/P:** [D, ?/–] **CI:** Coma, CNS depression, resp depression, NAG, severe uncontrolled pain, PRG **Disp:** Tabs 2, 5, 10 mg; soln 5 mg/mL; Inj 5 mg/mL; rectal gel 2.5, 5, 10, 20 mg/mL **SE:** Sedation, amnesia, ↓ HR, ↓ BP, rash, ↑ resp rate **Notes:** 5 mg/min IV max in adults or 1–2 mg/min in peds (resp arrest possible); IM absorption erratic; avoid abrupt D/C

Diazoxide (Proglycem) **Uses:** *Hypoglycemia d/t hyperinsulinism* **Acts:** ↓ Pancreatic insulin release; antihypertensive **Dose:** Repeat in 5–15 min until BP controlled; repeat q4–24h; monitor BP closely. *Hypoglycemia: Adults & Peds.* 3–8 mg/kg/24 h PO ÷ q8–12h. *Neonates.* 8–10 mg/kg/24 h PO in 2–3 equal doses **W/P:** [C, ?] ↓ Effect w/ phenytoin; ↑ effect w/ diuretics, warfarin **CI:** Allergy to thiazides or other sulfonamide-containing products; HTN associated w/ aortic coarctation, AV shunt, or pheochromocytoma **Disp:** PO susp 50 mg/mL

SE: Hyperglycemia, ↓ BP, dizziness, Na^+ & H_2O retention, N/V, weakness
Notes: Can give false(−) insulin response to glucagons

Dibucaine (Nupercainal) Uses: *Hemorrhoids & minor skin conditions*
Acts: Topical anesthetic **Dose:** Insert PR w/ applicator bid & after each bowel movement; apply sparingly to skin **W/P:** [C, ?] Topical use only **CI:** Component sensitivity
Disp: 1% oint w/ rectal applicator **SE:** Local irritation, rash

Diclofenac & Misoprostol (Arthrotec) **BOX:** May induce abortion, birth defects; do not take if PRG; may ↑ risk of CV events & GI bleeding; CI in postop CABG Uses: *OA and RA w/ ↑ risk GI bleed* **Acts:** NSAID w/ GI protective PGE_1
Dose: OA: 50–75 mg PO bid-tid; RA 50 mg bid-qid or 75 mg bid; w/ food or milk
W/P: [X, ?] CHF, HTN, renal/hepatic dysfunction, & Hx PUD, asthma; avoid w/ porphyria **CI:** PRG; GI bleed; renal/hepatic failure; severe CHF; NSAID/aspirin ASA allergy; following CABG **Disp:** Tabs *Arthrotec* 50: 50 mg diclofenac w/ 200 mcg misoprostol; *Arthrotec*: 75 mg diclofenac w/ 200 mcg misoprostol **SE:** *Oral:* Abd cramps, heartburn, GI ulcers, rash, interstitial nephritis **Notes:** Do not crush tabs; watch for GI bleed; ✓CBC, LFTs; PRG test females before use

Diclofenac, Ophthalmic (Voltaren Ophthalmic) Uses: *Inflammation postcataract or pain/photophobia post corneal refractive surgery* **Acts:** NSAID
Dose: *Postop cataract:* 1 gtt qid, start 24 h postop × 2 wk. *Postop refractive:* 1–2 gtt w/in 1 h preop and w/in 15 min postop then qid up to 3 d **W/P:** [C, ?] May ↑ bleed risk in ocular tissues **CI:** NSAID/ASA allergy **Disp:** Ophthal soln 0.1% 2.5-mL bottle **SE:** Burning/stinging/itching, keratitis, ↑ IOP, lacrimation, abnormal vision, conjunctivitis, lid swelling, discharge

Diclofenac, Oral (Cataflam, Voltaren, Voltaren-XR) **BOX:** May ↑ risk of CV events & GI bleeding; CI in postop CABG Uses: *Arthritis (RA/OA) & pain, oral and topical, actinic keratosis* **Acts:** NSAID **Dose:** RA/OA: 150–200 mg/d ÷ 2–4 doses DR; 100 mg/d XR; w/ food or milk **W/P:** [C (avoid after 30 wk), ?] CHF, HTN, renal/hepatic dysfunction, & Hx PUD, asthma **CI:** NSAID/aspirin ASA allergy; porphyria; following CABG **Disp:** Tabs 50 mg; tabs DR 25, 50, 75, 100 mg; XR tabs 100 mg **SE:** *Oral:* Abd cramps, heartburn, GI ulceration, rash, interstitial nephritis **Notes:** Do not crush tabs; watch for GI bleed; ✓CBC, LFTs periodically

Diclofenac, Topical (Flector Patch, Pennsaid, Solaraze, Voltaren Gel) **BOX:** May ↑ risk of CV events & GI bleeding; CI in postop CABG Uses: *Arthritis of the knee (Pennsaid); arthritis of knee/hands (Voltaren Gel); pain due to strain, sprain, and contusions (Flector Patch); actinic keratosis (Solaraze)* **Acts:** NSAID **Dose:** *Flector Patch:* 1 patch to painful area bid *Pennsaid:* 10 drops spread around knee; repeat until 40 drops applied. Usual **dose:** 40 drops/knee qid; wash hands; wait until dry before dressing. *Solaraze:* 0.5 g to each 5 × 5 cm lesion 60–90 d; apply bid; *Voltaren Gel:* upper extremity 2 g qid (max 8 g/d); lower extremity 4 g qid (max 16 g/d) **W/P:** [C < 30 wk gest; D > 30 wk; ?] avoid nonintact skin; CV events possible w/ CHF, ↑ BP, renal/hepatic dysfunct, w/ Hx PUD, asthma; avoid w/ PO NSAID **CI:** NSAID/ASA allergy; following CABG; component allergy **Disp:** *Flector Patch:* 180 mg (10 × 14 cm); *Voltaren Gel* 1%; *Solaraze* 3%; *Pennsaid* 1.5% soln **SE:** Pruritus, dermatitis, burning, dry skin, N, HA **Notes:** Do not apply patch/gel to damaged skin or while bathing; ✓CBC, LFTs periodically; no box warning on *Solaraze*

Dicloxacillin (Dynapen, Dycill) Uses: *Rx of pneumonia, skin, & soft-tissue Infxns, & osteomyelitis caused by penicillinase-producing staphylococci* **Acts:** Bactericidal; ↓ cell wall synth. *Spectrum: S. aureus & Streptococcus* **Dose:** *Adults.* 150–500 mg qid (2 g/d max) *Peds < 40 kg.* 12.5–100 mg/kg/d ÷ qid; take on empty stomach **W/P:** [B, ?] **CI:** Component or PCN sensitivity **Disp:** Caps 125, 250, 500 mg **SE:** N/D, Abd pain **Notes:** Monitor PTT if pt on warfarin

Dicyclomine (Bentyl) Uses: *Functional IBS* **Acts:** Smooth-muscle relaxant **Dose:** *Adults.* 20 mg PO qid; ↑ to 160 mg/d max or 20 mg IM q6h, 80 mg/d ÷ qid then ↑ to 160 mg/d, max 2 wk **W/P:** [B, –] **CI:** Infants < 6 mo, NAG, MyG, severe UC, BOO, GI obst, reflux esophagitis **Disp:** Caps 10 mg; tabs 20 mg; syrup 10 mg/5 mL; Inj 10 mg/mL **SE:** Anticholinergic SEs may limit dose **Notes:** Take 30–60 min ac; avoid EtOH, do not administer IV

Didanosine [ddI] (Videx) **BOX:** Allergy manifested as fever, rash, fatigue, GI/resp Sxs reported; stop drug immediately & do not rechallenge; lactic acidosis & hepatomegaly/steatosis reported Uses: *HIV Infxn in zidovudine-intolerant pts* **Acts:** NRTI **Dose:** *Adults. > 60 kg:* 400 mg/d PO or 200 mg PO bid. *< 60 kg:* 250 mg/d PO or 125 mg PO bid; adults should take 2 tabs/administration. *Peds 2 wk–8 mo.* 100 mg/m² PO *> 8 mo:* 120 mg/m² PO bid; on empty stomach; ↓ w/ renal impair **W/P:** [B, –] CDC rec: HIV-infected mothers not breast-feed **CI:** Component sensitivity **Disp:** Chew tabs 100, 150, 200 mg; DR caps 125, 200, 250, 400 mg; powder for soln 2, 4 g **SE:** Pancreatitis, peripheral neuropathy, D, HA **Notes:** Do not take w/ meals; thoroughly chew tabs, do not mix w/ fruit juice or acidic beverages; reconstitute powder w/ H₂O, many drug interactions

Diflunisal (Dolobid) **BOX:** May ↑ risk of CV events & GI bleeding; CI in postop CABG Uses: *Mild–mod pain; OA* **Acts:** NSAID **Dose:** *Pain:* 500 mg PO bid. *OA:* 500–1000/mg/d PO bid (max 1.5 g/d); ↓ in renal impair, take w/ food/ milk **W/P:** [C (D 3rd tri or near delivery), ?] CHF, HTN, renal/hepatic dysfunction, & Hx PUD **CI:** Allergy to NSAIDs or ASA, active GI bleed, post-CABG **Disp:** Tabs 500 mg **SE:** May ↑ bleeding time; HA, Abd cramps, heartburn, GI ulceration, rash, interstitial nephritis, fluid retention

Digoxin (Digitek, Lanoxin) Uses: *CHF, AF & A flutter, & PAT* **Acts:** Positive inotrope; AV node refractory period **Dose:** *Adults. PO digitalization:* 0.5–0.75 mg PO, then 0.25 mg PO q6–8h to total 1–1.5 mg. *IV or IM digitalization:* 0.25–0.5 mg IM or IV, then 0.25 mg q4–6h to total 0.125–0.5 mg/d PO, IM, or IV (average daily dose 0.125–0.25 mg). *Peds. Preterm infants: Digitalization:* 30 mcg/kg PO or 25 mcg/kg IV; give 1/2 of dose initial, then 1/4 of dose at 8–12 h intervals for 2 doses. *Maint:* 5–7.5 mcg/kg/24 h PO or 4–6 mcg/kg/24 h IV ÷ q12h.

Term infants: *Digitalization:* 25–35 mcg/kg PO or 20–30 mcg/kg IV; give 1/2 the initial dose, then 1/3 of dose at 8–12 h. *Maint:* 6–10 mcg/kg/24 h PO or 5–8 mcg/kg/24 h ÷ q12h. ***2–5 yo:*** *Digitalization:* 30–40 mcg/kg PO or 25–35 mcg/kg IV. *Maint:* 7.5–10 mcg/kg/24 h PO or 6–9 mcg/kg IV ÷ q12h. ***5–10 y:*** *Digitalization:* 25–35 mcg/kg PO or 15–30 mcg/kg IV; *Maint:* 5–10 mcg/kg/24 h PO or 4–8 mcg/kg q12 h. ***>10 y:*** 10–15 mcg/kg PO or 8–12 mcg/kg IV. *Maint:* 2.5-5 mcg/kg PO or 2–3 mcg/kg IV q 4 h; ↓ in renal impair **W/P:** [C, +] w/ K+, Mg2+, renal failure **CI:** AV block; IHSS; constrictive pericarditis **Disp:** Tabs 0.125, 0.25 mg; elixir 0.05 mg/mL; Inj 0.1, 0.25 mg/mL **SE:** Can cause heart block; ↓ K+ potentiates tox; N/V, HA, fatigue, visual disturbances (yellow-green halos around lights), cardiac arrhythmias **Notes:** Multiple drug interactions; IM Inj painful, has erratic absorption & should not be used. *Levels: Trough:* Just before next dose. *Therapeutic:* 0.8–2 ng/mL; *Toxic:* > 2 ng/mL; *Half-life:* 36 h

Digoxin Immune Fab (DigiFab) Uses: *Life-threatening digoxin intoxication* Acts: Antigen-binding fragments bind & inactivate digoxin Dose: *Adults & Peds.* Based on serum level & pt's Wt; see charts provided w/ drug W/P: [C, ?] CI: Sheep product allergy Disp: Inj 40 mg/vial SE: Worsening of cardiac output or CHF, ↓ K+, facial swelling, & redness Notes: Each vial binds ~ 0.5 mg of digoxin; renal failure may require redosing in several days

Diltiazem (Cardizem, Cardizem CD, Cardizem LA, Cartia XT, Dilacor XR, Diltia XT, Taztia XT, Tiazac) Uses: *Angina, prevention of reinfarction, HTN, A-fib & A-flutter, & PAT* Acts: CCB Dose: *Stable angina PO:* Initial, 30 mg PO qid; ↑ to 120–320 mg/d in 3–4 ÷ doses PRN; XR 120 mg/d (540 mg/d max), *LA:* 180–360 mg/d. *HTN:* SR: 60–120 mg PO bid; ↑ to 360 mg/d max. *CD or XR:* 120–360 mg/d (max 540 mg/d) or LA 180–360 mg/d. *A-Fib, A-Flutter, PSVT:* 0.25 mg/kg IV bolus over 2 min; may repeat in 15 min at 0.35 mg/kg; begin Inf 5–15 mg/h. *ECC 2010. Acute rate control:* 0.25 mg/kg (15–20 mg) over 2 min, followed in 15 min by 0.35 mg/kg (20–25 mg) over 2 min; maint Inf 5–15 mg/h W/P: [C, +] ↑ Effect w/ amiodarone, cimetidine, fentanyl, Li, cyclosporine, digoxin, β-blockers, theophylline CI: SSS, AV block, ↓ BP, AMI, pulm congestion Disp: *Cardizem CD:* Caps 120, 180, 240, 300, 360 mg; *Cardizem LA:* Tabs 120, 180, 240, 300, 360, 420 mg; *Cardizem SR:* Caps 60, 90, 120 mg; *Cardizem:* Tabs 30, 60, 90, 120 mg; *Cartia XT:* Caps 120, 180, 240, 300 mg; *Dilacor XR:* Caps 120, 180, 240 mg; *Diltia XT:* Caps 120, 180, 240 mg; *Tiazac:* Caps 120, 180, 240, 300, 360, 420 mg; Inj 5 mg/mL; *Taztia XT:* 120, 180, 240, 300, 360 mg SE: Gingival hyperplasia, ↓ HR, AV block, ECG abnormalities, peripheral edema, dizziness, HA Notes: *Cardizem CD, Dilacor XR, & Tiazac* not interchangeable

Dimenhydrinate (Dramamine, Others) Uses: *Prevention & Rx of N/V, dizziness, or vertigo of motion sickness* Acts: Antiemetic, action unknown Dose: *Adults.* 50–100 mg PO q4–6h, max 400 mg/d; 50 mg IM/IV PRN. *Peds 2–6 y.* 12.5–25 mg q6–8h max 75 mg/d. *6–12 y:* 25–50 mg q6–8h max 150 mg/d W/P: [B, ?]

CI: Component sensitivity **Disp:** Tabs 25, 50 mg; chew tabs 50 mg; Inj: 50 mg/mL **SE:** Anticholinergic SE **Notes:** Take 30 min before travel for motion sickness

Dimethyl Sulfoxide [DMSO] (Rimso-50) **Uses:** *Interstitial cystitis* **Acts:** Unknown **Dose:** Intravesical, 50 mL, retain for 15 min; repeat q2wk until relief **W/P:** [C, ?] **CI:** Component sensitivity **Disp:** 50% soln **SE:** Cystitis, eosinophilia, GI, & taste disturbance

Dinoprostone (Cervidil Vaginal Insert, Prepidil Vaginal Gel, Prostin E2) **BOX:** Should only be used by trained personnel in an appropriate hospital setting **Uses:** *Induce labor; terminate PRG (12–20 wk); evacuate uterus in missed abortion or fetal death* **Acts:** Prostaglandin, changes consistency, dilatation, & effacement of the cervix; induces uterine contraction **Dose:** *Gel:* 0.5 mg; if no cervical/uterine response, repeat 0.5 mg q6h (max 24-h dose 1.5 mg). *Vag insert:* 1 insert (10 mg = 0.3 mg dinoprostone/h over 12 h); remove w/ onset of labor or 12 h after insertion. *Vag supp:* 20 mg repeated q3–5h; adjust PRN supp: 1 high in vagina, repeat at 3–5-h intervals until abortion (240 mg max) **W/P:** [X, ?] **CI:** Ruptured membranes, allergy to prostaglandins, placenta previa or AUB, when oxytocic drugs CI or if prolonged uterine contractions are inappropriate (Hx C-section, cephalopelvic disproportion, etc) **Disp:** *Endocervical gel:* 0.5 mg in 3-g syringes (w/ 10- & 20-mm shielded catheter). *Vag gel:* 1 mg/3 g, 2 mg/3 g. *Vag supp:* 20 mg. *Vag insert, CR:* 10 mg **SE:** N/V/D, dizziness, flushing, HA, fever, abnormal uterine contractions

Diphenhydramine (Benadryl) [OTC] **Uses:** *Rx & prevent allergic Rxns, motion sickness, potentiate narcotics, sedation, cough suppression, & Rx of extrapyramidal Rxns* **Acts:** Antihistamine, antiemetic **Dose:** *Adults.* 25–50 mg PO, IV, or IM tid-qid. *Peds > 2 y.* 5 mg/kg/24 h PO or IM ÷ q6h (max 300 mg/d); ↑ dosing interval w/ mod–severe renal Insuff **W/P:** [B, –] Elderly, NAG, BPH, w/ MAOI **CI:** acute asthma **Disp:** Tabs & caps 25, 50 mg; chew tabs 12.5 mg; elixir 12.5 mg/ 5 mL; syrup 12.5 mg/5 mL; liq 12.5 mg/5 mL; Inj 50 mg/mL, cream, gel, liq 2% **SE:** Anticholinergic (xerostomia, urinary retention, sedation)

Diphenoxylate + Atropine (Lomotil, Lonox) [C-V] **Uses:** *D* **Acts:** Constipating meperidine congener, ↓ GI motility **Dose:** *Adults.* Initial, 5 mg PO tid-qid until controlled, then 2.5–5 mg PO bid; 20 mg/d max **Peds > 2 y.** 0.3–0.4 mg/kg/24 h (of diphenoxylate) bid-qid, 10 mg/d max **W/P:** [C, ?/–] Elderly, w/ renal impair **CI:** Obstructive jaundice, D d/t bacterial Infxn; children < 2 y **Disp:** Tabs 2.5 mg diphenoxylate/0.025 mg atropine; liq 2.5 mg diphenoxylate/0.025 mg atropine/5 mL **SE:** Drowsiness, dizziness, xerostomia, blurred vision, urinary retention, constipation

Diphtheria & Tetanus Toxoids (Td) (Decavac, Tenivac—for > 7 y) **Uses:** Primary immunization, booster (peds 7–9 y; peds 11–12 y if 5 y since last shot then q10yr); tetanus protection after wound. **Acts:** Active immunization **Dose:** 0.5 mL IM × 1 **W/P:** [C, ?/–] **CI:** Component sensitivity **Disp:** Single-dose syringes 0.5 mL **SE:** Inj site pain, redness, swelling; fever, fatigue, HA, malaise, neuro disorders rare **Notes:** If IM, use only preservative-free Inj; Use DTaP

(*Adacel*) rather than TT or Td all adults 19–64 y who have **not** previously received 1 dose of DTaP (protection adult pertussis) and Tdap for ages 10–18 y (*Boostrix*); do not confuse Td (for adults) w/ DT (for children < 7 y)

Diphtheria & Tetanus Toxoids (DT) (Generic Only for < 7 y)
Uses: Primary immunization ages < 7 y (DTaP is recommended vaccine) **Acts:** Active immunization **Dose:** 0.5 mL IM ×1, 5 dose series for primary immunization if DTaP CI **W/P:** [C, N/A] **CI:** Component sensitivity **Disp:** Single-dose syringes 0.5 mL **SE:** Inj site pain, redness, swelling; fever, fatigue, myalgias/arthralgias, N/V, Sz, other neurological SE rare; syncope, apnea in preemies **Notes:** If IM, use only preservative-free Inj. Do not confuse DT (for children < 7 y) w/ Td (for adults); DTaP is recommended for primary immunization

Diphtheria, Tetanus Toxoids, & Acellular Pertussis Adsorbed (Tdap) (Ages > 10–11 y) (Boosters: Adacel, Boostrix)
Acts: Active immunization, ages > 10–11 y **Uses:** "Catch-up" vaccination if 1 or more of the 5 childhood doses of DTP or DTaP missed; all adults 19–64 y who have **not** received 1 dose previously (adult pertussis protection) or if around infants < 12 mo; booster q10y; tetanus protection after fresh wound. **Actions:** Active immunization **Dose:** 0.5 mL IM ×1 **W/P:** [C, ?/–] w/ Latex allergy **CI:** Component sensitivity; if previous pertussis vaccine caused progressive neurologic disorder/encephalopathy w/in 7 d of shot **Disp:** Single-dose vials 0.5 mL **SE:** Inj site pain, redness, swelling; Abd pain, arthralgias/myalgias, fatigue, fever, HA, N/V/D, rash, tiredness **Notes:** If IM, use only preservative-free Inj; ACIP rec: Tdap for ages 10–18 y (*Boostrix*) or 11–64 y (*Adacel*); Td should be used in children 7–9 y; CDC rec pts > age 65 who have close contact w/ infants get a dose of Tdap (protection against pertussis).

Diphtheria, Tetanus Toxoids, & Acellular Pertussis Adsorbed (DTaP) (Ages < 7 y) (Daptacel, Infanrix, Tripedia)
Uses: Primary vaccination; 5 Inj at 2, 4, 6, 15–18 mo and 4–6 y **Acts:** Active immunization **Dose:** 0.5 mL IM ×1 as in previous above **W/P:** [C, N/A] **CI:** Component sensitivity; if previous pertussis vaccine caused progressive neurologic disorder/encephalopathy w/in 7 d of shot **Disp:** Single-dose vials 0.5 mL **SE:** Inj site nodule/pain/swelling/redness; drowsiness, fatigue, fever, fussiness, irritability, lethargy, V, prolonged crying; rare ITP and neurologic disorders **Notes:** If IM, use only preservative-free Inj; DTaP recommended for primary immunization age < 7 y, if age 7–9 y use Td, ages > 10–11 y use Tdap; if encephalopathy or other neurologic disorder w/in 7 d of previous dose DO NOT USE DTaP, use DT or Td depending on age

Diphtheria, Tetanus Toxoids, Acellular Pertussis Adsorbed, Inactivated Poliovirus Vaccine [IPV] & Haemophilus b Conjugate Vaccine Combined (Pentacel)
Uses: *Immunization against diphtheria, tetanus, pertussis, poliomyelitis and invasive Dz due to *Haemophilus influenzae* type b* **Acts:** Active immunization **Dose:** *Infants:* 0.5 mL IM at 2, 4, 6 and 15–18 mo

of age **W/P:** [C, N/A] w/ Fever > 40.5°C (105°F), hypotonic-hyporesponsive episode (HHE) or persistent, inconsolable crying > 3 h w/in 48 h after a previous pertussis-containing vaccine; Sz w/in 3 d after a previous pertussis-containing vaccine; Guillain-Barré w/in 6 wk of previous tetanus toxoid vaccine; w/ Hx Sz antipyretic may be administered w/ vaccine × 24 h w/ bleeding disorders **CI:** Allergy to any components; encephalopathy w/in 7 d of previous pertussis vaccine; w/ progressive neurologic disorders **Disp:** Single-dose vials 0.5 mL **SE:** Fussiness/irritability and inconsolable crying; fever > 38.0°C Inj site Rxn

Diphtheria, Tetanus Toxoids, & Acellular Pertussis Adsorbed, Hep B (Recombinant), & Inactivated Poliovirus Vaccine [IPV], Combined (Pediarix) **Uses:** *Vaccine against diphtheria, tetanus, pertussis, HBV, polio (types 1, 2, 3) as a 3-dose primary series in infants & children < 7 y, born to HBsAg(−) mothers* **Acts:** Active immunization **Dose:** *Infants:* Three 0.5-mL doses IM, at 6–8-wk intervals, start at 2 mo; child given 1 dose of hep B vaccine, same; previously vaccinated w/ 1 or more doses inactivated poliovirus vaccine, use to complete series **W/P:** [C, N/A] w/ Bleeding disorders **CI:** HBsAg(+) mother, adults, children > 7 y, immunosuppressed, component sensitivity or allergy to yeast/neomycin/polymyxin B; encephalopathy, or progressive neurologic disorders **Disp:** Single-dose syringes 0.5 mL **SE:** Drowsiness, restlessness, fever, fussiness, ↓ appetite, Inj site pain/swelling/nodule/redness **Notes:** If IM, use only preservative-free Inj

Dipivefrin (Propine) **Uses:** *Open-angle glaucoma* **Acts:** α-Adrenergic agonist **Dose:** 1 gtt in eye q12h **W/P:** [B, ?] **CI:** NAG **Disp:** 0.1% soln **SE:** HA, local irritation, blurred vision, photophobia, HTN

Dipyridamole (Persantine) **Uses:** *Prevent postop thromboembolic disorders, often in combo w/ ASA or warfarin (eg, CABG, vascular graft); w/ warfarin after artificial heart valve; chronic angina; w/ ASA to prevent coronary artery thrombosis; dipyridamole IV used in place of exercise stress test for CAD* **Acts:** Anti-plt activity; coronary vasodilator **Dose:** *Adults.* 75–100 mg PO qid; stress test 0.14 mg/kg/min (max 60 mg over 4 min). *Peds > 12 y.* 3–6 mg/kg/d ÷ tid (safety/efficacy not established) **W/P:** [B, ?/−] w/ Other drugs that affect coagulation **CI:** Component sensitivity **Disp:** Tabs 25, 50, 75 mg; Inj 5 mg/mL **SE:** HA, ↓ BP, N, Abd distress, flushing rash, dizziness, dyspnea **Notes:** IV use can worsen angina

Dipyridamole & Aspirin (Aggrenox) **Uses:** *↓ Reinfarction after MI; prevent occlusion after CABG; ↓ risk of stroke* **Acts:** ↓ Plt aggregation (both agents) **Dose:** 1 cap PO bid **W/P:** [D, ?] **CI:** Ulcers, bleeding diathesis **Disp:** Dipyridamole (XR) 200 mg/ASA 25 mg **SE:** ASA component: allergic Rxns, skin Rxns, ulcers/GI bleed, bronchospasm; dipyridamole component: dizziness, HA, rash **Notes:** Swallow caps whole

Disopyramide (Norpace, Norpace CR, NAPAmide, Rythmodan) **BOX:** Excessive mortality or nonfatal cardiac arrest rate w/ use in asymptomatic non–life-threatening ventricular arrhythmias w/ MI 6 d–2 y prior. Restrict use to life-threatening arrhythmias only **Uses:** *Suppression & prevention of VT* **Acts:**

Class IA antiarrhythmic; stabilizes membranes, ↓ action potential **Dose:** *Adults.* Immediate < 50 kg 200 mg, > 50 kg 300 mg, maint 400–800 mg/d ÷ q6h or q12h for CR, max 1600 mg/d. *Peds < 1 y.* 10–30 mg/kg/24 h PO (÷ qid). *1–4 y:* 10–20 mg/kg/24 h PO (÷ qid). *4–12 y:* 10–15 mg/kg/24 h PO (÷ qid). *12–18 y:* 6–15 mg/kg/24 h PO (÷ qid); ↓ in renal/hepatic impair **W/P:** [C, +] Elderly, w/ abnormal ECG, lytes, liver/renal impair, NAG **CI:** AV block, cardiogenic shock, ↓ BP, CHF **Disp:** Caps 100, 150 mg; CR caps 100, 150 mg **SE:** Anticholinergic SEs; negative inotrope, may induce CHF **Notes:** Levels: *Trough:* just before next dose; *Therapeutic:* 2–5 mcg/mL; *Toxic* > 7 mcg/mL; half-life: 4–10 h

Dobutamine (Dobutrex) Uses: *Short-term in cardiac decompensation secondary to ↓ contractility* **Acts:** Positive inotrope **Dose:** *Adults. ECC 2010.* 2.5–20 mcg/kg/min; titrate to HR **Peds. ECC 2010.** *Shock w/ high SVR:* 2–20 mcg/kg/min; titrate **W/P:** [B, ?/ –] w/ Arrhythmia, MI, severe CAD, ↓ vol **CI:** Sensitivity to sulfites, IHSS **Disp:** Inj 250 mg/20 mL, 500 mg/40 mL **SE:** CP, HTN, dyspnea **Notes:** Monitor PWP & cardiac output if possible; ✓ ECG for ↑ HR, ectopic activity; follow BP

Docetaxel (Taxotere) **BOX:** Do not administer if neutrophil count < 1500 cells/mm³; severe Rxns possible in hepatic dysfunction **Uses:** *Breast (anthracycline-resistant), ovarian, lung, & prostate CA* **Acts:** Antimitotic agent; promotes microtubular aggregation; semisynthetic taxoid **Dose:** 100 mg/m³ over 1 h IV q3wk (per protocols), dexamethasone 8 mg bid prior & continue for 3–4 d; ↓ dose w/ ↑ bili levels **W/P:** [D, –] **CI:** Sensitivity to meds w/ polysorbate 80, component sensitivity **Disp:** Inj 20 mg/0.5 mL, 80 mg/2 mL **SE:** ↓ BM, neuropathy, N/V, alopecia, fluid retention synd; cumulative doses of 300–400 mg/m² w/o steroid prep & post-Tx & 600–800 mg/m² w/ steroid prep; allergy possible (rare w/ steroid prep) **Notes:** ✓ Bili/SGOT/SGPT prior to each cycle; frequent CBC during Rx

Docusate Calcium (Surfak)/Docusate Potassium (Dialose)/ Docusate Sodium (DOSS, Colace) Uses: *Constipation; adjunct to painful anorectal conditions (hemorrhoids)* **Acts:** Stool softener **Dose:** *Adults.* 50–500 mg PO ÷ daily-qid. *Peds Infants–3 y.* 10–40 mg/24 h ÷ daily-qid. *3–6 y:* 20–60 mg/24 h ÷ daily-qid. *6–12 y:* 40–150 mg/24 h ÷ daily-qid **W/P:** [C, ?] **CI:** Use w/ mineral oil; intestinal obst, acute Abd pain, N/V **Disp:** *Ca:* Caps 50, 240 mg. *K:* Caps 100, 240 mg. *Na:* Caps 50, 100 mg; syrup 50, 60 mg/15 mL; liq 150 mg/15 mL; soln 50 mg/mL; enema 283 mg/mL **SE:** Rare Abd cramping, D **Notes:** Take w/ full glass of water; no laxative action; do not use > 1 wk

Dofetilide (Tikosyn) **BOX:** To minimize the risk of induced arrhythmia, hospitalize for minimum of 3 d to provide calculations of CrCl, cont ECG monitoring, & cardiac resuscitation **Uses:** *Maintain nl sinus rhythm in AF/A flutter after conversion* **Acts:** Class III antiarrhythmic, prolongs action potential **Dose:** Based on CrCl & QTc; CrCl > 60 mL/min 500 mcg PO q12h, ✓ QTc 2–3 h after, if QTc > 15% over baseline or > 500 ms, ↓ to 250 mcg q12h, ✓ after each dose;

if CrCl < 60 mL/min, see PI; D/C if QTc > 500 ms after dosing adjustments **W/P:** [C, –] w/ AV block, renal Dz, electrolyte imbalance **CI:** Baseline QTc > 440 ms, CrCl < 20 mL/min; w/ verapamil, cimetidine, trimethoprim, ketoconazole, quinolones, ACE inhib/HCTZ combo **Disp:** Caps 125, 250, 500 mcg **SE:** Ventricular arrhythmias, QT ↑, torsades de pointes, rash, HA, CP, dizziness **Notes:** Avoid w/ other drugs that ↑ QT interval; hold class I/III antiarrhythmics for 3 half-lives prior to dosing; amiodarone level should be < 0.3 mg/L before use, do not initiate if HR < 60 BPM; restricted to participating prescribers; correct K+ and Mg2+ before use

Dolasetron (Anzemet) Uses: *Prevent chemotherapy and postop-associated N/V* Acts: 5-HT₃ receptor antagonist Dose: *Adults.* PO: 100 mg PO as a single dose 1 h prior to chemotherapy. *Postop:* 12.5 mg IV, or 100 mg PO 2 h preop *Peds 2–16 y.* 1.8 mg/kg PO (max 100 mg) as single dose. *Postop.* 0.35 mg/kg IV or 1.2 mg/kg PO W/P: [B, ?] w/ Cardiac conduction problems CI: IV use w/ chemo component sensitivity Disp: Tabs 50, 100 mg; Inj 20 mg/mL SE: ↑ QT interval, D, HTN, HA, Abd pain, urinary retention, transient ↑ LFTs Notes: IV form no longer approved for chemo-induced N&V due to heart rhythm abnormalities.

Donepezil (Aricept) Uses: *Severe Alzheimer dementia*; ADHD; behavioral synds in dementia; dementia w/ Parkinson Dz; Lewy-body dementia Acts: ACH inhib Dose: *Adults.* 5 mg qhs, ↑ to 10 mg PO qhs after 4–6 wk Peds. ADHD: 5 mg/d W/P: [C, ?] Risk for ↓ HR w/ preexisting conduction abnormalities, may exaggerate succinylcholine-type muscle relaxation w/ anesthesia, ↑ gastric acid secretion CI: Hypersens Disp: Tabs 5, 10, 23 mg; ODT tab 5, 10 mg SE: N/V/D, insomnia, Infxn, muscle cramp, fatigue, anorexia Notes: N/V/D dose-related & resolves in 1–3 wk

Dopamine (Intropin) BOX: Tissue vesicant, give phentolamine w/ extrav Uses: *Short-term use in cardiac decompensation secondary to ↓ contractility; ↑ organ perfusion (at low dose)* Acts: Positive inotropic agent w/ dose response: 1–10 mcg/kg/min β effects (↑ CO); 10–20 mcg/kg/min β-effects (peripheral vasoconstriction, pressor); > 20 mcg/kg/min peripheral & renal vasoconstriction Dose: *Adults.* 5 mcg/kg/min by cont Inf, ↑ by 5 mcg/kg/min to 50 mcg/kg/min max to effect; *ECC 2010.* 2–20 mcg/kg/min Peds. *ECC 2010. Shock w/ adequate intravascular volume and stable rhythm:* 2–20 mcg/kg/min; titrate, if > 20 mcg/kg/min needed, consider alternative adrenergic W/P: [C, ?] ↓ Dose w/ MAOI CI: Pheochromocytoma, VF, sulfite sensitivity Disp: Inj 40, 80, 160 mg/mL, premixed 0.8, 1.6, 3.2 mg/mL SE: Tachycardia, vasoconstriction, ↓ BP, HA, N/V, dyspnea Notes: > 10 mcg/kg/min ↓ renal perfusion; monitor urinary output & ECG for ↑ HR, BP, ectopy; monitor PCWP & cardiac output if possible, phentolamine used for extrav 10–15 mL NS w/ 5–10 mg of phentolamine

Doripenem (Doribax) Uses: *Complicated intra-Abd Infxn and UTI including pyelo* Acts: Carbapenem, ↓ cell wall synth, a β-lactam Spectrum: Excellent gram(+) (except MRSA and *Enterococcus* sp), excellent gram(−) coverage including β-lactamase producers, good anaerobic **Dose:** 500 mg IV q8h, ↓ w/ renal impair **W/P:** [B, ?] **CI:** Carbapenem β-lactams hypersens **Disp:** 250, 500 mg vial **SE:** HA, N/D, rash, phlebitis **Notes:** May ↓ valproic acid levels; overuse may ↑ bacterial resistance; monitor for *C. difficile*-associated D

Dornase Alfa (Pulmozyme, DNase) Uses: *↓↓ Frequency of resp Infxns in CF* **Acts:** Enzyme cleaves extracellular DNA, ↓ mucous viscosity **Dose:** *Adults.* Inh 2.5 mg/bid dosing w/ FVC > 85% w/ recommended nebulizer *Peds > 5 y.* Inh 2.5 mg/daily-bid if forced vital capacity > 85% **W/P:** [B, ?] **CI:** Chinese hamster product allergy **Disp:** Soln for Inh 1 mg/mL **SE:** Pharyngitis, voice alteration, CP, rash

Dorzolamide (Trusopt) Uses: *Open-angle glaucoma, ocular hypertension* **Acts:** Carbonic anhydrase inhib **Dose:** 1 gtt in eye(s) tid **W/P:** [C, ?] w/ NAG, CrCl < 30 mL/min **CI:** Component sensitivity **Disp:** 2% soln **SE:** Irritation, bitter taste, punctate keratitis, ocular allergic Rxn

Dorzolamide & Timolol (Cosopt) Uses: *Open-angle glaucoma, ocular hypertension* **Acts:** Carbonic anhydrase inhib w/ β-adrenergic blocker **Dose:** 1 gtt in eye(s) bid **W/P:** [C, ?] CrCl < 30 mL/min **CI:** Component sensitivity, asthma, severe COPD, sinus bradycardia, AV block **Disp:** Soln dorzolamide 2% & timolol 0.5% **SE:** Irritation, bitter taste, superficial keratitis, ocular allergic Rxn

Doxazosin (Cardura, Cardura XL) Uses: *HTN & symptomatic BPH* **Acts:** α₁-Adrenergic blocker; relaxes bladder neck smooth muscle **Dose:** *HTN:* Initial 1 mg/d PO; may be ↑ to 16 mg/d PO. *BPH:* Initial 1 mg/d PO, may ↑ to 8 mg/d; XL 4–8 mg q A.M. **W/P:** [C, ?] w/ Liver impair **CI:** Component sensitivity; use w/ PDE5 inhib (eg, sildenafil) can cause ↓ BP **Disp:** Tabs 1, 2, 4, 8 mg; XL 4, 8 mg **SE:** Dizziness, HA, drowsiness, fatigue, malaise, sexual dysfunction, doses > 4 mg ↑ postural ↓ BP risk; intraoperative floppy iris synd **Notes:** 1st dose hs; syncope may occur w/in 90 min of initial dose

Doxepin (Adapin) BOX: Closely monitor for worsening depression or emergence of suicidality Uses: *Depression, anxiety, chronic pain* **Acts:** TCA; ↑ synaptic CNS serotonin or norepinephrine **Dose:** 25–150 mg/d PO, usually hs but can ÷ doses; up to 300 mg/d for depression; ↓ in hepatic impair **W/P:** [C, ?/–] w/ EtOH abuse, elderly, w/ MAOI **CI:** NAG, urinary retention, MAOI use w/in 14 d, in recovery phase of MI **Disp:** Caps 10, 25, 50, 75, 100, 150 mg; PO conc 10 mg/mL **SE:** Anticholinergic SEs, ↓ BP, tachycardia, drowsiness, photosens

Doxepin (Silenor) Uses: *Insomnia* **Acts:** TCA **Dose:** Take w/in 30 min HS 6 mg qd; 3 mg in elderly; 6 mg/d max; not w/in 3 h of a meal **W/P:** [C, ?/–] w/ EtOH abuse/elderly/sleep apnea/CNS depressants; may cause abnormal thinking and hallucinations; may worsen depression **CI:** NAG, urinary retention, MAOI w/in 14 d **Disp:** Tabs 3, 6 mg **SE:** Somnolence/sedation, N, URI

Doxepin, Topical (Prudoxin, Zonalon) Uses: *Short-term Rx pruritus (atopic dermatitis or lichen simplex chronicus)* **Acts:** Antipruritic; H₁- & H₂-receptor antagonism **Dose:** Apply thin coating tid-qid, 8 d max **W/P:** [B, ?/–] **CI:** Component sensitivity **Disp:** 5% cream **SE:** ↓ BP, tachycardia, drowsiness, photosens **Notes:** Limit application area to avoid systemic tox

Doxorubicin (Adriamycin, Rubex) **Uses:** *Acute leukemias; Hodgkin Dz & NHLs; soft tissue, osteo- & Ewing sarcoma; Wilms tumor; neuroblastoma; bladder, breast, ovarian, gastric, thyroid, & lung CAs* **Acts:** Intercalates DNA; ↓ DNA topoisomerase I & II **Dose:** 60–75 mg/m² q3wk; ↓ w/ hepatic impair; IV use only ↓ cardiotox w/ weekly (20 mg/m²/wk) or cont Inf (60–90 mg/m² over 96 h); (per protocols) **W/P:** [D, ?] **CI:** Severe CHF, cardiomyopathy, preexisting ↓ BM, previous Rx w/ total cumulative doses of doxorubicin, idarubicin, daunorubicin **Disp:** Inj 10, 20, 50, 150, 200 mg **SE:** ↓ BM, venous streaking & phlebitis, N/V/D, mucositis, radiation recall phenomenon, cardiomyopathy rare (dose-related) **Notes:** Limit of 550 mg/m² cumulative dose (400 mg/m² w/ prior mediastinal irradiation); dexrazoxane may limit cardiac tox; tissue damage w/ extrav; red/orange urine; tissue vesicant w/ extrav, Rx w/ dexrazoxane

Doxycycline (Adoxa, Periostat, Oracea, Vibramycin, Vibra-Tabs) **Uses:** *Broad-spectrum antibiotic* acne vulgaris, uncomplicated GC, chlamydia, PID, Lyme Dz, skin Infxns, anthrax, malaria prophylaxis **Acts:** Tetracycline; bacteriostatic; ↓ protein synth. **Spectrum:** Limited gram(+) and (–), *Rickettsia* sp, *Chlamydia, M. pneumoniae, B. anthracis* **Dose:** *Adults.* 100 mg PO q12h on 1st d, then 100 mg PO daily-bid or 100 mg IV q12h; acne q day, chlamydia × 7 d, Lyme × 21 d, PID × 14 d *Peds > 8 y.* 5 mg/kg/24 h PO, 200 mg/d max ÷ daily-bid **W/P:** [D, –] hepatic impair **CI:** Children < 8 y, severe hepatic dysfunction **Disp:** Tabs 20, 50, 75, 100, 150 mg; caps 50, 75, 100, 150 mg; Oracea 40 mg caps (30 mg timed release, 10 mg DR); syrup 50 mg/5 mL; susp 25 mg/5 mL; Inj 100/vial **SE:** D, GI disturbance, photosens **Notes:** ↓ Effect w/ antacids; tetracycline of choice w/in renal impair; for inhalational anthrax use w/ 1–2 additional antibiotics, not for CNS anthrax

Dronabinol (Marinol) [C-III] **Uses:** *N/V associated w/ CA chemotherapy; appetite stimulation* **Acts:** Antiemetic; ↓ V center in the medulla **Dose:** *Adults & Peds.* Antiemetic: 5–15 mg/m²/dose q4–6h PRN. *Adults.* Appetite stimulant: 2.5 mg PO before lunch & dinner; max 20 mg/d **W/P:** [C, ?] Elderly, Hx psychological disorder, Sz disorder, substance abuse **CI:** Hx schizophrenia, sesame oil hypersens **Disp:** Caps 2.5, 5, 10 mg **SE:** Drowsiness, dizziness, anxiety, mood change, hallucinations, depersonalization, orthostatic ↓ BP, tachycardia **Notes:** Principal psychoactive substance present in marijuana

Dronedarone (Multaq) **BOX:** CI w/ NYHA Class IV HF or NYHA Class II-III HF w/ decompensation; CI in A Fib if cannot be converted to NSR **Uses:** *A Fib/A flutter* **Acts:** Antiarrhythmic **Dose:** 400 mg PO bid w/ A.M. and P.M. meal **W/P:** [X, –] w/ Other drugs (see PI); increased risk of death and serious CV events **CI:** See Box; 2nd-/3rd-degree AV block or SSS (unless w/ pacemaker), HR < 50 BPM, w/ strong CYP3A inhib, w/ drugs/herbals that ↑ QT interval, QTc interval ≥ 500 ms, severe hepatic impair, PRG **Disp:** Tabs 400 mg **SE:** N/V/D, Abd pain, asthenia, heart failure, ↑ K⁺, ↑ Mg²⁺, ↑ QTc, ↓ HR, ↑ SCr, rash **Notes:** Avoid grapefruit juice

Droperidol (Inapsine) **BOX:** Cases of QT interval prolongation and torsades de pointes (some fatal) reported **Uses:** *N/V; anesthetic premedication* **Acts:** Tranquilizer, sedation, antiemetic **Dose:** *Adults.* **N:** initial max 2.5 mg IV/IM, may repeat 1.25 mg based on response. **Peds.** *Premed:* 0.01–0.15 mg/kg/dose (max 1.25 mg); *N Tx* 0.1 mg/kg/dose (max 2.5 mg) **W/P:** [C, ?] w/ Hepatic/renal impair **CI:** Component sensitivity **Disp:** Inj 2.5 mg/mL **SE:** Drowsiness, ↓ BP, occasional tachycardia & extrapyramidal Rxns, ↑ QT interval, arrhythmias **Notes:** Give IV push slowly over 2–5 min

Duloxetine (Cymbalta) **BOX:** Antidepressants may ↑ risk of suicidality; consider risks/benefits of use. Closely monitor for clinical worsening, suicidality, or behavior changes **Uses:** *Depression, DM peripheral neuropathic pain, generalized anxiety disorder (GAD), fibromyalgia, chronic OA & back pain* **Acts:** Selective serotonin & norepinephrine reuptake inhib (SSNRI) **Dose:** *Depression:* 40–60 mg/d PO ÷ bid. *DM neuropathy:* 60 mg/d PO; *GAD:* 60 mg/d, max 120 mg/d; *Fibromyalgia, OA/back pain:* 30–60 mg/d, 60 mg/d max **W/P:** [C, ?/–]; use in 3rd tri; avoid if CrCl < 30 mL/min, NAG, w/ fluvoxamine, inhib of CYP2D6 (Table 10, p 319), TCAs, phenothiazines, type class IC antiarrhythmics (Table 9, p 318) **CI:** ↑ risk serotonin synd w/ MAOIs [linezolid or IV meth blue] MAOI use w/in 14 d, w/ thioridazine, NAG, hepatic Insuff **Disp:** Caps delayed-release 20, 30, 60 mg **SE:** N, dry mouth, somnolence, fatigue, constipation, ↓ appetite, hyperhydrosis **Notes:** Swallow whole; monitor BP; avoid abrupt D/C

Dutasteride (Avodart) **Uses:** *Symptomatic BPH to improve Sxs, ↓ risk of retention and BPH surgery alone or in combo w/ tamsulosin* **Acts:** 5α-Reductase inhib; ↓ intracellular dihydrotestosterone (DHT) **Dose:** *Monotherapy:* 0.5 mg PO/d. *Combo:* 0.5 mg PO q day w/ tamsulosin 0.4 mg q day **W/P:** [X, –] Hepatic impair; pregnant women should not handle pills; R/O CA before starting **CI:** Women, peds **Disp:** Caps 0.5 mg **SE:** ↑ Testosterone, ↑ TSH, impotence, ↓ libido, gynecomastia, ejaculatory disturbance, may ↑ risk of high-grade prostate CA **Notes:** No blood donation until 6 mo after D/C; ✓ PSA, ✓ new baseline PSA at 6 mo (corrected PSA × 2); any PSA rise on dutasteride suspicious for CA; now available in fixed dose combination w/ tamsulosin (see *Jalyn*)

Dutasteride & Tamsulosin (Jalyn) **Uses:** *Symptomatic BPH to improve Sxs* **Acts:** 5α-Reductase inhib (↓ intracellular DHT) w/ α-blocker **Dose:** 1 capsule daily after same meal **W/P:** [X, –] w/ CYP3A4 and CYP2D6 inhib may ↑ SEs; pregnant women should not handle pills; R/O CA before starting; IFIS (tamsulosin) discuss w/ ophthalmologist before cataract surgery; rare priapism; w/ warfarin; may ↑ risk of high-grade prostate CA **CI:** Women, peds, component sens **Disp:** Caps 0.5 mg dutasteride w/ 0.4 mg tamsulosin **SE:** Impotence, decreased libido, ejaculation disorders, and breast disorders **Notes:** No blood donation until 6 mo after D/C; ↓ PSA, ✓ new baseline PSA at 6 mo (corrected PSA × 2); any PSA rise on dutasteride suspicious for CA (see also dutasteride and tamsulosin)

Ecallantide (Kalbitor) **BOX:** Anaphylaxis reported, administer in a setting able to manage anaphylaxis and HAE, monitor closely **Uses:** *Acute attacks of hereditary angioedema (HAE)* **Acts:** Plasma kallikrein inhibitor **Dose:** *Adult & > 16 y.* 30 mg SC in three 10-mg injections; if attack persists may repeat 30-mg dose w/in 24 h **W/P:** [C, ?/−] Hypersens Rxns **CI:** Hypersens to ecallantide **Disp:** Inj 10 mg/mL **SE:** HA, N/V/D, pyrexia, Inj site Rxn, nasopharyngitis, fatigue, Abd pain

Echothiophate Iodine (Phospholine Ophthalmic) **Uses:** *Glaucoma* **Acts:** Cholinesterase inhib **Dose:** 1 gtt eye(s) bid w/ 1 dose hs **W/P:** [C, ?] CI: Active uveal inflammation, inflammatory Dz of iris/ciliary body, glaucoma iridocyclitis **Disp:** Powder for reconstitution 6.25 mg/5 mL (0.125%) **SE:** Local irritation, myopia, blurred vision, ↓ BP, ↓ HR

Econazole (Spectazole) **Uses:** *Tinea, cutaneous Candida, & tinea versicolor Infxns* **Acts:** Topical antifungal **Dose:** Apply to areas bid *Candida;* (daily for tinea versicolor) for 2–4 wk **W/P:** [C, ?] **CI:** Component sensitivity **Disp:** Topical cream 1% **SE:** Local irritation, pruritus, erythema **Notes:** Early Sx/clinical improvement; complete course to avoid recurrence

Eculizumab (Soliris) **BOX:** ↑ Risk of meningococcal Infxns (give meningococcal vaccine 2 wk prior to 1st dose and revaccinate per guidelines) **Uses:** *Rx paroxysmal nocturnal hemoglobinuria* **Acts:** Complement inhib **Dose:** 600 mg IV q7d × 4 wk, then 900 mg IV 5th dose 7 d later, then 900 mg IV q14d **W/P:** [C, ?] **CI:** Active *N. meningitidis* Infxn; if not vaccinated against *N. meningitidis* **Disp:** 300-mg vial **SE:** Meningococcal Infxn, HA, nasopharyngitis, N, back pain, Infxns, fatigue, severe hemolysis on D/C **Notes:** IV over 35 min (2-h max Inf time); monitor for 1 h for S/Sx of Inf Rxn

Edrophonium (Enlon) **Uses:** *Diagnosis of MyG; acute MyG crisis; curare antagonist, reverse of nondepolarizing neuromuscular blockers* **Acts:** Anticholinesterase **Dose:** *Adults.* Test for MyG: 2 mg IV in 1 min; if tolerated, give 8 mg IV; (+) test is brief ↑ in strength. *Peds.* See label **W/P:** [C, ?] **CI:** GI or GU obst; allergy to sulfite **Disp:** Inj 10 mg/mL **SE:** N/V/D, excessive salivation, stomach cramps, ↑ aminotransferases **Notes:** Can cause severe cholinergic effects; keep atropine available, 0.4–0.5 mg IV to Rx muscarinic SE (fasciculations, muscle weakness)

Efavirenz (Sustiva) **Uses:** *HIV Infxns* **Acts:** Antiretroviral; nonnucleoside RT inhib **Dose:** *Adults.* 600 mg/d PO q hs *Peds ≥ 3 y 10–< 15 kg.* 200 mg PO q day; *15–< 20 kg:* 250 mg PO q day; *20–< 25 kg:* 300 mg PO q day; *25–< 32.5 kg:* 350 mg PO q day; *32.5–< 40 kg:* 400 mg PO q day ≥ *40 kg:* 600 mg PO q day; on empty stomach **W/P:** [D, ?] CDC rec: HIV-infected mothers not breast-feed **CI:** w/ Astemizole, bepridil, cisapride, midazolam, pimozide, triazolam, ergot derivatives, voriconazole **Disp:** Caps 50, 200; 600 mg tab **SE:** Somnolence, vivid dreams, depression, CNS Sxs, dizziness, rash, N/V/D **Notes:** ✓ LFTs (especially w/ underlying liver Dz), cholesterol; not for monotherapy

Efavirenz, Emtricitabine, Tenofovir (Atripla) **BOX:** Lactic acidosis and severe hepatomegaly w/ steatosis, including fatal cases, reported w/ nucleoside analogs alone or combo w/ other antiretrovirals **Uses:** *HIV Infxns* **Acts:** Triple fixed-dose combo nonnucleoside RT inhib/nucleoside analog **Dose:** *Adults.* 1 tab q day on empty stomach; hs dose may ↓ CNS SE **W/P:** [D, ?] CDC rec: HIV-infected mothers not breast-feed, w/ obesity **CI:** < 12 y or < 40 kg, w/ astemizole, midazolam, triazolam, or ergot derivatives (CYP3A4 competition by efavirenz could cause serious/life-threatening SE) **Disp:** Tab (efavirenz 600 mg/emtricitabine 200 mg/tenofovir 300 mg) **SE:** Somnolence, vivid dreams, HA, dizziness, rash, N/V/D, ↓ BMD **Notes:** Monitor LFTs, cholesterol; see individual agents for additional info, not for HIV/hep B coinfection

Eletriptan (Relpax) **Uses:** *Acute Rx of migraine* **Acts:** Selective serotonin receptor (5-HT$_{1B/1D}$) agonist **Dose:** 20–40 mg PO, may repeat in 2 h; 80 mg/24 h max **W/P:** [C, ?/–] **CI:** Hx ischemic heart Dz, coronary artery spasm, stroke or TIA, peripheral vascular Dz, IBD, uncontrolled HTN, hemiplegic or basilar migraine, severe hepatic impair, w/in 24 h of another 5-HT$_1$ agonist or ergot, w/in 72 h of CYP3A4 inhib **Disp:** Tabs 20, 40 mg **SE:** Dizziness, somnolence, N, asthenia, xerostomia, paresthesias; pain, pressure, or tightness in chest, jaw, or neck; serious cardiac events

Eltrombopag (Promacta) **BOX:** May cause hepatotox ✓ baseline ALT/AST1/bili, q2wk w/ dosage adjustment, then monthly. D/C if ALT is > 3× ULN w/ ↑ bili, or Sx of liver injury **Uses:** *Tx ↑ plt in idiopathic thrombocytopenia refractory to steroids, immune globulins, splenectomy* **Acts:** Thrombopoietin receptor agonist **Dose:** 50 mg PO daily, adjust to keep plt ≥ 50,000 cells/mm^3; 75 mg max; start 25 mg/d if East-Asian or w/ hepatic impair; on an empty stomach; not w/in 4 h of product w/ polyvalent cations **W/P:** [C, ?/–] ↑ Risk for BM reticulin fiber deposition, heme malignancies, rebound ↓ plt on D/C, thromboembolism **CI:** None **Disp:** Tabs 12.5, 25, 50, 75 mg **SE:** Rash, bruising, menorrhagia, N/V, dyspepsia, ↓ plt, ↑ ALT/AST, limb pain, myalgia, paresthesia, cataract, conjunctival hemorrhage **Notes:** D/C if no ↑ plt count after 4 wk; restricted distribution *Promacta Cares (1-877-9-PROMACTA)*

Emedastine (Emadine) **Uses:** *Allergic conjunctivitis* **Acts:** Antihistamine; selective H$_1$-antagonist **Dose:** 1 gtt in eye(s) up to qid **W/P:** [B, ?] **CI:** Allergy to ingredients (preservatives benzalkonium, tromethamine) **Disp:** 0.05% soln **SE:** HA, blurred vision, burning/stinging, corneal infiltrates/staining, dry eyes, foreign body sensation, hyperemia, keratitis, tearing, pruritus, rhinitis, sinusitis, asthenia, bad taste, dermatitis, discomfort **Notes:** Do not use contact lenses if eyes are red

Emtricitabine (Emtriva) **BOX:** Lactic acidosis & severe hepatomegaly w/ steatosis reported; not for HBV Infxn **Uses:** *HIV-1 Infxn* **Acts:** NRTI **Dose:** 200 mg caps or 240 mg soln PO daily; ↓ w/ renal impair **W/P:** [B, –] Risk of liver Dz **CI:** Component sensitivity **Disp:** Soln 10 mg/mL, caps 200 mg **SE:** HA, N/D, rash, rare hyperpigmentation of feet & hands, posttreatment exacerbation of hep **Notes:** 1st once-daily NRTI; caps/soln not equivalent; not OK as monotherapy; screen for hep B, do not use w/ HIV & HBV coinfection

Enalapril (Vasotec) BOX: ACE inhib used during PRG can cause fetal injury & death Uses: *HTN, CHF, LVD*, DN Acts: ACE inhib Dose: *Adults.* 2.5–40 mg/d PO; 1.25 mg IV q6h. *Peds.* 0.05–0.08 mg/kg/d PO q12–24h; ↓ w/ renal impair W/P: [C (1st tri; D 2nd & 3rd tri), +] D/C immediately w/ PRG, w/ NSAIDs, K⁺ supplements CI: Bilateral RAS, angioedema Disp: Tabs 2.5, 5, 10, 20 mg; IV 1.25 mg/mL (1, 2 mL) SE: ↓ BP w/ initial dose (especially w/ diuretics), ↑ K⁺, ↑ Cr nonproductive cough, angioedema Notes: Monitor Cr; D/C diuretic for 2–3 d prior to start

Enfuvirtide (Fuzeon) BOX: Rarely allergy; never rechallenge Uses: *w/ Antiretroviral agents for HIV-1 in Tx-experienced pts w/ viral replication despite ongoing Rx* Acts: Viral fusion inhib Dose: *Adults.* 90 mg (1 mL) SQ bid in upper arm, anterior thigh, or Abd; rotate site Peds. See PI W/P: [B, –] CI: Previous allergy to drug Disp: 90 mg/mL recons; pt kit w/ supplies × 1 mo SE: Inj site Rxns; pneumonia, D, N, fatigue, insomnia, peripheral neuropathy Notes: Available via restricted distribution system; use immediately on recons or refrigerate (24 h max)

Enoxaparin (Lovenox) BOX: Recent or anticipated epidural/spinal anesthesia, ↑ risk of spinal/epidural hematoma w/ subsequent paralysis Uses: *Prevention & Rx of DVT; Rx PE; unstable angina & non–Q-wave MI* Acts: LMW heparin; inhibit thrombin by complexing w/ antithrombin III Dose: *Adults. Prevention:* 30 mg SQ bid or 40 mg SQ q24h. *DVT/PE Rx:* 1 mg/kg SQ q12h or 1.5 mg/kg SQ q24h. *Angina:* 1 mg/kg SQ q12h; *Ancillary to AMI fibrinolysis:* 30 mg IV bolus, then 1 mg/kg SQ bid; CrCl < 30 mL/min ↓ to 1 mg/kg SQ q day Peds. *Prevention:* 0.5 mg/kg SQ q12h. *DVT/PE Rx:* 1 mg/kg SQ q12h; ↓ dose w/ CrCl < 30 mL/min W/P: [B, ?] Not for prophylaxis in prosthetic heart valves CI: Active bleeding, HIT Ab, heparin, pork sens Disp: Inj 10 mg/0.1 mL (30-, 40-, 60-, 80-, 100-, 120-, 150-mg syringes); 300-mg/mL multi-dose vial SE: Bleeding, hemorrhage, bruising, thrombocytopenia, fever, pain/hematoma at site, ↑ AST/ALT Notes: No effect on bleeding time, plt Fxn, PT, or aPTT; monitor plt for HIT, clinical bleeding; may monitor antifactor Xa; not for IM

Entacapone (Comtan) Uses: *Parkinson Dz* Acts: Selective & reversible catechol-O-methyltransferase inhib Dose: 200 mg w/ each levodopa/carbidopa dose; max 1600 mg/d; ↓ levodopa/carbidopa dose 25% w/ levodopa dose > 800 mg W/P: [C, ?] Hepatic impair CI: Use w/ MAOI Disp: Tabs 200 mg SE: Dyskinesia, hyperkinesia, N, D, dizziness, hallucinations, orthostatic ↓ BP, brown-orange urine Notes: ✓ LFTs; do not D/C abruptly

Enzalutamide (Xtandi) Uses: *Metastatic castration-resistant prostate cancer w/ previous docetaxel* Acts: Androgen receptor inhibitor Dose *(men only):* 160 mg daily, do not chew/open caps W/P: [X, –] Sz risk CI: PRG Disp: Caps 40 mg SE: HA, dizziness, insomnia, fatigue, anxiety, MS pain, muscle weakness, paresthesia, back pain, spinal cord compression, cauda equina synd, arthralgias, edema, URI, lower resp Infxn, hematuria, ↑ BP Notes: Avoid w/ strong CYP2C8 inhib, strong/mod CYP3A4 or CYP2C8 induc, avoid CPY3A4, CYP2C9, CYP2C19 substrates w/ narrow therapeutic index; if on warfarin ✓ INR

Ephedrine Uses: *Acute bronchospasm, bronchial asthma, nasal congestion*, ↓ BP, narcolepsy, enuresis, & MyG Acts: Sympathomimetic; stimulates alpha- & beta-receptors; bronchodilator Dose: *Adults. Congestion:* 12.5–25 mg PO q4h PRN w/ expectorant; ↓ *BP:* 25–50 mg IV q5–10min, 150 mg/d max. *Peds.* 0.2–0.3 mg/kg/dose IV q4–6h PRN W/P: [C, ?/–] CI: Arrhythmias; NAG Disp: Caps 25 mg; Inj 50 mg/mL; nasal spray 0.25% SE: CNS stimulation (nervousness, anxiety, trembling), tachycardia, arrhythmia, HTN, xerostomia, dysuria Notes: Protect from light; monitor BP, HR, urinary output; can cause false(+) amphetamine EMIT; take last dose 4–6 h before hs; abuse potential, OTC sales mostly banned/ restricted

Epinastine (Elestat) Uses: Itching w/ allergic conjunctivitis Acts: Antihistamine Dose: 1 gtt bid W/P: [C, ?/–] Disp: Soln 0.05% SE: Burning, folliculosis, hyperemia, pruritus, URI, HA, rhinitis, sinusitis, cough, pharyngitis Notes: Remove contacts before, reinsert in 10 min

Epinephrine (Adrenalin, EpiPen, EpiPen Jr., Others) Uses: *Cardiac arrest, anaphylactic Rxn, bronchospasm, open-angle glaucoma* Acts: Betaadrenergic agonist, some alpha-effects Dose: *Adults. ECC 2010.* 1-mg (10 mL of 1:1000 soln) IV/IO push, repeat q3–5min (0.2 mg/kg max) if 1-mg dose fails Inf: 0.1–0.5 mcg/kg/min, titrate. ET 2–2.5 mg in 5–10 mL NS. *Profound bradycardia/ hypotension:* 2–10 mcg/min (1 mg in 250 mL D5W). *Allergic Rxn:* 0.3–0.5 mg (0.3–0.5 mL of 1:1000 soln) SQ. *Anaphylaxis:* 0.3–0.5 (0.3–0.5 mL of 1:1000 soln) IV. *Asthma:* 0.1–0.5 mL SQ of 1:1000 dilution, repeat q20min to 4 h, or 1 Inh (metered-dose) repeat in 1–2 min, or susp 0.1–0.3 mL SQ for extended effect. *Peds. ECC 2010.* Pulseless arrest: (0.01 mL/kg 1:1000) IV/IO q3–5min; max dose 1 mg; OK via ET tube (0.01 mL/kg 1:1000) until IV/IO access. *Symptomatic bradycardia:* 0.01 mg/kg (0.1 mL/kg 1:1000) cont Inf: typical 0.1–1 mcg/kg/min, titrate. *Anaphylaxis/status asthmaticus:* 0.01 mg/kg (0.1 mL/kg 1:1000) IM, repeat PRN; max single dose 0.3 mg W/P: [C, ?] ↓ bronchodilation w/ β-blockers CI: Cardiac arrhythmias, NAG Disp: Inj 1:1000, 1:2000, 1:10,000; nasal inhal 0.1%; oral inhal 2.25% soln; EpiPen Autoinjector 1 dose = 0.30 mg; EpiPen Jr. 1 dose = 0.15 mg SE: CV (tachycardia, HTN, vasoconstriction), CNS stimulation (nervousness, anxiety, trembling), ↓ renal blood flow Notes: Can give via ET tube if no central line (use 2–2.5 × IV dose); EpiPen for pt self-use (www.EpiPen.com)

Epirubicin (Ellence) BOX: Do not give IM or SQ. Extrav causes tissue necrosis; potential cardiotox; severe myelosuppression; ↓ dose w/ hepatic impair Uses: *Adjuvant Rx for (+) axillary nodes after resection of primary breast CA secondary AML* Acts: Anthracycline cytotoxic agent Dose: Per protocols; ↓ dose w/ hepatic impair W/P: [D, –] CI: Baseline neutrophil count < 1500 cells/mm^3, severe cardiac Insuff, recent MI, severe arrhythmias, severe hepatic dysfunction, previous anthracyclines Rx to max cumulative dose **Disp:** Inj 50 mg/25 mL, 200 mg/100 mL **SE:** Mucositis, N/V/D, alopecia, ↓ BM, cardiotox, secondary AML, tissue necrosis w/ extrav (see Adriamycin for Rx), lethargy **Notes:** ✓ CBC, bili, AST, Cr, cardiac Fxn before/during each cycle

Eplerenone (Inspra) Uses: *↑HTN, ↑ survival after MI w/ LVEF < 40% and CHF* **Acts:** Selective aldosterone antagonist **Dose:** *Adults.* 50 mg PO daily-bid, doses > 100 mg/d no benefit w/ ↑ K^+; ↓ to 25 mg PO daily if giving w/ CYP3A4 inhib w/ ACE inhib, ARBs, NSAIDs, K^+-sparing diuretics; grapefruit juice; St. John's Wort **CI:** K^+ > 5.5 mEq/L; non–insulin-dependent diabetes mellitus (NIDDM) w/ microalbuminuria; SCr > 2 mg/dL (males), > 1.8 mg/dL (females); CrCl < 30 mL/min; w/ K^+ supls/K^+-sparing diuretics, ketoconazole **Disp:** Tabs 25, 50 mg **SE:** ↑ cholesterol/triglycerides, ↑ K^+, HA, dizziness, gynecomastia, D, orthostatic ↓ BP **Notes:** May take 4 wk for full effect

Epoetin Alfa [Erythropoietin, EPO] (Epogen, Procrit) BOX: ↑ Mortality, serious CV/thromboembolic events, and tumor progression. Renal failure pts experienced ↑ greater risks (death/CV events) on erythropoiesis-stimulating agents (ESAs) to target Hgb levels 11 g/dL. Maintain Hgb 10–12 g/dL. In CA pt, ESAs ↓ survival/time to progression in some CA when dosed Hgb ≥ 12 g/dL. Use lowest dose needed. Use only for myelosuppressive chemotherapy. D/C following chemotherapy. Preop ESA ↑ DVT. Consider DVT prophylaxis Uses: *CRF-associated anemia, zidovudine Rx in HIV-infected pts, CA chemotherapy; ↓ transfusions associated w/ surgery* **Acts:** Induces erythropoiesis **Dose:** *Adults & Peds.* 50–150 units/kg IV/SQ 3×/wk; adjust dose q4–6wk PRN. *Surgery:* 300 units/kg/d × 10 d before to 4 d after; ↓ dose if Hct ~36% or Hgb, ↑ > ≥ 12 g/dL or Hgb ↑ > 1 g/dL in 2-wk period; hold dose if Hgb > 12 g/dL **W/P:** [C, ?/–] CI: Uncontrolled HTN **Disp:** Inj 2000, 3000, 4000, 10,000, 20,000, 40,000 units/mL **SE:** HTN, HA, fatigue, fever, tachycardia, N/V **Notes:** Refrigerate; monitor baseline & posttreatment Hct/Hgb, BP, ferritin

Epoprostenol (Flolan, Veletri) Uses: *Pulm HTN* **Acts:** Dilates pulm/systemic arterial vascular beds; ↓ plt aggregation **Dose:** Initial 2 ng/kg/min; ↑ by 2 ng/kg/min q15min until dose-limiting SE (CP, dizziness, N/V, HA, ↓ BP, flushing); IV cont Inf 4 ng/kg/min < max tolerated rate; adjust based on response; see PI **W/P:** [B, ?] ↑ tox w/ diuretics, vasodilators, acetate in dialysis fluids, anticoagulants **CI:** Chronic use in CHF 2nd degree, if pt develops pulm edema w/ dose initiation, severe LVSD **Disp:** Inj 0.5, 1.5 mg **SE:** Flushing, tachycardia, CHF, fever, chills, nervousness, HA, N/V/D, jaw pain, flu-like Sxs **Notes:** Abrupt D/C can cause rebound pulm HTN; monitor bleeding w/ other antiplatelet/anticoagulants; watch ↓ BP w/ other vasodilators/diuretics

Eprosartan (Teveten) Uses: *HTN*, DN, CHF **Acts:** ARB **Dose:** 400–800 mg/d single dose or bid **W/P:** [C (1st tri); D (2nd & 3rd tri), D/C immediately when PRG detected] w/ Li, ↑ K^+ w/ K^+-sparing diuretics/supls/high-dose trimethoprim

CI: Bilateral RAS, 1st-degree aldosteronism **Disp:** Tabs 400, 600 mg **SE:** Fatigue, depression, URI, UTI, Abd pain, rhinitis/pharyngitis/cough, hypertriglyceridemia

Eptifibatide (Integrilin) Uses: *ACS, PCI* Acts: Glycoprotein IIb/IIIa inhib **Dose:** 180 mcg/kg IV bolus, then 2 mcg/kg/min cont Inf; ↓ in renal impair (CrCl < 50 mL/min: 180 mcg/kg, then 1 mcg/kg/min); *ECC 2010. ACS:* 180 mcg/kg/min IV bolus over 1–2 min, then 2 mcg/kg/min, then repeat bolus in 10 min; continue infusion 18–24 h post-PCI **W/P:** [B, ?] Monitor bleeding w/ other anticoagulants **CI:** Other glycoprotein IIb/IIIa inhib, Hx abnormal bleeding, hemorrhagic stroke (w/in 30 d), severe HTN, major surgery (w/in 6 wk), plt count < 100,000 cells/mm³, renal dialysis **Disp:** Inj 0.75, 2 mg/mL **SE:** Bleeding, ↓ BP, Inj site Rxn, thrombocytopenia **Notes:** Monitor bleeding, coagulants, plts, SCr, activated coagulation time (ACT) w/ prothrombin consumption index (keep ACT 200–300 s)

Eribulin (Halaven) Uses: *Met breast CA after 2 chemo regimens (including anthracycline & taxane)* Acts: Microtubule inhibitor **Dose:** *Adults.* 1.4 mg/m² IV (over 2–5 min) days 1 & 8 of 21-d cycle; ↓ dose w/ hepatic & mod renal impair; delay/ ↓ for tox (see label) **W/P:** [D, –] **CI:** None **Disp:** Inj 0.5 mg/mL **SE:** ↓ WBC/Hct/plt, fatigue/asthenia, neuropathy, N/V/D, constipation, pyrexia, alopecia, ↑ QT, arthralgia/myalgia, back/pain, cough, dyspnea, UTI **Notes:** ✓ CBC & monitor for neuropathy prior to dosing

Erlotinib (Tarceva) Uses: *NSCLC after failing 1 chemotherapy; maint NSCLC who have not progressed after 4 cycles cisplatin-based therapy, CA pancreas* Acts: HER2/EGFR TKI **Dose:** CA pancreas 100 mg, others 150 mg/d PO 1 h ac or 2 h pc; ↓ (in 50-mg decrements) w/ severe Rxn or w/ CYP3A4 inhib (Table 10, p 319); per protocols **W/P:** [D, ?/–] Avoid pregnancy; w/ CYP3A4 inhib (Table 10, p 319) **Disp:** Tabs 25, 100, 150 mg **SE:** Rash, N/V/D, anorexia, Abd pain, fatigue, cough, dyspnea, edema, stomatitis, conjunctivitis, pruritus, skin/nail changes, Infxn, ↑ LFTs, interstitial lung Dz **Notes:** May ↑ INR w/ warfarin, monitor INR

Ertapenem (Invanz) Uses: *Complicated intra-Abd, acute pelvic, & skin Infxns, pyelonephritis, CAP* Acts: α-carbapenem; β-lactam antibiotic, ↓ cell wall synth. *Spectrum:* Good gram(+/–) & anaerobic coverage, not *Pseudomonas*, PCN-resistant pneumococci, MRSA, *Enterococcus*, β-lactamase (+) *H. influenzae, Mycoplasma, Chlamydia* **Dose:** *Adults.* 1 g IM/IV daily; 500 mg/d in CrCl < 30 mL/min *Peds 3 mo–12 y.* 15 mg/kg bid IM/IV, max 1 g/d **W/P:** [B, ?/–] Sz Hx, CNS disorders, β-lactam & multiple allergies, probenecid ↓ renal clearance **CI:** component hypersens or amide anesthetics **Disp:** Inj 1 g/vial **SE:** HA, N/V/D, Inj site Rxns, thrombocytosis, ↑ LFTs **Notes:** Can give IM × 7 d, IV × 14 d; 137 mg Na⁺ (6 mEq)/g ertapenem

Erythromycin (E-Mycin, E.E.S., Ery-Tab, EryPed, Ilotycin) Uses: *Bacterial Infxns; bowel prep*; ↑ GI motility (prokinetic); *acne vulgaris* Acts: Bacteriostatic; interferes w/ protein synth. *Spectrum:* Group A streptococci (*S. pyogenes*), *S. pneumoniae, N. gonorrhoeae* (if PCN-allergic), *Legionella, M. pneumoniae* **Dose:** *Adults.* Base 250–500 mg PO q6–12h or ethylsuccinate 400–800 mg q6–12h; 500 mg–1 g IV q6h. *Prokinetic:* 250 mg PO tid 30 min ac. **Peds.** 30–50 mg/kg/d PO ÷ q6–8h or 20–40 mg/kg/d IV ÷ q6h, max 2 g/d **W/P:** [B, +] Pseudomembranous colitis risk, ↑ tox of carbamazepine, cyclosporine, digoxin, methylprednisolone, theophylline, felodipine, warfarin, simvastatin/lovastatin; ↓ sildenafil dose w/ use **CI:** Hepatic impair, preexisting liver Dz (estolate), use w/ pimozide ergotamine dihydroergotamine **Disp:** *Lactobionate (Ilotycin): Powder for Inj* 500 mg, 1 g. *Base:* Tabs 250, 333, 500 mg; caps 250 mg. *Stearate (Erythrocin):* Tabs 250, 500 mg. *Ethylsuccinate (EES, EryPed):* Chew tabs 200 mg; tabs 400 mg; susp 200, 400 mg/5 mL **SE:** HA, Abd pain, N/V/D; ↑ QT, torsades de pointes, ventricular arrhythmias/tachycardias (rarely); cholestatic jaundice (estolate) **Notes:** 400 mg ethylsuccinate = 250 mg base/estolate; w/ food minimizes GI upset; lactobionate contains benzyl alcohol (caution in neonates)

Erythromycin, Ophthalmic (Ilotycin Ophthalmic)   **Uses:** *Conjunctival/corneal Infxns* **Acts:** Macrolide antibiotic **Dose:** 1/2 in 2–6×/d **W/P:** [B, +] **CI:** Erythromycin hypersens **Disp:** 0.5% oint **SE:** Local irritation

Erythromycin, Topical (Akne-Mycin, Ery, Erythra-Derm, Generic) **Uses:** *Acne vulgaris* **Acts:** Macrolide antibiotic **Dose:** Wash & dry area, apply 2% product over area bid **W/P:** [B, +] Pseudomembranous colitis possible **CI:** Component sensitivity **Disp:** Soln 1.5%, 2%; gel 2%; pads & swabs 2% **SE:** Local irritation

Erythromycin/Benzoyl Peroxide (Benzamycin)   **Uses:** *Topical for acne vulgaris* **Acts:** Macrolide antibiotic w/ keratolytic **Dose:** Apply bid (A.M. & P.M.) **W/P:** [C, ?] **CI:** Component sensitivity **Disp:** Gel erythromycin 30 mg/benzoyl peroxide 50 mg/g **SE:** Local irritation, dryness

Erythromycin/Sulfisoxazole (E.S.P.)   **Uses:** *Upper & lower resp tract; bacterial Infxns; H. influenzae otitis media in children*; Infxns in PCN-allergic pts **Acts:** Macrolide antibiotic w/ sulfonamide **Dose:** **Adults.** Based on erythromycin content; 400 mg erythromycin/1200 mg sulfisoxazole PO q6h. **Peds > 2 mo.** 40–50 mg/kg/d erythromycin & 150 mg/kg/d sulfisoxazole PO ÷ q6h; max 2 g/d erythromycin or 6 g/d sulfisoxazole × 10 d; ↓ in renal impair **W/P:** [C (D if near term), +] w/ PO anticoagulants, hypoglycemics, phenytoin, cyclosporine **CI:** Infants < 2 mo **Disp:** Susp erythromycin ethylsuccinate 200 mg/sulfisoxazole 600 mg/5 mL (100, 150, 200 mL) **SE:** GI upset

Escitalopram (Lexapro, Generic)   **BOX:** Closely monitor for worsening depression or emergence of suicidality, particularly in ped pts **Uses:** Depression, anxiety **Acts:** SSRI **Dose:** **Adults.** 10–20 mg PO daily; 10 mg/d in elderly & hepatic impair **W/P:** [C, +/−] Serotonin synd (Table 11, p 321); use of escitalopram, w/ NSAID, ASA, or other drugs affecting coagulation associated w/ ↑ bleeding risk **CI:** w/in 14 d of MAOI **Disp:** Tabs 5, 10, 20 mg; soln 1 mg/mL **SE:** N/V/D, sweating, insomnia, dizziness, xerostomia, sexual dysfunction **Note:** Full effects may take 3 wk

Esmolol (Brevibloc, Generic) Uses: *SVT & noncompensatory sinus tachycardia, AF/A flutter* Acts: β₁-Adrenergic blocker; class II antiarrhythmic Dose: *Adults & Peds. ECC 2010.* 0.5 mg/kg (500 mcg/kg) over 1 min, then 0.05 mg/kg/min (50 mcg/kg/min) Inf; if inadequate response after 5 min, repeat 0.5 mg/kg bolus, then titrate Inf up to 0.2 mg/kg/min (200 mcg/kg/min); max 0.3 mg/kg/min (300 mcg/kg/min) W/P: [C (1st tri; D 2nd or 3rd tri), ?] CI: Sinus bradycardia, heart block, uncompensated CHF, cardiogenic shock, ↓ BP Disp: Inj 10, 20, 250 mg/mL; premix Inf 10 mg/mL SE: ↓ BP; ↓ HR, diaphoresis, dizziness, pain on Inj Notes: Hemodynamic effects back to baseline w/in 30 min after D/C Inf

Esomeprazole (Nexium) Uses: *Short-term (4–8 wk) for erosive esophagitis/GERD; H. pylori Infxn in combo w/ antibiotics* Acts: Proton pump inhib, ↓ gastric acid Dose: *Adults. GERD/erosive gastritis:* 20–40 mg/d PO × 4–8 wk; 20–40 mg IV 10–30 min Inf or > 3 min IV push, 10 d max; *Maint:* 20 mg/d PO. *H. pylori Infxn:* 40 mg/d PO, plus clarithromycin 500 mg PO bid & amoxicillin 1000 mg/bid for 10 d; W/P: [B, ?/–] CI: Component sensitivity; do not use w/ clopidogrel (↓ effect) Disp: Caps 20, 40 mg; IV 20, 40 mg SE: HA, D, Abd pain Notes: Do not chew; may open caps & sprinkle on applesauce; ? ↑ risk of fractures w/ all PPI; risk of hypomagnesemia w/ long-term use, monitor

Estazolam (ProSom, Generic) [C-IV] Uses: *Short-term management of insomnia* Acts: Benzodiazepine Dose: 1–2 mg PO qhs PRN; ↓ in hepatic impair/ elderly/debilitated W/P: [X, –] ↑ Effects w/ CNS depressants; cross-sensitivity w/ other benzodiazepines CI: PRG, component hypersens, w/ itraconazole or ketoconazole Disp: Tabs 1, 2 mg SE: Somnolence, weakness, palpitations, anaphylaxis, angioedema, amnesia Notes: May cause psychological/physical dependence; avoid abrupt D/C after prolonged use

Esterified Estrogens (Menest) [C-IV] BOX: ↑ Risk endometrial CA. Do not use in the prevention of CV Dz or dementia; ↑ risk of MI, stroke, breast CA, PE, DVT, in postmenopausal Uses: *Vasomotor Sxs or vulvar/Vag atrophy w/ menopause; female hypogonadism, PCa* Acts: Estrogen supl Dose: *Menopausal vasomotor Sx:* 0.3–1.25 mg/d, cyclically 3 wk on, 1 wk off; add progestin 10–14 d w/ 28-d cycle w/ uterus intact; *Vulvovaginal atrophy:* Same regimen except use 0.3–1.25 mg; *Hypogonadism:* 2.5–7.5 mg/d PO × 20 d, off × 10 d; add progestin 10–14 d w/ 28-d cycle w/ uterus intact W/P: [X, –] CI: Undiagnosed genital bleeding, breast CA, estrogen-dependent tumors, thromboembolic disorders, thrombophlebitis, recent MI, PRG, severe hepatic Dz Disp: Tabs 0.3, 0.625, 1.25, 2.5 mg SE: N, HA, bloating, breast enlargement/tenderness, edema, venous thromboembolism, hypertriglyceridemia, gallbladder Dz Notes: Use lowest dose for shortest time (see WHI data [www.whi.org])

Estradiol, Gel (Divigel) BOX: ↑ Risk endometrial CA. Do not use to prevent CV Dz or dementia; ↑ risk MI, stroke, breast CA, PE, and DVT in postmenopausal (50–79 y). ↑ Dementia risk in postmenopausal (≥ 65 y) Uses: *Vasomotor Sx in menopause* Acts: Estrogen Dose: 0.25 g q day on right or left upper thigh (alternate) W/P: [X, +/–] May ↑ thyroid binding globulin (TBD) w/ thyroid Dz CI:

Undiagnosed genital bleeding, breast CA, estrogen-dependent tumors, thromboembolic disorders, thrombophlebitis, recent MI, PRG, severe hepatic Dz **Disp:** 0.1% gel 0.25/0.5/1 g single-dose foil packets w/ 0.25-, 0.5-, 1-mg estradiol, respectively **SE:** N, HA, bloating, breast enlargement/tenderness, edema, venous thromboembolism, ↑ BP, hypertriglyceridemia, gallbladder Dz **Notes:** If person other than pt applies, glove should be used, keep dry immediately after, rotate site; contains alcohol, caution around flames until dry, not for Vag use

Estradiol, Metered Gel (Elestrin, Estrogel) **BOX:** ↑ Risk endometrial CA. Do not use to prevent CV Dz or dementia; ↑ risk MI, stroke, breast CA, PE, and DVT in postmenopausal (50–79 y). ↑ Dementia risk in postmenopausal (≥ 65 y) **Uses:** *Postmenopausal vasomotor Sxs* **Acts:** Estrogen **Dose:** Apply 0.87–1.7 g to upper arm skin q day; add progestin × 10–14 d/28-d cycle w/ intact uterus; use lowest effective estrogen dose **W/P:** [X, ?] **CI:** AUB, breast CA, estrogen-dependent tumors, hereditary angioedema, thromboembolic disorders, recent MI, PRG, severe hepatic Dz **Disp:** Gel 0.06%; metered dose/activation **SE:** Thromboembolic events, MI, stroke, ↑ BP, breast/ovarian/endometrial CA, site Rxns, Vag spotting, breast changes, Abd bloating, cramps, HA, fluid retention **Notes:** Wait > 25 min before sunscreen; avoid concomitant use for > 7 d; BP, breast exams

Estradiol, Oral (Delestrogen, Estrace, Femtrace) **BOX:** ↑ Risk endometrial CA. Do not use to prevent CV Dz or dementia; ↑ risk MI, stroke, breast CA, PE, and DVT in postmenopausal (50–79 y). ↑ Dementia risk in posmenopausal (≥ 65 y) **Uses:** *Atrophic vaginitis, menopausal vasomotor Sxs, prevent osteoporosis, ↑ low estrogen levels, palliation breast and PCa* **Acts:** Estrogen **Dose:** *PO:* 1–2 mg/d, adjust PRN to control Sxs. *Vag cream:* 2–4 g/d × 2 wk, then 1 g 1–3×/wk. *Vasomotor Sx/Vag atrophy:* 10–20 mg IM q4wk, D/C or taper at 3- to 6-mo intervals. *Hypoestrogenism:* 10–20 mg IM q4wk. *PCa:* 30 mg IM q12wk **W/P:** [X, −] **CI:** Genital bleeding of unknown cause, breast CA, porphyria, estrogen-dependent tumors, thromboembolic disorders, thrombophlebitis; recent MI; hepatic impair **Disp:** Tabs 0.5, 1, 2 mg; depot Inj (*Delestrogen*) 10, 20, 40 mg/mL **SE:** N, HA, bloating, breast enlargement/tenderness, edema, ↑ triglycerides, venous thromboembolism, gallbladder Dz **Notes:** When estrogen used in postmenopausal w/ uterus, use w/ progestin

Estradiol, Spray (Evamist) **BOX:** ↑ Risk endometrial CA. Do not use to prevent CV Dz or dementia; ↑ risk MI, stroke, breast CA, PE, and DVT in postmenopausal (50–79 y). ↑ Dementia risk in posmenopausal (≥ 65 y) **Uses:** *Vasomotor Sx in menopause* **Acts:** Estrogen supl **Dose:** 1 spray on inner surface of forearm **W/P:** [X, +/−] May ↑ PT/PTT/plt aggregation w/ thyroid Dz **CI:** Undiagnosed genital bleeding, breast CA, estrogen-dependent tumors, thromboembolic disorders, thrombophlebitis, recent MI, PRG, severe hepatic Dz **Disp:** 1.53 mg/spray (56-spray container) **SE:** N, HA, bloating, breast enlargement/tenderness, edema, venous thromboembolism, ↑ BP, hypertriglyceridemia, gallbladder Dz **Notes:** Contains alcohol, caution around flames until dry; not for Vag use

Estradiol, Transdermal (Alora, Climara, Estraderm, Vivelle Dot)
BOX: ↑ Risk endometrial CA. Do not use to prevent CV Dz or dementia; ↑ risk MI, stroke, breast CA, PE, and DVT in postmenopausal (50–79 y). ↑ Dementia risk in postmenopausal (≥ 65 y) **Uses:** *Severe menopausal vasomotor Sxs; female hypogonadism* **Acts:** Estrogen supl **Dose:** Start 0.0375–0.05 mg/d patch 1–2×/wk based on product (*Climara* 1×/wk; *Alora* 2×wk) adjust PRN to control Sxs; w/ intact uterus cycle 3 wk on 1 wk off or use cyclic progestin 10–14 d **W/P:** [X, –] See estradiol **CI:** PRG, AUB, porphyria, breast CA, estrogen-dependent tumors, Hx thrombophlebitis, thrombosis **Disp:** Transdermal patches (mg/24 h) 0.025, 0.0375, 0.05, 0.06, 0.075, 0.1 **SE:** N, bloating, breast enlargement/tenderness, edema, HA, hypertriglyceridemia, gallbladder Dz **Notes:** Do not apply to breasts, place on trunk, rotate sites; see estradiol, oral notes

Estradiol, Vaginal (Estring, Femring, Vagifem) BOX: ↑ Risk endometrial CA. Do not use to prevent CV Dz or dementia; ↑ risk MI, stroke, breast CA, PE, and DVT in postmenopausal (50–79 y). ↑ Dementia risk in postmenopausal (≥ 65 y) **Uses:** *Postmenopausal Vag atrophy (Estring)* *vasomotor Sxs and vulvar/Vag atrophy associated w/ menopause (Femring)* *atrophic vaginitis (Vagifem)* **Acts:** Estrogen supl **Dose:** *Estring:* Insert ring into upper third of Vag vault; remove and replace after 90 d; reassess 3–6 mo; *Femring:* Use lowest effective dose, insert vaginally, replace q3mo; *Vagifem:* 1 tab vaginally q day × 2 wk, then maint 1 tab 2×/ wk, D/C or taper at 3–6 mo **W/P:** [X, –] May ↑ PT/PTT/plt aggregation w/ thyroid Dz, toxic shock reported **CI:** Undiagnosed genital bleeding, breast CA, estrogen-dependent tumors, thromboembolic disorders, thrombophlebitis, recent MI, PRG, severe hepatic Dz **Disp:** *Estring ring:* 0.0075 mg/24 h; *Femring ring:* 0.05 and 0.1 mg/d *Vagifem tab (Vag):* 10 mcg **SE:** HA, leukorrhea, back pain, candidiasis, vaginitis, Vag discomfort/hemorrhage, arthralgia, insomnia, Abd pain; see estradiol, oral notes

Estradiol/Levonorgestrel, Transdermal (Climara Pro) BOX: ↑ Risk endometrial CA. Do not use to prevent CV Dz or dementia; ↑ risk MI, stroke, breast CA, PE, and DVT in postmenopausal (50–79 y). ↑ Dementia risk in postmenopausal (≥ 65 y) **Uses:** *Menopausal vasomotor Sx; prevent postmenopausal osteoporosis* **Acts:** Estrogen & progesterone **Dose:** 1 patch 1×/wk **W/P:** [X, –] w/ ↓ Thyroid **CI:** AUB, estrogen-sensitive tumors, Hx thromboembolism, liver impair, PRG, hysterectomy **Disp:** Estradiol 0.045 mg/levonorgestrel 0.015 mg day patch **SE:** Site Rxn, Vag bleed/spotting, breast changes, Abd bloating/ cramps, HA, retention fluid, edema, ↑ BP **Notes:** Apply lower Abd; for osteoporosis give Ca²⁺/vit D supl; follow breast exams

Estradiol/Norethindrone (Activella, Generic) BOX: ↑ Risk endometrial CA. Do not use to prevent CV Dz or dementia; ↑ risk MI, stroke, breast CA, PE, and DVT in postmenopausal (50–79 y). ↑ Dementia risk in postmenopausal (≥ 65 y) **Uses:** *Menopause vasomotor Sxs; prevent osteoporosis* **Acts:** Estrogen/progestin; plant derived **Dose:** 1 tab/d start w/ lowest dose combo **W/P:** [X, –] w/ ↓ Ca²⁺/thyroid **CI:** PRG; Hx breast CA; estrogen-dependent tumor; abnormal genital bleeding; Hx DVT, PE, or related disorders; recent (w/in past year) arterial thromboembolic Dz (CVA, MI) **Disp:** *Femhrt:* Tabs 2.5/0.5, 5 mcg/1 mg; *Activella:* Tabs 1/0.5, 0.5 mg/0.1 mg **SE:** Thrombosis, dizziness, HA, libido changes, insomnia, emotional instability, breast pain **Notes:** Use in women w/ intact uterus; caution in heavy smokers; combo also used as OCP

Estramustine Phosphate (Emcyt) **Uses:** *Advanced PCa* **Acts:** Estradiol w/ nitrogen mustard; exact mechanism unknown **Dose:** 14 mg/kg/d in 3–4 ÷ doses; on empty stomach, no dairy products **W/P:** [NA, not used in females] **CI:** Active thrombophlebitis or thromboembolic disorders **Disp:** Caps 140 mg **SE:** N/V, exacerbation of preexisting CHF, edema, hepatic disturbances, thrombophlebitis, MI, PE, gynecomastia in 20–100% **Notes:** Low-dose breast irradiation before may ↓ gynecomastia

Estrogen, Conjugated (Premarin) **BOX:** ↑ Risk endometrial CA. Do not use to prevent CV Dz or dementia; ↑ risk MI, stroke, breast CA, PE, and DVT in postmenopausal (50–79 y). ↑ Dementia risk in postmenopausal (≥ 65 y) **Uses:** *Mod–severe menopausal vasomotor Sxs; atrophic vaginitis, dyspareunia*; palliative advanced CAP; prevention & Tx of estrogen deficiency osteoporosis **Acts:** Estrogen replacement **Dose:** 0.3–1.25 mg/d PO; intravaginal cream 0.5–2g × 21 d, then off × 7 d or 0.5 mg twice weekly **W/P:** [X, –] **CI:** Severe hepatic impair, genital bleeding of unknown cause, breast CA, estrogen-dependent tumors, thromboembolic disorders, thrombosis, thrombophlebitis, recent MI **Disp:** Tabs 0.3, 0.45, 0.625, 0.9, 1.25 mg; Vag cream 0.625 mg/g **SE:** ↑ Risk of endometrial CA, gallbladder Dz, thromboembolism, HA, & possibly breast CA **Notes:** Generic products not equivalent

Estrogen, Conjugated + Medroxyprogesterone (Prempro, Premphase) **BOX:** ↑ Risk endometrial CA. Do not use to prevent CV Dz or dementia; ↑ risk MI, stroke, breast CA, PE, and DVT in postmenopausal (50–79 y). ↑ Dementia risk in postmenopausal (≥ 65 y) **Uses:** *Mod–severe menopausal vasomotor Sxs; atrophic vaginitis; prevent postmenopausal osteoporosis* **Acts:** Hormonal replacement **Dose:** *Prempro* 1 tab PO daily; *Premphase* 1 tab PO daily **W/P:** [X, –] **CI:** Severe hepatic impair, genital bleeding of unknown cause, breast CA, estrogen-dependent tumors, thromboembolic disorders, thrombosis, thrombophlebitis **Disp:** (As estrogen/ medroxyprogesterone) *Prempro:* Tabs 0.3/1.5, 0.45/1.5, 0.625/2.5, 0.625/5 mg; *Premphase:* Tabs 0.625/0 (d 1–14) & 0.625/5 mg (d 15–28) **SE:** Gallbladder Dz, thromboembolism, HA, breast tenderness **Notes:** See WHI (www.whi.org); use lowest dose/shortest time possible

Estrogen, Conjugated Synthetic (Cenestin, Enjuvia) **BOX:** ↑ Risk endometrial CA. Do not use to prevent CV Dz or dementia; ↑ risk MI, stroke, breast CA, PE, and DVT in postmenopausal (50–79 y). ↑ Dementia risk in postmenopausal (≥ 65 y) **Uses:** *Vasomotor menopausal Sxs, vulvovaginal atrophy* **Acts:** Multiple estrogen replacement **Dose:** For all w/ intact uterus progestin × 10–14 d/28-d cycle; *Vasomotor:* 0.3–1.25 mg (*Enjuvia*) 0.625–1.25 mg (*Cenestin*) PO daily; *Vag atrophy:* 0.3 mg/d; *Osteoporosis:* (*Cenestin*) 0.625 mg/d **W/P:** [X, –] **CI:** See Estrogen, conjugated **Disp:** Tabs, *Cenestin,* 0.3, 0.45, 0.625, 0.9, 1.25 mg; *Enjuvia* ER

0.3, 0.45, 0.625, 0.9, 1.25 mg **SE:** ↑ Risk endometrial/breast CA, gallbladder Dz, thromboembolism

Eszopiclone (Lunesta) [C-IV] Uses: *Insomnia* **Acts:** Nonbenzodiazepine hypnotic **Dose:** 2–3 mg/d hs *Elderly:* 1–2 mg/d hs; w/ hepatic impair use w/ CYP3A4 inhib (Table 10, p 319): 1 mg/d hs **W/P:** [C, ?/–] **Disp:** Tabs 1, 2, 3 mg **SE:** HA, xerostomia, dizziness, somnolence, hallucinations, rash, Infxn, unpleasant taste, anaphylaxis, angioedema **Notes:** High-fat meals ↓ absorption

Etanercept (Enbrel) BOX: Serious Infxns (bacterial sepsis, TB, reported); D/C w/ severe Infxn. Evaluate for TB risk; test for TB before use; lymphoma/other CA possible in children/adolescents possible Uses: *↓ Sxs of RA in pts who fail other DMARD*, Crohn Dz **Acts:** TNF-receptor blocker **Dose:** *Adults.* RA 50 mg SQ weekly or 25 mg SQ 2×/wk (separated by at least 72–96 h). *Peds 4–17 y.* 0.8 mg/kg/wk (max 50 mg/wk) or 0.4 mg/kg (max 25 mg/dose) 2×/wk 72–96 h apart **W/P:** [B, ?] w/ Predisposition to Infxn (ie, DM); may ↑ risk of malignancy in peds and young adults **CI:** Active Infxn **Disp:** Inj 25 mg/vial, 50 mg syringe **SE:** HA, rhinitis, Inj site Rxn, URI, new-onset psoriasis **Notes:** Rotate Inj sites

Ethambutol (Myambutol, Generic) Uses: *Pulm TB* & other mycobacterial Infxns, MAC **Acts:** ↓ RNA synth **Dose:** *Adults & Peds > 12 y.* 15–25 mg/kg/d PO single dose; ↓ in renal impair, take w/ food, avoid antacids **W/P:** [C, +] **CI:** Unconscious pts, optic neuritis **Disp:** Tabs 100, 400 mg **SE:** HA, hyperuricemia, acute gout, Abd pain, ↑ LFTs, optic neuritis, GI upset

Ethinyl Estradiol & Norelgestromin (Ortho Evra) BOX: Cigarette smoking ↑ risk of serious CV events. ↑ Risk w/ age & no. of cigarettes smoked. Hormonal contraceptives should not be used by women who are > 35 y and smoke. Different from OCP pharmacokinetics Uses: *Contraceptive patch* **Acts:** Estrogen & progestin **Dose:** Apply patch to Abd, buttocks, upper torso (not breasts), or upper outer arm at the beginning of the menstrual cycle; new patch is applied weekly for 3 wk; wk 4 is patch-free **W/P:** [X, +/–] **CI:** PRG, Hx or current DVT/ PE, stroke, MI, CV Dz, CAD; SBP ≥ 160 systolic mm Hg or DBP ≥ 100 diastolic mm Hg severe HTN; severe HA w/ focal neurologic Sx; breast/endometrial CA; estrogen-dependent neoplasms; hepatic dysfunction; jaundice; major surgery w/ prolonged immobilization; heavy smoking if > 35 y **Disp:** 20 cm² patch (6-mg norelgestromin [active metabolite norgestimate] & 0.75 mg of ethinyl estradiol) **SE:** Breast discomfort, HA, site Rxns, N, menstrual cramps; thrombosis risks similar to OCP **Notes:** Less effective in women > 90 kg; instruct pt does not protect against STD/HIV; discourage smoking

Ethosuximide (Zarontin, Generic) Uses: *Absence (petit mal) Szs* **Acts:** Anticonvulsant; ↑ Sz threshold **Dose:** *Adults & peds > 6 y.* Initial, 500 mg PO ÷ bid; ↑ by 250 mg/d q4–7d PRN (max 1500 mg/d) usual maint 20–30 mg/ kg. *Peds 3–6 y.* 250 mg/d; ↑ by 250 mg/d q4–7d PRN; maint 20–30 mg/kg/d ÷ bid; max 1500 mg/d **W/P:** [D, +] In renal/hepatic impair; antiepileptics may ↑ risk of suicidal behavior or ideation **CI:** Component sensitivity **Disp:** Caps 250 mg; syrup

250 mg/5 mL **SE:** Blood dyscrasias, GI upset, drowsiness, dizziness, irritability **Notes:** Levels: *Trough:* just before next dose; *Therapeutic: Peak:* 40–100 mcg/mL; *Toxic Trough:* > 100 mcg/mL; *Half-life:* 25–60 h

Etidronate Disodium (Didronel, Generic) Uses: *↑ Ca^{2+} of malignancy, Paget Dz, & heterotopic ossification* **Acts:** ↓ Nl & abnormal bone resorption **Dose:** *Paget Dz:* 5–10 mg/kg/d PO ÷ doses (for 3–6 mo). ↑ Ca^{2+}: 20 mg/kg/d IV × 30–90 d **W/P:** [B PO (C parenteral), ?] Bisphosphonates may cause severe musculoskeletal pain **CI:** Overt osteomalacia, SCr > 5 mg/dL **Disp:** Tabs 200, 400 mg **SE:** GI intolerance (↓ by ÷ daily doses); hyperphosphatemia, hypomagnesemia, bone pain, abnormal taste, fever, convulsions, nephrotox **Notes:** Take PO on empty stomach 2 h before or 2 h pc

Etodolac BOX: May ↑ risk of CV events & GI bleeding; may worsen ↑ BP Uses: *OA & pain*, RA **Acts:** NSAID **Dose:** 200–400 mg PO bid-qid (max 1200 mg/d) **W/P:** [C (D 3rd tri), ?] ↑ Bleeding risk w/ ASA, warfarin; ↑ nephrotox w/ cyclosporine; Hx CHF, HTN, renal/hepatic impair, PUD **CI:** Active GI ulcer **Disp:** Tabs 400, 500 mg; ER tabs 400, 500, 600 mg; caps 200, 300 mg **SE:** N/V/D, gastritis, Abd cramps, dizziness, HA, depression, edema, renal impair **Notes:** Do not crush tabs

Etomidate (Amidate, Generic) Uses: *Induce general or short-procedure anesthesia* **Acts:** Short-acting hypnotic **Dose:** *Adults & Peds > 10 y.* Induce anesthesia 0.2–0.6 mg/kg IV over 30–60 s; *Peds < 10 y.* Not recommended Peds. ECC 2010. *Rapid sedation:* 0.2–0.4 mg/kg IV/IO over 30–60 s; max dose 20 mg **W/P:** [C, ?] **CI:** Hypersens **Disp:** Inj 2 mg/mL **SE:** Inj site pain, myoclonus

Etonogestrel Implant (Implanon) Uses: *Contraception* **Acts:** Transforms endometrium from proliferative to secretory **Dose:** 1 implant subdermally q3y **W/P:** [X, +] Exclude PRG before implant **CI:** PRG, hormonally responsive tumors, breast CA, AUB, hepatic tumor, active liver Dz, Hx thromboembolic Dz **Disp:** 68-mg implant 4 cm long **SE:** Spotting, irregular periods, amenorrhea, dysmenorrhea, HA, tender breasts, N, Wt gain, acne, ectopic PRG, PE, ovarian cysts, stroke, ↑ BP **Notes:** 99% effective; remove implant and replace; restricted distribution; physician must register and train; does not protect against STDs; site nondominant arm 8–10 cm above medial epicondyle of humerus; implant must be palpable after placement

Etonogestrel/Ethinyl Estradiol Vaginal Insert (NuvaRing) BOX: Cigarette smoking ↑ risk of serious CV events. ↑ Risk w/ age & # cigarettes smoked. Hormonal contraceptives should not be used by women who are > 35 y and smoke. Different from OCP pharmacokinetics Uses: *Contraceptive* **Acts:** Estrogen & progestin combo **Dose:** Rule out PRG first; insert ring vaginally for 3 wk, remove for 1 wk; insert new ring 7 d after last removed (even if bleeding) at same time of day ring removed. 1st day of menses is day 1, insert before day 5 even if bleeding. Use other contraception for first 7 d of starting Rx. See PI if converting from other contraceptive; after delivery or 2nd trim Ab, insert 4 wk postpartum (if not breastfeeding) **W/P:** [X, ?/–] HTN, gallbladder Dz, ↑ lipids, migraines, sudden HA

CI: PRG, heavy smokers > 35 y, DVT, PE, cerebro-/CV Dz, estrogen-dependent neoplasm, undiagnosed abnormal genital bleeding, hepatic tumors, cholestatic jaundice **Disp:** Intravag ring: ethinyl estradiol 0.015 mg/d & etonogestrel 0.12 mg/d **Notes:** If ring removed, rinse w/ cool/lukewarm H_2O (not hot) & reinsert ASAP; if not reinserted w/in 3 h, effectiveness ↓; do not use w/ diaphragm

Etoposide [VP-16] (Etopophos, Toposar, Vepesid, Generic) Uses: *Testicular, NSCLC, Hodgkin Dz, & NHLs, peds ALL, & allogeneic/autologous BMT in high doses* **Acts:** Topoisomerase II inhib **Dose:** 50 mg/m^2/d IV for 3–5 d; 50 mg/m^2/d PO for 21 d (PO availability = 50% of IV); 2–6 g/m^2 or 25–70 mg/kg in BMT (per protocols); ↓ in renal/hepatic impair **W/P:** [D, –] **CI:** IT administration **Disp:** Caps 50 mg; Inj 20 mg/mL **SE:** N/V (emesis in 10–30%), ↓ BM, alopecia, ↓ BP w/ rapid IV, anorexia, anemia, leukopenia, ↑ risk secondary leukemias

Etravirine (Intelence) Uses: *HIV* **Acts:** Non-NRTI **Dose:** *Adult:* 200 mg PO bid after a meal. *Peds:* 16–20 kg: 100 mg, 20–25 kg: 125 mg, 25–30 kg: 150 mg, > 30 kg: 200 mg all PO bid after a meal **W/P:** [B, ±] Many interactions: substrate/inducer (CYP3A4), substrate/inhib (CYP2C9, CYP2C19); do not use w/ tipranavir/ritonavir, fosamprenavir/ritonavir, atazanavir/ritonavir, protease inhib w/o ritonavir, and non-NRTIs **CI:** None **Disp:** Tabs 100, 200 mg **SE:** N/V/D, rash, severe/potentially life-threatening skin Rxns, fat redistribution

Everolimus (Afinitor, Affinitor Disperz) Uses: *Advanced RCC w/ sunitinib or sorafenib failure, subependymal giant cell astrocytoma and PNET in nonsurgical candidates w/ tuberous sclerosis* **Acts:** mTOR inhib **Dose:** 10 mg PO daily, ↓ to 5 mg w/ SE or hepatic impair; avoid w/ high fat meal **W/P:** [D, ?] Avoid w/ or if received live vaccines; w/ CYP3A4 inhib **CI:** Compound/ rapamycin derivative hypersens **Disp:** Tabs 2.5, 5, 7.5, 10 mg; Disperz for suspen 2, 3, 5 mg **SE:** Noninfectious pneumonitis, ↑ Infxn risk, oral ulcers, asthenia, cough, fatigue, diarrhea, ↑ glucose/SCr/lipids; ↓ hemoglobin/WBC/plt **Notes:** Follow CBC, LFT, glucose, lipids; see also everolimus (*Zortress*)

Everolimus (Zortress) Uses: *Prevent renal and liver transplant rejection; combo w/ basiliximab w/ ↓ dose of steroids and cyclosporine* **Acts:** mTOR inhib (mammalian rapamycin target) **Dose:** 0.75 mg PO bid, adjust to trough levels 3–8 ng/mL **W/P:** [D, ?] **CI:** Compound/rapamycin-derivative hypersens **Disp:** Tabs 0.25, 0.5,0.75 mg **SE:** Peripheral edema, constipation, ↑ BP, N, ↓ Hct, UTI, ↑ lipids **Notes:** Follow CBC, LFT, glucose, lipids; see also everolimus (Afinitor); trough level 3–8 ng/mL w/ cyclosporine

Exemestane (Aromasin, Generic) Uses: *Advanced breast CA in postmenopausal women w/ progression after tamoxifen* **Acts:** Irreversible, steroidal aromatase inhib; ↓ estrogens **Dose:** 25 mg PO daily after a meal **W/P:** [D, ?/–] **CI:** PRG, component sensitivity **Disp:** Tabs 25 mg **SE:** Hot flashes, N, fatigue, ↑ alkaline phosphate

Exenatide (Byetta) Uses: Type 2 DM combined w/ metformin &/or sulfonylurea **Acts:** Incretin mimetic: ↑ insulin release, ↓ glucagon secretion, ↓ gastric emptying, promotes satiety **Dose:** 5 mcg SQ bid w/in 60 min before A.M. & P.M. meals; ↑ to 10 mcg SQ bid after 1 mo PRN; do not give pc **W/P:** [C, ?/–] May ↓ absorption of other drugs (take antibiotics/contraceptives 1 h before) **CI:** CrCl < 30 mL/min **Disp:** Soln 5, 10 mcg/dose in prefilled pen **SE:** Hypoglycemia, N/V/D, dizziness, HA, dyspepsia, ↓ appetite, jittery; acute pancreatitis **Notes:** Consider ↓ sulfonylurea to ↓ risk of hypoglycemia; discard pen 30 d after 1st use; monitor Cr

Exenatide ER (Bydureon) **BOX:** Causes thyroid C-cell tumors in rats, ? human relevance; CI in pts w/ Hx or family Hx medullary thyroid carcinoma (MTC) or multiple endocrine neoplasia synd type 2 (MEN2); counsel pts on thyroid tumor risk & Sx **Uses:** *Type 2 DM* **Acts:** Glucagon-like peptide-1 (GLP-1) receptor agonist **Dose:** *Adult.* 2 mg SQ 1 × wk; w/ or w/o meals **W/P:** [C, ?/–] w/ mod renal impair; w/ severe GI Dz; may cause acute pancreatitis and absorption of PO meds, may ↑ INR w/ warfarin **CI:** MTC, MEN2, hypersens; CrCl < 30 mL/min **Disp:** Inj 2 mg/vial **SE:** N/V/D/C, dyspepsia, ↓ appetite, hypoglycemia, HA, Inj site Rxn, pancreatitis, renal impair, hypersens

Ezetimibe (Zetia) **Uses:** *Hypercholesterolemia alone or w/ a HMG-CoA reductase inhib* **Acts:** ↓ Cholesterol & phytosterols absorption **Dose:** *Adults & Peds > 10 y.* 10 mg/d PO **W/P:** [C, +/–] Bile acid sequestrants ↓ bioavailability **CI:** Hepatic impair **Disp:** Tabs 10 mg **SE:** HA, D, Abd pain, ↑ transaminases w/ HMG-CoA reductase inhib, erythema multiforme **Notes:** See ezetimibe/simvastatin

Ezetimibe/Simvastatin (Vytorin) **Uses:** *Hypercholesterolemia* **Acts:** ↓ Absorption of cholesterol & phytosterols w/ HMG-CoA-reductase inhib **Dose:** 10/10–10/80 mg/d PO; w/ cyclosporine/ or danazol: 10/10 mg/d max; w/ diltiazem/ amiodarone or verapamil: 10/10 mg/d max; w/ amlodipine/ranolazine 10/20 max; ↓ w/ severe renal Insuff; give 2 h before or 4 h after bile acid sequestrants **W/P:** [X, –]; w/ CYP3A4 inhib (Table 10, p 319), gemfibrozil, niacin > 1 g/d, danazol, amiodarone, verapamil; avoid high dose w/ diltiazem; w/ Chinese pt on lipid-modifying meds **CI:** PRG/lactation; w/ cyclosporine & danazol; liver Dz, ↑ LFTs **Disp:** Tabs (mg ezetimibe/ mg simvastatin) 10/10, 10/20, 10/40, 10/80 **SE:** HA, GI upset, myalgia, myopathy (muscle pain, weakness, or tenderness w/ creatine kinase 10 × ULN, rhabdomyolysis), hep, Infxn **Notes:** Monitor LFTs, lipids; ezetimibe/simvastatin combo lowered LDL more than simvastatin alone in ENHANCE study, but was no difference in carotid-intima media thickness; pts to report muscle pain

Ezogabine (Potiga) **Uses:** *Partial-onset Szs* **Acts:** ↑ Transmembrane K^+ currents & augment GABA mediated currents **Dose:** *Adult.* 100 mg PO 3 × d; ↑ dose by 50 mg 3 × d qwk, max dose 400 mg 3 × d (1200 mg/d); ↓ dosage in elderly, renal/hepatic impair (see labeling); swallow whole **W/P:** [C, ?/–] May need to ↑ dose when used w/ phenytoin & carbamazepine; monitor digoxin levels **Disp:** Tabs 50, 200, 300, 400 mg **SE:** Dizziness, somnolence, fatigue, abnormal coordination, gait disturbance, confusion, psychotic Sxs, hallucinations, attention disturbance, memory impair, vertigo, tremor, blurred vision, aphasia, dysarthria, urinary retention, ↑ QT interval, suicidal ideation/behavior, withdrawal Szs **Notes:** Withdraw over min. of 3 wk

Famciclovir (Famvir, Generic) Uses: *Acute herpes zoster (shingles) & genital herpes* **Acts:** ↓ Viral DNA synth **Dose:** *Zoster:* 500 mg PO q8h × 7 d. *Simplex:* 125–250 mg PO bid; ↓ w/ renal impair **W/P:** [B, –] **CI:** Component sensitivity **Disp:** Tabs 125, 250, 500 mg **SE:** Fatigue, dizziness, HA, pruritus, N/D **Notes:** Best w/in 72 h of initial lesion

Famotidine (Fluxid, Pepcid, Pepcid AC, Generic) [OTC] Uses: *Short-term Tx of duodenal ulcer & benign gastric ulcer; maint for duodenal ulcer, hypersecretory conditions, GERD, & heartburn* **Acts:** H₂-antagonist; ↓ gastric acid **Dose:** *Adults. Ulcer:* 20 mg IV q12h or 20–40 mg PO qhs × 4–8 wk. *Hypersecretion:* 20–160 mg PO q6h. *GERD:* 20 mg PO bid × 6 wk; maint: 20 mg PO hs. *Heartburn:* 10 mg PO PRN q12h. *Peds.* 0.5–1 mg/kg/d; ↓ in severe renal Insuff **W/P:** [B, M] **CI:** Component sensitivity **Disp:** Tabs 10, 20, 40 mg; chew tabs 10 mg; susp 40 mg/5 mL; gelatin caps 10 mg; *Fluxid* ODT 20 mg; Inj 10 mg/2 mL **SE:** Dizziness, HA, constipation, N/V/D, ↓ plt, hepatitis **Notes:** Chew tabs contain phenylalanine

Febuxostat (Uloric) Uses: *Hyperuricemia and gout* **Acts:** Xanthine oxidase inhib (enzyme that converts hypoxanthine to xanthine to uric acid) **Dose:** 40 mg PO 1 × d, ↑ 80 mg if uric acid not < 6 mg/dL after 2 wk **W/P:** [C, ?/–] **CI:** Use w/ azathioprine, mercaptopurine, theophylline **Supplied:** Tabs 40, 80 mg **SE:** ↑ LFTs, rash, myalgia **Notes:** OK to continue w/ gouty flare or use w/ NSAIDs

Felodipine (Plendil) Uses: *HTN & CHF* **Acts:** CCB **Dose:** 2.5–10 mg PO daily; swallow whole; ↓ in hepatic impair **W/P:** [C, ?] ↑ Effect w/ azole antifungals, erythromycin, grapefruit juice **CI:** Component sensitivity **Disp:** ER tabs 2.5, 5, 10 mg **SE:** Peripheral edema, flushing, tachycardia, HA, gingival hyperplasia **Notes:** Follow BP in elderly & w/ hepatic impair

Fenofibrate (Antara, Lipofen, Lofibra, TriCor, Triglide, Generic) Uses: *Hypertriglyceridemia, hypercholesteremia* **Acts:** ↓ Triglyceride synth **Dose:** 43–160 mg/d; ↓ w/ renal impair; take w/ meals **W/P:** [C, ?] **CI:** Hepatic/severe renal Insuff, primary biliary cirrhosis, unexplained ↑ LFTs, gallbladder Dz **Disp:** Caps 35, 40, 43, 48, 50, 54, 67, 105, 107, 130, 134, 145, 160, 200 mg **SE:** GI disturbances, cholecystitis, arthralgia, myalgia, dizziness, ↑ LFTs **Notes:** Monitor LFTs

Fenofibric Acid (Fibricor, Trilipix) Uses: *Adjunct to diet for ↑ triglycerides, to ↓ LDL-C, cholesterol, triglycerides, and apo B, to ↑ HDL-C in hypercholesterolemia/mixed dyslipidemia; adjunct to diet w/ a statin to ↓ triglycerides and ↑ HDL-C w/ CHD or w/ CHD risk* **Acts:** Agonist of peroxisome proliferator-activated receptor-alpha (PPAR-α), causes ↑ VLDL catabolism, fatty acid oxidation, and clearing of triglyceride-rich particles w/ ↓ VLDL, triglycerides; ↑ HDL in some **Dose:** *Mixed dyslipidemia w/ a statin:* 135 mg PO × 1 d; *Hypertriglyceridemia:*

45–135 mg 1 × d; maint based on response; *Primary hypercholesterolemia/mixed dyslipidemia:* 135 mg PO 1 × d; 135 mg/d max; 35 mg w/ renal impair **W/P:** [C, /–] Multiple interactions, ↑ embolic phenomenon **CI:** Severe renal impair, pt on dialysis, active liver/gall bladder Dz, nursing **Disp:** DR Caps 35, 45, 105, 135 mg **SE:** HA, back pain, nasopharyngitis, URI, N/D, myalgia, gall stones, ✓ CBC (usually stabilizes), rare myositis/rhabdomyolysis **Notes:** ✓CBC, lipid panel, LFTs; D/C if LFT > 3× ULN

Fenoldopam (Corlopam, Generic) Uses: *Hypertensive emergency* **Acts:** Rapid vasodilator **Dose:** Initial 0.03–0.1 mcg/kg/min IV Inf, titrate q15min by 0.05–0.1 mcg/kg/min to max 1.6 mcg/kg/min **W/P:** [B, ?] ↓ BP w/ β-blockers **CI:** Allergy to sulfites **Disp:** Inj 10 mg/mL **SE:** ↓ BP, edema, facial flushing, N/V/D, atrial flutter/fibrillation, ↑ IOP **Notes:** Avoid concurrent β-blockers

Fenoprofen (Nalfon, Generic) **BOX:** May ↑ risk of CV events and GI bleeding Uses: *Arthritis & pain* **Acts:** NSAID **Dose:** 200–600 mg q4–8h, to 3200 mg/d max; w/ food **W/P:** [B (D 3rd tri), +/–] CHF, HTN, renal/hepatic impair, Hx PUD **CI:** NSAID sensitivity **Disp:** Caps 200, 400, 600 mg **SE:** GI disturbance, dizziness, HA, rash, edema, renal impair, hep **Notes:** Swallow whole

Fentanyl (Sublimaze, Generic) [C-II] Uses: *Short-acting analgesic* in anesthesia & PCA **Acts:** Narcotic analgesic **Dose:** *Adults.* 1–2 mcg/kg *or* 25–100 mcg/dose IV/IM titrated; *Anesthesia:* 5–15 mcg/kg; *Pain:* 200 mcg over 15 min, titrate to effect *Peds.* 1–2 mcg/kg IV/IM q1–4h titrate; ↓ in renal impair **W/P:** [B, +] **CI:** Paralytic ileus ↑ ICP, resp depression, severe renal/hepatic impair **Disp:** Inj 0.05 mg/mL **SE:** Sedation, ↓ BP, ↓ HR, constipation, N, resp depression, miosis **Notes:** 0.1 mg fentanyl = 10 mg morphine IM

Fentanyl, Transdermal (Duragesic, Generic) [C-II] **BOX:** Potential for abuse and fatal OD Uses: *Persistent mod–severe chronic pain in pts already tolerant to opioids* **Acts:** Narcotic **Dose:** Apply patch to upper torso q72h; dose based on narcotic requirements in previous 24 h; start 25 mcg/h patch q72h; ↓ in renal impair **W/P:** [B, +] w/ CYP3A4 inhib (Table 10, p 319) may ↑ fentanyl effect, w/ Hx substance abuse **CI:** Not opioid tolerant, short-term pain management, postop outpatient pain in outpatient surgery, mild pain, PRN use, ↑ ICP, resp depression, severe renal/hepatic impair, peds < 2 y **Disp:** Patches 12.5, 25, 50, 75, 100 mcg/h **SE:** Resp depression (fatal), sedation, ↓ BP, ↓ HR, constipation, N, miosis **Notes:** 0.1 mg fentanyl = 10 mg morphine IM; do not cut patch; peak level in PRG 24–72 h

Fentanyl, Transmucosal (Abstral, Actiq, Fentora, Lazanda, Onsolis, Generic) [C-II] **BOX:** Potential for abuse and fatal OD; use only in pts w/ chronic pain who are opioid tolerant; CI in acute/postop pain; do not substitute for other fentanyl products; fentanyl can be fatal to children, keep away; use w/ strong CYP3A4 inhib may ↑ fentanyl levels. *Abstral, Onsolis* restricted distribution Uses:

Breakthrough CA pain w/ tolerance to opioids **Acts:** Narcotic analgesic, transmucosal absorption **Dose:** Titrate to effect

- *Abstral:* Start 100 mcg SL, 2 doses max per pain breakthrough episode; wait 2 h for next breakthrough dose; limit to < 4 breakthrough doses w/ successful baseline dosing
- *Actiq:* Start 200 mcg PO × 1, may repeat × 1 after 30 min
- *Fentora:* Start 100 mcg buccal tab × 1, may repeat in 30 min, 4 tabs/dose max
- *Lazanda:* Through TIRF REMS Access Program; initial 1 × 100 mcg spray; if no relief, titrate for breakthrough pain as follows: 2 × 100 mcg spray (1 in each nostril); 1 × 400 mcg; 2 × 400 mcg (1 in each nostril); wait 2 h before another dose; max 4 doses/24h
- *Onsolis:* Start 200 mcg film, ↑ 200 mcg increments to max four 200-mcg films or single 1200-mcg film

W/P: [B, +] resp/CNS depression possible; CNS depressants/CYP3A4 inhib may ↑ effect; may impair tasks (driving, machinery); w/ severe renal/hepatic impair **CI:** Opioid intolerant pt, acute/postop pain **Disp:**

- *Abstral:* SL tabs 100, 200, 300, 400, 600, 800 mcg
- *Actiq:* Lozenges on stick 200, 400, 600, 800, 1200, 1600 mcg
- *Fentora:* Buccal tabs 100, 200, 400, 600, 800 mcg
- *Lazanda:* Nasal spray metered dose audible and visual counter, 8 doses/bottle, 100/400 mcg/spray
- *Onsolis:* Buccal soluble film 200, 400, 600, 1200 mcg

SE: Sedation, ↓ BP, ↓ HR, constipation, N/V, ↓ resp, dyspnea, HA, miosis, anxiety, confusion, depression, rash dizziness **Notes:** 0.1 mg fentanyl = 10 mg IM morphine

Ferrous Gluconate (Fergon [OTC], Others)

BOX: Accidental OD of iron-containing products is a leading cause of fatal poisoning in children < 6 y. Keep out of reach of children **Uses:** *Iron-deficiency anemia* & Fe supl **Acts:** Dietary supl **Dose:** *Adults.* 100–200 mg of elemental Fe/d ÷ doses. *Peds.* 4–6 mg/kg/d ÷ doses; on empty stomach (OK w/ meals if GI upset occurs); avoid antacids **W/P:** [A, ?] **CI:** Hemochromatosis, hemolytic anemia **Disp:** Tabs Fergon 240 (27 mg Fe), 246 (28 mg Fe), 300 (34 mg Fe), 324 mg (38 mg Fe) **SE:** GI upset, constipation, dark stools, discoloration of urine, may stain teeth **Notes:** 12% Elemental Fe; false(+) stool guaiac; keep away from children; severe tox in OD

Ferrous Gluconate Complex (Ferrlecit)

Uses: *Iron-deficiency anemia or supl to erythropoietin Rx therapy* **Acts:** Fe supl **Dose:** *Test dose:* 2 mL (25 mg Fe) IV over 1 h, if OK, 125 mg (10 mL) IV over 1 h. *Usual cumulative dose:* 1 g Fe over 8 sessions (until favorable Hct) **W/P:** [B, ?] **CI:** Non–Fe-deficiency anemia; CHF; Fe overload **Disp:** Inj 12.5 mg/mL Fe **SE:** ↓ BP, serious allergic Rxns, GI disturbance, Inj site Rxn **Notes:** Dose expressed as mg Fe; may infuse during dialysis

Ferrous Sulfate (OTC)

Uses: *Fe-deficiency anemia & Fe supl* **Acts:** Dietary supl **Dose:** *Adults.* 100–200 mg elemental Fe/d in ÷ doses. *Peds.* 1–6 mg/kg/d ÷

daily–tid; on empty stomach (OK w/ meals if GI upset occurs); avoid antacids **W/P:** [A, ?] ↑ Absorption w/ vit C; ↓ absorption w/ tetracycline, fluoroquinolones, antacids, H$_2$ blockers, proton pump inhib **CI:** Hemochromatosis, hemolytic anemia **Disp:** Tabs 187 (60 mg Fe), 200 (65 mg Fe), 324 (65 mg Fe), 325 mg (65 mg Fe); SR caplets & tabs 160 (50 mg Fe), 200 mg (65 mg Fe); gtt 75 mg/0.6 mL (15 mg Fe/0.6 mL); elixir 220 mg/5 mL (44 mg Fe/5 mL); syrup 90 mg/5 mL (18 mg Fe/5 mL) **SE:** GI upset, constipation, dark stools, discolored urine

Ferumoxytol (Feraheme)   Uses: *Iron-deficiency anemia in chronic kidney Dz* **Acts:** Fe replacement **Dose:** *Adults.* 510 mg IV × 1, then 510 mg IV × 1 3–8 d later; give 1 mL/s **W/P:** [C, ?/–] Monitor for hypersens & ↓ BP for 30 mins after dose, may alter MRI studies **CI:** Iron overload; hypersens to ferumoxytol **Disp:** IV soln 30 mg/mL (510 mg elemental Fe/17 mL) **SE:** N/D, constipation, dizziness, hypotension, peripheral edema, hypersens Rxn **Notes:** ✓ hematologic response 1 month after 2nd dose

Fesoterodine (Toviaz)   Uses: * OAB w/ urge urinary incontinence, urgency, frequency* **Acts:** Competitive muscarinic receptor antagonist, ↓ bladder muscle contractions **Dose:** 4 mg PO qd, ↑ to 8 mg PO daily PRN **W/P:** [C, /?] Avoid > 4 mg w/ severe renal Insuff or w/ CYP3A4 inhib (eg, ketoconazole, clarithromycin); w/ BOO, ↓ GI motility/constipation, NAG, MyG **CI:** Urinary/gastric retention, or uncontrolled NAG, hypersens to class **Disp:** Tabs 4, 8 mg **SE:** Dry mouth, constipation, ↓ sweating can cause heat prostration

Fexofenadine (Allegra, Allegra-D, Generic)   Uses: *Allergic rhinitis; chronic idiopathic urticaria* **Acts:** Selective antihistamine, antagonizes H$_1$-receptors; Allegra-D contains w/ pseudoephedrine **Dose:** *Adults & Peds > 12 y.* 60 mg PO bid or 180 mg/d; 12-h ER form bid, 24-h ER form qd. *Peds 2–11 y.* 30 mg PO bid; ↓ in renal impair **W/P:** [C, +] w/ Nevirapine **CI:** Component sensitivity **Disp:** Tabs 30, 60, 180 mg; susp 6 mg/mL; *Allegra-D* 12-h ER tab (60 mg fexofenadine/120 mg pseudoephedrine), *Allegra-D* 24-h *ER* (180 mg fexofenadine/240 mg pseudoephedrine) **SE:** Drowsiness (rare), HA, ischemic colitis

Fidaxomicin (Dificid)   Uses: **Clostridium difficile*-associated diarrhea* **Acts:** Macrolide antibiotic **Dose:** 200 mg PO bid × 10 d **W/P:** [B, +/–] Not for systemic Infxn or < 18 y; to ↓ resistance, use only when diagnosis suspected/proven **Disp:** Tabs 200 mg **SE:** N/V, Abd pain, GI bleed, anemia, neutropenia

Filgrastim [G-CSF] (Neupogen)   Uses: *↓ Incidence of Infxn in febrile neutropenic pts; Rx chronic neutropenia* **Acts:** Recombinant G-CSF **Dose:** *Adults & Peds.* 5 mcg/kg/d SQ or IV single daily dose; D/C when ANC > 10,000 cells/mm^3 **W/P:** [C, ?] w/ Drugs that potentiate release of neutrophils (eg, Li) **CI:** Allergy to *E. coli*-derived proteins or G-CSF **Disp:** Inj 300 mcg/mL, 480 mg/1.6 mL **SE:** Fever, alopecia, N/V/D, splenomegaly, bone pain, HA, rash **Notes:** ✓ CBC & plt; monitor for cardiac events; no benefit w/ ANC > 10,000 cells/mm^3

Finasteride (Proscar [Generic], Propecia)   Uses: *BPH & androgenetic alopecia* **Acts:** ↓ 5-alpha-reductase **Dose:** *BPH:* 5 mg/d PO. *Alopecia:* 1 mg/d

PO; food ↓ absorption **W/P:** [X, –] Hepatic impair **CI:** Pregnant women should avoid handling pills, teratogen to male fetus **Disp:** Tabs 1 mg (*Propecia*), 5 mg (*Proscar*) **SE:** ↓ Libido, vol ejaculate, ED, gynecomastia; may slightly ↑ risk of high grade prostate CA **Notes:** Both ↑ PSA by ~50%; reestablish PSA baseline 6 mo (double PSA for "true" reading); 3–6 mo for effect on urinary Sxs; continue to maintain new hair, not for use in women

Fingolimod (Gilenya) Uses: *Relapsing MS* **Acts:** Sphingosine 1-phosphate receptor modulator; ↓ lymphocyte migration into CNS **Dose:** *Adults.* 0.5 mg PO 1 × d; monitor for 6 h after 1st dose for bradycardia; monitor **W/P:** [C, –] Monitor w/ severe hepatic impair and if on Class 1a or III antiarrhythmics/beta-blockers/ CCBs (rhythm disturbances); avoid live vaccines during & 2 mo after D/C; ketoconazole ↑ level **Disp:** Caps 0.5 mg **SE:** HA, D, back pain, dizziness, bradycardia, AV block, HTN, Infxns, macular edema, ↑ LFTs, cough, dyspnea **Notes:** Obtain baseline ECG, CBC, LFTs & eye exam; women of childbearing potential should use contraception during & 2 mo after D/C

Flavoxate (Generic) Uses: *Relief of Sx of dysuria, urgency, nocturia, suprapubic pain, urinary frequency, incontinence* **Acts:** Antispasmodic **Dose:** 100–200 mg PO tid-qid **W/P:** [B, ?] **CI:** GI obst, GI hemorrhage, ileus, achalasia, BPH **Disp:** Tabs 100 mg **SE:** Drowsiness, blurred vision, xerostomia

Flecainide (Tambocor) BOX: ↑ Mortality in pts w/ ventricular arrhythmias and recent MI; pulm effects reported; ventricular proarrhythmic effects in AF/A flutter, not OK for chronic AF Uses: *Prevent AF/A flutter & PSVT, *prevent/suppress life-threatening ventricular arrhythmias* **Acts:** Class 1C antiarrhythmic **Dose:** *Adults.* Start 50 mg PO q12h; ↑ by 50 mg q12h q4d, to max 400 mg/d max *Peds.* 3–6 mg/kg/d in 3 ÷ doses; ↓ w/ renal impair, **W/P:** [C, +] Monitor w/ hepatic impair, ↑ conc w/ amiodarone, digoxin, quinidine, ritonavir/amprenavir, β-blockers, verapamil; may worsen arrhythmias **CI:** 2nd-/3rd-degree AV block, right BBB w/ bifascicular or trifascicular block, cardiogenic shock, CAD, ritonavir/amprenavir, alkalinizing agents **Disp:** Tabs 50, 100, 150 mg **SE:** Dizziness, visual disturbances, dyspnea, palpitations, edema, CP, tachycardia, CHF, HA, fatigue, rash, N **Notes:** Initiate Rx in hospital; dose q8h if pt is intolerant/uncontrolled at q12h; *Levels: Trough:* Just before next dose; *Therapeutic:* 0.2–1 mcg/mL; *Toxic:* > 1 mcg/mL; *half-life:* 11–14 h

Floxuridine (Generic) BOX: Administration by experienced physician only; pts should be hospitalized for 1st course d/t risk for severe Rxn Uses: *GI adenoma, liver, renal CAs* **Acts:** Converted to 5-FU; colon & pancreatic CAs **Acts:** Converted to 5-FU; inhibits thymidylate synthase; ↓ DNA synthase (S-phase specific) **Dose:** 0.1–0.6 mg/kg/d for 1–6 wk (per protocols) usually intraarterial for liver mets **W/P:** [D, –] Interaction w/ vaccines **CI:** BM suppression, poor nutritional status, serious Infxn, PRG, component sensitivity **Disp:** Inj 500 mg **SE:** ↓ BM, anorexia, Abd cramps, N/V/D, mucositis, alopecia, skin rash, & hyperpigmentation; rare neurotox (blurred vision, depression, nystagmus, vertigo, & lethargy); intraarterial catheter-related problems (ischemia, thrombosis, bleeding, & Infxn) **Notes:** Need effective birth control; palliative Rx for inoperable/incurable pts

Fluconazole (Diflucan, Generic) **Uses:** *Candidiasis (esophageal, oropharyngeal, urinary tract, Vag, prophylaxis); cryptococcal meningitis, prophylaxis w/ BMT* **Acts:** Antifungal; ↓ cytochrome P-450 sterol demethylation. *Spectrum:* All *Candida* sp except *C. krusei* **Dose:** *Adults.* 100–400 mg/d PO or IV. *Vaginitis:* 150 mg PO daily. *Crypto:* Doses up to 800 mg/d reported; 400 mg d 1, then 200 mg × 10–12 wk after CSF (−). *Peds.* 3–6 mg/kg/d PO or IV; 12 mg/kg/d/systemic Infxn; ↓ in renal impair **W/P:** [C, Vag candidiasis (D high or prolonged dose), −] Do not use w/ clopidogrel (↓ effect) **CI:** None **Disp:** Tabs 50, 100, 150, 200 mg; susp 10, 40 mg/mL; Inj 2 mg/mL **SE:** HA, rash, GI upset, ↓ K⁺, ↑ LFTs **Notes:** PO (preferred) = IV levels; cong anomalies w/ high dose 1st tri

Fludarabine (Generic) **BOX:** Administer only under supervision of qualified physician experienced in chemotherapy. Can ↓ BM and cause severe CNS effects (blindness, coma, and death). Severe/fatal autoimmune hemolytic anemia reported; monitor for hemolysis. Use w/ pentostatin not OK (fatal pulm tox) **Uses:** *Autoimmune hemolytic anemia, CLL, cold agglutinin hemolysis*, low-grade lymphoma, mycosis fungoides **Acts:** ↓ Ribonucleotide reductase; blocks DNA polymerase-induced DNA repair **Dose:** 18–30 mg/m²/d for 5 d, as a 30-min Inf (per protocols); ↓ w/ renal impair **W/P:** [D, −] Give cytarabine before fludarabine (↓ its metabolism) **CI:** w/ Pentostatin, severe Infxns, CrCl < 30 mL/min, hemolytic anemia **Disp:** Inj 50 mg **SE:** ↓ BM, N/V/D, ↑ LFTs, edema, CHF, fever, chills, fatigue, dyspnea, nonproductive cough, pneumonitis, severe CNS tox rare in leukemia, autoimmune hemolytic anemia

Fludrocortisone Acetate (Florinef, Generic) **Uses:** *Adrenocortical Insuff, Addison Dz, salt-wasting synd* **Acts:** Mineralocorticoid **Dose:** *Adults.* 0.1–0.2 mg/d PO. *Peds.* 0.05–0.1 mg/d PO **W/P:** [C, ?] **CI:** Systemic fungal Infxns; known allergy **Disp:** Tabs 0.1 mg **SE:** HTN, edema, CHF, HA, dizziness, convulsions, acne, rash, bruising, hyperglycemia, hypothalamic-pituitary-adrenal suppression, cataracts **Notes:** For adrenal Insuff, use w/ glucocorticoid; dose changes based on plasma renin activity

Flumazenil (Romazicon, Generic) **Uses:** *Reverse sedative effects of benzodiazepines & general anesthesia* **Acts:** Benzodiazepine receptor antagonist **Dose:** *Adults.* 0.2 mg IV over 15 s; repeat PRN, to 1 mg max (5 mg max in benzodiazepine OD). *Peds.* 0.01 mg/kg (0.2 mg/dose max) IV over 15 s; repeat 0.005 mg/kg at 1-min intervals to max 1 mg total; ↓ in hepatic impair **W/P:** [C, ?] **CI:** TCA OD; if pts given benzodiazepines to control life-threatening conditions (ICP/ status epilepticus) **Disp:** Inj 0.1 mg/mL **SE:** N/V, palpitations, HA, anxiety, nervousness, hot flashes, tremor, blurred vision, dyspnea, hyperventilation, withdrawal synd **Notes:** Does not reverse narcotic Sx or amnesia, use associated w/ Szs

Fluorouracil, Injection [5-FU] (Generic) **BOX:** Administration by experienced chemotherapy physician only; pts should be hospitalized for 1st course d/t risk for severe Rxn **Uses:** *Colorectal, gastric, pancreatic, breast, basal cell*, head, neck, bladder CAs **Acts:** Inhibits thymidylate synthetase ($\downarrow$ DNA synth, S-phase specific) **Dose:** 370–1000 mg/m^2/d × 1–5 d IV push to 24-h cont Inf; protracted venous Inf of 200–300 mg/m^2/d (per protocol); 800 mg/d max **W/P:** [D, ?] $\uparrow$ Tox w/ allopurinol; do not give live vaccine before 5-FU **CI:** Poor nutritional status, depressed BM Fxn, thrombocytopenia, major surgery w/in past mo, G6PD enzyme deficiency, PRG, serious Infxn, bili > 5 mg/dL **Disp:** Inj 50 mg/mL **SE:** Stomatitis, esophago-phar-yngitis, N/V/D, anorexia, $\downarrow$ BM, rash/dry skin/photosens, tingling in hands/feet w/ pain (palmar-plantar erythrodysesthesia), phlebitis/discoloration at Inj sites **Notes:** $\uparrow$ Thiamine intake; contraception OK

Fluorouracil, Topical [5-FU] (Carac, Efudex, Fluoroplex, Generic)

Uses: *Basal cell carcinoma (when standard therapy impractical); actinic/solar keratosis* **Acts:** Inhibits thymidylate synthetase ($\downarrow$ DNA synth, S-phase specific) **Dose:** 5% cream bid × 2–6 wk **W/P:** [D, ?] Irritant chemotherapy **CI:** Component sensitivity **Disp:** Cream 0.5, 1, 5%; soln 1, 2, 5% **SE:** Rash, dry skin, photosens **Notes:** Healing may not be evident for 1–2 mo; wash hands thoroughly; avoid occlusive dressings; do not overuse

Fluoxetine (Gaboxetine, Prozac, Prozac Weekly, Sarafem, Generic) BOX: Closely monitor for worsening depression or emergence of sui-cidality, particularly in ped pt

Uses: *Depression, OCD, panic disorder, bulimia (Prozac)* *PMDD (Sarafem)* **Acts:** SSRI **Dose:** 20 mg/d PO (max 80 mg/d ÷ dose); weekly 90 mg/wk after 1–2 wk of standard dose. *Bulimia:* 60 mg q A.M. *Panic disorder:* 20 mg/d. *OCD:* 20–80 mg/d. *PMDD:* 20 mg/d or 20 mg intermittently, start 14 d prior to menses, repeat w/ each cycle; $\downarrow$ in hepatic failure **W/P:** [C, ?/–] Sero-tonin synd w/ MAOI, SSRI, serotonin agonists, linezolid; QT prolongation w/ pheno-thiazines; do not use w/ clopidogrel ($\downarrow$ effect) **CI:** w/ MAOI/thioridazine (wait 5 wk after D/C before MAOI) **Disp:** *Prozac:* Caps 10, 20, 40 mg; scored tabs 10, 20 mg; SR weekly caps 90 mg; soln 20 mg/5 mL. *Sarafem:* Caps 10, 15, 20 mg **SE:** N, ner-vousness, Wt loss, HA, insomnia

Fluoxymesterone (Androxy) [C-III]

Uses: Androgen-responsive meta-static *breast CA, hypogonadism* **Acts:** $\downarrow$ Secretion of LH & FSH (feedback inhi-bition) **Dose:** *Breast CA:* 10–40 mg/d ÷ × 1–3 mo. *Hypogonadism:* 5–20 mg/d **W/P:** [X, ?/–] $\uparrow$ Effect w/ anticoagulants, cyclosporine, insulin, Li, narcotics **CI:** Serious cardiac, liver, or kidney Dz; PRG **Disp:** Tabs 10 mg **SE:** Priapism, edema, virilization, amenorrhea & menstrual irregularities, hirsutism, alopecia, acne, N, cholestasis; suppression of factors II, V, VII, & X, & polycythemia; $\uparrow$ libido, HA, anxiety **Notes:** Radiographic exam of hand/wrist q6mo in prepubertal children; $\downarrow$ total T$_4$ levels

Flurazepam (Dalmane, Generic) [C-IV]

Uses: *Insomnia* **Acts:** Ben-zodiazepine **Dose:** *Adults & Peds > 15 y.* 15–30 mg PO qhs PRN; $\downarrow$ in elderly **W/P:** [X, ?/–] Elderly, low albumin, hepatic impair **CI:** NAG; PRG **Disp:** Caps 15, 30 mg **SE:** "Hangover" d/t accumulation of metabolites, apnea, anaphylaxis, angioedema, amnesia **Notes:** May cause dependency

Flurbiprofen (Ansaid, Ocufen, Generic) **BOX:** May ↑ risk of CV events and GI bleeding **Uses:** *Arthritis, ocular surgery* **Acts:** NSAID **Dose:** *Ansaid* 50–300 mg/d ÷ bid-qid, max 300 mg/d w/ food; *Ocufen:* Ocular 1 gtt q30 min × 4, beginning 2 h preop **W/P:** [C (D in 3rd tri); ?/–] **CI:** PRG (3rd tri); ASA allergy **Disp:** Tabs 50, 100 mg; Ocufen 0.03% opthal soln **SE:** Dizziness, GI upset, peptic ulcer Dz, ocular irritation

Flutamide (Generic) **BOX:** Liver failure & death reported. Measure LFTs before, monthly, & periodically after; D/C immediately if ALT 2 × ULN or jaundice develops **Uses:** Advanced *PCa* (w/ LHRH agonists, eg, leuprolide or goserelin); w/ radiation & GnRH for localized CAP **Acts:** Nonsteroidal antiandrogen **Dose:** 250 mg PO tid (750 mg total) **W/P:** [D, ?] **CI:** Severe hepatic impair **Disp:** Caps 125 mg **SE:** Hot flashes, loss of libido, impotence, N/V/D, gynecomastia, hepatic failure **Notes:** ✓ LFTs, avoid EtOH

Fluticasone Furoate, Nasal (Veramyst) **Uses:** *Seasonal allergic rhinitis* **Acts:** Topical steroid **Dose:** *Adults & Peds > 12 y.* 2 sprays/nostril/d, then 1 spray/d maint. *Peds 2–11 y.* 1–2 sprays/nostril/d **W/P:** [C, M] Avoid w/ ritonavir, other steroids, recent nasal surgery/trauma **CI:** None **Disp:** Nasal spray 27.5 mcg/actuation **SE:** HA, epistaxis, nasopharyngitis, pyrexia, pharyngolaryngeal pain, cough, nasal ulcers, back pain, anaphylaxis

Fluticasone Propionate, Inhalation (Flovent HFA, Flovent Diskus) **Uses:** *Chronic asthma* **Acts:** Topical steroid **Dose:** *Adults & Peds > 12 y.* 2–4 puffs bid. *Peds 4–11 y.* 44 or 50 mcg bid **W/P:** [C, M] **CI:** Status asthmaticus **Disp:** *Diskus* dry powder: 50, 100, 250 mcg/action; HFA; MDI 44/110/220 mcg/Inh **SE:** HA, dysphonia, oral candidiasis **Notes:** Risk of thrush, rinse mouth after; counsel on use of devices

Fluticasone Propionate, Nasal (Flonase, Generic) **Uses:** *Seasonal allergic rhinitis* **Acts:** Topical steroid **Dose:** *Adults & Peds > 12 y.* 2 sprays/nostril/d *Peds 4–11 y.* 1–2 sprays/nostril/d **W/P:** [C, M] **CI:** Primary Rx of status asthmaticus **Disp:** Nasal spray 50 mcg/actuation **SE:** HA, dysphonia, oral candidiasis

Fluticasone Propionate & Salmeterol Xinafoate (Advair Diskus, Advair HFA) **BOX:** ↑ Risk of worsening wheezing or asthma-related death w/ long-acting β2-adrenergic agonists; use only if asthma not controlled on agent such as inhaled steroid **Uses:** *Maint Rx for asthma & COPD* **Acts:** Corticosteroid w/ LA bronchodilator β2 agonist **Dose:** *Adults & Peds > 12 y.* 1 Inh bid q12h; titrate to lowest effective dose (4 Inh or 920/84 mcg/d max) **W/P:** [C, M] **CI:** Acute asthma attack; conversion from PO steroids; w/ phenothiazines **Disp:** Diskus = metered-dose Inh powder (fluticasone/salmeterol in mcg) 100/50, 250/50, 500/50; HFA = aerosol 45/21, 115/21, 230/21 mg **SE:** URI, pharyngitis, HA **Notes:** Combo of Flovent & Serevent; do not wash mouthpiece, do not exhale into device; Advair HFA for pts not controlled on other meds (eg, low-medium dose Inh steroids) or whose Dz severity warrants 2 maint therapies

Fluvastatin (Lescol, Generic) Uses: *Atherosclerosis, primary hypercholesterolemia, heterozygous familial hypercholesterolemia, hypertriglyceridemia* **Acts:** HMG-CoA reductase inhib **Dose:** 20–40 mg bid PO or XL 80 mg/d ↓ w/ hepatic impair **W/P:** [X, –] **CI:** Active liver Dz, ↑ LFTs, PRG, breast-feeding **Disp:** Caps 20, 40 mg; XL 80 mg **SE:** HA, dyspepsia, N/D, Abd pain **Notes:** Dose no longer limited to hs; ✓ LFTs; OK w/ grapefruit

Fluvoxamine (Luvox CR, Generic) **BOX:** Closely monitor for worsening depression or emergence of suicidality, particularly in ped pts Uses: *OCD, SAD* **Acts:** SSRI **Dose:** Initial 50-mg single qhs dose, ↑ to 300 mg/d in ÷ doses; *CR:* 100–300 mg PO qhs, may ↑ by 50 mg/d qwk, max 300 mg/d ↓ in elderly/hepatic impair, titrate slowly; ÷ doses > 100 mg **W/P:** [C, ?/–] Multiple interactions (see PI: MAOIs, phenothiazines, SSRIs, serotonin agonists, others); do not use w/ clopidogrel **CI:** MAOI w/in 14 d, w/ alosetron, tizanidine, thioridazine, pimozide **Disp:** Tabs 25, 50, 100 mg; caps ER 100, 150 mg **SE:** HA, N/D, somnolence, insomnia, ↓ Na⁺, **Notes:** Gradual taper to D/C

Folic Acid, Injectable, Oral (Generic) Uses: *Megaloblastic anemia; folate deficiency* **Acts:** Dietary suppl **Dose:** *Adults.* Supl: 0.4 mg/d PO. *PRG:* 0.8 mg/d PO. *Folate deficiency:* 1 mg PO daily–tid. *Peds.* Supl: 0.04–0.4 mg/24 h PO, IM, IV, or SQ. *Folate deficiency:* 0.5–1 mg/24 h PO, IM, IV, or SQ **W/P:** [A, +] **CI:** Pernicious, aplastic, normocytic anemias **Disp:** Tabs 0.4, 0.8, 1 mg, Inj 5 mg/mL **SE:** Well tolerated **Notes:** OK for all women of childbearing age; ↓ fetal neural tube defects by 50%; no effect on normocytic anemias

Fondaparinux (Arixtra) **BOX:** When epidural/spinal anesthesia or spinal puncture is used, pts anticoagulated or scheduled to be anticoagulated w/ LMW heparins, heparinoids, or fondaparinux are at risk for epidural or spinal hematoma, which can result in long-term or permanent paralysis Uses: *DVT prophylaxis* w/ hip fracture, hip or knee replacement, Abd surgery; w/ DVT or PE in combo w/ warfarin **Acts:** Synth inhib of activated factor X; a pentasaccharide **Dose:** *Prophylaxis* 2.5 mg SQ daily, up to 5–9 d; start > 6 h postop; Tx: 7.5 mg SQ daily (< 50 kg: 5 mg SQ daily; > 100 kg: 10mg SQ daily); ↓ w/ renal impair **W/P:** [B, ?] ↑ Bleeding risk w/ anticoagulants, anti-plts, drotrecogin alfa, NSAIDs **CI:** Wt < 50 kg, CrCl < 30 mL/min, active bleeding, SBE ↓ plt w/ anti-plt Ab **Disp:** Prefilled syringes w/ 27-gauge needle: 2.5/0.5, 5/0.4, 7.5 /0.6, 10/0.8 mg/mL **SE:** Thrombocytopenia, anemia, fever, N **Notes:** D/C if plts < 100,000 cells/mcL; only give SQ; may monitor antifactor Xa levels

Formoterol Fumarate (Foradil, Perforomist) **BOX:** May ↑ risk of asthma-related death Uses: *Long-term Rx of bronchoconstriction in COPD, EIB (only Foradil)* **Acts:** LA β₂-agonist **Dose:** *Adults. Perforomist:* 20-mcg Inh q12h; *Foradil:* 12-mcg Inh q12h, 24 mcg/d max; *EIB:* 12 mcg 15 min before exercise *Peds > 5y.* (Foradil) See Adults **W/P:** [C, M] Not for acute Sx, w/ CV Dz, w/ adrenergic meds, xanthine derivatives meds that ↑ QT; β-blockers may ↓ effect, D/C w/ ECG change **CI:** None **Disp:** *Foradil* caps 12 mcg for Aerolizer inhaler (12 & 60 doses),

Performomist: 20 mcg/2 mL for inhaler **SE:** N/D, nasopharyngitis, dry mouth, angina, HTN, ↓ BP, tachycardia, arrhythmias, nervousness, HA, tremor, muscle cramps, palpitations, dizziness **Notes:** Excess use may ↑ CV risks; not for oral use

Fosamprenavir (Lexiva)   BOX: Do not use w/ severe liver dysfunction, reduce dose w/ mild–mod liver impair (fosamprenavir 700 mg bid w/o ritonavir) **Uses:** HIV Infxn **Acts:** Protease inhib **Dose:** 1400 mg bid w/o ritonavir; fosamprenavir 1400 mg + ritonavir 200 mg daily or fosamprenavir 700 mg + ritonavir 100 mg bid; w/ efavirenz & ritonavir: fosamprenavir 1400 mg + ritonavir 300 mg daily **W/P:** [C, ?/–] Do not use w/ salmeterol, colchicine (w/ renal/hepatic failure); adjust dose w/ bosentan, tadalafil for PAH **CI:** w/ CYP3A4 drugs (Table 10, p 319) such as w/ rifampin, lovastatin, simvastatin, delavirdine, ergot alkaloids, midazolam, triazolam, or pimozide; sulfa allergy; w/ alpha 1-adrenoceptor antagonist (alfuzosin); w/ PDE5 inhibitor sildenafil **Disp:** Tabs 700 mg; susp 50 mg/mL **SE:** N/V/D, HA, fatigue, rash **Notes:** Numerous drug interactions cause of hepatic metabolism; replaced amprenavir

Fosaprepitant (Emend, Injection) Uses: *Prevent chemotherapy-associated N/V* **Acts:** Substance P/neurokinin 1 receptor antagonist **Dose:** *Chemotherapy:* 150 mg IV 30 min before chemotherapy on d 1 (followed by aprepitant [*Emend, Oral*] 80 mg PO days 2 and 3) in combo w/ other antiemetics **W/P:** [B, ?/–] Potential for drug interactions, substrate and mod CYP3A4 inhib (dose-dependent); ↓ effect of OCP and warfarin **CI:** w/ Pimozide, terfenadine, astemizole, or cisapride **Disp:** Inj 115 mg **SE:** N/D, weakness, hiccups, dizziness, HA, dehydration, hot flushing, dyspepsia, Abd pain, neutropenia, ↑ LFTs, Inj site discomfort **Notes:** See also aprepitant (Emend, Oral)

Foscarnet (Foscavir, Generic) Uses: *CMV retinitis*; acyclovir-resistant *herpes Infxns* **Acts:** ↓ Viral DNA polymerase & RT **Dose:** *CMV retinitis: Induction:* 90 mg/kg IV q12h or 60 mg/kg q8h × 14–21 d. *Maint:* 90–120 mg/kg/d IV (Mon–Fri). *Acyclovir-resistant HSV: Induction:* 40 mg/kg IV q8–12h × 14–21 d; use central line; ↓ w/ renal impair **W/P:** [C, –] ↑ Sz potential w/ fluoroquinolones; avoid nephrotoxic Rx (cyclosporine, aminoglycosides, amphotericin B, protease inhib) **CI:** CrCl < 0.4 mL/min/kg **Disp:** Inj 24 mg/mL **SE:** Nephrotox, electrolyte abnormalities **Notes:** Sodium loading (500 mL 0.9% NaCl) before & after helps minimize nephrotox; monitor-ionized Ca^{2+}

Fosfomycin (Monurol, Generic) Uses: *Uncomplicated UTI* **Acts:** ↓ Cell wall synth *Spectrum:* gram(+) *Enterococcus,* staphylococci, pneumococci; gram(–) (*E. coli, Salmonella, Shigella, H. influenzae, Neisseria,* indole(–) *Proteus, Providencia*); *B. fragilis* & anaerobic gram(–) cocci are resistant **Dose:** 3 g PO in 90–120 mL of H_2O single dose; ↓ in renal impair **W/P:** [B, ?] ↓ Absorption w/ antacids/Ca salts **CI:** Component sensitivity **Disp:** Granule packets 3 g **SE:** HA, GI upset **Notes:** May take 2–3 d for Sxs to improve

Fosinopril (Monopril, Generic) Uses: *HTN, CHF*, DN **Acts:** ACE inhib **Dose:** 10 mg/d PO initial; max 40 mg/d PO; ↓ in elderly; ↓ in renal impair **W/P:** [D, +]

↑ K^+ w/ K^+ supls, ARBs, K^+-sparing diuretics; ↑ renal after effects w/ NSAIDs, diuretics, hypovolemia **CI:** Hereditary/idiopathic angioedema or angioedema w/ ACE inhib, bilateral RAS **Disp:** Tabs 10, 20, 40 mg **SE:** Cough, dizziness, angioedema, ↑ K^+

Fosphenytoin (Cerebyx, Generic) **Uses:** *Status epilepticus* **Acts:** ↓ Sz spread in motor cortex **Dose:** As phenytoin equivalents (PE). *Load:* 15–20 mg PE/kg. *Maint:* 4–6 mg PE/kg/d; ↓ dosage, monitor levels in hepatic impair **W/P:** [D, +] May ↑ phenobarbital **CI:** Sinus bradycardia, SA block, 2nd-/3rd-degree AV block, Adams-Stokes synd, rash during Rx **Disp:** Inj 75 mg/mL **SE:** ↓ BP, dizziness, ataxia, pruritus, nystagmus **Notes:** 15 min to convert fosphenytoin to phenytoin; administer < 150 mg PE/min to prevent ↓ BP; administer w/ BP monitoring

Frovatriptan (Frova) **Uses:** *Rx acute migraine* **Acts:** Vascular serotonin receptor agonist **Dose:** 2.5 mg PO repeat in 2 h PRN; max 7.5 mg/d **W/P:** [C, ?/–] **CI:** Angina, ischemic heart Dz, coronary artery vasospasm, hemiplegic or basilar migraine, uncontrolled HTN, ergot use, MAOI use w/in 14 d **Supplied:** Tabs 2.5 mg **SE:** N, V, dizziness, hot flashes, paresthesias, dyspepsia, dry mouth, hot/cold sensation, CP, skeletal pain, flushing, weakness, numbness, coronary vasospasm, HTN

Fulvestrant (Faslodex) **Uses:** *HR(+) metastatic breast CA in postmenopausal women w/ progression following antiestrogen Rx therapy* **Acts:** Estrogen receptor antagonist **Dose:** 500 mg days 1, 15, & 29, maint 500 mg IM mo Inj in buttocks **W/P:** [X, ?/–] ↑ Effects w/ CYP3A4 inhib (Table 10, p 319); w/ hepatic impair **CI:** PRG **Disp:** Prefilled syringes 50 mg/mL (single 5 mL, dual 2.5 mL) **SE:** N/V/D, constipation, Abd pain, HA, back pain, hot flushes, pharyngitis, Inj site Rxns **Notes:** Only use IM

Furosemide (Lasix, Generic) **Uses:** *CHF, HTN, edema*, ascites **Acts:** Loop diuretic; ↓ Na & Cl reabsorption in ascending loop of Henle & distal tubule **Dose:** *Adults* 20–80 mg PO or IV bid. *Peds.* 1 mg/kg/dose IV q6–12h; 2 mg/kg/dose PO q12–24h (max 6 mg/kg/dose); ↑ doses w/ renal impair **W/P:** [C, +] ↓ K^+, ↑ risk digoxin tox & ototox w/ aminoglycosides, cisplatin (especially in renal dysfunction) **CI:** Sulfonylurea allergy; anuria; hepatic coma; electrolyte depletion **Disp:** Tabs 20, 40, 80 mg; soln 10 mg/mL, 40 mg/5 mL; Inj 10 mg/mL **SE:** ↓ BP, hyperglycemia, ↓ K^+ **Notes:** ✓ Lytes, renal Fxn; high doses IV may cause ototox

Gabapentin (Neurontin, Generic) **Uses:** Adjunct in *partial Szs; postherpetic neuralgia (PHN)*; chronic pain synds **Acts:** Anticonvulsant; GABA analog **Dose:** *Adults & Peds > 12 y. Anticonvulsant:* 300 mg PO tid, ↑ max 3600 mg/d. *PHN:* 300 mg day 1, 300 mg bid day 2, 300 mg tid day 3, titrate (1800–3600 mg/d); *Peds 3–12 y.* 10–15 mg/kg/d ÷ tid, ↑ over 3 d: *3–4 y:* 40 mg/kg/d given ≥5 y: 25–35 mg/kg/d ÷ tid, 50 mg/kg/d max; ↓ w/ renal impair **W/P:** [C, ?] Use in peds 3–12 y w/ epilepsy may ↑ CNS-related adverse events **CI:** Component sensitivity **Disp:** Caps 100, 300, 400 mg; soln 250 mg/5 mL; scored tab 600, 800 mg **SE:** Somnolence, dizziness, ataxia, fatigue **Notes:** Not necessary to monitor levels; taper ↑ or ↓ over 1 wk

Gabapentin Enacarbil (Horizant) Uses: **RLS** Acts: GABA analog; ? mechanism **Dose:** *Adult.* CrCl > 60 mL/min: 600 mg PO 1 × d; 30–59 mL/min: 300 mg 1 × d (max 600 mg/d); 15–29 mL/min: 300 mg 1 × d; < 15 mL/min: 300 mg q other day; not recommended w/ hemodialysis; take w/ food at 5 P.M.; swallow whole **W/P:** [C, ?/–] **Disp:** Tabs ER 300, 600 mg **SE:** Somnolence, sedation, fatigue, dizziness, HA, blurred vision, feeling drunk, disorientation, ↓ libido, depression, suicidal thoughts/behaviors, multiorgan hypersens

Galantamine (Razadyne, Razadyne ER, Generic) Uses: **Mild–mod Alzheimer Dz** Acts: ? Acetylcholinesterase inhib **Dose:** *Razadyne* 4 mg PO bid, ↑ to 8 mg bid after 4 wk; may ↑ to 16 mg bid in 4 wk; target 16–24 mg/d ÷ bid. *Razadyne ER* Start 8 mg/d, ↑ to 16 mg/d after 4 wk, then to 24 mg/d after 4 more wk; give q A.M. w/ food **W/P:** [B, ?] w/ Heart block, ↑ effect w/ succinylcholine, bethanechol, amiodarone, diltiazem, verapamil, NSAIDs, digoxin; ↓ effect w/ anticholinergics; ↑ risk of death w/ mild impair **CI:** Severe renal/hepatic impair **Disp:** *Razadyne* Tabs 4, 8, 12 mg; soln 4 mg/mL. *Razadyne ER* Caps 8, 16, 24 mg **SE:** GI disturbances, ↓ Wt, sleep disturbances, dizziness, HA **Notes:** Caution w/ urinary outflow obst, Parkinson Dz, severe asthma/COPD, severe heart Dz or ↓ BP

Gallium Nitrate (Ganite) **BOX:** ↑ Risk of severe renal Insuff w/ concurrent use of nephrotoxic drugs (eg, aminoglycosides, amphotericin B). D/C if use of potentially nephrotoxic drug is indicated; hydrate several d after administration. D/C w/ SCr > 2.5 mg/dL Uses: **↑ Ca²⁺ of malignancy**; bladder CA Acts: ↓ Bone resorption of Ca²⁺ **Dose:** ↑ *Ca²⁺:* 100–200 mg/m²/d × 5 d. *CA:* 350 mg/m² cont Inf × 5 d to 700 mg/m² rapid IV Inf q2wk in antineoplastic settings (per protocols), Inf over 24 h **W/P:** [C, ?] Don't give w/ live or rotavirus vaccine **CI:** SCr > 2.5 mg/dL **Disp:** Inj 25 mg/mL **SE:** Renal Insuff, ↓ Ca²⁺, hypophosphatemia, ↓ bicarb, < 1% acute optic neuritis **Notes:** Bladder CA, use in combo w/ vinblastine & ifosfamide

Ganciclovir (Cytovene, Vitrasert, Generic) Uses: **Rx & prevent CMV retinitis, prevent CMV Dz** in transplant recipients Acts: ↓ viral DNA synth **Dose:** *Adults & Peds.* **IV:** 5 mg/kg IV q12h for 14–21 d, then maint 5 mg/kg/d IV × 7 d/wk or 6 mg/kg/d IV × 5 d/wk. *Ocular implant:* 1 implant q5–8mo. *Adults.* **PO:** Following induction, 1000 mg PO tid. *Prevention:* 1000 mg PO tid; w/ food; ↓ in renal impair **W/P:** [C, –] ↑ Effect w/ immunosuppressives, imipenem/cilastatin, zidovudine, didanosine, other nephrotoxic Rx **CI:** ANC < 500 cells/mm³, plt < 25,000 cells/mm³, intravitreal implant **Disp:** Caps 250, 500 mg; Inj 500 mg, ocular implant 4.5 mg **SE:** Granulocytopenia & thrombocytopenia, fever, rash, GI upset **Notes:** Not a cure for CMV; handle Inj w/ cytotoxic cautions; no systemic benefit w/ implant

Ganciclovir, Ophthalmic Gel (Zirgan) Uses: **Acute herpetic keratitis (dendritic ulcers)** Acts: ↓ Viral DNA synth **Dose:** *Adult & Peds ≥2 y.* 1 gtt affected eye/s 5 × d (q3h while awake) until ulcer heals, then 1 gtt tid × 7 d **W/P:** [C, ?/–] Remove contacts during therapy **CI:** None **Disp:** Gel, 5-g tube **SE:**

Blurred vision, eye irritation, punctate keratitis, conjunctival hyperemia **Notes:** Correct ↓ Ca²⁺ before use; ✓ Ca²⁺

Gemcitabine (Gemzar, Generic) Uses: *Pancreatic CA (single agent), breast CA w/ paclitaxel, NSCLC w/ cisplatin, ovarian CA w/ carboplatin*, gastric CA **Acts:** Antimetabolite; nucleoside metabolic inhibitor; ↓ ribonucleotide reductase; produces false nucleotide base-inhibiting DNA synth **Dose:** 1000–1250 mg/m² over 30 min–1 h IV Inf/wk × 3–4 wk or 6–8 wk; modify dose based on hematologic Fxn (per protocol) **W/P:** [D, ?/–] **CI:** PRG **Disp:** Inj 200 mg, 1 g **SE:** ↓ BM, N/V/D, drug fever, skin rash **Notes:** Reconstituted soln 38 mg/mL; monitor hepatic/renal Fxn

Gemfibrozil (Lopid, Generic) Uses: *Hypertriglyceridemia, coronary heart Dz* **Acts:** Fibric acid **Dose:** 1200 mg/d PO ÷ bid 30 min ac A.M. & P.M. **W/P:** [C, ?] ↑ Warfarin effect, sulfonylureas; ↑ risk of myopathy w/ HMG-CoA reductase inhib; ↑ effects w/ cyclosporine **CI:** Renal/hepatic impair (SCr > 2.0 mg/dL), gallbladder Dz, primary biliary cirrhosis, use w/ repaglinide (↓ glucose) **Disp:** Tabs 600 mg **SE:** Cholelithiasis, GI upset **Notes:** Avoid w/HMG-CoA reductase inhib; ✓ LFTs & serum lipids

Gemifloxacin (Factive) Uses: *CAP, acute exacerbation of chronic bronchitis* **Acts:** ↓ DNA gyrase & topoisomerase IV; *Spectrum; S. pneumoniae* (including multidrug-resistant strains), *H. influenzae, H. parainfluenzae, M. catarrhalis, M. pneumoniae, C. pneumoniae, K. pneumoniae* **Dose:** 320 mg PO daily × 5–7 d; CrCl < 40 mL/min: 160 mg PO/d **W/P:** [C, ?/–]; Peds < 18 y; Hx of ↑ QTc interval, electrolyte disorders, w/ class IA/III antiarrhythmics, erythromycin, TCAs, antipsychotics, ↑ INR and bleeding risk w/ warfarin **CI:** Fluoroquinolone allergy **Disp:** Tab 320 mg **SE:** Rash, N/V/D, *C. difficile* enterocolitis, ↑ risk of Achilles tendon rupture, tendonitis, Abd pain, dizziness, xerostomia, arthralgia, allergy/anaphylactic Rxns, peripheral neuropathy, tendon rupture **Notes:** Take 3 h before or 2 h after Al/Mg antacids, Fe²⁺, Zn²⁺ or other metal cations; ↑ rash risk w/ ↑ duration of Rx

Gentamicin, Injectable (Generic) Uses: *Septicemia, serious bacterial Infxn of CNS, urinary tract, resp tract, GI tract, including peritonitis, skin, bone, soft tissue, including burns; severe Infxn P. aeruginosa w/ carbenicillin; group D streptococci endocarditis w/ PCN-type drug; serious staphylococcal Infxns, but not the antibiotic of 1st choice; mixed Infxn w/ staphylococci and gram(–)* **Acts:** Aminoglycoside, bactericidal; ↓ protein synth *Spectrum:* gram(–) (not *Neisseria, Legionella, Acinetobacter*); weaker gram(+) but synergy w/ PCNs **Dose:** *Adults. Standard:* 1–2 mg/kg IV q8–12h or daily dosing 4–7 mg/kg q24h IV. *Gram(+) Synergy:* 1 mg/kg q8h **Peds.** *Infants < 7 d < 1200 g.* 2.5 mg/kg/dose q18–24h. *Infants > 1200 g:* 2.5 mg/kg/dose q12–18h. *Infants > 7 d:* 2.5 mg/kg/dose IV q8–12h. *Children:* 2.5 mg/kg/d IV q8h; ↓ w/ renal Insuff; if obese, dose based on IBW **W/P:** [C, +/–] Avoid other nephrotoxics **CI:** Aminoglycoside sensitivity **Disp:** Premixed Inf 40, 60, 70, 80, 90, 100, 120 mg; ADD-Vantage Inj vials 10 mg/mL; Inj 40 mg/mL;

IT preservative-free 2 mg/mL **SE:** Nephro-/oto-/neurotox **Notes:** Follow CrCl, SCr, & serum conc for dose adjustments; use IBW for dose adjusted if obese > 30% IBW); OK to use intraperitoneal for peritoneal dialysis-related Infxns **Levels:** *Peak:* 30 min after Inf; *Trough:* < 0.5 h before next dose; *Therapeutic: Peak:* 5–8 mcg/mL, *Trough:* < 2 mcg/mL, if > 2 mcg/mL associated w/ renal tox

Gentamicin, Ophthalmic (Garamycin, Genoptic, Gentak, Generic) **Uses:** *Conjunctival Infxns* **Acts:** Bactericidal; ↓ protein synth **Dose:** *Oint:* Apply 1/2 in bid-tid. *Soln:* 1–2 gtt q2–4h, up to 2 gtt/h for severe Infxn **W/P:** [C, ?] **CI:** Aminoglycoside sensitivity **Disp:** Soln & oint 0.1% and 0.3% **SE:** Local irritation **Notes:** Do not use other eye drops w/in 5–10 min; do not touch dropper to eye

Gentamicin, Topical (Generic) **Uses:** *Skin Infxns* caused by susceptible organisms **Acts:** Bactericidal; ↓ protein synth **Dose:** *Adults & Peds > 1 y.* Apply tid-qid **W/P:** [C, ?] **CI:** Aminoglycoside sensitivity **Disp:** Cream & oint 0.1% **SE:** Irritation

Gentamicin/Prednisolone (Pred-G Ophthalmic) **Uses:** *Steroid-responsive ocular & conjunctival Infxns* sensitive to gentamicin **Acts:** Bactericidal; ↓ protein synth w/ anti-inflammatory. *Spectrum: Staphylococcus, E. coli, H. influenzae, Klebsiella, Neisseria, Pseudomonas, Proteus,* & *Serratia* sp **Dose:** *Oint:* 1/2 in conjunctival sac daily-tid. *Susp:* 1 gtt bid-qid, up to 1 gtt/h for severe Infxns **CI:** Aminoglycoside sensitivity **W/P:** [C, ?] **Disp:** Oint, ophthal: Prednisolone acetate 0.6% & gentamicin sulfate 0.3% (3.5 g). *Susp, ophthal:* Prednisolone acetate 1% & gentamicin sulfate 0.3% (2, 5, 10 mL) **SE:** Local irritation

Glimepiride (Amaryl, Generic) **Uses:** *Type 2 DM* **Acts:** Sulfonylurea; ↑ pancreatic insulin release; ↑ peripheral insulin sensitivity; ↓ hepatic glucose output/ production **Dose:** 1–4 mg/d, max 8 mg **W/P:** [C, –] **CI:** DKA **Disp:** Tabs 1, 2, 4 mg **SE:** HA, N, hypoglycemia **Notes:** Give w/ 1st meal of day

Glimepiride/Pioglitazone (Duetact) **BOX:** Thiazolidinediones, including pioglitazone, cause or exacerbate CHF. Not recommended in pts w/ symptomatic heart failure. CI w/ NYHA Class III or IV heart failure **Uses:** *Adjunct to exercise type 2 DM not controlled by single agent* **Acts:** Sulfonylurea (↓ glucose) w/ agent that ↑ insulin sensitivity & ↓ gluconeogenesis **Dose:** Initial 30 mg/2 mg PO q A.M.; 45 mg pioglitazone/8 mg glimepiride/d max; w/ food **W/P:** [C, ?/–] w/ Liver impair, elderly, w/ Hx bladder CA **CI:** Component hypersens, DKA **Disp:** Tabs 30/2, 30 mg/4 mg **SE:** Hct, ↑ ALT, ↓ glucose, URI, ↑ Wt, edema, HA, N/D, may ↑ CV mortality **Notes:** Monitor CBC, ALT, Cr, Wt

Glipizide (Glucotrol, Glucotrol XL, Generic) **Uses:** *Type 2 DM* **Acts:** Sulfonylurea; ↑ pancreatic insulin release; ↑ peripheral insulin sensitivity; ↓ hepatic glucose output/production; ↓ intestinal glucose absorption **Dose:** 5 mg initial, ↑ by 2.5–5 mg/d, max 40 mg/d; XL max 20 mg; 30 min ac; hold if NPO **W/P:** [C, ?/–] Severe liver Dz **CI:** DKA, type 1 DM, sulfonamide sensitivity **Disp:** Tabs 5, 10 mg; XL tabs 2.5, 5, 10 mg **SE:** HA, anorexia, N/V/D, constipation, fullness, rash, urticaria, photosens **Notes:** Counsel about DM management; wait several days before adjusting dose; monitor glucose

Glucagon, Recombinant (GlucaGen) **Uses:** Severe *hypoglycemic Rxns in DM*, radiologic GI tract diagnostic aid; β-blocker/CCB OD **Acts:** Accelerates liver gluconeogenesis **Dose:** *Adults.* 0.5–1 mg SQ, IM, or IV; repeat in 20 min PRN. *ECC 2010.* β-Blocker or CCB overdose: 3–10 mg slow IV over 3–5 min; follow w/ Inf of 3–5 mg/h; Hypoglycemia: 1 mg IV, IM, or SQ. *Peds. Neonates.* 30 mcg/kg/dose SQ, IM, or IV q4h PRN. *Children.* 0.025–0.1 mg/kg/dose SQ, IM, or IV; repeat in 20 min PRN **W/P:** [B, M] **CI:** Pheochromocytoma **Disp:** Inj 1 mg **SE:** N/V, ↓ BP **Notes:** Administration of dextrose IV necessary; ineffective in starvation, adrenal Insuff, or chronic hypoglycemia

Glucarpidase (Voraxaze) **Uses:** *Tx toxic plasma MTX conc (> 1 micromole/L) in pts w/ ↓ clearance* **Acts:** Carboxypeptidase enzyme converts MTX to inactive metabolites **Dose:** 50 units/kg IV over 5 min × 1 **W/P:** [C, ?/–] serious allergic/anaphylactic Rxns; do not administer leucovorin w/in 2 h before/after dose **Disp:** Inj (powder) 1000 units/vial **SE:** N/V/D, HA, ↓/↑ BP, flushing, paracsthesias, hypersens, blurred vision, rash, tremor, throat irritation **Notes:** Measure MTX conc by chromatographic method w/in 48 h of admin; continue leucovorin until methotrexate conc below leucovorin Tx threshold × 3 d; hydrate & alkalinize urine

Glyburide (DiaBeta, Glynase, Generic) **Uses:** *Type 2 DM* **Acts:** Sulfonylurea; ↑ pancreatic insulin release; ↑ peripheral insulin sensitivity; ↓ hepatic glucose output/production; ↓ intestinal glucose absorption **Dose:** 1.25–10 mg daily-bid, max 20 mg/d. Micronized: 0.75–6 mg daily or bid, max 12 mg/d **W/P:** [C, ?] Renal impair, sulfonamide allergy, ? ↑ CV risk **CI:** DKA, type 1 DM **Disp:** Tabs 1.25, 2.5, 5 mg; micronized tabs (*Glynase*) 1.5, 3, 6 mg **SE:** HA, hypoglycemia, cholestatic jaundice, and hepatitis may cause liver failure **Notes:** Not OK for CrCl < 50 mL/min; hold dose if NPO; hypoglycemia may be difficult to recognize; many medications can enhance hypoglycemic effects

Glyburide/Metformin (Glucovance, Generic) **Uses:** *Type 2 DM* **Acts:** *Sulfonylurea:* ↑ Pancreatic insulin release. *Metformin:* ↑ Peripheral insulin sensitivity; ↓ hepatic glucose output/production; ↓ intestinal glucose absorption **Dose:** 1st line (naïve pts), 1.25/250 mg PO daily-bid; 2nd line, 2.5/500 or 5/500 mg bid (max 20/2000 mg); take w/ meals, slowly ↑ dose; hold before & 48 h after ionic contrast media **W/P:** [C, –] **CI:** SCr > 1.4 mg/dL in females or > 1.5 mg/dL in males; hypoxemic conditions (sepsis, recent MI); alcoholism; metabolic acidosis; liver Dz; **Disp:** Tabs (glyburide/metformin) 1.25/250, 2.5/500, 5/500 mg **SE:** HA, hypoglycemia, lactic acidosis, anorexia, N/V, rash **Notes:** Avoid EtOH; hold dose if NPO; monitor folate levels (megaloblastic anemia)

Glycerin Suppository **Uses:** *Constipation* **Acts:** Hyperosmolar laxative **Dose:** *Adults.* 1 Adult supp PR PRN. *Peds.* 1 Infant supp PR daily-bid PRN **W/P:** [C, ?] **Disp:** Supp (adult, infant); liq 4 mL/applicator full **SE:** D

Golimumab (Simponi)　　**BOX:** Serious Infxns (bacterial, fungal, TB, opportunistic) possible. D/C w/ severe Infxn/sepsis, test and monitor for TB w/ Tx; lymphoma/other CA possible in children/adolescents **Uses:** *Mod–severe RA w/ methotrexate, psoriatic arthritis w/ or w/o methotrexate, ankylosing spondylitis* **Acts:** TNF blocker **Dose:** 50 mg SQ 1 × mo **W/P:** [B, ?/–] Do use w/ active Infxn; w/ malignancies, CHF, demyelinating Dz; do use w/ abatacept, anakinra, live vaccines **CI:** None **Disp:** Prefilled syringe & SmartJect auto-injector 50 mg/0.5 mL **SE:** URI, nasopharyngitis, Inj site Rxn, ↑ LFTs, Infxn, hep B reactivation, new-onset psoriasis

Goserelin (Zoladex)　　**Uses:** *Advanced CA prostate & w/ radiation and flutamide for localized high-risk Dz,*endometriosis, breast CA **Acts:** LHRH agonist, transient ↑ then ↓ in LH, w/ ↓ testosterone **Dose:** 3.6 mg SQ (implant) q28d or 10.8 mg SQ q3mo; usually upper Abd wall **W/P:** [X, –] **CI:** PRG, breast-feeding, 10.8-mg implant not for women **Disp:** SQ implant 3.6 (1 mo), 10.8 (3 mo) **SE:** Hot flashes, ↓ libido, gynecomastia, & transient exacerbation of CA-related bone pain ("flare Rxn") 7–10 d after 1st dose) **Notes:** Inject SQ into fat in Abd wall; do not aspirate; females must use contraception

Granisetron (Generic)　　**Uses:** *Rx and Prevention of N/V (chemo/radiation/postoperation)* **Acts:** Serotonin (5-HT₃) receptor antagonist **Dose:** *Adults & Peds. Chemotherapy:* 10 mcg/kg/dose IV 30 min prior to chemotherapy **Adults.** *Chemotherapy:* 2 mg PO qd 1 h before chemotherapy, then 12 h later. *Postop N/V:* 1 mg IV over 30 s before end of case **W/P:** [B, +/–] St. John's wort ↓ levels **CI:** Liver Dz, children < 2 y **Disp:** Tabs 1 mg; Inj 1 mg/mL; soln 2 mg/10 mL **SE:** HA, asthenia, somnolence, D, constipation, Abd pain, dizziness, insomnia, ↑ LFTs

Guaifenesin (Robitussin, Others, Generic)　　**Uses:** *Relief of dry, non-productive cough* **Acts:** Expectorant **Dose:** *Adults.* 200–400 mg (10–20 mL) PO q4h SR 600–1200 mg PO bid (max 2.4 g/d). *Peds 2–5 y.* 50–100 mg (2.5–5 mL) PO q4h (max 600 mg/d). *6–11 y:* 100 mg (5–10 mL) PO q4h (max 1.2 g/d) **W/P:** [C, ?] **Disp:** Tabs 100, 200 mg; SR tabs 600, 1200 mg; caps 200 mg; SR caps 300 mg; liq 100 mg/5 mL **SE:** GI upset **Notes** Give w/ large amount of water; some dosage forms contain EtOH

Guaifenesin/Codeine (Robafen AC, Others, Generic) [C-V]　　**Uses:** *Relief of dry cough* **Acts:** Antitussive w/ expectorant **Dose:** *Adults.* 5–10 mL q4–6h (max 30 mL/24 h) q6–8h (max 60 mL/24 h). *Peds > 6 y.* 1–1.5 mg/kg codeine/d ÷ dose q4–6h (max 30 mg/24 h). *6–12 y:* 5 mL q4h (max 30 mL/24 h) **W/P:** [C, +] **Disp:** Brontex tab 10 mg codeine/300 mg guaifenesin; liq 2.5 mg codeine/75 mg guaifenesin/5 mL; others 10 mg codeine/100 mg guaifenesin/5 mL **SE:** Somnolence, constipation **Notes:** Not recommended for children < 6 y

Guaifenesin/Dextromethorphan (Many OTC Brands)　　**Uses:** *Cough* d/t upper resp tract irritation **Acts:** Antitussive w/ expectorant **Dose:** *Adults & Peds > 12 y.* 10 mL PO q6–8h (max 40 mL/24 h). *Peds 2–6 y.* Dextromethorphan 1–2 mg/kg/24 h ÷ 3–4 × d (max 10 mL/d). *6–12 y:* 5 mL q6–8h (max

20 mL/d) **W/P:** [C, +] **CI:** Administration w/ MAOI **Disp:** Many OTC formulations **SE:** Somnolence **Notes:** Give w/ plenty of fluids; some forms contain EtOH

Guanfacine (Intuniv, Tenex, Generic)
Uses: *ADHD (peds > 6 y)*; *HTN (adults)* **Acts:** Central α_{2a}-adrenergic agonist **Dose:** *Adults.* 1–3 mg/d IR PO h (*Tenex*), ↑ by 1 mg q3–4wk PRN 3 mg/d max; *Peds.* 1–4 mg/d XR PO (*Intuniv*), ↑ by 1 mg q1wk PRN 4 mg/d max **W/P:** [B, +/–] **Disp:** Tabs IR 1, 2 mg; tabs XR 1, 2, 3, 4 mg **SE:** Somnolence, dizziness, HA, fatigue, constipation, Abd pain, xerostomia, hypotension, bradycardia, syncope **Notes:** Rebound ↑ BP, anxiety, nervousness w/ abrupt D/C; metabolized by CYP3A4

Haemophilus B Conjugate Vaccine (ActHIB, HibTITER, Hiberix, PedvaxHIB, Others)
Uses: *Immunize children against H. influenzae type B Dzs* **Acts:** Active immunization **Dose:** *Peds.* 0.5 mL (25 mg) IM (deltoid or vastus lateralis muscle) 2 doses 2 and 4 mo; booster 12–15 mo or 2, 4, and 6 mo booster at 12–15 mo depending on formulation; **W/P:** [C, +] **CI:** Component sensitivity, febrile illness, immunosuppression, thimerosal allergy **Disp:** Inj 7.5, 10, 15, 25 mcg/0.5 mL **SE:** Fever, restlessness, fussiness, anorexia, pain/redness Inj site; observe for anaphylaxis; edema, ↑ risk of *Haemophilus* B Infxn the wk after vaccination **Notes:** *Prohibit* and *TriHIBit* cannot be used in children < 12 mo. *Hiberix* approved ages 15 mo–4 y, single dose; booster beyond 5 y old not required; report SAE to Vaccine Adverse Events Reporting System (VAERS: 1-800-822-7967); dosing varies, check w/ each product

Haloperidol (Haldol, Generic)
BOX: ↑ Mortality in elderly w/ dementia-related psychosis. Risk for torsade de pointes and QT prolongation, death w/ IV administration at higher doses **Uses:** *Psychotic disorders, agitation, Tourette disorders, hyperactivity in children* **Acts:** Butyrophenone; antipsychotic, neuroleptic **Dose:** *Adults. Mod Sxs:* 0.5–2 mg PO bid-tid. *Severe Sxs/agitation:* 3–5 mg PO bid-tid or 1–5 mg IM q4h PRN (max 100 mg/d). *ICU psychosis:* 2–10 mg IV q 30 min to effect, the 25% max dose q6h *Peds 3–6 y:* 0.01–0.03 mg/kg/24 h PO daily. *6–12 y:* Initial, 0.5–1.5 mg/24 h PO; ↑ by 0.5 mg/24 h to maint of 2–4 mg/24 h (0.05–0.1 mg/kg/24 h) or 1–3 mg/dose IM q4–8h to 0.1 mg/kg/24 h max; Tourette Dz may require up to 15 mg/24 h PO; ↓ in elderly **W/P:** [C, ?] ↑ Effects w/ SSRIs, CNS depressants, TCA, indomethacin, metoclopramide; avoid levodopa (↓ antiparkinsonian effects) **CI:** NAG, severe CNS depression, coma, Parkinson Dz, ↓ BM suppression, severe cardiac/hepatic Dz **Disp:** Tabs 0.5, 1, 2, 5, 10, 20 mg; conc liq 2 mg/mL; Inj 5 mg/mL; decanoate Inj 50, 100 mg/mL **SE:** Extrapyramidal Sxs (EPS), tardive dyskinesia, neuroleptic malignant synd, ↓ BP, anxiety, dystonias, risk for torsades de pointes and QT prolongation; leukopenia, neutropenia and agranulocytosis **Notes:** Do not give decanoate IV; dilute PO conc liq w/ H₂O/juice; monitor for EPS; ECG monitoring w/ off-label IV use; follow CBC if WBC counts decreased

Heparin (Generic)
Uses: *Rx & prevention of DVT & PE*, unstable angina, AF w/ emboli, & acute arterial occlusion **Acts:** Acts w/ antithrombin III to inactivate

thrombin & ↓ thromboplastin formation **Dose: *Adults. Prophylaxis:*** 3000–5000 units SQ q8–12h. ***DVT/PE Rx:*** Load 50–80 units/kg IV (max 10,000 units), then 10–20 units/kg IV qh (adjust based on PTT); ***ECC 2010. STEMI:*** Bolus 60 units/kg (max 4000 units); then 12 units/kg/h (max 1000 units/h) round to nearest 50 units; keep aPTT 1.5–2 × control 48 h or until angiography. ***Peds Infants.*** Load 50 units/kg IV bolus, then 20 units/kg IV by cont Inf. ***Children:*** Load 50 units/kg IV, then 15–25 units/kg cont Inf or 100 units/kg/dose q4h IV intermittent bolus (adjust based on PTT) **W/P:** [C, +] ↑ Risk of hemorrhage w/ anticoagulants, ASA, anti-plt, cephalosporins w/ MTT side chain **CI:** Uncontrolled bleeding, severe thrombocytopenia, suspected ICH **Disp:** Unfractionated Inj 10, 100, 1000, 2000, 2500, 5000, 7500, 10,000, 20,000, 40,000 units/mL **SE:** Bruising, bleeding, thrombocytopenia **Notes:** Follow PTT, thrombin time, or activated clotting time; little PT effect; therapeutic PTT 1.5–2 control for most conditions; monitor for HIT w/ plt counts; new "USP" formulation heparin is approximately 10% less effective than older formulations

Hepatitis A (Inactivated) & Hepatitis B (Recombinant) Vaccine (Twinrix) **Uses:** *Active immunization against hep A/B in pts > 18 y* **Acts:** Active immunity **Dose:** 1 mL IM at 0, 1, & 6 mo; accelerated regimen 1 mL IM day 0, 7 and 21–30 then booster at 12 mo; 720 ELISA EL.U. units hep A antigen, 20 mcg/mL hep B surface antigen **W/P:** [C, +/−] **CI:** Component sensitivity **Disp:** Single-dose vials, syringes **SE:** Fever, fatigue, HA, pain/redness at site **Notes:** Booster OK 6–12 mo after vaccination; report SAE to Vaccine Adverse Events Reporting System (VAERS: 1-800-822-7967)

Hepatitis A Vaccine (HAVRIX, VAQTA) **Uses:** *Prevent hep A* in high-risk individuals (eg, travelers, certain professions, day-care workers if 1 or more children or workers are infected, high-risk behaviors, children at ↑ risk); in chronic liver Dz **Acts:** Active immunity **Dose: *Adults.* HAVRIX** 1.0-mL IM w/ 1.0-mL booster 6–12 mo later; *VAQTA:* 1.0 mL IM w/ 1.0 mL IM booster 6–18 mo later *Peds > 12 mo.* HAVRIX 0.5-mL IM, w/ 0.5-mL booster 6–18 mo later; VAQTA 0.5 mL IM w/ booster 0.5 mL 6–18 mo later **W/P:** [C, +] **CI:** Component sensitivity; syringes contain latex **Disp:** *HAVRIX:* Inj 720 EL.U./0.5 mL, 1440 EL.U./1 mL; *VAQTA* 50 units/mL **SE:** Fever, fatigue, HA, Inj site pain **Notes:** Give primary at least 2 wk before anticipated exposure; do not give HAVRIX in gluteal region; report SAE to VAERS (1-800-822-7967)

Hepatitis B Immune Globulin (HyperHep, HepaGam B, Nabi-HB, H-BIG) **Uses:** *Exposure to HBsAg(+) material (eg, blood, accidental needlestick, mucous membrane contact, PO or sexual contact), prevent hep B in HBsAg(+) liver Tx pt* **Acts:** Passive immunization **Dose: *Adults & Peds.*** 0.06 mL/kg IM 5 mL max; w/in 24 h of exposure; w/in 14 d of sexual contact; repeat 1 mo if nonresponder or refused initial Tx; liver Tx per protocols **W/P:** [C, ?] **CI:** Allergies to γ-globulin, anti-immunoglobulin Ab, or thimerosal; IgA deficiency **Disp:** Inj **SE:** Inj site pain, dizziness, HA, myalgias, arthralgias, anaphylaxis **Notes:** IM in gluteal or deltoid; w/ continued exposure, give hep B vaccine; not for active hep B; ineffective for chronic hep B

Hepatitis B Vaccine (Engerix-B, Recombivax HB) Uses: *Prevent hep B*: men who have sex w/ men, people who inject street drugs; chronic renal/ liver Dz, healthcare workers exposed to blood, body fluids; sexually active not in monogamous relationship, people seeking evaluation for or w/ STDs; household contacts and partners of hep B infected persons, travelers to countries w/ ↑ hep B prevalence, clients/staff working w/ people w/ developmental disabilities Acts: Active immunization; recombinant DNA Dose: *Adults*. 3 IM doses 1 mL each; first 2 doses 1 mo apart; the third 6 mo after the first. *Peds*, 0.5 mL IM adult schedule W/P: [C, +] ↓ Effect w/ immunosuppressives CI: Yeast allergy, component sensitivity Disp: *Engerix-B*: Inj 20 mcg/mL; peds 10 mcg/0.5 mL. *Recombivax HB*: Inj 10 & 40 mcg/mL; peds Inj 5 mcg/0.5 mL SE: Fever, HA, Inj site pain Notes: Deltoid IM Inj adults/older peds; younger peds, use anterolateral thigh

Hetastarch (Hespan) Uses: *Plasma vol expansion* adjunct for leukapheresis Acts: Synthetic colloid; acts similar to albumin Dose: *Vol expansion:* 500–1000 mL (1500 mL/d max) IV (20 mL/kg/h max rate). *Leukapheresis:* 250–700 mL; ↓ in renal failure W/P: [C, +] CI: Severe bleeding disorders, CHF, oliguric/anuric renal failure Disp: Inj 6 g/100 mL SE: Bleeding (↑ PT, PTT, bleeding time) Notes: Not blood or plasma substitute

Histrelin Acetate (Supprelin LA, Vantas) Uses: *Advanced PCa, precocious puberty* Acts: GNRH agonist; paradoxically ↑ release of GnRH w/ ↓ LH from anterior pituitary; in men ↓ testosterone Dose: *Vantas:* 50 mg SQ implant q12mo inner aspect of the upper arm; *Supprelin LA:* 1 implant q12mo W/P: [X, –] Transient "flare Rxn" at 7–14 d after 1st dose [LH/testosterone surge before suppression]); w/ impending cord compression or urinary tract obstruction; ↑ risk DM, CV Dz, MI CI: GNRH sensitivity, PRG Disp: 50 mg 12-mo SQ implant SE: Hot flashes, fatigue, implant site Rxn, testis atrophy, gynecomastia Notes: Nonsteroidal antiandrogen (eg, bicalutamide) may block flare in men w/ PCa

Human Papillomavirus Recombinant Vaccine (Cervarix [Types 16, 18], Gardasil [Types 6, 11, 16, 18]) Uses: *Prevent cervical CA, precancerous genital lesions (Cervarix and Gardasil), genital warts, anal CA and oral CA (Gardasil)* d/t to HPV types 16, 18 (*Cervarix*) and types 6, 11, 16, 18 (*Gardasil*) in females 9–26 y*; prevent genital warts, anal CA, and anal intraepithelial neoplasia in males 9–26 y (*Gardasil*)* Acts: Recombinant vaccine, passive immunity Dose: 0.5 mL IM, then 1 and 6 mo (*Cervarix*), or 2 and 6 mo (*Gardasil*) (upper thigh or deltoid) W/P: [B, ?/–] Disp: Single-dose vial & prefilled syringe: 0.5 mL SE: Erythema, pain at Inj site, fever, syncope, venous thromboembolism Notes: 1st CA prevention vaccine, 90% effective in preventing CIN 2 or more severe Dz in HPV naive populations; report adverse events to Vaccine Adverse Events Reporting System (VAERS: 1-800-822-7967); continue cervical CA screening. Hx of genital warts, abn Pap smear, or + HPV DNA test is **not** CI to vaccination

Hydralazine (Apresoline, Others, Generic) Uses: *Mod–severe HTN, CHF* (w/ Isordil) Acts: Peripheral vasodilator Dose: *Adults*. Initial 10 mg PO

3–4×/d, ↑ to 25 mg 3–4×/d, 300 mg/d max. **Peds.** 0.75–3 mg/kg/24 h PO ÷ q6–12h; ↓ in renal impair; ✓ CBC & ANA before **W/P:** [C, +] ↓ Hepatic Fxn & CAD; ↑ tox w/ MAOI, indomethacin, β-blockers **Disp:** Dissecting aortic aneurysm, mitral valve/rheumatic heart Dz **Disp:** Tabs 10, 25, 50, 100 mg; Inj 20 mg/mL **SE:** SLE-like synd w/ chronic high doses; SVT following IM route; peripheral neuropathy **Notes:** Compensatory sinus tachycardia eliminated w/ β-blocker

Hydrochlorothiazide (HydroDIURIL, Esidrix, Others, Generic) **Uses:** *Edema, HTN* prevent stones in hypercalcuria **Acts:** Thiazide diuretic; ↓ distal tubule Na⁺ reabsorption **Dose:** **Adults.** 25–100 mg/d PO single or ÷ doses; 200 mg/d max. **Peds** < 6 mo. 2–3 mg/kg/d in 2 ÷ doses. > 6 mo: 2 mg/kg/d in 2 ÷ doses **W/P:** [D, +] **CI:** Anuria, sulfonamide allergy, renal Insuff **Disp:** Tabs 25, 50, mg; caps 12.5 mg; PO soln 50 mg/5 mL **SE:** ↓ K⁺, hyperglycemia, hyperuricemia, ↓ Na⁺; sun sensitivity **Notes:** Follow K⁺, may need supplementation

Hydrochlorothiazide/Amiloride (Moduretic, Generic) **Uses:** *HTN* **Acts:** Combined thiazide & K⁺-sparing diuretic **Dose:** 1–2 tabs/d PO **W/P:** [D, ?] **CI:** Renal failure, sulfonamide allergy **Disp:** Tabs (amiloride/HCTZ) 5 mg/50 mg **SE:** ↓ BP, photosens, ↑ K⁺/ ↓ K⁺, hyperglycemia, ↓ Na⁺, hyperlipidemia, hyperuricemia

Hydrochlorothiazide/Spironolactone (Aldactazide, Generic) **Uses:** *Edema, HTN* **Acts:** Thiazide & K⁺-sparing diuretic **Dose:** 25–200 mg each component/d, ÷ doses **W/P:** [D, +] **CI:** Sulfonamide allergy **Disp:** Tabs (HCTZ/ spironolactone) 25/25, 50/50 mg **SE:** Photosens, ↓ BP, ↑ or ↓ K⁺, ↓ Na⁺, hyperglycemia, hyperlipidemia, hyperuricemia

Hydrochlorothiazide/Triamterene (Dyazide, Maxzide, Generic) **Uses:** *Edema & HTN* **Acts:** Combo thiazide & K⁺-sparing diuretic **Dose:** Dyazide: 1–2 caps PO daily-bid. Maxzide: 1 tab/d PO **W/P:** [D, +/–] **CI:** Sulfonamide allergy **Disp:** (Triamterene/HCTZ) 37.5/25, 75/50 mg **SE:** Photosens, ↓ BP, ↑ or ↓ K⁺, ↓ Na⁺, hyperglycemia, hyperlipidemia, hyperuricemia **Notes:** HCTZ component in Maxzide more bioavailable than in Dyazide

Hydrocodone/Acetaminophen (Hycet, Lorcet, Vicodin, Others) [C-III] **Uses:** *Mod–severe pain* **Acts:** Narcotic analgesic w/ nonnarcotic analgesic **Dose:** **Adults.** 1–2 caps or tabs PO q4–6h PRN; soln 15 mL q4–6h **Peds.** Soln (Hycet) 0.27 mL/kg q4–6h **W/P:** [C, M] **CI:** CNS depression, severe resp depression **Disp:** Many formulations; specify hydrocodone/APAP dose; caps 5/500 mg; tabs 2.5/500, 5/300, 5/325, 5/500, 7.5/300, 7.5/325, 7.5/500, 7.5/650, 7.5/750, 10/300, 10/325, 10/500, 10/650, 10/660, 10/750 mg; soln Hycet (fruit punch) 7.5 mg hydrocodone/325 mg acetaminophen/15 mL **SE:** GI upset, sedation, fatigue **Notes:** Do not exceed > 4 g APAP/d; see Acetaminophen note p 36

Hydrocodone & Homatropine (Hycodan, Hydromet, Generic) [C-III] **Uses:** *Relief of cough* **Acts:** Combo antitussive **Dose:** (Based on hydrocodone) **Adults.** 5–10 mg q4–6h. **Peds.** 0.6 mg/kg/d ÷ tid-qid **W/P:** [C, M] **CI:** NAG, ↑ ICP, depressed ventilation **Disp:** Syrup 5 mg hydrocodone/5 mL; tabs 5 mg hydrocodone **SE:** Sedation, fatigue, GI upset **Notes:** Do not give < q4h; see individual drugs

Hydrocodone & Ibuprofen (Vicoprofen, Generic) [C-III] Uses: *Mod–severe pain (< 10 d)* **Acts:** Narcotic w/ NSAID **Dose:** 1–2 tabs q4–6h PRN **W/P:** [C, M] Renal Insuff; ↓ effect w/ ACE inhib & diuretics; ↑ effect w/ CNS depressants, EtOH, MAOI, ASA, TCA, anticoagulants **CI:** Component sensitivity **Disp:** Tabs 7.5 mg hydrocodone/200 mg ibuprofen **SE:** Sedation, fatigue, GI upset

Hydrocodone & Pseudoephedrine (Detussin, Histussin-D, Others, Generic) [C-III] Uses: *Cough & nasal congestion* **Acts:** Narcotic cough suppressant w/ decongestant **Dose:** 5 mL qid, PRN **W/P:** [C, M] **CI:** MAOIs **Disp:** hydrocodone/pseudoephedrine 5/60, 3/15 mg 5 mL; tab 5/60 mg **SE:** ↑ BP, GI upset, sedation, fatigue

Hydrocortisone, Rectal (Anusol-HC Suppository, Cortifoam Rectal, Proctocort, Others, Generic) Uses: *Painful anorectal conditions*, radiation proctitis, UC **Acts:** Anti-inflammatory steroid **Dose:** *Adults.* UC: 10–100 mg PR daily-bid for 2–3 wk **W/P:** [B, ?/–] **CI:** Component sensitivity **Disp:** *Hydrocortisone acetate:* Rectal aerosol 90 mg/applicator; supp 25 mg. *Hydrocortisone base:* Rectal 0.5%, 1%, 2.5%; rectal susp 100 mg/60 mL **SE:** Minimal systemic effect

Hydrocortisone, Topical & Systemic (Cortef, Solu-Cortef, Generic) See Steroids Systemic p 259 and Topical p 260 *Peds. ECC 2010.* Adrenal insufficiency: 2 mg/kg IV/IO bolus; max dose 100 mg **W/P:** [B, –] **CI:** Viral, fungal, or tubercular skin lesions; serious Infxns (except septic shock or TB meningitis) **SE:** *Systemic:* ↑ Appetite, insomnia, hyperglycemia, bruising **Notes:** May cause hypothalamic-pituitary-adrenal axis suppression

Hydromorphone (Dilaudid, Dilaudid HP, Generic) [C-II] **BOX:** A potent Schedule II opioid agonist; highest potential for abuse and risk of resp depression. HP formula is highly concentrated; do not confuse w/ standard formulations, OD and death could result. Alcohol, other opioids, CNS depressants ↑ resp depressant effects Uses: *Mod–severe pain* **Acts:** Narcotic analgesic **Dose:** 1–4 mg PO, IM, IV, or PR q4–6h PRN; 3 mg PR q6–8h PRN; ↓ w/ hepatic failure **W/P:** [B (D if prolonged use or high doses near term), ?] ↑ Resp depression and CNS effects, CNS depressants, phenothiazines, TCA **CI:** CNS lesion w/ ↑ ICP, COPD, cor pulmonale, emphysema, kyphoscoliosis, status asthmaticus; HP-Inj form in OB analgesia **Disp:** Tabs 2, 4, 8 mg scored; liq 5 mg/5 mL or 1 mg/mL; Inj 1, 2, 4 mg, *Dilaudid HP* Inj 10 mg/mL; supp 3 mg **SE:** Sedation, dizziness, GI upset **Notes:** Morphine 10 mg IM = hydromorphone 1.5 mg IM

Hydromorphone, Extended-Release (Exalgo) [C-II] **BOX:** Use in opioid tolerant only; high potential for abuse, criminal diversion and resp depression. Not for postop pain or PRN use. OD and death especially in children. Do not break/crush/chew tabs, may result in OD Uses: *Mod–severe chronic pain requiring around-the-clock opioid analgesic* *Acts:* Narcotic analgesic **Dose:** 8–64 mg PO/d titrate to effect; ↓ w/ hepatic/renal impair and elderly **W/P:** [C, –] Abuse potential;

↑ resp depression and CNS effects, w/ CNS depressants, pts susceptible to intracranial effects of CO_2 retention **CI:** Opioid-intolerant pts, ↓ pulmonary function, ileus, GI tract narrowing/obstr, component hypersens; w/in 14 d of MAOI; anticholinergics may ↑ SE **Disp:** Tabs 8, 12, 16 mg **SE:** constipation, N/V, somnolence, HA, dizziness **Notes:** See label for opioid conversion

Hydroxocobalamin (Cyanokit) Uses: *Cyanide poisoning* **Acts:** Binds cyanide to form nontoxic cyanocobalamin excreted in urine **Dose:** 5 g IV over 15 min, repeat PRN 5 g IV over 15 min–2 h, total dose 10 g **W/P:** [C, ?] **CI:** None known **Disp:** Kit- 2- to 2.5-g vials w/ Inf set **SE:** ↑ BP (can be severe) anaphylaxis, chest tightness, edema, urticaria, rash, chromaturia, N, HA, Inj site Rxns

Hydroxychloroquine (Plaquenil, Generic) **BOX:** Physicians should completely familiarize themselves w/ the complete contents of the FDA package insert before prescribing **Uses:** *Malaria: Plasmodium vivax, malariae, ovale, and falciparum* (**NOT** all strains of *falciparum*); malaria prophylaxis; discoid lupus, SLE, RA* **Acts:** Unknown/antimalarial **Dose:** *Acute Malaria: Adults.* 800 mg, 600 mg 6–8 h later then 400 mg daily × 2 d **Peds.** 32 mg base/kg over 3 d (200 mg = 155 mg base) 10 mg/kg day 1 (max 620 mg), then 5 mg/kg 6 h after 1st dose (max 310 mg), then 5 mg/kg 18 h after 2nd dose and then 5 mg/kg 24 h after 3rd dose. *Suppression Malaria: Adults.* 400 mg daily same day of wk, 2 wk before travel through 8 wk leaving endemic area **Peds.** 5 mg base/kg, same dosing schedule; *Lupus,* 400 mg daily or bid, reevaluate at 4–12 wk, then 200–400 mg daily *RA: Adults.* 400–600 mg daily, reevaluate at 4–12 wk, reduce by 50%; take w/ milk or food **W/P:** [D, ?/–] **CI:** Hx eye changes from any 4-aminoquinoline, hypersens **Disp:** Tabs 200 mg **SE:** HA, dizziness, N/V/D, Abd pain, anorexia, irritability, mood changes, psychosis, Szs, myopathy, blurred vision, corneal changes, visual field defects, retinopathy, aplastic anemia, leukopenia, derm Rxns including SJS **Notes:** Do not use long-term in children; cardiomyopathy rare

Hydroxyurea (Droxia, Hydrea, Generic) Uses: *CML, head & neck, ovarian & colon CA, melanoma, ALL, sickle cell anemia, polycythemia vera, HIV* **Acts:** ↓ Ribonucleotide reductase **Dose:** (per protocol) 50–75 mg/kg for WBC > 100,000 cells/mL; 20–30 mg/kg in refractory CML. *HIV:* 1000–1500 mg/d in single or ÷ doses; ↓ in renal Insuff **W/P:** [D, –] ↑ Effects w/ zidovudine, zalcitabine, didanosine, stavudine, fluorouracil DI: Severe anemia, BM suppression, WBC < 2500 cells/mm or plt < 100,000 cells/mm³, PRG **Disp:** Caps 200, 300, 400, 500 mg **SE:** ↓ BM (mostly leukopenia), N/V, rashes, facial erythema, radiation recall Rxns, renal impair **Notes:** Empty caps into H_2O

Hydroxyzine (Atarax, Vistaril, Generic) Uses: *Anxiety, sedation, itching* **Acts:** Antihistamine, antianxiety **Dose:** *Adults.* Anxiety/sedation: 50–100 mg PO or IM qid or PRN (max 600 mg/d). Itching: 25–50 mg PO or IM tid-qid. *Peds.* 0.5–1.0 mg/kg/24 h PO or IM q6h; ↓ w/ hepatic impair **W/P:** [C, +/–] ↑ Effects w/ CNS depressants, anticholinergics, EtOH **CI:** Component sensitivity **Disp:** Tabs 10, 25, 50 mg; caps 25, 50, mg; syrup 10 mg/5 mL; susp 25 mg/5 mL;

Inj 25, 50 mg/mL **SE:** Drowsiness, anticholinergic effects **Notes:** Used to potentiate narcotic effects; not for IV/SQ (thrombosis & digital gangrene possible)

Hyoscyamine (Anaspaz, Cystospaz, Levsin, Others, Generic)

Uses: *Spasm w/ GI & bladder disorders* **Acts:** Anticholinergic **Dose:** *Adults.* 0.125–0.25 mg (1–2 tabs) SL/PO tid-qid, ac & hs; 1 SR caps q12h **W/P:** [C, +] ↑ Effects w/ amantadine, antihistamines, antimuscarinics, haloperidol, phenothiazines, TCA, MAOI **CI:** BOO, GI obst, NAG, MyG, paralytic ileus, UC, MI **Disp:** (*Cystospaz-M, Levsinex*) time-release caps 0.375 mg; elixir (EtOH); soln 0.125 mg/5 mL; Inj 0.5 mg/mL; tab 0.125 mg; tab (*Cystospaz*) 0.15 mg; XR tab (*Levbid*) 0.375 mg; SL (*Levsin SL*) 0.125 mg **SE:** Dry skin, xerostomia, constipation, anticholinergic SE, heat prostration w/ hot weather **Notes:** Administer tabs ac

Hyoscyamine, Atropine, Scopolamine, & Phenobarbital (Donnatal, Others, Generic)

Uses: *Irritable bowel, spastic colitis, peptic ulcer, spastic bladder* **Acts:** Anticholinergic, antispasmodic **Dose:** 0.125–0.25 mg (1–2 tabs) tid-qid, 1 caps q12h (SR), 5–10 mL elixir tid-qid or q8h **W/P:** [D, M] **CI:** NAG **Disp:** Many combos/manufacturers. Caps (*Donnatal, others*): Hyoscyamine 0.1037 mg/atropine 0.0194 mg/scopolamine 0.0065 mg/phenobarbital 16.2 mg. Tabs (*Donnatal, others*): Hyoscyamine 0.1037 mg/atropine 0.0194 mg/scopolamine 0.0065 mg/phenobarbital 16.2 mg. *LA (Donnatal):* Hyoscyamine 0.311 mg/atropine 0.0582 mg/scopolamine 0.0195 mg/phenobarbital 48.6 mg. Elixirs (*Donnatal, others*): Hyoscyamine 0.1037 mg/atropine 0.0194 mg/scopolamine 0.0065 mg/phenobarbital 16.2 mg/5 mL **SE:** Sedation, xerostomia, constipation

Ibandronate (Boniva, Generic)

Uses: *Rx & prevent osteoporosis in postmenopausal women* **Acts:** Bisphosphonate, ↓ osteoclast-mediated bone resorption **Dose:** 2.5 mg PO daily or 150 mg 1 × mo on same day (do not lie down for 60 min after); 3 mg IV over 15–30 s q3mo **W/P:** [C, ?/–] Avoid w/ CrCl < 30 mL/min **CI:** Uncorrected ↓ Ca²⁺; inability to stand/sit upright for 60 min (PO) **Disp:** Tabs 2.5, 150 mg, Inj IV 3 mg/3 mL **SE:** Jaw osteonecrosis (avoid extensive dental procedures) N/D, HA, dizziness, asthenia, HTN, Infxn, dysphagia, esophagitis, esophageal/gastric ulcer, musculoskeletal pain **Notes:** Take 1st thing in A.M. w/ water (6–8 oz) > 60 min before 1st food/beverage & any meds w/ multivalent cations; give adequate Ca²⁺ & vit D supls; possible association between bisphosphonates & severe muscle/bone/joint pain; may ↑ atypical subtrochanteric femur fractures

Ibuprofen, Oral (Advil, Motrin, Motrin IB, Rufen, Others, Generic) [OTC]

BOX: May ↑ risk of CV events & GI bleeding **Uses:** *Arthritis, pain, fever* **Acts:** NSAID **Dose:** *Adults.* 200–800 mg PO bid-qid (max 2.4 g/d). *Peds.* 30–40 mg/kg/d in 3–4 ÷ doses (max 40 mg/kg/d); w/ food **W/P:** [C (D ≥ 30 wk gestation), +] May interfere w/ ASAs anti-plt effect if given < 8 h before ASA **CI:** 3rd-tri PRG, severe hepatic impair, allergy, use w/ other NSAIDs, upper GI bleeding, ulcers **Disp:** Tabs 100, 200, 400, 600, 800 mg; chew tabs 50, 100 mg; caps 200 mg; susp 50 mg/1.25 mL, 100 mg/2.5 mL, 100 mg/5 mL, 40 mg/mL (Motrin IB & Advil OTC 200 mg are the OTC forms) **SE:** Dizziness, peptic ulcer, plt inhibition, worsening of renal Insuff

Ibuprofen, Parenteral (Caldolor) **BOX:** May ↑ risk of CV events & GI bleeding **Uses:** *Mild–mod pain, as adjunct to opioids, ↓ fever* **Acts:** NSAID **Dose:** *Pain:* 400–800 mg IV over 30 min q6h PRN; *Fever:* 400 mg IV over 30 min, the 400 mg q4–6h plus 100–200 mg q4–6h PRN **W/P:** [C < 30 wk, D after 30 wk, ?/–] May ↓ ACE effects; avoid w/ ASA, and < 17 y **CI:** Hypersens NSAIDs; asthma, urticaria, or allergic Rxns w/ NSAIDs, periop CABG **Disp:** Vials 400 mg/4 mL, 800 mg/8 mL **SE:** N/V, HA, flatulence, hemorrhage, dizziness **Notes:** Make sure pt well hydrated; use lowest dose/shortest duration possible

Ibutilide (Corvert, Generic) **Uses:** *Rapid conversion of AF/A flutter* **Acts:** Class III antiarrhythmic **Dose:** *Adults > 60 kg.* 1 mg IV over 10 min; may repeat × 1; < 60 kg use 0.01 mg/kg *ECC 2010. SVT (AFib and AFlutter): Adults > 60 kg.* 1 mg (10 mL) over 10 min; a 2nd dose may be used; < 60 kg 0.01 mg/kg over 10 min. Consider DC cardioversion **W/P:** [C, –] **CI:** w/ Class I/III antiarrhythmics (Table 9, p 318); QTc > 440 ms **Disp:** Inj 0.1 mg/mL **SE:** Arrhythmias, HA **Notes:** Give w/ ECG monitoring; ✓ K⁺, Mg²⁺; wait 10 min between doses

Icatibant (Firazyr) **Uses:** *Hereditary angioedema* **Acts:** Bradykinin B₂ receptor antag **Dose:** *Adult.* 30 mg SQ in Abd; repeat q6h × 3 doses/max/24 h **W/P:** [C, ?/–] Seek medical attn after Tx of laryngeal attack **Disp:** Inj 10 mg/mL (30 mg/syringe) **SE:** Inj site Rxns, pyrexia, ↑ LFTs, dizziness, rash

Icosapent Ethyl (Vascepa) **Uses:** *Hypertriglyceridemia w/ triglycerides > 500 mg/dL* **Acts:** ↓ Hepatic VLDL-triglyceride synth/secretion & ↑ triglyceride clearance **Dose:** *Adults.* 2 caps bid w/ food **W/P:** [C, M] If hepatic Dx ✓ ALT/AST; caution w/ fish/shellfish allergy; may ↑ bleeding time **CI:** Component hypersens **Disp:** Caps 1 g **SE:** Arthralgias **Notes:** (Ethyl ester of eicosapentaenoic); ↓ risk of pancreatitis or CV morbidity/mortality not proven

Idarubicin (Idamycin, Generic) **BOX:** Administer only under supervision of an MD experienced in leukemia and in an institution w/ resources to maintain a pt compromised by drug tox **Uses:** *Acute leukemias* (AML, ALL), *CML in blast crisis, breast CA* **Acts:** DNA-intercalating agent; ↓ DNA topoisomerase I & II **Dose:** (Per protocol) 10–12 mg/m²/d for 3–4 d; ↓ in renal/hepatic impair **W/P:** [D, –] **CI:** Bilirubin > 5 mg/dL, PRG **Disp:** Inj 1 mg/mL (5-, 10-, 20-mg vials) **SE:** ↓ BM, cardiotox, N/V, mucositis, alopecia, & IV site Rxns, rarely ↓ renal/hepatic Fxn **Notes:** Avoid extrav, potent vesicant; IV only

Ifosfamide (Ifex, Generic) **BOX:** Administer only under supervision by an MD experienced in chemotherapy; hemorrhagic cystitis, myelosupp; confusion, coma possible **Uses:** *Testis*, lung, breast, pancreatic, & gastric CA, Hodgkin lymphoma/NHL, soft-tissue sarcoma **Acts:** Alkylating agent **Dose:** (Per protocol) 1.2 g/m²/d for 5-d bolus or cont Inf; 2.4 g/m²/d for 3 d; w/ mesna uroprotection; ↓ in renal/hepatic impair **W/P:** [D, M] ↑ Effect w/ phenobarbital, carbamazepine, phenytoin; St. John's wort may ↓ levels **CI:** ↓ BM Fxn, PRG **Disp:** Inj 1, 3 g **SE:** Hemorrhagic cystitis, nephrotox, N/V, mild–mod leukopenia, lethargy & confusion, alopecia, ↑ LFT **Notes:** Administer w/ mesna to prevent hemorrhagic cystitis; WBC nadir 10–14 d; recovery 21–28 d

Iloperidone (Fanapt) **BOX:** Risk for torsades de pointes and ↑ QT. Elderly pts at ↑ risk of death, CVA **Uses:** *Acute schizophrenia* **Acts:** Atypical antipsychotic **Dose:** *Initial:* 1 mg PO bid then ↑ daily to goal 6–12 mg bid, max titration 4 mg/d **W/P:** [?/–] **CI:** Component hypersens **Disp:** Tabs 1, 2, 4, 6, 8, 10, 12 mg **SE:** Orthostatic ↓ BP, dizziness, dry mouth, ↑ Wt **Notes:** Titrate to ↓ BP risk. Monitor QT interval

Iloprost (Ventavis) **BOX:** Associated w/ syncope; may require dosage adjustment **Uses:** *NYHA class III/IV pulm arterial HTN* **Acts:** Prostaglandin analog **Dose:** Initial 2.5 mcg; if tolerated, ↑ to 5 mcg Inh 6–9×/d at least 2 h apart while awake **W/P:** [C, ?/–] Anti-plt effects, ↑ bleeding risk w/ anticoagulants; additive hypotensive effects **CI:** SBP < 85 mm Hg **Disp:** Inh soln 10, 20 mcg/mL **SE:** Syncope, ↓ BP, vasodilation, cough, HA, trismus, D, dysgeusia, rash, oral irritation **Notes:** Requires *Pro-Dose AAD* or *I-neb ADD* system nebulizer; counsel on syncope risk; do not mix w/ other drugs; monitor vitals during initial Rx

Imatinib (Gleevec) **Uses:** *Rx CML Ph (+), CML blast crisis, ALL Ph(+), myelodysplastic/myeloproliferative Dz, aggressive systemic mastocytosis, chronic eosinophilic leukemia, GIST, dermatofibrosarcoma protuberans* **Acts:** ↓ BCL-ABL; TKI **Dose:** *Adults.* Typical dose 400–600 mg PO daily; w/ meal **Peds.** CML Ph(+) newly diagnosed 340 mg/m²/d, 600 mg/d max; recurrent 260 mg/m²/d PO daily-bid, to 340 mg/m²/d max **W/P:** [D, ?/–] w/ CYP3A4 meds (Table 10, p 319), warfarin **CI:** Component sensitivity **Disp:** Tab 100, 400 mg **SE:** GI upset, fluid retention, muscle cramps, musculoskeletal pain, arthralgia, rash, HA, neutropenia, thrombocytopenia **Notes:** Follow CBCs & LFTs baseline & monthly; w/ large glass of H₂O & food to ↓ GI irritation

Imipenem/Cilastatin (Primaxin, Generic) **Uses:** *Serious Infxns* d/t susceptible bacteria **Acts:** Bactericidal; ↓ cell wall synth. *Spectrum:* Gram(+) (*S. aureus*, group A & B streptococci), gram(–) (not *Legionella*), anaerobes **Dose:** *Adults.* 250–1000 mg (imipenem) IV q6–8h, 500–750 mg IM. *Peds.* 60–100 mg/kg/24 h IV ÷ q6h; ↓ if CrCl is < 70 mL/min **W/P:** [C, +/–] Probenecid ↑ tox **CI:** Peds pts w/ CNS Infxn (↑ Sz risk) & < 30 kg w/ renal impair **Disp:** Inj (imipenem/cilastatin) 250/250, 500/500 mg **SE:** Szs if accumulates, GI upset, thrombocytopenia

Imipramine (Tofranil, Generic) **BOX:** Close observation for suicidal thinking or unusual changes in behavior **Uses:** *Depression, enuresis*, panic attack, chronic pain **Acts:** TCA; ↑ CNS synaptic serotonin or norepinephrine **Dose:** *Adults.* Hospitalized: Initial 100 mg/24 h PO in ÷ doses; ↑ over several wk 300 mg/d max. *Outpatient:* Maint 50–150 mg PO hs, 300 mg/24 h max. *Peds. Antidepressant:* 1.5–5 mg/kg/24 h ÷ daily-qid. *Enuresis: > 6 y:* 10–25 mg PO qhs; ↑ by 10–25 mg at 1- to 2-wk intervals (max 50 mg for 6–12 y, 75 mg for > 12 y); Rx for 2–3 mo, then taper **W/P:** [D, ?/–]

CI: Use w/ MAOIs, NAG, recovery from AMI, PRG, CHF, angina, CV Dz, arrhythmias **Disp:** Tabs 10, 25, 50 mg; caps 75, 100, 125, 150 mg **SE:** CV Sxs, dizziness, xerostomia, discolored urine **Notes:** Less sedation than amitriptyline

Imiquimod Cream (Aldara, Zyclara) **Uses:** *Anogenital warts, HPV, condylomata acuminata (*Aldara, Zyclara*); actinic keratosis (*Zyclara*); basal cell carcinoma (*Aldara*)* **Acts:** Unknown; ? cytokine induction **Dose:** *Adults/Peds > 12 yr.* *Warts:* 1 × day up to 8 wk (*Zyclara*); apply 3×/wk, leave on 6–10 h & wash off w/ soap & water, continue 16 wk max (*Aldara*); *Actinic keratosis:* apply daily two 2 × wk cycle separate by 2 wk; *Basal cell:* apply 5 d/wk × 6 wk, dose based on lesion size (see label) **W/P:** [B, ?] Topical only, not intravaginal or intra-anal **CI:** Component sensitivity **Disp:** 2.5% packet, 3.75% packet or pump (*Zyclara);* single-dose packets 5% (250-mg cream *Aldara*) **SE:** Local skin Rxns, flu-like synd **Notes:** Not a cure; may weaken condoms/Vag diaphragms, wash hands before & after use

Immune Globulin, IV (Gamimune N, Gammaplex, Gammar IV, Sandoglobulin, Others) **Uses:** *IgG deficiency Dz states, B-cell CLL, CIDP, HIV, hep A prophylaxis, ITP*, Kawasaki Dz, travel to ↑ prevalence area, and hep A vaccination w/in 2 wk of travel **Acts:** IgG supl **Dose:** *Adults & Peds. Immunodeficiency:* 200-(300 *Gammaplex*)-800 mg/kg/mo IV at 0.01–0.04 (0.08 *Gammaplex*) mL/kg/min; initial dose 0.01 mL/kg/min. *B-cell CLL:* 400 mg/kg/dose IV q3wk, *CIDP:* 2000 mg/kg ÷ doses over 2–4 d *ITP:* 400 mg/kg/dose IV daily × 5 d. *BMT:* 500 mg/kg/wk; ↓ in renal Insuff **W/P:** [C, ?] Separate live vaccines by 3 mo **CI:** IgA deficiency w/ Abs to IgA, severe ↓ plt, coag disorders **Disp:** Inj **SE:** Associated mostly w/ Inf rate; GI upset, thrombotic events, hemolysis, renal failure/dysfun, TRALI **Notes:** Monitor vitals during Inf; do not give if volume depleted; hep A prophylaxis w/ immunoglobulin is no better than w/ vaccination; advantages to using vaccination, cost similar

Immune Globulin, Subcutaneous (Hizentra) **Uses:** *Primary immunodeficiency* **Acts:** IgG supl **Dose:** See label for dosage calculation/adjustment; for SQ Inf only **W/P:** [C, ?] **CI:** Hx anaphylaxis w/ immune globulin; severe IgA deficiency **Disp:** Soln for SQ Inj 0.2 g/mL (20%) **SE:** Inj site Rxns, HA, GI complaint, fatigue, fever, N, D, rash, sore throat **Notes:** May instruct in home administration; keep refrigerated; discard unused drug; use up to 4 Inj sites, max flow rate not > 50 mL/h all sites combined

Inamrinone [Amrinone] (Inocor) **Uses:** *Acute CHF, ischemic cardiomyopathy* **Acts:** Inotrope w/ vasodilator **Dose:** *Adults.* IV bolus 0.75 mg/kg over 2–3 min; maint 5–10 mcg/kg/min, 10 mg/kg/d max; ↓ if CrCl < 30 mL/min *Peds. ECC 2010. CHF in postop CV surg pts, shock w/ ↑ SVR:* 0.75–1 mg/kg IV/IO load over 5 min; repeat × 2 PRN; max 3 mg/kg; cont Inf 5–10 mcg/kg/min **W/P:** [C, ?] **CI:** Bisulfite allergy **Disp:** Inj 5 mg/mL **SE:** Monitor fluid, lyte, & renal changes **Notes:** Incompatible w/ dextrose solns, ✓ LFTs, observe for arrhythmias

Indacaterol Inhalation Powder (Arcapta Neohaler) BOX: LABA increase risk of asthma related deaths. Considered a class effect of all LABA. Uses: *Daily maint of COPD (chronic bronchitis/emphysema)* Acts: Long-acting β_2-adrenergic agonist (LABA) Dose: 75-mcg capsule inhaled 1×/day w/ Neohaler inhaler only W/P: [C, ?/–] Not for acute deterioration of COPD or asthma; paradoxical bronchospasm possible; excessive use or use w/ other LABA can cause cardiac effects and can be fatal; caution w/ Sz disorders, thyrotoxicosis or sympathomimetic sensitivity; w/ meds that can ↓ K^+ or ↑ QTc; β-blockers may ↓ effect CI: All LABA CI in asthma w/o use of long term asthma control med; not indicated for asthma Disp: Inhal hard cap 75 mcg (30 blister pack w/ 1 Neohaler) SE: Cough, oropharyngeal pain, nasopharyngitis, HA, N Notes: Inform patient not to swallow caps

Indapamide (Lozol, Generic) Uses: *HTN, edema, CHF* Acts: Thiazide diuretic; ↑ Na, Cl, & H_2O excretion in distal tubule Dose: 1.25–5 mg/d PO W/P: [D, ?] ↑ Effect w/ loop diuretics, ACE inhib, cyclosporine, digoxin, Li CI: Anuria, thiazide/sulfonamide allergy, renal Insuff, PRG Disp: Tabs 1.25, 2.5 mg SE: ↓ BP, dizziness, photosens Notes: No additional effects w/ doses > 5 mg; take early to avoid nocturia; use sunscreen; OK w/ food/milk

Indinavir (Crixivan) Uses: *HIV Infxn* Acts: Protease inhib; ↓ maturation of noninfectious virions to mature infectious virus Dose: Typical 800 mg PO q8h in combo w/ other antiretrovirals (dose varies); on empty stomach; ↓ w/ hepatic impair W/P: [C, ?] Numerous interactions, especially CYP3A4 inhib (Table 10, p 319) CI: Triazolam, midazolam, pimozide, ergot alkaloids, simvastatin, lovastatin, sildenafil, St. John's wort, amiodarone, salmeterol, PDE5 inhib, alpha 1-adrenoreceptor antagonist (alfuzosin); colchicine Disp: Caps 200, 400 mg SE: Nephrolithiasis, dyslipidemia, lipodystrophy, N/V, ↑ bili Notes: Drink six 8-oz glasses of water/d

Indomethacin (Indocin, Generic) BOX: May ↑ risk of CV events & GI bleeding Uses: *Arthritis; close ductus arteriosus; ankylosing spondylitis* Acts: ↓ Prostaglandins Dose: **Adults.** 25–50 mg PO bid-tid, max 200 mg/d **Infants:** 0.2–0.25 mg/kg/dose IV; may repeat in 12–24 h max 3 doses; w/ food W/P: [C, +] CI: ASA/NSAID sensitivity, peptic ulcer/active GI bleed, precipitation of asthma/urticaria/rhinitis by NSAIDs/ASA, premature neonates w/ NEC, ↓ renal Fxn, active bleeding, thrombocytopenia, 3rd tri PRG Disp: Inj 1 mg/vial; caps 25, 50 mg; SR caps 75 mg; susp 25 mg/5 mL SE: GI bleeding or upset, dizziness, edema Notes: Monitor renal Fxn

Infliximab (Remicade) BOX: TB, invasive fungal Infxns, & other opportunistic Infxns reported, some fatal; perform TB skin testing prior to use; possible association w/ rare lymphoma Uses: *Mod–severe Crohn Dz; fistulizing Crohn Dz; UC; RA (w/ MTX) psoriasis, ankylosing spondylitis* Acts: IgG1K neutralizes TNF-α Dose: **Adults.** Crohn Dz: Induction: 5 mg/kg IV Inf, w/ doses 2 & 6 wk after. *Maint:* 5 mg/kg IV Inf q8wk. *RA:* 3 mg/kg IV Inf at 0, 2, 6 wk, then q8wk. **Peds > 6 y.** 5 mg/kg IV q8wk **W/P:** [B, ?/–] Active Infxn, hepatic impair, Hx or risk of TB, hep B **CI:** Murine allergy, mod–severe CHF, w/ live vaccines (eg, smallpox) **Disp:** 100-mg Inj **SE:** Allergic Rxns; HA, fatigue, GI upset, Inf Rxns; hepatotox; reactivation hep B, pneumonia, BM suppression, systemic vasculitis, pericardial effusion, new psoriasis **Notes:** Monitor LFTs, PPD at baseline, monitor hep B carrier, skin exam for malignancy w/ psoriasis; can premedicate w/ antihistamines, APAP, and/or steroids to ↓ Inf Rxns

Influenza Vaccine, Inactivated, Quadrivalent (IIV₄) (Fluarix Quadrivalent, Fluzone Quadrivalent) See Table 13, p 324 **Uses:** *Prevent influenza* all ≥ 6 mo **Acts:** Active immunization **Dose: *Adults and Peds > 9 y.*** 0.5 mL/dose IM annually **Peds 6–35 mo.** (*Fluzone*) 0.25 mL IM annually; 0.25 mL IM × 2 doses 4 wk apart for 1st vaccination; give 2 doses in 2nd vaccination year if only 1 dose given in 1st year. **3–8 y.** 0.5 mL IM annually; 0.5 mL IM × 2 doses 4 wk apart for 1st vaccination **W/P:** [C, +] Hx Guillain-Barré synd w/in 6 wk of previous flu vaccine; syncope may occur w/ admin; immunocompromised w/ ↓ immune response **CI:** Hx allergy to egg protein, latex (*Fluarix*); egg protein (*Fluzone*) **Disp:** Based on manufacturer, 0.25-, 0.5-mL prefilled syringe, single-dose vial **SE:** Inj site soreness, fever, chills, HA, insomnia, myalgia, malaise, rash, urticaria, anaphylactoid Rxns, Guillain-Barré synd **Notes:** US Oct-Nov best, protection 1–2 wk after, lasts up to 6 mo; given yearly, vaccines based on predictions of flu season (Nov-April in US, w/ sporadic cases all year); refer to ACIP annual recs (*www.cdc.gov/vaccines/acip*)

Influenza Vaccine, Inactivated, Trivalent (IIV₃) (Afluria, Fluarix, Flucelvax, FluLaval, Fluvirin, Fluzone, Fluzone High Dose, Fluzone Intradermal) See Table 13, p 324 **Uses:** *Prevent influenza* all persons ≥ 6 mo **Acts:** Active immunization **Dose:** *Adult/Peds > 9 y.* 0.5 mL/dose IM annually; or 0.1 mL intradermal Inj annually (*Fluzone Intradermal* for adults 18–64 y). **Peds 6–35 mo.** 0.25 mL IM annually; 0.25 mL IM × 2 doses 4 wk apart for 1st vaccination; give 2 doses in 2nd vaccination year if only 1 dose given in 1st year. **3–8 y.** 0.5 mL IM annually; 0.5 mL IM × 2 doses 4 wk apart for 1st vaccination **W/P:** [B, +] Hx Guillain-Barré synd w/in 6 wk of previous influenza vaccine; syncope may occur w/ admin; immunocompromised w/ ↓ immune response **CI:** Hx allergy to egg protein, neomycin, polymyxin (*Afluria*); egg protein, latex, gentamicin (*Fluarix*); latex (*Flucelvax*); egg protein, latex (*FluLaval*); egg protein, latex, polymyxin, neomycin (*Fluvirin*); egg protein, latex (*Fluzone*); thimerosal allergy (*FluLaval, Fluvirin,* & multi-dose *Afluria, Fluzone*); single-/multi-dose vials latex free; acute resp or febrile illness **Disp:** Based on manufacturer, 0.25-, 0.5-mL prefilled syringe, single-/multi-dose vial **SE:** Inj site soreness, fever, chills, HA, insomnia, myalgia, malaise, rash, urticaria, anaphylactoid Rxns, Guillain-Barré synd **Notes:** US Oct-Nov best, protection 1–2 wk after, lasts up to

6 mo; given yearly, vaccines based on predictions of flu season (Nov–April in US, w/ sporadic cases all year); refer to ACIP annual recs (*www.cdc.gov/vaccines/acip*)

Influenza Vaccine, Live Attenuated, Quadrivalent (LAIV₄) (FluMist)
See Table 13, p 324 Uses: *Prevent influenza* Acts: Live attenuated vaccine Dose: *Adults and Peds 9–49 y.* 0.1 mL each nostril annually *Peds 2–8 y.* 0.1 mL each nostril annually; initial 0.1 mL each nostril × 2 doses 4 wk apart in 1st vaccination yr W/P: [B, ?/–] Hx Guillain-Barré synd w/in 6 wk of previous influenza vaccine; ↑ risk of wheezing w/ asthma; use w/ influenza A/B antiviral drugs may ↓ efficacy CI: Hx allergy to egg protein, gentamicin, gelatin, or arginine; peds 2–17 y on ASA, PRG, known/suspected immune deficiency, asthma/reactive airway Dz, acute febrile illness Disp: Single-dose, nasal sprayer 0.2 mL; shipped frozen, store 35–46°F SE: Runny nose, nasal congestion, HA, cough, fever, sore throat Notes: Do not give w/ other vaccines; avoid contact w/ immunocompromised individuals for 21 d; live influenza vaccine more effective in children than inactivated flu vaccine; refer to ACIP annual recs (*www.cdc.gov/vaccines/acip*)

Influenza Vaccine, Recombinant, Trivalent (RIV₃) (FluBlok) See Table 13, p 324 Uses: *Prevent influenza* Acts: Active immunization Dose: *Adults 18–49 y.* 0.5 mL/dose IM annually W/P: [B, ?/–] Hx Guillain-Barré synd w/in 6 wk of previous flu vaccine; immunocompromised w/ ↓ immune response CI: Hx component allergy (contains no egg protein, antibiotics, preservatives, latex) Disp: 0.5-mL single-dose vial SE: Inj site soreness, HA, fatigue, myalgia Notes: US Oct-Nov best, protection 1–2 wk after, lasts up to 6 mo; given yearly, vaccines based on predictions of flu season (Nov-April in US, w/sporadic cases all year); refer to ACIP annual recs (*www.cdc.gov/vaccines/acip*)

Ingenol Mebutate (Picato) Uses: *Actinic keratosis* Acts: Necrosis by neutrophil activation Dose: *Adults.* 25 cm² area (1 tube), evenly spread; 0.015% to face daily × 3 d; 0.05% to trunk/neck daily × 2 d W/P: [C, ?/–] CI: None Disp: Gel; 0.015%, 0.25 g/tube × 3 tubes; 0.05% 0.25 g/tube × 2 tubes SE: Local skin reactions Notes: From plant sap Euphorbia peplus; allow to dry × 15 min; do not wash/ touch × 6 h; avoid eye contact

Insulin, Injectable (See Table 4, p 305) Uses: *Type 1 or type 2 DM refractory to diet or PO hypoglycemic agents; acute life-threatening ↑ K⁺* Acts: Insulin supl Dose: Based on serum glucose; usually SQ (upper arms, Abd wall [most rapid absorption site], upper legs, buttocks); can give IV (only regular)/IM; type 1 typical start dose 0.5–1 units/kg/d; type 2 0.3–0.4 units/kg/d; renal failure ↓ insulin needs W/P: [B, +] CI: Hypoglycemia Disp: Table 4, p 305. Some can dispensed w/ preloaded insulin cartridge pens w/ 29-, 30-, or 31-gauge needles and dosing adjustments. SE: Hypoglycemia. Highly purified insulins ↑ free insulin; monitor for several weeks when changing doses/agents Notes: Specific agent/regimen based on pt and physician choices that maintain glycemic control. Typical type 1 regimens use a basal daily insulin w/ premeal Inj of rapidly acting insulins. Insulin pumps may achieve basal insulin levels. ↑ malignancy risk w/ glargine controversial

Interferon Alfa-2b (Intron-A) BOX: Can cause or aggravate fatal or life-threatening neuropsychiatric autoimmune, ischemic, and infectious disorders. Monitor closely **Uses:** *HCL, Kaposi sarcoma, melanoma, CML, chronic hep B & C, follicular NHL, condylomata acuminata* **Acts:** Antiproliferative; modulates host immune response; ↓ viral replication in infected cells **Dose:** Per protocols. *Adults.* Per protocols. *HCL:* 2 mill units/m² IM/SQ 3×/wk for 2–6 mo. *Chronic hep B:* 5 mill units/d or 10 mill units 3×/wk IM/SQ × 16 wk. *Follicular NHL:* 5 mill units SQ 3×/wk × 18 mo. *Melanoma:* 20 mill units/m² IV × 5 d/wk × 4 wk, then 10 mill units/m² SQ 3×/wk × 48 wk. *Kaposi sarcoma:* 30 mill units/m² IM/SQ 3×/wk until Dz progression or maximal response achieved. *Chronic hep C* (Intron-A): 3 mill units IM/SQ 3×/wk × 16 wk (continue 18–24 mo if response). *Condyloma:* 1 mill units/lesion (max 5 lesions) 3×/wk (on alternate days) for 3 wk. *Peds.* Chronic hep B: 3 mill units/m² SQ 3×/wk × 1 wk, then 6 mill units/m² max 10 mill units/dose 3×/wk × 16–24 wk. **CI:** Benzyl alcohol sensitivity, decompensated liver Dz, autoimmune hep immunosuppressed, PRG, CrCl < 50 mL/min in combo w/ ribavirin **Disp:** Inj forms: powder 10/18/50 mill Int units; soln 6/10 mill Int units/mL (see also polyethylene glycol [PEG]-interferon) **SE:** Flu-like Sxs, fatigue, anorexia, neurotox at high doses; up to 40% neutralizing Ab w/ Rx

Interferon Alfacon-1 (Infergen) BOX: Can cause or aggravate fatal or life-threatening neuropsychiatric, autoimmune, ischemic, & infectious disorders; combo therapy w/ ribavirin. Monitor closely **Uses:** *Chronic hep C* **Acts:** Biologic response modifier **Dose:** *Monotherapy:* 9 mcg 3 × wk × 24 wk (initial Rx) or 15 mcg 3×/wk up to 48 wk (retreatment). *Combo:* 15 mcg/d w/ ribavirin 1000 or 1200 mg (Wt < 75 kg and ≥ 75 kg) qd up to 48 wk (retreatment); ↓ dose w/ SAE **W/P:** [C, M] **CI:** E. coli product allergy, decompensated liver Dz, autoimmune hep **Disp:** Inj 30 mcg/mL **SE:** Flu-like synd, depression, blood dyscrasias, colitis, pancreatitis, hepatic decompensation, ↑ SCr, eye disorders, ↓ thyroid **Notes:** Allow > 48 h between Inj; monitor CBC, plt, SCr, TFT

Interferon Beta-1a (Avonex, Rebif) **Uses:** *MS, relapsing* **Acts:** Biologic response modifier **Dose:** *(Rebif)* Give SQ for target dose 44 mcg 3×/wk: start 8.8 mcg 3×/wk × 2 wk then 22 mcg 3×/wk × 2 wk then 44 mcg 3×/wk × 2 wk; target dose 22 mcg: 4.4 mcg 3×/wk × 2 wk, then 11 mcg 3×/wk × 2 wk then 22 mcg SQ 3×/wk; *(Avonex)* 30 mcg SQ 1×/wk **W/P:** [C, ?/–] w/ Hepatic impair, depression, Sz disorder, thyroid Dz **CI:** Human albumin allergy **Disp:** 0.5-mL prefilled syringes w/ 29-gauge needle *Titrate Pak* 8.8 and 22 mcg; 22 or 44 mcg **SE:** Inj site Rxn, HA, flu-like Sx, malaise, fatigue, rigors, myalgia, depression w/ suicidal ideation, hepatotox, ↓ BM **Notes:** Dose > 48 h between Inj; ✓ CBC 1, 3, 6 mo; ✓ TFTs q6mo w/ Hx thyroid Dz

Interferon Beta-1b (Betaseron, Extavia) Uses: *MS, relapsing/remitting/ secondary progressive* **Acts:** Biologic response modifier **Dose:** 0.0625 mg (2 mill units) (0.25 mL) q other day SQ, ↑ by 0.0625 mg q2wk to target dose 0.25 mg (1 mL) q other day **W/P:** [C, –] **CI:** Human albumin sensitivity **Disp:** Powder for Inj 0.3 mg (9.6 mill units interferon [IFN]) **SE:** Flu-like synd, depression, suicide, blood dyscrasias, ↑ AST/ALT/GGT, Inj site necrosis, anaphylaxis **Notes:** Teach pt self-injection, rotate sites; ✓ LFTs, CBC 1, 3, 6 mo; TFT q6mo; consider stopping w/ depression

Interferon Gamma-1b (Actimmune) Uses: *↑↓ Incidence of serious Infxns in chronic granulomatous Dz (CGD), severe malignant osteopetrosis* **Acts:** Biologic response modifier **Dose:** 50 mcg/m² SQ (1.5 mill units/m²) BSA > 0.5 m²; if BSA < 0.5 m², give 1.5 mcg/kg/dose; given 3×/wk **W/P:** [C, –] **CI:** Allergy to *E. coli*-derived products **Disp:** Inj 100 mcg (2 mill units) **SE:** Flu-like synd, depression, blood dyscrasias, dizziness, altered mental status, gait disturbance, hepatic tox **Notes:** may ↑ deaths in interstitial pulm fibrosis

Ipilimumab (Yervoy) **BOX:** Severe fatal immune Rxns possible; D/C and Tx w/ high-dose steroids w/ severe Rxn; assess for enterocolitis, dermatitis, neuropathy, endocrinopathy before each dose Uses: *Unresectable/metastatic melanoma* **Acts:** Human cytotoxic T-lymphocyte antigen 4 (CTLA-4)-blocking Ab; ↑ T cell proliferation/activation **Dose:** 3 mg/kg IV q3wk × 4 doses; Inf over 90 min **W/P:** [C, –] Can cause immune-mediated adverse Rxns; endocrinopathies may require Rx; hep dermatologic tox, heuramuscular tox, opthalmic tox **CI:** None **Disp:** IV 50 mg/10 mL, 200 mg/40 mL **SE:** Fatigue, D, pruritus, rash, colitis **Notes:** ✓ LFTs, TFT, chemistries baseline/pre/Inf

Ipratropium (Atrovent HFA, Atrovent Nasal) Uses: *Bronchospasm w/ COPD, rhinitis, rhinorrhea* **Acts:** Synthetic anticholinergic similar to atropine; antagonizes acetylcholine receptors, inhibits mucous gland secretions **Dose:** *Adults & Peds > 12 y.* 2–4 puffs qid, max 12 Inh/d *Nasal:* 2 sprays/nostril bid-tid; *Nebulization:* 500 mcg 3–4 ×/d; *ECC 2010. Asthma:* 250–500 mcg by neb/ MDI q20min × 3 **W/P:** [B, ?/M] w/ Inhaled insulin **CI:** Allergy to soya lecithin-related foods **Disp:** *HFA* Metered-dose inhaler 17 mcg/dose; Inh soln 0.02%; nasal spray 0.03, 0.06% **SE:** Nervousness, dizziness, HA, cough, bitter taste, nasal dryness, URI, epistaxis **Notes:** Not for acute bronchospasm unless used w/ inhaled β-agonist

Irbesartan (Avapro) **BOX:** D/C immediately if PRG detected Uses: *HTN, DN* **Acts:** Angiotensin II receptor antagonist **Dose:** 150 mg/d PO, may ↑ to 300 mg/d **W/P:** [C (1st tri); D 2nd/3rd tri), ?/–] **CI:** PRG, component sensitivity **Disp:** Tabs 75, 150, 300 mg **SE:** Fatigue, ↓ BP, ↑ K

Irinotecan (Camptosar, Generic) **BOX:** D & myelosuppression administered by experienced physician Uses: *Colorectal* & *lung CA* **Acts:** Topoisomerase I inhib; ↓ DNA synth **Dose:** Per protocol; 125–350 mg/m² qwk–q3wk (↓ hepatic dysfunction, as tolerated per tox) **W/P:** [D, –] **CI:** Allergy to component **Disp:** Inj

20 mg/mL **SE:** ↓ BM, N/V/D, Abd cramping, alopecia; D is dose limiting; Rx acute D w/ atropine; Rx subacute D w/ loperamide **Notes:** D correlated to levels of metabolite SN-38

Iron Dextran (Dexferrum, INFeD) **BOX:** Anaphylactic Rxn w/ death reported; proper personnel and equipment should be available. Use test dose on only if PO iron not possible **Uses:** *Iron-deficiency anemia where PO administration not possible* **Dose:** See also label for tables/formula to calculate dose. Estimate Fe deficiency; total dose (mL) = [0.0442 × (desired Hgb − observed Hgb) × lean body Wt] + (0.26 × lean body Wt); Fe replacement, blood loss: total dose (mg) = blood loss (mL) × Hct (as decimal fraction) max 100 mg/d. **IV use:** *Test dose:* 0.5 mL IV over 30 s, if OK, 2 mL or less daily IV over 1 mL/min to calculated total dose **IM use:** *Test dose* 0.5 mL deep IM in buttock. Administer calculated total dose not to exceed daily doses as follows: Infants < 5 kg: 1.0 mL; children < 10 kg; all others 2.0 mL (100 mg of iron). **W/P:** [C, M] w/Hx allergy/asthma. Keep Epi available (1:1000) for acute Rxn **CI:** Component hypersens, non–Fe-deficiency anemia **Disp:** Inj 50 mg Fe/mL in 2 mL vials (*INFeD*) and 1 & 2 mL vials (*Dexferrum*) **Notes:** Not rec in infants < 4 mo. ✓ Hgb/Hct. Also Fe, TIBC, and % saturation transferrin may be used to monitor. Reticulocyte count best early indicator of response (several days). IM use "Z-track" technique

Iron Sucrose (Venofer) **Uses:** *Iron-deficiency anemia in CKD, w/ wo dialysis, w/ wo erythropoietin* **Acts:** Fe supl **Dose:** 100 mg on dialysis; 200 mg slow IV over 25 min × 5 doses over 14 d. Total cum dose 1000 mg **W/P:** [B, M] Hypersens, ↓ BP, Fe overload, may interfere w/ MRI **CI:** Non–Fe-deficiency anemia; Fe overload; component sens **Disp:** Inj 20 mg Fe/mL, 2.5, 5, 10 mL vials **SE:** Muscle cramps, N/V, strange taste in the mouth, diarrhea, constipation, HA, cough, back/jt pain, dizziness, swelling of the arms/legs **Notes:** Safety in peds not established

Isoniazid (INH) **BOX:** Severe & sometimes fatal hep may occur usually w/in 1st 3 mo of Tx, although may develop after mo of Tx **Uses:** *Rx & prophylaxis of TB* **Acts:** Bactericidal; interferes w/ mycolic acid synth, disrupts cell wall **Dose:** *Adults. Active TB:* 5 mg/kg/24 h PO or IM (usually 300 mg/d) or *DOT:* 15 mg/kg (max 900 mg) 3×/wk. *Prophylaxis:* 300 mg/d PO for 6–12 mo or 900 mg 2×/wk. *Peds. Active TB:* 10–15 mg/kg/d daily PO or IM 300 mg/d max. *Prophylaxis:* 10 mg/kg/24 h PO; ↓ in hepatic/renal dysfunction **W/P:** [C, +] Liver Dz, dialysis; avoid EtOH **CI:** Acute liver Dz, Hx INH hep **Disp:** Tabs 100, 300 mg; syrup 50 mg/5 mL; Inj 100 mg/ mL **SE:** Hep, peripheral neuropathy, GI upset, anorexia, dizziness, skin Rxn **Notes:** Use w/ 2–3 other drugs for active TB, based on INH resistance patterns when TB acquired & sensitivity results; prophylaxis usually w/ INH alone. IM rarely used. ↓ Peripheral neuropathy w/ pyridoxine 50–100 mg/d. See CDC guidelines (http://www. cdc.gov/tb/) for current TB recommendations

Isoproterenol (Isuprel) **Uses:** *Shock, cardiac arrest, AV nodal block* **Acts:** β_1- & β_2-receptor stimulants **Dose:** *Adults.* 2–10 mcg/min IV Inf; titrate;

2–10 mcg/min titrate (*ECC 2005*) **Peds.** 0.2–2 mcg/kg/min IV Inf; titrate **W/P:** [C, ?] **CI:** Angina, tachyarrhythmias (digitalis-induced or others) **Disp:** 0.02 mg/mL, 0.2 mg/mL **SE:** Insomnia, arrhythmias, HA, trembling, dizziness **Notes:** Pulse > 130 BPM may induce arrhythmias

Isosorbide Dinitrate (Dilatrate-SR, Isordil, Sorbitrate, Generic) **Uses:** *Rx & prevent angina*, CHF (w/ hydralazine) **Acts:** Relaxes vascular smooth muscle **Dose:** *Acute angina:* 5–10 mg PO (chew tabs) q2–3h or 2.5–10 mg SL PRN q5–10 min; do not give > 3 doses in a 15- to 30-min period. *Angina prophylaxis:* 5–40 mg PO q6h; do not give nitrates on a chronic q6h or qid basis > 7–10 d; tolerance may develop; provide 10- to 12-h drug-free intervals; *dose in CHF:* initial 20 mg 3–4×/d, target 120–160 mg/d **W/P:** [C, ?] **CI:** Severe anemia, NAG, postural ↓ BP, cerebral hemorrhage, head trauma (can ↑ ICP), w/ sildenafil, tadalafil, vardenafil **Disp:** Tabs 5, 10, 20, 30; SR tabs 40 mg; SL tabs 2.5, 5 mg; SR caps 40 mg **SE:** HA, ↓ BP, flushing, tachycardia, dizziness **Notes:** Higher PO dose needed for same results as SL forms

Isosorbide Mononitrate (Ismo, Imdur, Monoket) **Uses:** *Prevention/Rx of angina pectoris* **Acts:** Relaxes vascular smooth muscle **Dose:** 5–20 mg PO bid, w/ doses 7 h apart or XR (Imdur) 30–60 mg/d PO, max 240 mg **W/P:** [B, ?] Severe hypotension w/ paradoxical bradycardia, hypertrophic cardiomyopathy; head trauma/cerebral hemorrhage (can ↑ ICP) **CI:** w/ Sildenafil, tadalafil, vardenafil **Disp:** Tabs 10, 20 mg; XR 30, 60, 120 mg **SE:** HA, dizziness, ↓ BP

Isotretinoin (Amnesteem, Claravis, Myorisan, Sotret, Zentane, Generic) **BOX:** Do not use in pts who are/may become PRG; ↑ risk severe birth defects; available only through iPLEDGE restricted distribution program; pts, prescribers, pharmacies, and distributors must enroll **Uses:** *Severe nodular acne resistant to other Tx* **Acts:** Inhib sebaceous gland Fxn & keratinization **Dose:** *Adults and Peds ≥ 12 y:* 0.5–1 mg/kg/d ÷ doses × 15–20 wk, do NOT take only 1×/d; PRG test prior to Rx each mo, end of Tx, and 1 mo after D/C **W/P:** [X, –] Micro-dosed progesterone BCPs NOT an acceptable method of birth control; depression, suicidal thoughts and behaviors, psychosis/aggressive/violent behavior; pseudotumor cerebri; TEN, SJS; ↓ hearing, corneal opacities, ↓ night vision; IBD, pancreatitis, hepatic toxicity, ✓ lipids/LFTs regularly; back/joint pain, osteopenia, premature epiphyseal closure; ↑ chol, ↑ triglycerides, ↓ HDL; ↑ CK; ↑ glu **CI:** PRG, hypersens **Disp:** Caps 10, 20, 30, 40 mg **SE:** Dry/chapped lips, cheilitis, dry skin, dermatitis, dry eye, ↓ vision, HA, epistaxis, nasopharyngitis, URI, back pain **Notes:** ✓ Lipids/LFTs before; vit A may ↑ adverse events; avoid tetracyclines and any meds that may interfere w/ BCP effectiveness

Isradipine (DynaCirc) **Uses:** *HTN* **Acts:** CCB **Dose:** 2.5–5 mg PO bid; IR 2.5–10 mg bid; CR 5–20 qd **W/P:** [C, ?/–] **CI:** Severe heart block, sinus bradycardia, CHF, dosing w/in several hours of IV β-blockers **CI:** Hypotension < 90 mm Hg systolic **Disp:** Caps 2.5, 5 mg; tabs CR 5, 10 mg **SE:** HA, edema, flushing, fatigue, dizziness, palpitations

Itraconazole (Onmel, Sporanox, Generic) **BOX:** CI w/ cisapride, pimozide, quinidine, dofetilide, or levacetylmethadol. Serious CV events (eg, ↑ QT, torsades de pointes, VT, cardiac arrest, and/or sudden death) reported w/ these meds and other CYP3A4 inhib. Do not use for onychomycosis w/ ventricular dysfunction. Negative inotropic effects have been observed following IV administration D/C/reasses use if S/Sxs of HF occur during Tx **Uses:** *Fungal Infxns (aspergillosis, blastomycosis, histoplasmosis, candidiasis, onychomycosis)* **Acts:** Azole antifungal, ↓ ergosterol synth **Dose:** Dose based on indication. 200 mg PO daily-tid (caps w/ meals or cola/grapefruit juice); PO soln on empty stomach; avoid antacids **W/P:** [C, –] Numerous interactions **CI:** See Box; PRG or considering PRG; ventricular dysfunction CHF **Disp:** Caps 100 mg; soln 10 mg/mL **SE:** N/V, rash, hepatotoxic, ↓ K⁺, CHF, ↑ BP, neuropathy **Notes:** Soln & caps not interchangeable; useful in pts who cannot take amphotericin B; follow LFTs

Ivacaftor (Kalydeco) **Uses:** *Cystic fibrosis w/ G551D mutation transmembrane conductance regulator (CFTR) gene* **Acts:** ↑ Chloride transport **Dose:** *Adult & Peds > 6 y.* 150 mg bid; w/ fatty meal; ↓ hepatic impair or w CYP3A inhib **W/P:** [B, ?/–] w/ CYP3A inhib (ketoconazole, itraconazole, clarithromycin); may ↑ digoxin, cyclosporin, tacrolimus, benzodiazepine levels; w/ hepatic impair Child-Pugh Class C; severe renal impair **CI:** None **Disp:** Tabs 150 mg **SE:** HA, URI, oropharyngeal pain, Abd pain, N/D **Notes:** ✓ LFTs q3mo × 4, then yearly; D/C if AST/ALT 5 × ULN

Ivermectin, Oral (Stromectol) **Uses:** *Strongyloidiasis (intestinal), onchocerciasis* **Acts:** Binds glutamate-gated chloride channels in nerve and muscle cells, paralysis and death of nematodes **Dose:** *Adults & Peds.* Based on Wt and condition: *intestinal strongyloidiasis* 1 tab 15–24 kg, 2 tabs 25–35 kg, 3 tabs 36–50 kg, 4 tabs 51–65 kg, 5 tabs 66–79 kg, 80 or > 200 mcg/kg; *onchocerciasis* repeat dose × 1 in 2 wk, 1 tab 15–25 kg, 2 tabs 26–44 kg, 3 tabs 45–64 kg, 4 tabs 65–84 kg; 85 or > 150/mcg/kg; on empty stomach **W/P:** [C, ?/–] Potential severe allergic/inflammatory Rxn Tx of onchocerciasis **CI:** Hypersensitivity **Disp:** Tabs 3 mg **SE:** N/V/D, dizziness, pruritus ↑ AST/ALT; ↓ WBC, RBC **Notes:** From fermented *Streptomyces avermitilis*; does not kill adult onchocerca, requires redosing

Ivermectin, Topical (Sklice) **Uses:** *Head lice* **Acts:** Binds to glutamate-gated chloride channels in nerve and muscle cells, paralysis and death of lice **Dose:** *Adult & Peds > 6 mo.* Coat hair/scalp **W/P:** [C, ?/–] **CI:** None **Disp:** Lotion 0.5%, 4-oz tube **SE:** Conjunctivitis, red eye, dry skin **Notes:** From fermented *Streptomyces avermitilis*; coat dry hair and scalp thoroughly; avoid eye contact; use w/ lice management plan

Ixabepilone Kit (Ixempra) **BOX:** CI in combo w/ capecitabine w/ AST/ALT > 2.5 × ULN or bili > 1× ULN d/t ↑ tox and neutropenia-related death **Uses:** *Metastatic/locally advanced breast CA after failure of an anthracycline, a taxane, and capecitabine* **Acts:** Microtubule inhib **Dose:** 40 mg/m² IV over 3 h q3wk 88 mg max **W/P:** [D, ?/–] **CI:** Hypersens to Cremophor EL; baseline ANC < 1500 cells/mm³ or plt < 100,000 cells/mm³; AST/ or ALT > 2.5 × ULN, bili > 1 × ULN capecitabine **Disp:** Inj 15, 45 mg (use supplied diluent) **SE:** Neutropenia, leukopenia, anemia, thrombocytopenia, peripheral sensory neuropathy, fatigue/asthenia, myalgia/arthralgia, alopecia, N/V/D, stomatitis/mucositis **Notes:** Substrate CYP3A4, adjust dose w/ strong CYP3A4 inhib/inducers

Japanese Encephalitis Vaccine, Inactivated, Adsorbed (Ixiaro, Je-Vax)
Uses: *Prevent Japanese encephalitis* **Acts:** Inactivated vaccine **Dose:** *Adults.* 0.5 mL IM, repeat 28 d later given at least 1 wk prior to exposure *Peds.* Use Je-Vax, 1–3 y: Three 0.5 mL SQ doses day 0, 7, 30; > 3 y: Three 1 mL SQ doses on day 0, 7, 30 **W/P:** [B (Ixiaro)/ ?] Severe urticaria or angio edema may occur up to 10 d after vaccination **SE:** HA, fatigue, Inj site pain, flu-like syndrome, hypersens Rxns **Notes:** Abbrev admin schedules of 3 doses on day 0, 7, and 14; booster dose recommended after 2 y. Avoid EtOH 48 h after dose, use is not recommended for all travelling to Asia

Ketamine (Ketalar, Generic) [C-III]
Uses: *Induction/maintenance of anesthesia* (in combo w/ sedatives), sedation, analgesia **Acts:** Dissociative anesthesia; IV onset 30 s, duration 5–10 min **Dose:** *Adults.* 1–4.5 mg/kg IV, typical 2 mg/kg; 3–8 mg/kg IM **Peds.** 0.5–2 mg/kg IV; 0.5–1 mg/kg for minor procedures (also IM/PO regimens) **W/P:** w/ CAD, ↑ BP, tachycardia, EtOH use/abuse [C, ?/–] **CI:** When ↑ BP hazardous **Disp:** Soln 10, 50, 100 mg/mL **SE:** Arrhythmia, ↑/↓ HR, ↑/↓ BP, N/V, resp depression, emergence Rxn, ↑ CSF pressure. CYP2B6 inhibs w/ ↓ metabolism **Notes:** Used in RSI protocols; street drug of abuse

Ketoconazole (Nizoral, Generic)
BOX: (Oral use) Risk of fatal hepatotox. Concomitant terfenadine, astemizole, and cisapride are CI d/t serious CV adverse events **Uses:** *Systemic fungal Infxns (Candida, blastomycosis, histoplasmosis, etc); refractory topical dermatophyte Infxn*; PCa when rapid ↓ testosterone needed or hormone refractory **Acts:** Azole, ↓ fungal cell wall synth; high dose blocks P450, to ↓ testosterone production **Dose:** *PO:* 200 mg PO daily; ↑ to 400 mg PO daily for serious Infxn. *PCa:* 400 mg PO tid; best on empty stomach **W/P:** [C, –/–] w/ Any agent that ↑ gastric pH (↓ absorption); may enhance anticoagulants; w/ EtOH (disulfiram-like Rxn); numerous interactions including statins, niacin; do not use w/ clopidogrel (↓ effect) **CI:** CNS fungal Infxns, w/ astemizole, triazolam **Disp:** Tabs 200 mg **SE:** N, rashes, hair loss, HA, ↑ Wt gain, dizziness, disorientation, fatigue, impotence, hepatox, adrenal suppression, acquired cutaneous adherence ("sticky skin synd") **Notes:** Monitor LFTs; can rapidly ↓ testosterone levels

Ketoconazole, Topical (Extina, Nizoral A-D Shampoo, Xolegel) [Shampoo—OTC]
Uses: *Topical for seborrheic dermatitis, shampoo for dandruff* local fungal Infxns d/t dermatophyte & yeast **Acts:** Azole, ↓ fungal cell wall synth **Dose:** *Topical:* Apply qd-bid **W/P:** [C, +/–] **Disp:** Topical cream 2%; (*Xolegel*) gel 2%, (*Extina*) foam 2%, shampoo 2% **SE:** Irritation, pruritus, stinging **Notes:** Do not dispense foam into hands

Ketoprofen (Orudis, Oruvail) **BOX:** May ↑ risk of fatal CV events & GI bleeding; CI for perioperative pain in CABG surgery Uses: *Arthritis (RA/OA), pain* **Acts:** NSAID; ↓ prostaglandins **Dose:** 25–75 mg PO tid-qid, 300 mg/d/max; SR 200 mg/d; w/ food; ↓ w/ hepatic/renal impair, elderly **W/P:** [C (D 3rd tri), −] w/ ACE, diuretics; ↑ warfarin, Li, MTX, avoid EtOH **CI:** NSAID/ASA sensitivity **Disp:** Caps 50, 75 mg; caps, SR 200 mg **SE:** GI upset, peptic ulcers, dizziness, edema, rash, ↑ BP, ↑ LFTs, renal dysfunction

Ketorolac (Toradol) **BOX:** For short-term (≤ 5 d) Rx of mod–severe acute pain; CI w/ PUD, GI bleed, post CABG, anticipated major surgery, severe renal Insuff, bleeding diathesis, L&D, nursing, and w/ ASA/NSAIDs. NSAIDs may cause ↑ risk of CV/thrombotic events (MI, stroke). PO CI in peds < 16 y, dose adjustments for < 50 kg Uses: *Pain* **Acts:** NSAID; ↓ prostaglandins **Dose:** *Adults.* 15–30 mg IV/IM q6h; 10 mg PO qid only as continuation of IV/IM; max IV/IM 120 mg/d, max PO 40 mg/d. *Peds 2–16 y.* 1 mg/kg IM × 1 dose; 30 mg max; IV: 0.5 mg/kg, 15 mg max; do not use for > 5 d; ↓ if > 65 y, elderly, w/ renal impair, < 50 kg **W/P:** [C (D 3rd tri), −] w/ ACE inhib, diuretics, BP meds, warfarin **CI:** See Box **Disp:** Tabs 10 mg; Inj 15 mg/mL, 30 mg/mL **SE:** Bleeding, peptic ulcer Dz, ↑ Cr & LFTs, ↑ BP, edema, dizziness, allergy

Ketorolac, Nasal (Sprix) **BOX:** For short-term (5 d) use; CI w/ PUD, GI bleed, suspected bleeding risk, postop CABG, advanced renal Dz or risk of renal failure w/ vol depletion; can ↑ CV thrombotic events (MI, stroke). Not indicated for use in children Uses: *Short-term (< 5 d) Rx pain requiring opioid level analgesia* **Acts:** NSAID; ↓ prostaglandins **Dose:** *< 65 y.* 31.5 mg (one 15.75-mg spray each nostril) q6–8h; max 126 mg/d. *≥ 65 y, w/ renal impair or < 50 kg.* 15.75 mg (one 15.75-mg spray in only 1 nostril) q6–8h; max 63 mg/d **W/P:** [C (D 3rd tri), −] Do not use w/ other NSAIDs; can cause severe skin Rxns; do not use w/ critical bleeding risk; w/ CHF **CI:** See Box; prophylactic to major surgery/L&D, w/ Hx allergy to other NSAIDs recent or Hx of GI bleed or perforation **Disp:** Nasal spray 15.75-mg ketorolac/100-mcL soln (8 sprays/bottle) **SE:** Nasal discomfort/rhinitis, ↑ lacrimation, throat irritation, oliguria, rash, ↓ HR, ↓ urine output, ↑ ALT/AST, ↑ BP Notes: Discard open bottle after 24 h

Ketorolac Ophthalmic (Acular, Acular LS, Acular PF, Acuvail) Uses: *Ocular itching w/ seasonal allergies; inflammation w/ cataract extraction*; pain/ photophobia w/ incisional refractive surgery (Acular PF); pain w/ corneal refractive surgery (Acular LS) **Acts:** NSAID **Dose:** 1 gtt qid **W/P:** [C, +] Possible cross-sensitivity to NSAIDs, ASA **CI:** Hypersens **Disp:** *Acular LS:* 0.4% 5 mL; *Acular:* 0.5% 3, 5, 10 mL; *Acular PF:* Soln 0.5% Acuvail soln 0.45% **SE:** Local irritation, ↑ bleeding ocular tissues, hyphemas, slow healing, keratitis **Notes:** Do not use w/ contacts

Ketotifen (Alaway, Claritin Eye, Zaditor, Zyrtec Itchy Eye) [OTC] Uses: *Allergic conjunctivitis* **Acts:** Antihistamine H₁-receptor antagonist, mast cell stabilizer **Dose:** *Adults & Peds > 3 y.* 1 gtt in eye(s) q8–12h **W/P:** [C, ?/−]

Disp: Soln 0.025%/5 & 10 mL **SE:** Local irritation, HA, rhinitis, keratitis, mydriasis **Notes:** Wait 10 min before inserting contacts

Kunecatechins [Sinecatechins] (Veregen) Uses: *External genital/perianal warts* **Acts:** Unknown; green tea extract **Dose:** Apply 0.5-cm ribbon to each wart 3×/d until all warts clear; not > 16 wk **W/P:** [C, ?] **Disp:** Oint 15% **SE:** Erythema, pruritus, burning, pain, erosion/ulceration, edema, induration, rash, phimosis **Notes:** Wash hands before/after use; not necessary to wipe off prior to next use; avoid on open wounds, may weaken condoms & Vag diaphragms, use in combo is not recommended

Labetalol (Trandate) Uses: *HTN* & hypertensive emergencies (IV) **Acts:** α- & β-Adrenergic blockers **Dose:** *Adults. HTN:* Initial, 100 mg PO bid, then 200–400 mg PO bid. *Hypertensive emergency:* 20–80 mg IV bolus, then 2 mg/min IV Inf, titrate up to 300 mg; *ECC 2010.* 10 mg IV over 1–2 min; repeat or double dose q10min (150 mg max); or initial bolus, then 2–8 mg/min **Peds.** *PO:* 1–3 mg/kg/d in ÷ doses, 1200 mg/d max. *Hypertensive emergency:* 0.4–1.5 mg/kg/h IV cont Inf **W/P:** [C (D in 2nd or 3rd tri), +] **CI:** Asthma/COPD, cardiogenic shock, uncompensated CHF, heart block, sinus brady **Disp:** Tabs 100, 200, 300 mg; Inj 5 mg/mL **SE:** Dizziness, N, ↓ BP, fatigue, CV effects

Lacosamide (Vimpat) Uses: *Adjunct in partial-onset Szs* **Acts:** Anticonvulsant **Dose:** *Initial:* 50 mg IV or PO bid, ↑ weekly; *Maint.* 200–400 mg/d; 300 mg/d max if CrCl < 30 mL/min or mild–mod hepatic Dz **W/P:** [C, ?] DRESS ↑ PR [C–V] Antiepileptics associated w/ ↑ risk of suicide ideation **CI:** None **Disp:** *IV:* 200 mg/20 mL; Tabs: 50, 100, 150, 200 mg; oral soln 10 mg/mL **SE:** Dizziness, N/V, ataxia **Notes:** ✓ ECG before dosing

Lactic Acid & Ammonium Hydroxide [Ammonium Lactate] (LacHydrin) [OTC] Uses: *Severe xerosis & ichthyosis* **Acts:** Emollient moisturizer, humectant **Dose:** Apply bid **W/P:** [B, ?] **Disp:** Cream, lotion, lactic acid 12% w/ ammonium hydroxide **SE:** Local irritation, photosens **Notes:** Shake well before use

Lactobacillus (Lactinex Granules) [OTC] Uses: *Control of D*, especially after antibiotic Rx **Acts:** Replaces nl intestinal flora, lactase production; *Lactobacillus acidophilus* and *Lactobacillus helveticus.* **Dose:** *Adults & Peds > 3 y.* 1 packet, 1–2 caps, or 4 tabs qd-qid **W/P:** [A, +] Some products may contain whey **CI:** Milk/lactose allergy **Disp:** Tabs, caps; granules in packets (all OTC) **SE:** Flatulence **Notes:** May take granules on food

Lactulose (Constulose, Generlac, Enulose, Others) Uses: *Hepatic encephalopathy; constipation* **Acts:** Acidifies the colon, allows ammonia to diffuse into colon; osmotic effect to ↑ peristalsis **Dose:** *Acute hepatic encephalopathy:* 30–45 mL PO q1h until soft stools, then tid-qid, adjust 2–3 stool/d. *Constipation:* 15–30 mL/d, ↑ to 60 mL/d 1–2 ÷ doses, adjust to 2–3 stools. *Rectally:* 200 g in 700 mL of H₂O PR, retain 30–60 min q4–6h **Peds Infants.** 2.5–10 mL/24 h ÷ tid-qid **Other Peds.** 40–90 mL/24 h ÷ tid-qid. *Peds constipation:* 1–3 mL/kg/d ÷ doses (max 60 mL/d) PO after breakfast **W/P:** [B, ?] **CI:** Galactosemia **Disp:** Syrup 10 g/15 mL, soln

10 g/15 mL, 10, 20 g/packet **SE:** Severe D, N/V, cramping, flatulence; life-threatening lyte disturbances

Lamivudine (Epivir, Epivir-HBV, 3TC [Many Combo Regimens])

BOX: Lactic acidosis & severe hepatomegaly w/ steatosis reported w/ nucleoside analogs do not use Epivir-HBV for Tx of HIV, monitor pts closely following D/C of therapy for hep B **Uses:** *HIV Infxn, chronic hep B* **Acts:** NRTI, ↓ HIV RT & hep B viral polymerase, causes viral DNA chain termination **Dose:** *HIV: Adults & Peds > 16 y.* 150 mg PO bid or 300 mg PO daily *Peds able to swallow pills. 14–21 kg:* 75 mg bid; *22–29 kg:* 75 mg q A.M., 150 mg q P.M. *> 30 kg:* 150 mg bid *Neonates < 30 d:* 2 mg/kg bid; infants 1–3 mo 4 mg/kg/dose > 3 mo & child < 16 y 4 mg/kg/dose bid (max 150 mg bid) *Epivir-HBV: Adults.* 100 mg/d PO. *Peds 2–17 y.* 3 mg/kg/d PO, 100 mg max; ↓ w/ CrCl < 50 mL/min **W/P:** [C, ?] w/ Interferon-α and ribavirin may cause liver failure; do not use w/ zalcitabine or w/ ganciclovir/valganciclovir **Disp:** Tabs 100 mg (Epivir-HBV) 150 mg, 300 mg; soln 5 mg/mL (Epivir-HBV), 10 mg/mL **SE:** Malaise, fatigue, N/V/D, HA, pancreatitis, lactic acidosis, peripheral neuropathy, fat redistribution, rhabdomyolysis hyperglycemia, nasal Sxs **Notes:** Differences in formulations; do not use Epivir-HBV for hep in pt w/ unrecognized HIV d/t rapid emergence of HIV resistance

Lamotrigine (Lamictal)

BOX: Life-threatening rashes, including Stevens-Johnson synd and toxic epidermal necrolysis, and/or rash-related death reported; D/C at 1st sign of rash **Uses:** *Epilepsy adjunct ≥ 2 y or monoRx ≥ 16 y old; bipolar disorder ≥ 18 y old* **Acts:** Phenyltriazine antiepileptic, ↓ glutamate, stabilize neuronal membrane **Dose:** *Adults. Szs:* Initial 50 mg/d PO, then 50 mg PO bid × 1–2 wk, maint 300–500 mg/d in 2 ÷ doses. *Bipolar:* Initial 25 mg/d PO × 1–2 wk, 50 mg PO daily for 2 wk, 100 mg PO daily for 1 wk, maint 200 mg/d. *Peds.* 0.6 mg/kg in 2 ÷ doses for wk 1 & 2, then 1.2 mg/kg for wk 3 & 4, q1–2wk to maint 5–15 mg/kg/d (max 400 mg/d) in 1–2 ÷ doses; ↓ hepatic Dz or w/ enzyme inducers or valproic acid **W/P:** [C, –] ↑ suicide risk, higher for those w/ epilepsy vs psych use. Interact w/ other antiepileptics, estrogen, rifampin **Disp:** (color-coded for use w/interacting meds); starter titrate kits; tabs 25, 100, 150, 200 mg; chew tabs 2, 5, 25 mg; ODT 25, 50, 100, 200 mg **SE:** Photosens, HA, GI upset, dizziness, diplopia, blurred vision, blood dyscrasias, ataxia, rash (more lifethreatening in peds vs adults), aseptic meningitis **Notes:** Value of therapeutic monitoring uncertain, taper w/ D/C

Lamotrigine, Extended-Release (Lamictal XR)

BOX: Life-threatening rashes, including Stevens-Johnson synd and toxic epidermal necrolysis, and/or rash-related death reported; D/C at 1st sign of rash **Uses:** *Adjunct primary generalized tonic-clonic Sz, conversion to monoRx in pt > 13 y w/ partial Szs* **Acts:** Phenyltriazine antiepileptic, ↓ glutamate, stabilize neuronal membrane **Dose:** Adjunct target 200–600 mg/d; *monoRx* conversion target dose 250–300 mg/d *Adults. w/ Valproate:* wk 1–2 25 mg qod, wk 3–4 25 mg qd, wk 5 50 mg qd, wk 6 100 mg qd, wk 7 150 mg qd, then maint 200–250 mg qd. *w/o Carbamazepine, phenytoin, phenobarbital, primidone, or valproate:* wk 1–2 25 mg qd, wk 3–4 50 mg qd, wk 5 100 mg qd, wk 6 150 mg qd, wk 7 200 mg qd, then maint 300–400 mg qd. *Convert IR to ER tabs:* Initial dose = total daily dose of IR. *Convert adjunctive to monoRx:* Maint: 250–300 mg qd. See label. w/*OCP:* See insert. **Peds > 13 y.** See adult **W/P:** [C, –] Interacts w/ other antiepileptics, estrogen (OCP), rifampin; valproic acid ↑ levels at least 2×; ↑ suicidal ideation; withdrawal Szs **CI:** Component hypersens (see Box) **Disp:** Tabs 25, 100, 150, 200 mg **SE:** Dizziness, tremor/intention tremor, V, diplopia, rash (more lifethreatening in peds than adults), aseptic meningitis, blood dyscrasias **Notes:** Taper over 2 wk w/ D/C

Lansoprazole (Prevacid, Prevacid 24HR [OTC]) Uses: *Duodenal ulcers, prevent & Rx NSAID gastric ulcers, active gastric ulcers, *H. pylori* Infxn, erosive esophagitis, & hypersecretory conditions, GERD* Acts: Proton pump inhib Dose: 15–30 mg/d PO, *NSAID ulcer prevention:* 15 mg/d PO = 12 wk. *NSAID ulcers:* 30 mg/d PO × 8 wk; *hypersecretory condition:* 60 mg/d before food doses of 90 mg bid have been used; ↓ w/ severe hepatic impair **W/P:** [B, ?/–] w/ Clopidogrel **Disp:** *Prevacid: DR* caps 15, 30 mg; *Prevacid 24HR* [OTC] 15 mg; *Prevacid SoluTab* (ODT) 15 mg (contains phenylalanine) **SE:** N/V, Abd pain, HA, fatigue **Notes:** Do not crush/chew; granules can be given w/ applesauce or apple juice (NG tube) only; ? ↑ risk of fractures w/ all PPI; caution w/ ODT in feeding tubes; risk of hypomagnesemia w/ long-term use; monitor

Lanthanum Carbonate (Fosrenol) Uses: *Hyperphosphatemia in end-stage renal Dz* Acts: Phosphate binder Dose: 750–1500 mg PO daily in ÷ doses, w/ or immediately after meal; titrate q2–3wk based on PO₄⁻ levels **W/P:** [C, ?/–] No data in GI Dz; not for peds **CI:** Bowel obstruction, fecal impaction, ileus **Disp:** Chew tabs 500, 750, 1000 mg **SE:** N/V, graft occlusion, HA, ↓ BP **Notes:** Chew tabs before swallowing; separate from meds that interact w/ antacids by 2 h

Lapatinib (Tykerb) BOX: Hepatotox has been reported (severe or fatal) Uses: *Advanced breast CA w/ capecitabine w/ tumors that over express HER2 and failed w/ anthracycline, taxane, & trastuzumab* and in combo w/ letrozole in postmenopausal women Acts: TKI Dose: Per protocol, 1250 mg PO days 1–21 w/ capecitabine 2000 mg/m²/d ÷ 2 doses/d on days 1–14; 1500 mg PO daily in combo w/ letrozole ↓ w/ severe cardiac or hepatic impair **W/P:** [D, ?/+] Avoid CYP3A4 inhib/inducers **CI:** Component hypersens **Disp:** Tabs 250 mg **SE:** N/V/D, anemia, ↓ plt, neutropenia, ↑ QT interval, hand-foot synd, ↑ LFTs, rash, ↓ left ventricular ejection fraction, interstitial lung Dz and pneumonitis **Notes:** Consider baseline LVEF & periodic ECG; LFTs at baseline & during Tx

Latanoprost (Xalatan) Uses: *Open-angle glaucoma, ocular HTN* Acts: Prostaglandin, ↑ outflow of aqueous humor Dose: 1 gtt eye(s) hs **W/P:** [C, M] **Disp:** 0.005% soln **SE:** May darken light irides; blurred vision, ocular stinging, & itching, ↑ number & length of eyelashes **Notes:** Wait 15 min before using contacts; separate from other eye products by 5 min

Leflunomide (Arava) BOX: PRG must be excluded prior to start of Rx; hepatotox; Tx should not be initiated in pts w/ acute or chronic liver Dz Uses:

Active RA, orphan drug for organ rejection **Acts:** DMARD, ↓ pyrimidine synth **Dose:** Initial 100 mg/d PO for 3 d, then 10–20 mg/d **W/P:** [X, –] w/ Bile acid sequestrants, warfarin, rifampin, MTX; not rec in pts w/ preexisting liver Dz **CI:** PRG **Disp:** Tabs 10, 20 mg **SE:** D, Infxn, HTN, alopecia, rash, N, jt pain, hep, interstitial lung Dz, immunosuppression peripheral neuropathy **Notes:** Monitor monthly & @ baseline LFTs, D/C therapy if ALT > 3 × ULN & begin drug elimination procedure, CBC, PO⁴⁻ during initial Rx; vaccine should be up-to-date, do not give w/ live vaccines

Lenalidomide (Revlimid) **BOX:** Significant teratogen; pt must be enrolled in RevAssist risk-reduction program; hematologic tox, DVT & PE risk **Uses:** *MDS, combo w/ dexamethasone in multiple myeloma in pt failing one prior Rx* **Acts:** Thalidomide analog, immune modulator **Dose:** *Adults.* MDS: 10 mg PO daily; swallow whole w/ water; multiple myeloma 25 mg/d days 1–21 of 28-d cycle w/ protocol dose of dexamethasone **W/P:** [X, –] w/ Renal impair **CI:** PRG **Disp:** Caps 5, 10, 15, 25 mg **SE:** D, pruritus, rash, fatigue, night sweats, edema, nasopharyngitis, ↓ BM (plt, WBC), ↑ K⁺, ↑ LFTs, thromboembolism **Notes:** Monitor CBC and for thromboembolism, hepatotox; routine PRG tests required; Rx only in 1-mo increments; limited distribution network; males must use condom and not donate sperm; use at least 2 forms contraception > 4 wk beyond D/C; see pkg insert for dose adjustments based on nonhematologic & hematologic tox

Lepirudin (Refludan) **Uses:** *HIT* **Acts:** Direct thrombin inhib **Dose:** *Bolus:* 0.4 mg/kg IV push then 0.15 mg/kg/h Inf; if > 110 kg 44 mg of Inf 16.5 mg/h max; ↓ dose & Inf rate w/ if CrCl < 60 mL/min or if used w/ thrombolytics **W/P:** [B, ?/–] Hemorrhagic event or severe HTN **CI:** Active bleeding **Disp:** Inj 50 mg **SE:** Bleeding, anemia, hematoma, anaphylaxis **Notes:** Adjust based on aPTT ratio, maintain aPTT 1.5–2.5 × control; S/Sxs of bleeding

Letrozole (Femara) **Uses:** *Breast CA:* Adjuvant w/postmenopausal hormone receptor positive early Dz; adjuvant in postmenopausal women w/ early breast CA w/ prior adjuvant tamoxifen therapy; 1st/2ndline in postmenopausal w/ hormone receptor positive or unknown* **Acts:** Nonsteroidal aromatase inhib **Dose:** 2.5 mg/d PO; q other day w/ severe liver Dz or cirrhosis **W/P:** [D, ?] [X, ?/–] **CI:** PRG, women who may become pregnant **Disp:** Tabs 2.5 mg **SE:** Anemia, N, hot flashes, arthralgia, hypercholesterolemia, decreased BMD, CNS depression **Notes:** Monitor CBC, thyroid Fxn, lytes, LFTs, SCr, BP, bone density, cholesterol

Leucovorin (Generic) **Uses:** *OD of folic acid antagonist; megaloblastic anemia, augment 5-FU, impaired MTX elimination; w/ 5-FU in colon CA* **Acts:** Reduced folate source; circumvents action of folate reductase inhib (eg, MTX) **Dose:** *Leucovorin rescue:* 10 mg/m² PO/IM/IV q6h; start w/in 24 h after dose or 15 mg PO/IM/IV q6h, for 10 doses until MTX level < 0.05 micromole/L *Folate antagonist OD (eg, Pemetrexed)* 100 mg/m² IM/IV × 1 then 50 mg/m² IM/IV q6h × 8 d;

5-FU adjuvant Tx, colon CA per protocol; low dose: 20 mg/m²/d IV × 5 d w/ 5-FU 425 mg/m²/d IV × 5 d, repeat q4–5wk × 6; *high dose:* 200 mg/m² in combo w/ 5-FU 370 mg/m² *Megaloblastic anemia:* 1 mg IM/IV daily **W/P:** [C, ?/–] **CI:** Pernicious anemia or vit B_{12} deficient megaloblastic anemias **Disp:** Tabs 5, 10, 15, 25 mg; Inj 50, 100, 200, 350, 500 mg **SE:** Allergic Rxn, N/V/D, fatigue, wheezing, ↑ liver enzymes **Notes:** Monitor Cr, methotrexate levels q24h w/ leucovorin rescue; do not use intrathecally/intraventricularly; w/ 5-FU CBC w/ diff, plt, LFTs, lytes

Leuprolide (Eligard, Lupron, Lupron DEPOT, Lupron DEPOT-Ped, Generic)

Uses: *Advanced PCa (all except Depot-Ped), endometriosis (Lupron), uterine fibroids (Lupron), & precocious puberty (Lupron-Ped)* **Acts:** LHRH agonist; paradoxically ↓ release of GnRH w/ ↓ LH from anterior pituitary; in men ↓ testosterone, in women ↓ estrogen **Dose:** *Adults. PCa: Lupron DEPOT:* 7.5 mg IM q28d or 22.5 mg IM q3mo or 30 mg IM q4mo or 45 mg IM q6mo. *Eligard:* 7.5 mg SQ q28d or 22.5 mg SQ q3mo or 30 mg SQ q4mo or 45 mg SQ 6 mo. *Endometriosis (Lupron DEPOT):* 3.75 mg IM qmo × 6 or 11.25 IM q3mo × 2. *Fibroids:* 3.75 mg IM qmo × 3 or 11.25 mg IM × 1. *Peds. CPP (Lupron DEPOT-Ped):* 50 mcg/kg/d SQ Inj; ↑ by 10 mcg/kg/d until total downregulation achieved. *Lupron DEPOT: < 25 kg:* 7.5 mg IM q4wk; *> 25–37.5 kg:* 11.25 mg IM q4wk; *> 37.5 kg:* 15 mg IM q4wk, ↑ by 3.75 mg q4wk until response **W/P:** [X, –] w/ Impending cord compression in PCa, ↑ QT w/ meds or preexisting CV Dz **CI:** AUB, implant in women/peds; PRG **Disp:** Inj 5 mg/mL; *Lupron DEPOT:* 3.75 mg (1 mo for fibroids, endometriosis); *Lupron DEPOT* for PCa: 7.5 mg (1 mo), 11.25 (3 mo), 22.5 (3 mo), 30 mg (4 mo), 45 mg (6 mo); *Eligard depot* for PCA: 7.5 (1 mo); 22.5 (3 mo), 30 (4 mo), 45 mg (6 mo); *Lupron DEPOT-Ped:* 7.5, 11.25, 15, 30 mg **SE:** Hot flashes, gynecomastia, N/V, alopecia, anorexia, dizziness, HA, insomnia, paresthesias, depression exacerbation, peripheral edema, & bone pain (transient "flare Rxn" at 7–14 d after the 1st dose [LH/testosterone surge before suppression]); ↓ BMD w/ > 6 mo use, bone loss possible, abnormal menses, hyperglycemia **Notes:** Nonsteroidal antiandrogen (eg, bicalutamide) may block flare in men w/ PCa; Viadur unavail to new Rx

Levalbuterol (Xopenex, Xopenex HFA)

Uses: *Asthma (Rx & prevention of bronchospasm)* **Acts:** Sympathomimetic bronchodilator; *R*-isomer of albuterol β_2-agonist **Dose:** Based on NIH Guidelines 2007 *Adults.* Acute–severe exacerbation Xopenex HFA 4–8 puffs q20min up to 4 h, the q1–4h PRN or nebulizer 1.25–2.5 mg q20min × 3, then 1.25–5 mg q1–4h PRN; *Peds < 5 y.* Quick relief 0.31–1.25 mg q4–6h PRN, severe 1.25 mg q20min × 3, then 0.075–0.15 mg/kg q1–4h PRN, 5 mg max. *5–11 y:* Acute–severe exacerbation 1.25 mg q20min × 3, then 0.075–0.15 mg/kg q1–4h PRN, 5 mg max, quick relief: 0.31–0.63 q8h PRN. *> 12 y:* 0.63–1.25 mg nebulizer q8h **W/P:** [C, M] w/ Non-K⁺-sparing diuretics, CAD, HTN, arrhythmias, ↓ K⁺, hyperthyroidism, glaucoma, diabetes **CI:** Component hypersens **Disp:** Multidose inhaler (Xopenex HFA) 45 mcg/puff (15 g); soln nebulizer Inh 0.31, 0.63, 1.25 mg/3 mL; concentrate 1.25 mg/0.5 mL **SE:** Paradox bronchospasm, anaphylaxis, angioedema, tachycardia, nervousness, V, ↓ K+ **Notes:** May ↓ CV SEs compared w/ albuterol; do not mix w/ other nebs or dilute

Levetiracetam (Keppra, Keppra XR) Uses: *Adjunctive PO Rx in partial onset Sz (adults & peds ≥ 4 y), myoclonic Szs (adults & peds ≥ 12 y) w/ juvenile myoclonic epilepsy (JME), primary generalized tonic-clonic (PGTC) Szs (adults & peds ≥ 6 y) w/ idiopathic generalized epilepsy. Adjunctive Inj Rx partial-onset Szs in adults w/ epilepsy; myoclonic Szs in adults w/ JME. Inj alternative for adults (≥ 16 y) when PO not possible* **Acts:** Unknown **Dose:** *Adults & Peds >16 y.* 500 mg PO bid, titrate q2wk, may ↑ 3000 mg/d max. *Peds 4–15 y.* 10 mg/kg/d ÷ in 2 doses to max 60 mg/kg/d (↓ in renal Insuff) **W/P:** [C, ?/–] Elderly, w/ renal impair, psychological disorders; ↑ suicidality risk for antiepileptic drugs, higher for those w/ epilepsy vs those using drug for psychological indications; Inj not for < 16 y **CI:** Component allergy **Disp:** Tabs 250, 500, 750, 1000 mg, ER 500, 750 mg soln 100 mg/mL; Inj 100 mg/mL **SE:** Dizziness, somnolence, HA, N/V, hostility, aggression, hallucinations, hematologic abnormalities, impaired coordination **Notes:** Do not D/C abruptly; postmarket hepatic failure and pancytopenia reported

Levobunolol (A-K Beta, Betagan) Uses: *Open-angle glaucoma, ocular HTN* **Acts:** β-Adrenergic blocker **Dose:** 1 gtt daily-bid **W/P:** [C, M] w/ Verapamil or systemic β-blockers **CI:** Asthma, COPD, sinus bradycardia, heart block (2nd-, 3rd-degree) CHF **Disp:** Soln 0.25, 0.5% **SE:** Ocular stinging/burning, ↓ HR, ↓ BP **Notes:** Possible systemic effects if absorbed

Levocetirizine (Xyzal) Uses: *Perennial/seasonal allergic rhinitis, chronic urticaria* **Acts:** Antihistamine **Dose:** *Adults.* 5 mg qd **Peds.** 6 mo–5 y: 1.25 mg once daily *6–11 y* 2.5 mg qd **W/P:** [B, ?/–] ↓ Adult dose w/ renal impair, CrCl 50–80 mL/min 2.5 mg daily, 30–50 mL/min 2.5 mg q other day, 10–30 mL/min 2.5 mg 2x/wk **CI:** Peds 6–11 y, w/ renal impair, adults w/ ESRD **Disp:** Tab 5 mg, soln 0.5 mL/mL (150 mL) **SE:** CNS depression, drowsiness, fatigue, xerostomia **Notes:** Take in evening

Levofloxacin (Levaquin, Generic) **BOX:** ↑ Risk Achilles tendon rupture and tendonitis, may exacerbate muscle weakness related to myasthenia gravis Uses: *Skin/skin structure Infxn (SSSI), UTI, chronic bacterial prostatitis, acute pyelo, acute bacterial sinusitis, acute bacterial exacerbation of chronic bronchitis, CAP, including multidrug-resistant S. pneumoniae, nosocomial pneumonia; Rx inhalational anthrax in adults & peds ≥ 6 mo* **Acts:** Quinolone, ↓ DNA gyrase. *Spectrum:* Excellent gram(+) except MRSA & *E. faecium;* excellent gram(−) except *Stenotrophomonas maltophilia & Acinetobacter* sp; poor anaerobic **Dose:** *Adults ≥ 18 y:* IV/PO: *Bronchitis:* 500 mg qd × 7 d. *CAP:* 500 mg qd × 7–14 d or 750 mg qd × 5 d. *Sinusitis:* 500 mg qd × 10–14 d or 750 mg qd × 5 d. *Prostatitis:* 500 mg qd × 28 d. *Uncomp SSSI:* 500 mg qd × 7–10 d. *Comp SSSI/nosocomial pneumonia:* 750 mg qd × 7–14 d. *Anthrax:* 500 mg qd × 60 d; *Uncomp UTI:* 250 mg qd × 3 d. *Comp UTI/acute pyelo:* 250 mg qd × 10 d or 750 mg qd × 5 d. CrCl 10–19 mL/min: 500 mg then 250 mg q other day or 750 mg, then 500 mg q48h.

Hemodialysis: 750 mg, then 500 mg q48h. *Peds ≥ 6 mo. Anthrax > 50 kg:* 500 mg q 24h × 60 d, < 50 kg 8 mg/kg (250 mg/dose max) q12h for 60 d ↓ w/ renal impair avoid antacids w/ PO; oral soln 1 h before, 2 h after meals *CAP:* ≥ 6 mo— ≤ 4 y 8 mg/kg/dose q12h (max 750 mg/d), 5–16 y 8 mg/kg/dose once daily (750 mg/d) **W/P:** [C, –] w/ Cation-containing products (eg, antacids), w/ drugs that ↑ QT interval **CI:** Quinolone sensitivity **Disp:** Tabs 250, 500, 750 mg; premixed IV 250, 500, 750 mg, Inj 25 mg/mL; Leva-Pak 750 mg × 5 d **SE:** N/D, dizziness, rash, GI upset, photosens, CNS stimulant w/ IV use, *C. difficile* enterocolitis; rare fatal hepatox, peripheral neuropathy risk **Notes:** Use w/ steroids ↑ tendon risk; only for anthrax in peds

Levofloxacin Ophthalmic (Quixin, Iquix) Uses: *Bacterial conjunctivitis* **Acts:** See levofloxacin **Dose:** *Ophthal:* 1–2 gtt in eye(s) q2h while awake up to 8×/d × 2 d, then q4h while awake × 5 d **W/P:** [C, –] **CI:** Quinolone sensitivity **Disp:** 25 mg/mL ophthal soln 0.5% (Quixin), 1.5% (Iquix) **SE:** Ocular burning/pain, ↓ vision, fever, foreign body sensation, HA, pharyngitis, photophobia

Levonorgestrel (Next Choice, Plan B One-Step, Generic [OTC]) Uses: *Emergency contraceptive ("morning-after pill")* **Acts:** Prevents PRG if taken < 72 h after unprotected sex/contraceptive failure; progestin, alters tubal transport & endometrium to implantation **Dose:** *Adults & Peds (postmenarche ♀)* w/in 72 h of unprotected intercourse: *Next Choice* 0.75 mg q12h × 2, *Plan B One-Step* 1.5 mg × 1 **W/P:** [X, M] w/ AUB; may ↑ ectopic PRG risk **CI:** Known/ suspected PRG **Disp:** *Next Choice* tab, 0.75 mg, 2 blister packs; *Plan B One-Step* tab, 1.5 mg, 1 blister pack **SE:** N/V/D, Abd pain, fatigue, HA, menstrual changes, dizziness, breast changes **Notes:** Will not induce Ab w/ PRG; federal court ruling in 2013 made these emergency contraceptives OTC w/o age or point-of-sale restrictions (label update pending)

Levonorgestrel IUD (Mirena) Uses: *Contraception, long-term* **Acts:** Progestin, alters endometrium, thicken cervical mucus, inhibits ovulation and implantation **Dose:** Up to 5 y, insert w/in 7 d menses onset or immediately after 1st-tri Ab; wait 6 wk if postpartum; replace any time during menstrual cycle **W/P:** [X, M] **CI:** PRG, w/ active hepatic Dz or tumor, uterine anomaly, breast CA, acute/ Hx of PID, postpartum endometriosis, infected Ab last 3 mo, gynecological neoplasia, abnormal Pap, AUB, untreated cervicitis/vaginitis, multiple sex partners, ↑ susceptibility to Infxn **Disp:** 52 mg IUD **SE:** Failed insertion, ectopic PRG, sepsis, PID, infertility, PRG comps w/ IUD left in place, Ab, embedment, ovarian cysts, perforation uterus/cervix, intestinal obst/perforation, peritonitis, N, Abd pain, ↑ BP, acne, HA **Notes:** Inform pt does not protect against STD/HIV; see PI for insertion instructions; reexamine placement after 1st menses; 80% PRG w/in 12 mo of removal

Levorphanol (Levo-Dromoran) [C-II] Uses: *Mod–severe pain; chronic pain* **Acts:** Narcotic analgesic, morphine derivative **Dose:** 2–4 mg PO PRN q6–8h; ↓ in hepatic impair **W/P:** [B/D (prolonged use/high doses at term), ?/–] w/ ↑ ICP, head trauma, adrenal Insuff **CI:** Component allergy, PRG **Disp:** Tabs 2 mg **SE:** Tachycardia, ↓ BP, drowsiness, GI upset, constipation, resp depression, pruritus

Levothyroxine (Synthroid, Levoxyl, Others) **BOX:** Not for obesity or Wt loss; tox w/ high doses, especially when combined w/ sympathomimetic amines **Uses:** *Hypothyroidism, pituitary thyroid-stimulating hormone (TSH) suppression, myxedema coma* **Acts:** T_4 supl l-thyroxine **Dose:** *Adults. Hypothyroid* titrate until euthyroid > 50 y w/o heart Dz or < 50 w/ heart Dz 25–50 mcg/d, ↑ q6–8wk; > 50 y w/ heart Dz 12.5–25 mcg/d, ↑ q6–8wk; usual 100–200 mcg/d. *Myxedema:* 200–500 mcg IV, then 100–300 mcg/d. *Peds. Hypothyroid: 1–3 mo:* 10–15 mcg/kg/24 h PO; *3–6 mo:* 8–10 mcg/kg/d PO; *6–12 mo:* 6–8 mcg/kg/d PO; *1–5 y:* 5–6 mcg/kg/d PO; *6–12 y:* 4–5 mcg/kg/d PO; *> 12 y:* 2–3 mcg/kg/d PO; if growth and puberty complete 1.7 mcg/kg/d; ↓ dose by 50% if IV; titrate based on response & thyroid tests; dose can ↑ rapidly in young/middle-aged; best on empty stomach **W/P:** [A, M] Many drug interactions; in elderly w/ CV Dz; thyrotoxicosis; w/ warfarin monitor INR **CI:** Recent MI, uncorrected adrenal Insuff; **Disp:** Tabs 25, 50, 75, 88, 100, 112, 125, 137, 150, 175, 200, 300 mcg; Inj 100, 500 mcg **SE:** Insomnia, Wt loss, N/V/D, ↑ LFTs, irregular periods, ↓ BMD, alopecia, arrhythmia **Notes:** Take w/ full glass of water (prevents choking); PRG may ↑ need for higher doses; takes 6 wk to see effect on TSH; wait 6 wk before checking TSH after dose change

Linagliptin (Tradjenta) **Uses:** *Type 2 DM* **Acts:** Dipeptidyl peptidase-4 (DPP-4) inhibitor; ↑ active incretin hormones (↑ insulin release, ↓ glucagon) **Dose:** *Adults.* 5 mg daily **W/P:** [B, ?/–] **CI:** Hypersensitivity **Disp:** Tabs 5 mg **SE:** Hypoglycemia w/ sulfonylurea; nasopharyngitis, pancreatitis **Notes:** Inhibitor of CYP3A4

Lidocaine, Systemic (Xylocaine, Others) **Uses:** *Rx cardiac arrhythmias* **Acts:** Class IB antiarrhythmic **Dose:** *Adults. Antiarrhythmic, ET:* 5 mg/kg; follow w/ 0.5 mg/kg in 10 min if effective. *IV load:* 1 mg/kg/dose bolus over 2–3 min; repeat in 5–10 min; 200–300 mg/h max; cont Inf 20–50 mcg/min or 1–4 mg/min; *ECC 2010. Cardiac arrest from VF/VT refractory VF: Initial:* 1–1.5 mg/kg IV/IO, additional 0.5–0.75 mg/kg IV push, repeat in 5–10 min, max total 3 mg/kg. ET: 2–4 mg/kg as last resort. *Reperfusing stable VT, wide complex tachycardia, or ectopy:* Doses of 0.5–0.75 mg/kg to 1–1.5 mg/kg may be used initially; repeat 0.5–0.75 mg/kg q5–10min; max dose 3 mg/kg. *Peds. ECC 2010. VF/pulseless VT, wide-complex tach (w/ pulses):* 1 mg/kg IV/IO, then maint 20–50 mcg/kg/min (repeat bolus if Inf started > 15 min after initial dose); RSI: 1–2 mg/kg IV/IO **W/P:** [B, M] ↓ Dose in severe hepatic impairment **CI:** Adams-Stokes synd; heart block; corn allergy **Disp:** Inj IV: 1% (10 mg/mL), 2% (20 mg/mL); admixture 4, 10, 20%. *IV Inf:* 0.2, 0.4% **SE:** Dizziness, paresthesias, & convulsions associated w/ tox **Notes:** 2nd line to amiodarone in ECC; dilute ET dose 1–2 mL w/ NS; for IV forms, or CHF; *Systemic levels:* steady state 6–12 h; *Therapeutic:* 1.2–5 mcg/mL; *Toxic:* > 6 mcg/mL; *half-life:* 1.5 h; constant ECG monitoring is necessary during IV admin

Lidocaine; Lidocaine w/ Epinephrine (Anestacon Topical, Xylocaine, Xylocaine Viscous, Xylocaine MPF, Others) Uses: *Local anesthetic, epidural/caudal anesthesia, regional nerve blocks, topical on mucous membranes (mouth/pharynx/urethra)* Acts: Anesthetic; stabilizes neuronal membranes; inhibits ionic fluxes required for initiation and conduction Dose: *Adults. Local Inj anesthetic:* 4.5 mg/kg max total dose or 300 mg; w/ epi 7 mg/kg or total 500 mg max dose. *Oral:* 15 mL viscous swish and spit or *pharyngeal* gargle and swallow, do not use < 3-h intervals or > 8 x in 24 h. *Urethra:* Jelly 5–30 mL (200–300 mg) jelly in men, 3–5 mL female urethra; 600 mg/24 h max. *Peds. Topical:* Apply max 3 mg/kg/dose. *Local Inj anesthetic:* Max 4.5 mg/kg (Table 1, p 300) W/P: [B, +] Epi-containing soln may interact w/ TCA or MAOI and cause severe ↑ BP CI: Do not use lidocaine w/ epi on digits, ears, or nose (vasoconstriction & necrosis) Disp: *Inj local:* 0.5, 1, 1.5, 2, 4, 10, 20%; Inj w/ epi 0.5%/1:200,000, 1%/1:100,000, 2%/1:100,000; (MPF) 1%/1:200,000, 1.5%/1:200,000, 2%/1:200,000; *Dental formulations:* 2%/1:50,000, 2%/1:100,000; cream 2, 3, 2%; lotion 30%; jelly 2%, gel 2, 2.5, 4, 5%; oint 5%; liq 2.5%; soln 2, 4%; viscous 2% topical spray 9.6% SE: Dizziness, paresthesias, & convulsions associated w/ tox Notes: See Table 1, p 300

Lidocaine/Prilocaine (EMLA, Oraq IX) Uses: *Topical anesthetic for intact skin or genital mucous membranes*; adjunct to phlebotomy or dermal procedures Acts: Amide local anesthetics Dose: *Adults. EMLA cream,* thick layer 2–2.5 g to intact skin over 20–25 cm² of skin surface, cover w/ occlusive dressing (eg, Tegaderm) for at least 1 h. *Anesthetic disc:* 1 g/10 cm² for at least 1 h. *Peds. Max dose: < 3 mo or < 5 kg:* 1 g/10 cm² for 1 h. *3–12 mo & > 5 kg:* 2 g/20 cm² for 4 h. *1–6 y & > 10 kg.* 10 g/100 cm² for 4 h. *7–12 y & > 20 kg:* 20 g/200 cm² for 4 h W/P: [B, +] CI: Methemoglobinemia use on mucous membranes, broken skin, eyes; allergy to amide-type anesthetics Disp: Cream 2.5% lidocaine/2.5% prilocaine; anesthetic disc (1 g); periodontal gel 2.5/2.5% SE: Burning, stinging, methemoglobinemia Notes: Longer contact time ↑ effect

Lidocaine/Tetracaine, Transdermal (Synera) Uses: Topical anesthetic; adjunct to phlebotomy or dermal procedures Acts: Topical anesthetic Dose: *Adults & Children > 3 y. Phlebotomy:* Apply to intact skin 20–30 min prior to venipuncture *Dermal procedures:* Apply to intact skin 30 min prior to procedure W/P: [B, ±] w/ liver Dz CI: Allergy to lidocaine/tetracaide/amide & ester-type anesthetics; corn allergy, use on mucous membranes, broken skin, eyes; pts w/ PABA hypersens Disp: TD patch: lidocaine 70 mg/tetracaine 70 mg SE: Erythema, blanching, edema, rash, burning, dizziness, HA, paresthesias

Linaclotide (Linzess) BOX: CI peds < 6 y; avoid in peds 6–17 y; death in juvenile mice Uses: *IBS w/ constipation, chronic idiopathic constipation* Acts: Guanylate cyclase-C agonist Dose: *IBS-C:* 290 mcg PO daily; *CIC:* 145 mcg PO daily; on empty stomach 30 min prior to 1st meal of the day; swallow whole W/P: [C, ?/–] CI: Pts < 6 y; GI obstruction Disp: Caps 145, 290 mcg SE: D, Abd pain/distention, flatulence

Lindane (Generic) BOX: Only for pts intolerant/failed 1st-line Rx w/ safer agents. Szs and deaths reported w/ repeated/prolonged use. Caution d/t increased risk of neurotox in infants, children, elderly, w/ other skin conditions, and if < 50 kg. Instruct pts on proper use and inform that itching occurs after successful killing of scabies or lice Uses: *Head lice, pubic "crab" lice, body lice, scabies*\ Acts: Ectoparasiticide & ovicide Dose: *Adults & Peds. Cream or lotion:* Thin layer to dry skin after bathing, leave for 8–12 h, rinse; also use on laundry. *Shampoo:* Apply 30 mL to dry hair, develop a lather w/ warm water for 4 min, comb out nits W/P: [C, –] CI: Premature infants, uncontrolled Sz disorders, norwegian scabies open wounds Disp: Lotion 1%; shampoo 1% SE: Arrhythmias, Szs, local irritation, GI upset, ataxia, alopecia, N/V, aplastic anemia Notes: Caution w/ overuse (may be absorbed); caution w/ hepatic in pts may repeat Rx in 7 d; try OTC first w/ pyrethrins (*Pronto, Rid,* others)

Linezolid (Zyvox) Uses: *Infxns caused by gram(+) bacteria (including VRE), pneumonia, skin Infxns*\ Acts: Unique, binds ribosomal bacterial RNA; bactericidal for streptococci, bacteriostatic for enterococci & staphylococci. *Spectrum:* Excellent gram(+) including VRE & MRSA Dose: *Adults.* 600 mg IV or PO q12h. *Peds ≤ 11 y.* 10 mg/kg IV or PO q8h (q12h in preterm neonates) W/P: [C, ?/–] CI: Concurrent MAOI use or w/in 2 wk, uncontrolled HTN, thyrotoxicosis, vasopressive agents, carcinoid tumor, SSRIs, tricyclics, w/ MAOI (may cause serotonin syndrome when used w/ these psych meds), avoid foods w/ tyramine & cough/cold products w/ pseudoephedrine; w/ ↓ BM Disp: Inj 200, 600 mg; tabs 600 mg; susp 100 mg/5 mL SE: Lactic acidosis, peripheral/optic neuropathy, HTN, N/D, HA, insomnia, GI upset, ↓ BM, tongue discoloration prolonged use-C. diff Infxn Notes: ✓ Weekly CBC; not for gram(–) Infxn, ↑ deaths in catheter-related Infxns; MAOI activity

Liothyronine (Cytomel, Triostat, T₃) BOX: Not for obesity or Wt loss Uses: *Hypothyroidism, nontoxic goiter, myxedema coma*\ Acts: T_3 replacement Dose: *Adults.* Initial 25 mcg/24 h, titrate q1–2wk to response & TFT; maint of 25–100 mcg/d PO. *Myxedema coma:* 25–50 mcg IV. *Myxedema:* 5 mcg/d, PO ↑ 5–10 mcg/d q1–2wk; maint 50–100 mcg/d. *Nontoxic goiter:* 5 mcg/d PO, ↑ 5–10 mcg/d q1–2wk, usual dose 75 mcg/d. *T₃ suppression test:* 75–100 mcg/d × 7d; ↓ in elderly & CV Dz Peds. Initial 5 mcg/24 h, titrate by 50-mcg/24-h increments at q3–4d intervals; maint. *Infants–12 mo:* 20 mcg/d Peds 1–3 y: 50 mcg/d *> 3 y:* Adult dose W/P: [A, +] CI: Recent MI, uncorrected adrenal Insuff, uncontrolled HTN, thyrotoxicosis, artificial rewarming Disp: Tabs 5, 25, 50 mcg; Inj 10 mcg/mL SE: Alopecia, arrhythmias, CP, HA, sweating, twitching, ↑ HR, ↑ BP, MI, CHF, fever Notes: Monitor TFT; separate antacids by 4 h; monitor glucose w/ DM meds; when switching from IV to PO, taper IV slowly

Liraglutide, Recombinant (Victoza) BOX: CI w/ personal or fam Hx of medullary thyroid CA (MTC) or w/ multiple endocrine neoplasia synd type 2 (MEN2) Uses: *Type 2 DM*\ Acts: Glucagon-like peptide-1 receptor agonist Dose: 1.8 mg/d;

begin 0.6 mg/d any time of day SQ (Abd/thigh/upper arm), ↑ to 1.2 mg after 1 wk, may ↑ to 1.8 mg after **W/P:** [C, ?/–] **CI:** See Box **Disp:** Multidose pens, 0.6, 1.2, 1.8 mg/dose, 6 mg/mL **SE:** Pancreatitis, MTC, ↓ glucose w/ sulfonylurea, HA, N/D, Wt loss **Notes:** Delays gastric emptying

Lisdexamfetamine Dimesylate (Vyvanse) [C-II] **BOX:** Amphetamines have ↑ potential for abuse; prolonged administration may lead to dependence; may cause sudden death and serious CV events in pts w/ preexisting structure cardiac abnormalities **Uses:** *ADHD* **Acts:** CNS stimulant **Dose:** *Adults & Peds 6–12 y.* 30 mg daily, ↑ qwk 10–20 mg/d, 70 mg/d max **W/P:** [C, ?/–] w/ Potential for drug dependency in pt w/ psychological or Sz disorder, Tourette synd, HTN **CI:** Severe arteriosclerotic CV Dz, mod–severe ↑ BP, ↑ thyroid, sensitivity to sympathomimetic amines, NAG, agitated states, Hx drug abuse, w/ or w/in 14 d of MAOI **Disp:** Caps 20, 30, 40, 50, 60, 70 mg **SE:** HA, insomnia, decreased appetite **Notes:** AHA statement April 2008: All children diagnosed w/ ADHD who are candidates for stimulant meds should undergo CV assessment prior to use; may be inappropriate for geriatric use

Lisinopril (Prinivil, Zestril) **BOX:** ACE inhib can cause fetal injury/death in 2nd/3rd tri; D/C w/ PRG **Uses:** *HTN, CHF, prevent DN & AMI* **Acts:** ACE inhib **Dose:** 5–40 mg/24 h PO daily-bid, CHF target 40 mg/d. *AMI:* 5 mg w/in 24 h of MI, then 5 mg after 24 h, 10 mg after 48 h, then 10 mg/d; ↓ in renal Insuff; use low dose, ↑ slowly in elderly **W/P:** [C (1st tri) D (2nd, 3rd tri), –] w/ Aortic stenosis/cardiomyopathy **CI:** PRG, ACE inhib sensitivity, idiopathic or hereditary angioedma **Disp:** Tabs 2.5, 5, 10, 20, 30, 40 mg **SE:** Dizziness, HA, cough, ↓ BP, angioedema, ↑ K+, ↑ Cr, rare ↓ BM **Notes:** To prevent DN, start when urinary microalbuminuria begins; ✓ BUN, Cr, K+, WBC

Lisinopril & Hydrochlorothiazide (Prinzide, Zestoretic, Generic) **BOX:** ACE inhib can cause fetal injury/death in 2nd/3rd tri, D/C w/ PRG **Uses:** *HTN* **Acts:** ACE inhib w/ diuretic (HCTZ) **Dose:** Initial 10 mg lisinopril/12.5mg HCTZ, titrate upward to effect; > 80 mg/d lisinopril or > 50 mg/day HCTZ are not recommended; ↓ in renal Insuff; use low dose, ↑ slowly in elderly **W/P:** [C 1st tri, D after, –] w/ Aortic stenosis/cardiomyopathy, bilateral RAS **CI:** PRG, ACE inhib, idiopathic or hereditary angioedema, sensitivity (angioedema) **Disp:** Tabs (mg lisinopril/mg HCTZ) 10/12.5, 20/12.5; Zestoretic also available as 20/25 **SE:** Anaphylactoid Rxn (rare), dizziness, HA, cough, fatigue, ↓ BP, angioedema, ↑ / ↓ K+, ↑ Cr, rare ↓ BM/cholestatic jaundice **Notes:** Use only when monotherapy fails; ✓ BUN, Cr, K+, WBC

Lithium Carbonate, Citrate (Generic) **BOX:** Li tox related to serum levels and can be seen at close to therapeutic levels **Uses:** *Manic episodes of bipolar Dz*, augment antidepressants, aggression, PTSD **Acts:** ?, Effects shift toward intraneuronal metabolism of catecholamines **Dose:** *Adults. Bipolar, acute mania:* 1800 mg/d PO in 2–3 ÷ doses (target serum 1–1.5 mEq/L ✓ 2×/wk until stable). *Bipolar maint:* 900–1800/d PO in 2–3 ÷ doses (target serum 0.6–1.2 mEq/L).

Peds ≥ *12 y.* See Adults; ↓ in renal Insuff, elderly **W/P:** [D, –] Many drug interactions; avoid ACE inhib or diuretics; thyroid Dz, caution in pts at risk of suicide **CI:** Severe renal impair or CV Dz, severe debilitation, dehydration, PRG, sodium depletion **Disp:** Carbonate: caps 150, 300, 600 mg; tabs 300, 600 mg; SR tabs 300 mg, CR tabs 450 mg; citrate: syrup 300 mg/5 mL **SE:** Polyuria, polydipsia, nephrogenic DI, long-term may affect renal conc ability and cause fibrosis; tremor; Na⁺ retention or diuretic use may ↑ tox; arrhythmias, dizziness, alopecia, goiter ↓ thyroid, N/V/D, ataxia, nystagmus, ↓ BP **Notes:** Levels: *Trough:* Just before next dose: *Therapeutic:* 0.8–1.2 mEq/mL; *Toxic:* > 1.5 mEq/mL *half-life:* 18–20 h. Follow levels q1–2mo on maint, draw concentrations 8–12 h postdose

Lodoxamide (Alomide)   **Uses:** *Vernal conjunctivitis/keratitis* **Acts:** Stabilizes mast cells **Dose:** *Adults & Peds > 2 y.* 1–2 gtt in eye(s) qid = 3 mo **W/P:** [B, ?] **Disp:** Soln 0.1% **SE:** Ocular burning, stinging, HA **Notes:** Do not use soft contacts during use

Lomitapide (Juxtapid)   **BOX:** May cause ↑ transaminases and/or hepatic steatosis. Monitor ALT/AST & bili at baseline & regularly; adjust dose if ALT/AST > 3× ULN (see label); D/C w/ significant liver tox **Uses:** *Homozygous familial hypercholesterolemia* **Acts:** Microsomal triglyceride transfer protein inhib **Dose:** *Adults.* 5 mg PO daily; ↑ to 10 mg after 2 wk, then at 4-wk intervals to 20, 40 mg; 60 mg max based on safety/tolerability; swallow whole w/ water > 2 h after evening meal; 40 mg max w/ ESRD on dialysis or mild hepatic impair; 30 mg max w/ weak CYP3A4 inhib (see label) **W/P:** [X, –] Avoid grapefruit; adjust w/ warfarin, P-glycoprotein substrates, simvastatin, lovastatin **CI:** PRG, w/ strong-mod CYP3A4 inhibitors, mod-severe hepatic impair **Disp:** Caps 5, 10, 20 mg **SE:** N/V/D, hepatotox, dyspepsia, Abd pain, flatulence, CP, influenza, fatigue, ↓ Wt, ↓ abs fat-soluble vits **Notes:** Limited distribution JUXTAPID REMS Program; PRG test before; use w/ low-fat diet (< 20% fat energy); take daily vit E, linoleic acid, ALA, EPA, DHA supl

Loperamide (Diamode, Imodium) [OTC]   **Uses:** *D* **Acts:** Slows intestinal motility **Dose:** *Adults.* Initial 4 mg PO, then 2 mg after each loose stool, up to 16 mg/d. *Peds 2–5 y, 13–20 kg.* 1 mg PO tid; *6–8 y, 20–30 kg:* 2 mg PO bid; *8–12 y, > 30 kg:* 2 mg PO tid **W/P:** [C, –] Not for acute D caused by *Salmonella, Shigella,* or *C. difficile;* w/ HIV may cause toxic megacolon **CI:** *Pseudomembranous colitis,* bloody D, Abd pain w/o D, < 2 y **Disp:** Caps 2 mg; tabs 2 mg; liq 1 mg/5 mL, 1 mg/7.5 mL (OTC) **SE:** Constipation, sedation, dizziness, Abd cramp, N

Lopinavir/Ritonavir (Kaletra)   **Uses:** *HIV Infxn* **Acts:** Protease inhib **Dose:** *Adults.* TX naïve: 800/200 mg PO daily or 400/100 mg PO bid; *TX Tx-experienced pt:* 400/100 mg PO bid (↑ dose if w/ amprenavir, efavirenz, fosamprenavir, nelfinavir, nevirapine); do not use qd dosing w/ concomitant Rx. *Peds 7–15 kg.* 12/3 mg/kg PO bid. *15–40 kg.* 10/2.5 mg/kg PO bid. *> 40 kg:* Adult dose; w/ food **W/P:** [C, ?/–] Numerous interactions, w/ hepatic impair; do not use w/ salmeterol, colchicine (w/ renal/hepatic failure); adjust dose w/ bosentan, tadalafil for PAH, ↑ QT w/ QT-prolonging drugs, hypokalemia, congenital long QT syndrome, immune reconstitution syndrome **CI:** w/ Drugs dependent on CYP3A/CYP2D6 (Table 10, p 319), lovastatin, rifampin, statins, St. John's wort, fluconazole; w/ alpha 1-adrenoreceptor antagonist (alfuzosin); w/ PDE5 inhibitor sildenafil **Disp:** (mg lopinavir/mg ritonavir) Tab 100/25, 200/50, soln 400/100/5 mL **SE:** Avoid disulfiram (soln has EtOH), metronidazole; GI upset, asthenia, ↑ cholesterol/triglycerides, pancreatitis; protease metabolic synd

Loratadine (Claritin, Alavert) **Uses:** *Allergic rhinitis, chronic idiopathic urticaria* **Acts:** Nonsedating antihistamine **Dose:** *Adults.* 10 mg/d PO. *Peds 2–5 y.* 5 mg PO daily. *> 6 y:* Adult dose; on empty stomach; ↓ in hepatic Insuff; q other day dose w/ CrCl < 30 mL/min **W/P:** [B, +/–] **CI:** Component allergy **Disp:** Tabs 10 mg (OTC); rapidly disintegrating RediTabs 10 mg; chew tabs 5 mg; syrup 1 mg/mL **SE:** HA, somnolence, xerostomia, hyperkinesis in peds

Lorazepam (Ativan, Others) [C-IV] **Uses:** *Anxiety & anxiety w/ depression; sedation; control status epilepticus*; EtOH withdrawal; antiemetic **Acts:** Benzodiazepine; antianxiety agent; works via postsynaptic GABA receptors **Dose:** *Adults.* Anxiety: 1–10 mg/d PO in 2–3 ÷ doses. *Preop.* 0.05 mg/kg–4 mg max IM 2 h before or 0.044 mg/kg 2 mg dose max IV 15–20 min before surgery. *Insomnia:* 2–4 mg PO hs *Status epilepticus:* 4 mg/dose slow over 2–5 min IV PRN q10–15min; usual total dose 8 mg. *Antiemetic:* 0.5–2 mg IV or PO q4–6h PRN. *EtOH withdrawal:* 1–4 mg IV or 2 mg PO initial depending on severity; titrate. *Peds, Status epilepticus:* 0.05–0.1 mg/kg/dose IV over 2–5 min, max 4 mg/dose repeat at 10- to 15-min intervals × 2 PRN. *Antiemetic, 2–15 y:* 0.05 mg/kg (to 2 mg/dose) prechemotherapy; ↓ in elderly; do not administer IV > 2 mg/min or 0.05 mg/kg/min **W/P:** [D, –] w/ Hepatic impair, other CNS depressant, COPD; ↓ dose by 50% w/ valproic acid and probenecid **CI:** Severe pain, severe ↓ BP, sleep apnea, NAG, allergy to propylene glycol or benzyl alcohol, severe resp Insuff (except mechanically ventilated) **Disp:** Tabs 0.5, 1, 2 mg; soln, PO conc 2 mg/mL; Inj 2, 4 mg/mL **SE:** Sedation, memory impair, EPS, dizziness, ataxia, tachycardia, ↓ BP, constipation, resp depression, paradoxical reactions, fall risk, abuse potential, rebound/withdrawal after abrupt D/C **Notes:** ~10 min for effect if IV; IV Inf requires inline filter

Lorcaserin (Belviq) **Uses:** *Manage Wt w/ BMI ≥ 30 kg/m² or ≥ 27 kg/m² w/ Wt-related comorbidity* **Acts:** Serotonin 2C receptor agonist **Dose:** *Adults.* 10 mg PO bid; D/C if not 5% Wt loss by wk 12 **W/P:** [X, –] √ glucose w/ diabetic meds; monitor for depression/suicidal thoughts, serotonin or neuroleptic malignant synd, cognitive impair, psych disorders, valvular heart Dz, priapism; risk of serotonin synd when used w/ other serotonergic drugs; caution w/ drugs that are CYP2D6 substrates **CI:** PRG **Disp:** Tabs 10 mg **SE:** HA, N, dizziness, fatigue, dry mouth, constipation, back pain, cough, hypoglycemia, euphoria, hallucination, dissociation, ↓ HR, ↑ prolactin

Losartan (Cozaar) **BOX:** Can cause fetal injury and death if used in 2nd & 3rd tri. D/C Rx if PRG detected **Uses:** *HTN, DN, prevent CVA in HTN and LVH*

Acts: Angiotensin II receptor antagonist **Dose:** *Adults.* 25–50 mg PO daily-bid, max 100 mg; ↓ in elderly/hepatic impair. *Peds ≥ 6 y.* HTN: Initial 0.7 mg/kg qd, ↑ to 50 mg/d PRN; 1.4 mg/kg/d or 100 mg/d max **W/P:** [C (1st tri, D 2nd & 3rd tri); ?/−] w/ NSAIDs; w/ K⁺-sparing diuretics, supl may cause ↑ K⁺; w/ RAS, hepatic impair **CI:** PRG, component sensitivity **Disp:** Tabs 25, 50, 100 mg **SE:** ↓ BP in pts on diuretics; ↑ K⁺; GI upset, facial/angioedema, dizziness, cough, weakness, ↓ renal Fxn

Loteprednol (Alrex, Lotemax) Uses: **Lotemax:* Steroid responsive inflammatory disorders of conjunctiva/cornea/anterior globe (keratitis, iritis, postop); *Alrex:* seasonal allergic conjunctivitis* **Acts:** Anti-inflammatory/steroid **Dose:** *Adults. Lotemax:* 1 drop conjunctival sac qid up to every h initially; Alrex 1 drop qid **W/P:** [C, ?/−] glaucoma **CI:** Viral Dz corneal and conjunctiva, varicella, mycobacterial and fungal Infxns; hypersens **Disp:** *Lotemax* 0.5% susp, 2.5, 5, 10, 15 mL; *Alrex* 0.2% susp, 2.5, 5, 10 mL **SE:** Glaucoma; ↑ risk Infxns; cornea/sclera thinning; HA, rhinitis **Notes:** May delay cataract surg healing; avoid use > 10 d; shake before use

Lovastatin (Altoprev, Mevacor) Uses: **Hypercholesterolemia to ↓ risk of MI, angina** **Acts:** HMG-CoA reductase inhib **Dose:** *Adults.* 20 mg/d PO w/ P.M. meal; may ↑ at 4-wk intervals to 80 mg/d max or 60 mg/d ER tab; take w/ meals. See pkg insert for dose limits w/ concurrent therapy (amiodarone, verapamil, diltiazem) *Peds 10–17 y (at least 1-y postmenarchal). Familial ↑ cholesterol:* 10 mg PO qd, ↑ q4wk PRN to 40 mg/d max (immediate release w/ P.M. meal) **W/P:** [X, −] Avoid w/ grapefruit juice, gemfibrozil; use caution, carefully consider doses > 20 mg/d w/ renal impair **CI:** Active liver Dz, PRG, lactation **Disp:** Tabs generic 10, 20, 40 mg; *Mevacor* 20,40 mg; *Altoprev* ER tabs 20, 40, 60 mg **SE:** HA & GI intolerance common; promptly report any unexplained muscle pain, tenderness, or weakness (myopathy) **Notes:** Maintain cholesterol-lowering diet; LFTs q12wk × 1 y, then q6mo; may alter TFT

Lubiprostone (Amitiza) Uses: **Chronic idiopathic constipation in adults, IBS w/ constipation in females > 18 y** **Acts:** Selective Cl⁻ channel activator; ↑ intestinal motility **Dose:** *Adults. Constipation:* 24 mcg PO bid w/ food. *IBS:* 8 mcg bid; w/ food **CI:** Mechanical GI obst **W/P:** [C, ?/−] Severe D, ↓ dose mod–severe hepatic impair **Disp:** Gelcaps 8, 24 mcg **SE:** N/D, may adjust dose based on tox (N), HA, GI distention, Abd pain **Notes:** Not approved in males; requires (−) PRG test before; use contraception; periodically reassess drug need; not for chronic use; may experience severe dyspnea w/in 1 h of dose, usually resolves w/in 3 h

Lucinactant (Surfaxin) Uses: **Prevention of RDS** **Acts:** Pulmonary surfactant **Dose:** *Peds.* 5.8 mL/kg birth Wt intratracheally no more often than q6h; max 4 doses in first 48 h of life **W/P:** [N/A, N/A] Frequent clinical assessments; interrupt w/ adverse Rxns and assess/stabilize infant; not for ARDS **CI:** None **Disp:** Susp 8.5 mL/vial **SE:** ET tube reflux/obstruction, pallor, bradycardia, oxygen desaturation, anemia, jaundice, metabolic/respiratory acidosis, hyperglycemia,

↓ Na, pneumonia, ↓ BP **Notes:** Warm vial for 15 min; shake prior to use; discard if not used w/in 2 h of warming

Lurasidone (Latuda) BOX: Elderly w/ dementia-related psychosis at ↑ death risk. Not approved for dementia-related psychosis. **Uses:** *Schizophrenia* **Acts:** Atypical antipsychotic: central D type 2 (D2) and serotonin type 2 (5HT2A) receptor antagonist **Dose:** 40–80 mg/d PO w/ food; 40 mg max w/ CrCl 10–49 mL/min OR mod–severe hepatic impair **W/P:** [B, –] **CI:** w/ Strong CYP3A4 inhib/inducer **Disp:** Tabs 20, 40, 80, 120 mg **SE:** Somnolence, agitation, tardive dyskinesia, akathisia, parkinsonism, stroke, TIAs, Sz, orthostatic hypotension, syncope, dysphagia, neuroleptic malignant syndrome, body temp dysregulation, N, ↑ Wt, type 2 DM, ↑ lipids, hyperprolactinemia, ↓ WBC **Notes:** w/ DM risk ✓ glucose

Lymphocyte Immune Globulin [Antithymocyte Globulin, ATG] (Atgam) BOX: Should only be used by physician experienced in immunosuppressive therapy or management of solid-organ and/or BMT pts. Adequate lab and supportive resources must be readily available **Uses:** *Allograft rejection in renal transplant pts; aplastic anemia if not candidates for BMT*, prevent rejection of other solid-organ transplants, GVHD after BMT **Acts:** ↓ Circulating antigen-reactive T lymphocytes; human, & equine product **Dose:** *Adults. Prevent rejection:* 15 mg/kg/d IV × 14 d, then q other day × 7 d for total 21 doses in 28 d; initial w/in 24 h before/after transplant. *Rx rejection:* Same but use 10–15 mg/kg/d; max 21 doses in 28 d, qd first 14 d. *Aplastic anemia:* 10–20 mg/kg/d × 8–14 d, then q other day × 7 doses for total 21 doses in 28 d. *Peds. Prevent renal allograft rejection:* 5–25 mg/kg/d IV; *aplastic anemia* 10–20 mg/kg/day IV 8–14 d then q other day for 7 more doses **W/P:** [C, ?/–] D/C if severe unremitting thrombocytopenia, leukopenia **CI:** Hx previous Rxn or Rxn to some γ globulin prep, ↓ plt and WBC **Disp:** Inj 50 mg/mL **SE:** D/C w/ severe ↓ plt and WBC; rash, fever, chills, ↓ BP, HA, CP, edema, N/V/D, lightheadedness **Notes:** Test dose: 0.1 mL 1:1000 dilution in NS, a systemic Rxn precludes use; give via central line; pretreat w/ antipyretic, antihistamine, and steroids; monitor WBC, plt; plt counts usually return to nl w/o D/C Rx 4 h Inf

Magaldrate & Simethicone (Riopan-Plus) [OTC] Uses: *Hyperacidity associated w/ peptic ulcer, gastritis, & hiatal hernia* **Acts:** Low-Na⁺ antacid **Dose:** 5–10 mL PO between meals & hs, on empty stomach **W/P:** [C, ?/+] **CI:** UC, diverticulitis, appendicitis, ileostomy/colostomy, renal Insuff (d/t Mg²⁺ content) **Disp:** Susp magaldrate/simethicone 540/20 mg/5 mL (OTC) **SE:** ↑ Mg²⁺, ↓ PO₄, white-flecked feces, constipation, N/V/D **Notes:** < 0.3 mg Na¹⁺/tab or tsp

Magnesium Citrate (Citroma, Others) [OTC] Uses: *Vigorous bowel prep*; constipation **Acts:** Cathartic laxative **Dose:** *Adults.* 150–300 mL PO PRN. *Peds. < 6 y:* 2–4 mL/kg ✕/ or in ÷ doses *6–12 y:* 100–150 mL ✕/ or in ÷ doses *≥ 12 y:* 150–300 mL ✕/or in ÷ doses **W/P:** [B, +] w/ Neuromuscular Dz & renal impairment **CI:** Severe renal Dz, heart block, N/V, rectal bleeding, intestinal obst/perforation/impaction, colostomy, ileostomy, UC, diverticulitis, DM **Disp:** soln 290 mg/5 mL (300 mL); 100 mg tabs **SE:** Abd cramps, gas, ↓ BP, ↑ Mg^{2+}, resp depression **Notes:** Only for occasional use w/ constipation

Magnesium Hydroxide (Milk of Magnesia) [OTC]
Uses: *Constipation*, hyperacidity, Mg^{2+} replacement **Acts:** NS laxative **Dose:** *Adults. Antacid:* 5–15 mL (400 mg/5 mL) or 2–4 tabs (311 mg) PO PRN up to qid. *Laxative:* 30–60 mL (400 mg/5 mL) or 15–30 mL (800 mg/5 mL) or 8 tabs (311 mg) PO qhs or ÷ doses. *Peds. Antacid and < 12 y not OK. Laxative:* < 2 y not OK. *2–5 y:* 5–15 mL (400 mg/5 mL) PO qhs or ÷ doses. *6–11 y:* 15–30 mL (400 mg/5 mL) or 7.5–15 mL (800 mg/5 mL) PO qhs or ÷ doses. *3–5 y:* 2 (311 mg) tabs PO qhs or ÷ doses. *6–11 y:* 4 (311 mg) tabs PO qhs or ÷ doses **W/P:** [B, +] w/ Neuromuscular Dz or renal impair **CI:** Component hypersens **Disp:** Chew tabs 311, 400 mg; liq 400, 800 mg/5 mL (OTC) **SE:** D, Abd cramps **Notes:** For occasional use in constipation, different forms may contain Al^{2+}

Magnesium Oxide (Mag-Ox 400, Others) [OTC]
Uses: *Replace low Mg^{2+} levels* **Acts:** Mg^{2+} supl **Dose:** 400–800 mg/d or ÷ w/ food in full glass of H$_2$O; ↓ w/ renal impair **W/P:** [B, +] w/ Neuromuscular Dz & renal impair, w/ bisphosphonates, calcitriol, CCBs, neuromuscular blockers, tetracyclines, quinolones **CI:** Component hypersens **Disp:** Caps 140, 250, 500, 600 mg; tabs 400 mg (OTC) **SE:** D, N

Magnesium Sulfate (Various)
Uses: *Replace low Mg^{2+}; preeclampsia, eclampsia, & premature labor, cardiac arrest, AMI arrhythmias, cerebral edema, barium poisoning, Szs, pediatric acute nephritis*; refractory ↓ K$^+$ & ↓ Ca^{2+} **Acts:** Mg^{2+} supl, bowel evacuation, ↓ acetylcholine in nerve terminals, ↓ rate of sinoatrial node firing **Dose:** *Adults.* 1 gm q6h IM ×4 doses & PRN 1–2 gm q3–6h IV then PRN to correct deficiency. *Preeclampsia/premature labor:* 4-g load then 1–2 g/h IV Inf. *ECC 2010. VF/pulseless VT arrest w/ torsade de pointes:* 1–2 g IV push (2–4 mL 50% soln) in 10 mL D5W. If pulse present, then 1–2 g in 50–100 mL D5W over 5–60 min. *Peds & Neonates.* 25–50 mg/kg/dose IV, repeat PRN; max 2 g single dose *ECC 2010. Pulseless VT w/ torsades:* 25–50 mg/kg IV/IO bolus; max dose 2 g; *Pulseless VT w/ torsades or hypomagnesemia:* 25–50 mg/kg IV/IO over 10–20 min; max dose 2 g; *Status asthmaticus:* 25–50 mg/kg IV over 15–30 min **W/P:** [A/C (manufacturer specific), +] w/ Neuromuscular Dz; interactions see Magnesium Oxide and aminoglycosides **CI:** Heart block, myocardial damage **Disp:** Premix Inj: 10, 20, 40, 80 mg/mL; Inj 125, 500 mg/mL; oral/topical powder 227, 454, 1810, 2720 g **SE:** CNS depression, D, flushing, heart block, ↓ BP, vasodilation **Notes:** Different formulation may contain Al^{2+}, monitor Mg^{2+} levels

Mannitol, Inhalation (Aridol)
BOX: Powder for Inh; use may result in severe bronchospasm, testing only done by trained professionals **Uses:** *Assess bronchial hyperresponsiveness in pts w/o clinically apparent asthma* **Acts:** Bronchoconstrictor, ? mechanism **Dose:** *Adults, Peds > 6 y.* Inhal caps ↑ dose (see disp)

until + test (15% ↓ FEV1 or 10% ↓ FEV1 between consecutive doses) or all caps inhaled **W/P:** [C, ?/M] Pt w/ comorbid cond that may ↑ effects **CI:** Mannitol/gelatin hypersens **Disp:** Dry powder caps graduated doses: 0, 5, 10, 20, 40 mg **SE:** HA, pharyngeal pain, irritation, N, cough, rhinorrhea, dyspnea, chest discomfort, wheezing, retching, dizziness **Notes:** Not a stand-alone test or screening test for asthma

Mannitol, Intravenous (Generic) Uses: *Cerebral edema, ↑ IOP, renal impair, poisonings* **Acts:** Osmotic diuretic **Dose:** *Test dose:* 0.2 g/kg/dose IV over 3–5 min; if no diuresis w/in 2 h, D/C. *Oliguria:* 50–100 g IV over 90 min ↑ *IOP:* 0.25–2 g/kg IV over 30 min. *Cerebral edema:* 0.25–1.5 g/kg/dose IV q6–8h PRN, maintain serum osmolality < 300–320 mOsm/kg **W/P:** [C, ?/M] w/ CHF or vol overload w/ nephrotoxic drugs & lithium **CI:** Anuria, dehydration, heart failure, PE, intracranial bleeding **Disp:** Inj 5, 10, 15, 20, 25% **SE:** May exacerbate CHF, N/V/D, ↓ / ↑ BP, ↑ HR **Notes:** Monitor for vol depletion

Maraviroc (Selzentry) BOX: Possible drug-induced hepatotox Uses: *Tx of CCR5-tropic HIV Infxn* **Acts:** Antiretroviral, CCR5 coreceptor antagonist **Dose:** 300 mg bid **W/P:** [B, –] w/ Concomitant CYP3A inducers/inhib and ↓ renal function, caution in mild–mod hepatic impair **CI:** Pts w/ severe renal impairment/ESRD taking potent CYP3A4 inhib/inducer **Disp:** Tab 150, 300 mg **SE:** Fever, URI, cough, rash; HIV attaches to the CCR5 receptor to infect CD4+ T cells

Measles, Mumps, & Rubella Vaccine Live [MMR] (M-M-R II) Uses: *Vaccination against measles, mumps, & rubella 12 mo and older* **Acts:** Active immunization, live attenuated viruses **Dose:** 1 (0.5-mL) SQ Inj, 1st dose 12 mo 2nd dose 4–6 y, at least 3 mo between doses (28 d if > 12 y), adults born after 1957 unless CI, Hx measles & mumps or documented immunity and childbearing age women w/ rubella immunity documented **W/P:** [C, ?/M] Hx of cerebral injury, Szs (febrile Rxn), ↓ plt **CI:** Component and gelatin sensitivity, Hx anaphylaxis to neomycin, blood dyscrasia, lymphoma, leukemia, malignant neoplasias affecting BM, immunosuppression, fever, PRG, Hx of active untreated TB **Disp:** Inj, single dose **SE:** Fever, febrile Szs (5–12 d after vaccination), Inj site Rxn, rash, ↓ plt **Notes:** Per FDA, CDC ↑ of febrile Sz (2×) w/ MMRV vs MMR and varicella separately; preferable use 2 separate vaccines; allow 1 mo between Inj & any other measles vaccine or 3 mo between any other varicella vaccine; limited avail of MMRV; avoid those who have not been exposed to varicella for 6 wk post-Inj; may contain albumin or trace egg antigen; avoid salicylates for 6 wk postvaccination; avoid PRG for 3 mo following vaccination; do not give w/in 3 mo of transfusion or immune globulin

Measles, Mumps, Rubella, & Varicella Virus Vaccine Live [MMRV] (ProQuad) Uses: *Vaccination against measles, mumps, rubella, & varicella* **Acts:** Active immunization, live attenuated viruses **Dose:** 1 (0.5-mL) vial SQ Inj 12 mo–12 y or for 2nd dose of measles, mumps, & rubella (MMR)*, at least 3 mo between doses (28 d if > 12 y) **W/P:** [C, ?/M] Hx of cerebral injury or Szs w/ fam Hx

Szs (febrile Rxn), ↓ plt **CI:** Component and gelatin sensitivity, Hx anaphylaxis to neomycin, blood dyscrasia, lymphoma, leukemia, malignant neoplasias affecting BM, immunosuppression, fever, active untreated TB, PRG **Disp:** Inj **SE:** Fever, febrile Szs, (5–12 d after vaccination), Inj site Rxn, rash, ↓ plt, **Notes:** Per FDA, CDC ↑ of febrile Sz (2 × risk) w/ combo vaccine (MMRV) vs MMR and varicella separately; preferable to use 2 separate vaccines; allow 1 mo between Inj & any other measles vaccine or 3 mo between any other varicella vaccine; limited avail of MMRV; substitute MMR II and/or Varivax; avoid those not been exposed to varicella for 6 wk post-Inj; may contain albumin or trace egg antigen; avoid salicylates

Mecasermin (Increlex, Iplex) **Uses:** *Growth failure in severe primary IGF-1 deficiency or human growth hormone (HGH) antibodies* **Acts:** Human IGF-1 (recombinant DNA origin) **Dose:** *Peds.* Increlex ≥ 2 y 0.04–0.08 mg/kg SQ bid; may ↑ by 0.04 mg/kg per dose to 0.12 mg/kg bid; take w/in 20 min of meal d/t insulin-like hypoglycemic effect; Iplex ≥ 3 y 0.5 mg/kg once daily ↑ to 1–2 mg/kg/day hold if hypoglycemia **W/P:** [C, ?/M] Contains benzyl alcohol **CI:** Closed epiphysia, neoplasia, not for IV **Disp:** Vial 10 mg/mL (40 mL) **SE:** Tonsillar hypertrophy, ↑ AST, ↑ LDH, HA, Inj site Rxn, V, hypoglycemia **Notes:** Rapid dose ↑ may cause hypoglycemia; initial funduscopic exam and during Tx; consider monitoring glucose until dose stable; limited distribution; rotate Inj site

Mechlorethamine (Mustargen) **BOX:** Highly toxic, handle w/ care, limit use to experienced physicians; avoid exposure during PRG; vesicant **Uses:** *Hodgkin Dz (stages III, IV), cutaneous T-cell lymphoma (mycosis fungoides), lung CA, CML, malignant pleural effusions, CLL, polycythemia vera*, psoriasis **Acts:** Alkylating agent, nitrogen analog of sulfur mustard **Dose:** Per protocol; 0.4 mg/kg single dose or 0.1 mg/kg/d for 4 d, or 0.2 mg/kg/d for 2 d, repeat at 4- to 6-wk intervals; *MOPP:* 6 mg/m^2 IV on days 1 & 8 of 28-d cycle; *Intracavitary:* 0.2–0.4 mg/kg × 1, may repeat PRN; *Topical:* 0.01–0.02% soln, lotion, oint **W/P:** [D, ?/–] Severe myleosuppression **CI:** PRG, known infect Dz **Disp:** Inj 10 mg; topical soln, lotion, oint, oint **SE:** ↓ BM, thrombosis, thrombophlebitis at site; tissue damage w/ extrav (Na thiosulfate used topically to Rx); N/V/D, skin rash/allergic dermatitis w/ contact, amenorrhea, sterility (especially in men), secondary leukemia if treated for Hodgkin Dz, chromosomal alterations, hepatotox, peripheral neuropathy **Notes:** Highly volatile and emetogenic; give w/in 30–60 min of prep

Meclizine (Antivert, Generic) (Dramamine [OTC]) **Uses:** *Motion sickness, vertigo* **Acts:** Antiemetic, anticholinergic, & antihistaminic properties **Dose:** *Adults & Peds > 12 y. Motion sickness:* 12.5–25 mg PO 1 h before travel, repeat PRN q12–24h. *Vertigo:* 25–100 mg/d ÷ doses **W/P:** [B, ?/–] NAG, BPH, BOO, elderly, asthma **Disp:** Tabs 12.5, 25, 50 mg; chew tabs 25 mg; caps 12.5 mg (OTC) **SE:** Drowsiness, xerostomia, blurred vision, thickens bronchial secretions

Medroxyprogesterone (Provera, Depo-Provera, Depo-Sub Q Provera, Generic) **BOX:** Do not use in the prevention of CV Dz or dementia; ↑ risk MI, stroke, breast CA, PE, & DVT in postmenopausal women (50–79 y).

↑ Dementia risk in postmenopausal women (≥ 65 y). Risk of sig bone loss; does not prevent against STD or HIV, long-term use > 2 y should be limited to situations where other birth control methods are inadequate **Uses:** *Contraception; secondary amenorrhea; endometrial CA, ↓ endometrial hyperplasia* AUB caused by hormonal imbalance **Acts:** Progestin supl **Dose:** *Contraception:* 150 mg IM q3mo depo or 104 mg SQ q3mo (depo SQ). *Secondary amenorrhea:* 5–10 mg/d PO for 5–10 d. *AUB:* 5–10 mg/d PO for 5–10 d beginning on the 16th or 21st d of menstrual cycle. *Endometrial CA:* 400–1000 mg/wk IM. *Endometrial hyperplasia:* 5–10 mg/d × 12–14 d on day 1 or 16 of cycle; ↓ in hepatic Insuff **W/P:** *Provera* [X, –] *Depo Provera* [X, +] **CI:** Thrombophlebitis/embolic disorders, cerebral apoplexy, severe hepatic dysfunction, CA breast/genital organs, undiagnosed Vag bleeding, missed Ab, PRG, as a diagnostic test for PRG **Disp:** Provera tabs 2.5, 5, 10 mg; depot Inj 150, 400 mg/mL; depo SQ Inj 104 mg/0.65 mL **SE:** Breakthrough bleeding, spotting, altered menstrual flow, breast tenderness, galactorrhea, depression, insomnia, jaundice, N, Wt gain, acne, hirsutism, vision changes **Notes:** Perform breast exam & Pap smear before contraceptive Rx; obtain PRG test if last Inj > 3 mo

Megestrol Acetate (Megace, Megace-ES, Generic)
Uses: *Breast/endometrial CAs; appetite stimulant in cachexia (CA & HIV)* **Acts:** Hormone; antileutinizing; progesterone analog **Dose:** *Appetite:* 800 mg/d PO ÷ dose or *Megace-ES* 625 mg/d **W/P:** [D (tablet)/X (suspension), –] Thromboembolism; handle w/ care **CI:** PRG **Disp:** Tabs 20, 40 mg; susp 40 mg/ mL, Megace-ES 125 mg/mL **SE:** DVT, edema, menstrual bleeding, photosens, N/V/D, HA, mastodynia, ↑ Ca, ↑ glucose, insomnia, rash, ↓ BM, ↑ BP, CP, palpitations, **Notes:** Do not D/C abruptly; Megace-ES not equivalent to others mg/mg; Megace-ES approved only for anorexia

Meloxicam (Mobic, Generic)
BOX: May ↑ risk of CV events & GI bleeding; CI in postop CABG **Uses:** *OA, RA, JRA* **Acts:** NSAID w/ ↑ COX-2 activity **Dose:** *Adults.* 7.5–15 mg/d PO. *Peds ≥ 2 y.* 0.125 mg/kg/d, max 7.5 mg; ↓ in renal Insuff; take w/ food **W/P:** [C, D (3rd tri), ?/–] w/ Severe renal Insuff, CHF, ACE inhib, diuretics, Li²⁺, MTX, warfarin, ↑ K⁺ Peptic ulcer, NSAID, or ASA sensitivity, PRG, postop CABG **Disp:** Tabs 7.5, 15 mg; susp. 7.5 mg/5 mL **SE:** HA, dizziness, GI upset, GI bleeding, edema, ↑ BP, renal impair, rash (SJS), ↑ LFTs

Melphalan [L-PAM] (Alkeran, Generic)
BOX: Administer under the supervision of a qualified physician experienced in the use of chemotherapy; severe BM depression, leukemogenic, & mutagenic hypersens (including anaphylaxis in ~2%) **Uses:** *Multiple myeloma, ovarian CAs*, breast & testicular CA, melanoma; allogenic & ABMT (high dose), neuroblastoma, rhabdomyosarcoma **Acts:** Alkylating agent, nitrogen mustard **Dose:** *Adults. Multiple myeloma:* 16 mg/ m² IV q2wk × 4 doses then at 4-wk intervals after tox resolves; w/ renal impair ↓ IV dose 50% or 6 mg PO qd × 2–3 wk, then D/C up to 4 wk, follow counts then 2 mg qd. *Ovarian CA:* 0.2 mg/kg qd × 5 d, repeat q4–5wk based on counts, ↓ in

renal Insuff **W/P:** [D, ?/–] w/ Cisplatin, digitalis, live vaccines extravasation, need central line **CI:** Allergy or resistance **Disp:** Tabs 2 mg; Inj 50 mg **SE:** N/V, secondary malignancy, AF, ↓ LVEF, ↓ BM, secondary leukemia, alopecia, dermatitis, stomatitis, pulm fibrosis; rare allergic Rxns, thrombocytopenia **Notes:** Take PO on empty stomach, false(+) direct Coombs test

Memantine (Namenda) Uses: *Mod–severe Alzheimer Dz*, mild–mod vascular dementia, mild cognitive impair **Acts:** N-methyl-D-aspartate (NMDA) receptor antagonist **Dose:** *Namenda:* Target 20 mg/d, start 5 mg/d, ↑ 5–20 mg/d, wait > 1 wk before ↑ dose; use bid if > 5 mg/d. *Vascular dementia:* 10 mg PO bid; *Namenda XR* (Alzheimer) 7 mg inital 1× qd, ↑ by 7 mg /wk each week to maint 28 mg/d × 1; ↓ to 14 mg w/ severe renal impair **W/P:** [B, ?/m] Hepatic/mod renal impair; Sx disorders, cardiac Dz **Disp:** *Namenda* tabs 5, 10 mg, combo pack: 5 mg × 28 + 10 mg × 21; soln 2 mg/mL **CI:** Component hypersens **SE:** Dizziness, HA, D **Notes:** Renal clearance ↓ by alkaline urine (↓ 80% at pH 8)

Meningococcal Conjugate Vaccine [Quadrivalent, MCV4] (Menactra, Menveo) Uses: *Immunize against N. meningitidis (meningococcus) high-risk 2–10 and 19–55 y and everyone 11–18 y* high-risk (college freshmen, military recruits, travel to endemic areas, terminal complement deficiencies, asplenia); if given age 11–12 y, give booster at 16, should have booster w/in 5 y of college **Acts:** Active immunization; N. meningitidis A, C, Y, W-135 polysaccharide conjugated to diphtheria toxoid (*Menactra*) or lyophilized conjugate component (*Menveo*) **Dose:** *Adults 18–55 y & Peds > 2 y.* 0.5 mL IM × 1 **W/P:** [B/C, (manufacturer dependent) ?/m] w/ Immunosuppression (↓ response) and bleeding disorders, Hx Guillain-Barré **CI:** Allergy to class/diphtheria toxoid/compound/latex **Disp:** Inj **SE:** Inj site Rxns, HA, N/V/D, anorexia, fatigue, irritability, arthralgia, Guillain-Barré **Notes:** IM only, reported accidental SQ; keep epi available for Rxns; use polysaccharide *Menomune* (MPSV4) if > 55 y; do not confuse w/ *Menactra, Menveo*; ACIP rec: MCV4 for 2–55 y, ↑ local Rxn compared to *Menomune* (MPSV4) but ↑ Ab titers; peds 2–10, Ab levels ↓ 3 y w/ MPSV4, revaccinate in 2–3 y, use MCV4 revaccination

Meningococcal Groups C and Y and Haemophilus b Tetanus Toxoid Conjugate Vaccine (Menhibrix) Uses: *Prevent meningococcal Dz and Haemophilus influenzae type b (Hib) in infants/young children* **Acts:** Active immunization; antibodies specific to organisms **Dose:** *Peds 6 wk–18 mo.* 4 doses 0.5 mL IM at 2, 4, 6, and 12–15 mo **W/P:** [C, N/A] Apnea in some infants reported; w/ Hx Guillain Barré; fainting may occur **CI:** Severe allergy to similar vaccines **Disp:** Inj 40 mg/mL/vial **SE:** Inj pain, redness; irritability; drowsiness; ↓ appetite; fever **Notes:** New in 2012

Meningococcal Polysaccharide Vaccine [MPSV4] (Menomune A/C/Y/W-135) Uses: *Immunize against N. meningitidis (meningococcus) in highrisk (college freshmen, military recruits, travel to endemic areas, terminal complement deficiencies, asplenia) **Acts:** Active immunization **Dose:** *Adults & Peds > 2 y.*

0.5 mL SQ only; Children < 2 y not recommended; 2 doses 3 mo apart may repeat in 3–5 y if high risk; repeat in 2–3 y if 1st dose given 2–4 y **W/P:** [C, ?/M] if immunocompromised (↓ response) **CI:** Thimerosal/latex sensitivity; w/ pertussis or typhoid vaccine, < 2 y **Disp:** Inj **SE:** Peds 2–10 y: Inj site Rxns, drowsiness, irritability 11–55 y: Inj site Rxns, HA, fatigue, malaise, fever, jt **Notes:** Keep epi (1:1000) available for Rxns. Recommended > 55 y, but also alternative to MCV4 in 2–55 y if no MCV4 available (MCV4 is preferred). Active against serotypes A, C, Y, & W-135 but not group B; antibody levels ↓ 3 y; high risk: revaccination q3–5y (use MCV4)

Meperidine (Demerol, Meperitab, Generic) [C–II] Uses: *Mod–severe pain*, postoperative shivering, rigors from amphotericin B **Acts:** Narcotic analgesic **Dose:** Adults. 50–150 mg PO or IV/IM/SQ q3–4h PRN. Peds. 1–1.5 mg/kg/dose PO or IM/SQ q3–4h PRN, up to 100 mg/dose; hepatic impair, avoid in renal impair, avoid use in elderly **W/P:** [C, –] ↓ Sz threshold, adrenal Insuff, head injury, ↑ ICP, hepatic impair, not OK in sickle cell Dz **CI:** w/ MAOIs **Disp:** Tabs 50, 100 mg; syrup/soln 50 mg/5 mL; Inj 25, 50, 75, 100 mg/mL **SE:** Resp/CNS depression, Szs, sedation, constipation, ↓ BP, rash N/V, biliary and urethral spasms, dyspnea **Notes:** Analgesic effects potentiated w/ hydroxyzine; 75 mg IM − 10 mg morphine IM; not best in elderly; do not use oral for acute pain; not OK for repetitive use in ICU setting, naloxone does not reverse neurotox, used as analgesic not recommended, limit Tx to < 48 h

Meprobamate (Generic) [C–IV] Uses: *Short-term relief of anxiety* muscle spasm, TMJ relief **Acts:** Mild tranquilizer; antianxiety **Dose:** Adults. 400 mg PO tid-qid, max 2400 mg/d. Peds 6–12 y. 100–200 mg PO bid-tid; ↓ in renal impair **W/P:** [D, +/−] Elderly, Sz Dz, caution w/ depression or suicidal tendencies **CI:** Acute intermittent prophyria **Disp:** Tabs 200, 400 mg **SE:** Drowsiness, syncope, tachycardia, edema, rash (SJS), N/V/D, ↓ WBC, agranulocytosis **Notes:** Do not abruptly D/C

Mercaptopurine [6-MP] (Purinethol, Generic) Uses: *ALL* 2nd-line Rx for CML & NHL, maint ALL in children, immunosuppressant w/ autoimmune Dzs (Crohn Dz, UC) **Acts:** Antimetabolite, mimics hypoxanthine **Dose:** Adults. ALL induction: 1.5–2.5 mg/kg/d; maint 60 mg/m²/d w/ allopurinol use 67–75% ↓ dose of 6-MP (interference w/ xanthine oxidase metabolism). Peds. ALL induction: 1.5–2.5 mg/kg/d maint 1.5–2.5 mg/kg/d PO or 60 mg/m²/d w/ renal/hepatic Insuff; take on empty stomach **W/P:** [D, ?] w/ Allopurinol, immunosuppression, TMP-SMX, warfarin, salicylates, severe BM Dz, PRG **CI:** Prior resistance, PRG **Disp:** Tabs 50 mg **SE:** Mild hematotoxicity, mucositis, stomatitis, D, rash, fever, eosinophilia, jaundice, hep, hyperuricemia, hyperpigmentation, alopecia **Notes:** Handle properly; limit use to experienced physicians; ensure adequate hydration; for ALL, evening dosing may ↓ risk of relapse; low emetogenicity, TPMT deficiency ↑ immunosuppressive effect

Meropenem (Merrem, Generic) Uses: *Intra-Abd Infxns, bacterial meningitis, skin Infxn* **Acts:** Carbapenem; ↓ cell wall synth. *Spectrum:* Excellent gram(+) (except MRSA, methicillin-resistant *S. epidermidis* [MRSE] & *E. faecium*); excellent gram(−) including extended-spectrum β-lactamase producers; good anaerobic **Dose:** *Adults. Abd Infxn:* 1–2 g IV q8h. *Skin Infxn:* 500 mg IV q8h. *Meningitis:* 2 g IV q8h. *Peds > 3 mo, < 50 kg. Abd Infxn:* 20 mg/kg IV q8h. *Skin Infxn:* 10 mg/kg IV q8h. *Meningitis:* 40 mg/kg IV q8h; *Peds > 50 kg.* Use adult dose; max 2 g IV q8h; ↓ in renal Insuff (see PI) **W/P:** [B, ?/M] w/ Probenecid, VPA **CI:** β-Lactam anaphylaxis **Disp:** Inj 1 g, 500 mg **SE:** Less Sz potential than imipenem; *C. difficile* enterocolitis, D, ↓ plt **Notes:** Overuse ↑ bacterial resistance

Mesalamine (Apriso, Asacol, Asacol HD, Canasa, Lialda, Pentasa, Rowasa, Generic)
Uses: *Rectal: mild–mod distal UC, proctosigmoiditis, proctitis; oral: treat/maint of mild–mod ulcerative colitis* **Acts:** 5-ASA derivative, may inhibit prostaglandins, may ↓ leukotrienes and TNF-α **Dose:** *Rectal:* 60 mL qhs, retain 8 h (enema), *PO:* Caps: 1 g PO qid; tab: 1.6–2.4 g/d ÷ doses (tid-qid) × 6 wk; DR 2.4–4.8 g PO daily 8 wk max, do not cut/crush/chew w/ food; ↓ initial dose in elderly, maint: depends on formulation **W/P:** [B/C (product specific), M] w/ Digitalis, PUD, pyloric stenosis, renal Insuff, elderly **CI:** Salicylate sensitivity **Disp:** Tabs ER (*Asacol*) 400, (*Asacol HD*) 800 mg; ER caps (*Pentasa*) 250, 500 mg, (*Apriso*) 375 mg; DR tab (*Lialda*) 1.2 g; supp (*Canasa*) 1000 mg; (*Rowasa*) rectal susp 4 g/60 mL **SE:** Yellow-brown urine, HA, malaise, Abd pain, flatulence, rash, pancreatitis, pericarditis, dizziness, rectal pain, hair loss, intolerance synd (bloody D) **Notes:** Retain rectally 1–3 h; ✓ CBC, Cr, BUN; Sx may ↑ when starting

Mesna (Mesnex [Oral], Generic [Inf])
Uses: *Prevent hemorrhagic cystitis d/t ifosfamide or cyclophosphamide* **Acts:** Antidote, reacts w/ acrolein and other metabolites to form stable compounds **Dose:** Per protocol; dose as % of ifosfamide or cyclophosphamide dose. *IV bolus:* 20% (eg, 10–12 mg/kg) IV at 0, 4, & 8 h; *IV Inf:* 20% prechemotherapy, 40% w/ chemotherapy for 12–24 h; *Oral:* 100% ifosfamide dose given as 20% IV at hour 0 then 40% PO at hours 4 & 8; if PO dose vomited repeat or give dose IV; mix PO w/ juice **W/P:** [B; ?/−] **CI:** Thiol sensitivity **Disp:** Inj 100 mg/mL; (*Mesnex*) tabs 400 mg **SE:** ↓ BP, ↓ plt, ↑ HR, ↑ RR allergic Rxns, HA, GI upset, taste perversion **Notes:** Hydration helps ↓ hemorrhagic cystitis; higher dose for BMT; IV contains benzyl alcohol

Metaproterenol (Generic)
Uses: *Asthma & reversible bronchospasm, COPD* **Acts:** Sympathomimetic bronchodilator **Dose:** *Adults. Nebulized:* 5% 2.5 mL q4–6h or PRN. *MDI:* 1–3 Inh q3–4h, 12 Inh max/24 h; wait 2 min between Inh. *PO:* 20 mg q6–8h. *Peds ≥ 12 y. MDI:* 2–3 Inh q3–4h, 12 Inh/d max. *Nebulizer:* 2.5 mL (soln 0.4, 0.6%) qid, up to q4h. *Peds > 9 y or ≥ 27 kg.* 20 mg PO tid-qid; *6–9 y or < 27 kg.* 10 mg PO tid-qid; ↓ in elderly **W/P:** [C, ?/−] w/ MAOI, TCA, sympathomimetics; avoid w/ β-blockers **CI:** Tachycardia, other arrhythmias **Disp:** Aerosol 0.65 mg/Inh; soln for Inh 0.4%, 0.6%; tabs 10, 20 mg; syrup 10 mg/5 mL **SE:** Nervousness, tremor, tachycardia, HTN, ↑ glucose, ↓ K⁺, ↑ IOP **Notes:** Fewer β₁ effects than isoproterenol & longer acting, but not a 1st-line

β-agonist. Use w/ face mask < 4 y; oral ↑ ADR; contains ozone-depleting CFCs; will be gradually removed from US market

Metaxalone (Skelaxin) Uses: *Painful musculoskeletal conditions* Acts: Centrally acting skeletal muscle relaxant Dose: 800 mg PO tid-qid W/P: [C, ?/–] w/ Elderly, EtOH & CNS depression, anemia CI: Severe hepatic/renal impair; drug-induced, hemolytic, or other anemias Disp: Tabs 800 mg SE: N/V, HA, drowsiness, hep

Metformin (Fortmet, Glucophage, Glucophage XR, Glumetza, Riomet, Generic) BOX: Associated w/ lactic acidosis, risk ↑ w/ sepsis, dehydration, renal/hepatic impair, ↑ alcohol, acute CHF; Sxs include myalgias, malaise, resp distress, Abd pain, somnolence; Labs: ↓ pH, ↑ anion gap, ↑ blood lactate; D/C immediately & hospitalize if suspected Uses: *Type 2 DM*, polycystic ovary synd (PCOS), HIV lipodystrophy Acts: Biguanide; ↓ hepatic glucose production & intestinal absorption of glucose; ↑ insulin sensitivity Dose: *Adults.* Initial: 500 mg PO bid; or 850 mg daily, titrate 1- to 2-wk intervals may ↑ to 2550 mg/d max; take w/ A.M. & P.M. meals; can convert total daily dose to daily dose of XR. *Peds 10–16 y.* 500 mg PO bid, ↑ 500 mg/wk to 2000 mg/d max in ÷ doses; do not use XR formulation in peds W/P: [B, +/–] Avoid EtOH; hold dose before & 48 h after ionic imaging contrast; hepatic impair, elderly CI: SCr ≥ 1.4 mg/dL in females or ≥ 1.5 mg/dL in males; hypoxemic conditions (eg, acute CHF/sepsis); metabolic acidosis, abnormal CrCl from any cause (AMI, shock) Disp: Tabs 500, 850, 1000 mg; XR tabs 500, 750, 1000 mg; (*Riomet*) soln 100 mg/mL SE: Anorexia, N/V/D, flatulence, weakness, myalgia, rash

Methadone (Dolophine, Methadose, Generic) [C-II] BOX: Deaths reported during initiation and conversion of pain pts to methadone Rx from Rx w/ other opioids. For PO only; tabs contain excipient. Resp depression and QT prolongation, arrhythmias observed. Only dispensed by certified opioid Tx programs for addiction. Analgesic use must outweigh risks Uses: *Severe pain not responsive to non-narcotics; detox w/ input of narcotic addiction* Acts: Narcotic analgesic Dose: *Adults.* 2.5 mg IM/IV/SQ q8–12h or PO q8h; titrate as needed; see PI for conversion from other opioids. *Peds.* (Not FDA approved) 0.1 mg/kg q4–12h IV; ↑ slowly to avoid resp depression; ↓ in renal impair W/P: [C, –] Avoid w/ severe liver Dz CI: Resp depression, acute asthma, ileus w/, selegiline Disp: Tabs 5, 10 mg; tab dispersible 40 mg; PO soln 5, 10 mg/5 mL; PO conc 10 mg/mL; Inj 10 mg/mL SE: Resp depression, sedation, constipation, urinary retention, ↑ QT interval, arrhythmias, ↓ HR, syncope, ↓ K⁺, ↓ Mg²⁺ Notes: Parenteral:oral 1:2; equianalgesic w/ parenteral morphine; longer 1/2; resp depression occurs later and lasts longer than analgesic effect, use w/ caution to avoid iatrogenic OD

Methenamine Hippurate (Hiprex), Methenamine Mandelate (Urex, Uroquid-Acid No. 2) Uses: *Suppress recurrent UTI long-term. Use only after Infxn cleared by antibiotics* Acts: Converted to formaldehyde & ammonia in acidic urine; nonspecific bactericidal action Dose: *Adults.* Hippurate:

1 g PO bid. *Mandelate:* initial 1 g qid PO pc & hs, maint 1–2 g/d. *Peds 6–12 y.* *Hippurate:* 0.5–1 g PO bid PO ÷ bid. *> 2 y: Mandelate:* 50–75 mg/kg/d PO ÷ qid; take w/ food, ascorbic acid w/ hydration **W/P:** [C, +] **CI:** Renal Insuff, severe hepatic Dz, & severe dehydration w/ sulfonamides (may precipitate in urine) **Disp:** *Methenamine hippurate:* Tabs 1 g. *Methenamine mandelate:* 500 mg, 1 g EC tabs **SE:** Rash, GI upset, dysuria, ↑ LFTs, super Infxn w/ prolonged use, *C. difficile*-associated diarrhea. **Notes:** Hippurate not indicated in peds < 6 y. Not for pts w/ indwelling catheters as dwell time in bladder required for action; "Urex" used internationally for many meds

Methenamine, Phenyl Salicylate, Methylene Blue, Benzoic Acid, Hyoscyamine (Prosed)

Uses: *Lower urinary tract discomfort* **Acts:** Methenamine in acid urine releases formaldehyde (antiseptic), phenyl salicylate mild analgesic methylene blue/benzoic acid mild antiseptic, hyoscyamine parasympatholytic ↓ muscle spasm **Dose:** *Adults Peds > 12 y.* 1 tab PO qid w/ liberal fluid intake. **W/P:** [C, ?/–] Avoid w/ sulfonamides, NAG, pyloric/duodenal obst, BOO, coronary artery spasm **CI:** Component hypersens **Disp:** Tabs **SE:** Rash, dry mouth, flushing, ↑ pulse, dizziness, blurred vision, urine/feces discoloration, voiding difficulty/retention **Notes:** Take w/ plenty of fluid, can cause crystalluria; not rec in peds ≤ 6 y

Methimazole (Tapazole, Generic)

Uses: *Hyperthyroidism, thyrotoxicosis*, prep for thyroid surgery or radiation **Acts:** Blocks T_3 & T_4 formation, but does not inactivate circulating T_3, T_4 **Dose:** *Adults.* Initial based on severity: 15–60 mg/d PO q8h. *Maint:* 5–15 mg PO daily. *Peds.* Initial: 0.4–0.7 mg/kg/24 h PO q8h. *Maint:* 0.2 mg/kg/d ÷ in 3 doses; take w/ food **W/P:** [D, –] w/ Other meds **CI:** Breast-feeding **Disp:** Tabs 5, 10 mg **SE:** GI upset, dizziness, blood dyscrasias, dermatitis, fever, hepatic Rxns, lupus-like synd **Notes:** Follow clinically & w/ TFT, CBC w/ diff

Methocarbamol (Robaxin, Generic)

Uses: *Relief of discomfort associated w/ painful musculoskeletal conditions* **Acts:** Centrally acting skeletal muscle relaxant **Dose:** *Adults & Peds ≥ 16 y.* 1.5 g PO qid for 2–3 d, then 1-g PO qid maint. *Tetanus:* 1–2 g IV q6h × 3 d, then use PO, max dose 24 g/d; *< 16 y:* 15 mg/kg/dose or 500 mg/m²/dose IV, may repeat PRN (tetanus only), max 1.8 g/m²/d × 3 d **W/P:** Sz disorders, hepatic & renal impair [C, ?/M] **CI:** MyG, renal impair w/ IV **Disp:** Tabs 500, 750 mg; Inj 100 mg/mL **SE:** Can discolor urine, lightheadedness, drowsiness, GI upset, ↓ HR, ↓ BP **Notes:** Tabs can be crushed and added to NG, do not operate heavy machinery; max rate IV = 3 mL/min

Methotrexate (Rheumatrex Dose Pack, Trexall, Generic)

BOX: Administration only by experienced physician; do not use in women of childbearing age unless absolutely necessary (teratogenic); impaired elimination w/ impaired renal Fxn, ascites, pleural effusion; severe ↓ BM w/ NSAIDs; hepatotox, occasionally fatal; can induce life-threatening pneumonitis; D and ulcerative stomatitis require D/C; lymphoma risk; may cause tumor lysis synd; can cause severe skin Rxn, opportunistic Infxns; w/ RT can ↑ tissue necrosis risk. Preservatives make this agent unsuitable for intrathecal IT or higher dose use **Uses:** *ALL, AML, leukemic meningitis, trophoblastic tumors (choriocarcinoma, hydatidiform mole), breast, lung, head, & neck CAs, Burkitt lymphoma, mycosis fungoides, osteosarcoma, Hodgkin Dz & NHL, psoriasis; RA, JRA, SLE*, chronic Dz **Acts:** ↓ Dihydrofolate reductase-mediated prod of tetrahydrofolate, causes ↓ DNA synth **Dose:** *Adults. CA:* Per protocol. *RA:* 7.5 mg/wk PO 1/wk or 2.5 mg q12h PO for 3 doses/wk. *Psoriasis:* 2.5–5 mg PO q12h × 3d/wk or 10–25 mg PO/IM qwk. *Chronic:* 15–25 mg IM/SQ qwk, then 15 mg/wk. *Peds.* JIA: 10 mg/m² PO/IM qwk, then 5–14 mg/m² × 1 or as 3 divided doses 12 h apart; ↓ elderly, w/ renal/hepatic impair **W/P:** [X, –] w/ Other nephro-/hepatotoxic meds, multiple interactions, w/ Sz, profound ↓ BM other than CA related **CI:** Severe renal/hepatic impair, PRG/lactation **Disp:** Dose pack 2.5 mg in 8, 12, 16, 20, or 24 doses; tabs 2.5, 5, 7.5, 10, 15 mg; Inj 25 mg/mL; Inj powder 20 mg, 1 g **SE:** ↓ BM, N/V/D, anorexia, mucositis, hepatotox (transient & reversible; may progress to atrophy, necrosis, fibrosis, cirrhosis), rashes, dizziness, malaise, blurred vision, alopecia, photosens, renal failure, pneumonitis; rare pulm fibrosis; chemical arachnoiditis & HA w/ IT delivery **Notes:** Monitor CBC, LFTs, Cr, MTX levels & CXR; "high dose" > 500 mg/m² requires leucovorin rescue to ↓ tox; w/ IT, use preservative-/alcohol-free soln; systemic levels: *Therapeutic:* > 0.01 micromole; *Toxic:* > 10 micromole over 24 h

Methyldopa (Generic) **Uses:** *HTN* **Acts:** Centrally acting antihypertensive, ↓ sympathetic outflow **Dose:** *Adults.* 250–500 mg PO bid-tid (max 2.5 g/d) or 250 mg–1 g IV q6–8h. *Peds Neonates.* 2.5–5 mg/kg PO/IV q8h. *Other peds.* 10 mg/kg/24 h PO in 2–3 ÷ doses or 5–10 mg/kg/dose IV q6–8h to max 65 mg/kg/24 h; ↓ in renal Insuff/elderly **W/P:** [B, +] **CI:** Liver Dz, w/ MAOIs, bisulfate allergy **Disp:** Tabs 250, 500 mg; Inj 50 mg/mL **SE:** Initial transient sedation/drowsiness, edema, hemolytic anemia, hepatic disorders, fevers, nightmares **Notes:** Tolerance may occur, false(+) Coombs test; often considered DOC for PRG

Methylene Blue (Urolene Blue, Various) **Uses:** *Methemoglobinemia, vasoplegic synd, ifosamide-induced encephalopathy, cyanide poisoning, dye in therapeutics/diagnosis* **Acts:** Low IV dose converts methemoglobin to hemoglobin; excreted, appears in urine as green/green-blue color; MAOI activity **Dose:** 1–2 mg/kg or 25–50 mg/m² IV over 5–10 min, repeat q1h; direct instillation into fistulous tract **W/P:** [X, –] w/ Severe renal impair w/ psych meds such as SSRI, SNRI, TCAs (may cause serotonin synd), w/ G6PD deficiency **CI:** Intra spinal Inj, severe renal Insuff **Disp:** 1, 10 mL Inj **SE:** *IV use:* N, Abd, GP, sweating, fecal/urine discoloration, hemolytic anemia **Notes:** Component of other medications; stains tissue blue, limits repeat use in surgical visualization

Methylergonovine (Methergine) **Uses:** *Postpartum bleeding (atony, hemorrhage)* **Acts:** Ergotamine derivative, rapid and sustained uterotonic effect **Dose:** 0.2 mg IM after anterior shoulder delivery or puerperium, may repeat in

2- to 4-h intervals or 0.2–0.4 mg PO q6–12h for 2–7 d **W/P:** [C, ?] w/ Sepsis, obliterative vascular Dz, hepatic/renal impair, w/ CYP3A4 inhib (Table 10, p 319) **CI:** HTN, PRG, toxemia **Disp:** Inj 0.2 mg/mL; tabs 0.2 mg **SE:** HTN, N/V, CP, ↓ BP, Sz **Notes:** Give IV only if absolutely necessary over > 1 min w/ BP monitoring

Methylnaltrexone Bromide (Relistor) Uses: *Opioid-induced constipation in pt w/ advanced illness such as CA* **Acts:** Peripheral opioid antagonist **Dose:** *Adults.* Wt-based < 38 kg: 0.15 mg/kg SQ; 38–61 kg: 8 mg SQ; 62–114 kg: 12 mg SQ >114 kg: 0.15 mg/kg, round to nearest 0.1 mL, dose q other day PRN, max 1 dose q24h **W/P:** [B, ?/M] w/ CrCl < 30 mL/min ↓ dose 50% **Disp:** Inj 12 mg/0.6 mL **SE:** N/D, Abd pain, dizziness **Notes:** Does not affect opioid analgesic effects or induce withdrawal

Methylphenidate, Oral (Concerta, Metadate CD, Metadate SR, Methylin, Ritalin, Ritalin LA, Ritalin SR, Quillivant XR) [C-II] BOX: w/ Hx of drug or alcohol dependence, avoid abrupt D/C; chronic use can lead to dependence or psychotic behavior; observe closely during withdrawal of drug Uses: *ADHD, narcolepsy*, depression **Acts:** CNS stimulant, blocks reuptake of norepinephrine and DA **Dose:** *Adults.* Narcolepsy: 10 mg PO 2–3×/d, 60 mg/d max. *Depression:* 2.5 mg q A.M.; ↑ slowly, 20 mg/d max, ÷ bid 7 A.M. & 12 P.M.; use regular release only. *Adults & Peds > 6 y.* ADHD: 5 mg PO bid, ↑ 5–10 to 60 mg/d, max (2 mg/kg/d), ER/SR use total IR dose qd. CD/LA 20 mg PO qd, ↑ 10–20 mg qwk to 60 mg/d max. Concerta: 18 mg PO q A.M. Rx naïve or already on 20 mg/d, 36 mg PO q A.M. if on 30–45 mg/d, 54 mg PO q A.M. if on 40–60 mg/d, 72 mg PO q A.M. **W/P:** [C, M] w/ Hx EtOH/drug abuse, CV Dz, HTN, bipolar Dz, Sz; separate from MAOIs by 14 d **Disp:** Chew tabs 2.5, 5, 10 mg; tabs scored IR (Ritalin) 5, 10, 20 mg; Caps ER (Ritalin LA) 10, 20, 30, 40 mg Caps ER (Metadate CD) 10, 20, 30, 40, 50, 60 mg (Methylin ER) 10, 20 mg; Tabs SR (Metadate SR, Ritalin SR) 20 mg; ER tabs (Concerta) 18, 27, 36, 54 mg. Oral soln 5, 10 mg/5 mL; (QuilliVant XR) ER Susp 5 mg/mL **SE:** CV/CNS stimulation, growth retard, GI upset, pancytopenia, ↑ LFTs **CI:** Marked anxiety, tension, agitation, NAG, motor tics, family Hx or diagnosis of Tourette synd, severe HTN, angina, arrhythmias, CHF, recent MI, ↑ thyroid; w/ or w/in 14 d of MAOI **Notes:** See also transdermal form; titrate dose; take 30–45 min ac; do not chew or crush; Concerta "ghost tablet" in stool, avoid w/ GI narrowing; Metadate contains sucrose, avoid w/ lactose/galactose problems. Do not use these meds w/ halogenated anesthetics; abuse and diversion concerns; AHA rec: all ADHD peds need CV assessment and consideration for ECG before Rx

Methylphenidate, Transdermal (Daytrana) [C-II] BOX: w/ Hx of drug or alcohol dependence; chronic use can lead to dependence or psychotic behavior; observe closely during withdrawal of drug Uses: *ADHD in children 6–17 y* **Acts:** CNS stimulant, blocks reuptake of norepinephrine and DA **Dose:** *Adults & Peds 6–17 y.* Apply to hip in A.M. (2 h before or desired effect), remove 9 h later; titrate 1st wk 10 mg/9 h, 2nd wk 15 mg/9 h, 3rd wk 20 mg/9 h, 4th wk 30 mg/9 h **W/P:** [C, +/–] See methylphenidate, oral; sensitization may preclude subsequent use of oral forms; abuse and diversion concerns **CI:** Significant anxiety, agitation; component allergy; glaucoma; w/ or w/in 14 d of MAOI; tics or family Hx Tourette synd **Disp:** Patches 10, 15, 20, 30 mg **SE:** Local Rxns, N/V, nasopharyngitis, ↓ Wt, ↓ appetite, lability, insomnia, tic **Notes:** Titrate dose weekly; effects last hours after removal; evaluate BP, HR at baseline and periodically; avoid heat exposure to patch, may cause OD, AHA rec: all ADHD peds need CV assessment and consideration for ECG before Rx

Methylprednisolone (A-Methapred, Depo-Medrol, Medrol, Medrol Dosepak, Solu-Medrol, Generic) [See Steroids, p 259 and Table 2 & 3 pp 301 & 302] Uses: *Steroid responsive conditions (endocrine, rheumatic, collagen, dermatologic, allergic, ophthalmic, respiratory, hematologic, neoplastic, edematous, GI, CNS, others)* **Acts:** Glucocorticoid **Dose: See Steroids** *Peds. ECC 2010. Status asthmaticus, anaphylactic shock:* 2 mg/kg IV/IO/IM (max 60 mg). *Maint:* 0.5 mg/kg IV q6h or 1 mg/kg q12h to 120 mg **W/P:** [C, ?/M] may mask Infx, cataract w/ prolonged use; avoid vaccines **CI:** Fungal Infx, component allergy **Disp:** Oral (*Medrol*) 4, 8, 16, 32 mg, (*Medrol Dosepak*) 21 4-mg tabs taken over 6 d; Inj acetate (*Depo-Medrol*) 20, 40, 80 mg/mL; Inj succinate (*Solu-Medrol*) 40, 125, 500 mg, 1, 2 g **SE:** Fluid and electrolyte disturbances, muscle weakness/loss, ulcers, impaired wound healing, others (see label) **Notes:** Taper dose to avoid adrenal Insuff

Metoclopramide (Metozolv, Reglan, Generic) BOX: Chronic use may cause tardive dyskinesia; D/C if Sxs develop; avoid prolonged use (> 12 wk) Uses: *Diabetic gastroparesis, symptomatic GERD; chemo & postop N/V, facilitate small-bowel intubation & upper GI radiologic exam*, *GERD, diabetic gastroparesis (Metozolv)* stimulate gut in prolonged postop ileus* **Acts:** ↑ Upper GI motility; blocks dopamine in chemoreceptor trigger zone, sensitized tissues to ACH **Dose: Adults.** *Gastroparesis (Reglan):* 10 mg PO 30 min ac & hs for 2–8 wk PRN, or same dose IM/IV for 10 d, then PO. *Reflux:* 10–15 mg PO 30 min ac & hs. *Chemo antiemetic:* 1–2 mg/kg/dose IV 30 min before chemo, then q2h × 2 doses, then q3h × 3 doses. *Postop:* 10–20 mg IV/IM q4–6h PRN. **Adults & Peds > 14 y.** *Intestinal intubation:* 10 mg IV × 1 over 1–2 min *Peds. Reflux:* 0.1–0.2 mg/kg/dose PO 30 min ac & hs. *Chemo antiemetic:* 1–2 mg/kg/dose IV as adults. *Postop:* 0.25 mg/kg IV q6–8h PRN. *Peds. Intestinal intubation:* **6–14 y:** 2.5–5 mg IV × 1 over 1–2 min; *< 6 y:* Use 0.1 mg/kg IV × 1 **W/P:** [B, M] Drugs w/ extrapyramidal ADRs, MAOIs, TCAs, sympathomimetics **CI:** w/ EPS meds, GI bleeding, pheochromocytoma, Sz disorders, GI obst **Disp:** Tabs 5, 10 mg; syrup 5 mg/5 mL; ODT (*Metozolv*) 5, 10 mg; Inj 5 mg/mL **SE:** Dystonic Rxns common w/ high doses (Rx w/ IV diphenhydramine), fluid retention, restlessness, D, drowsiness **Notes:** ↓ w/ Renal impair/elderly; ✓ baseline Cr

Metolazone (Zaroxolyn, Generic) Uses: *Mild–mod essential HTN & edema of renal Dz or cardiac failure* **Acts:** Thiazide-like diuretic; ↓ distal tubule Na reabsorption **Dose:** *HTN:* 2.5–5 mg/d PO qd *Edema:* 2.5–20 mg/d PO. **W/P:**

[B, –] Avoid w/ Li, gout, digitalis, SLE, many interactions **CI:** Anuria, hepatic coma or precoma **Disp:** Tabs 2.5, 5, 10 mg **SE:** Monitor fluid/lytes; dizziness, ↓ BP, ↓ K⁺, ↑ HR, ↑ uric acid, CP, photosens

Metoprolol Succinate (Toprol XL, Generic), Metoprolol Tartrate (Lopressor, Generic) BOX: Do not acutely stop Rx as marked worsening of angina can result; taper over 1–2 wk Uses: *HTN, angina, AMI, CHF (XL form)*

Acts: β₁-Adrenergic receptor blocker **Dose:** *Adults.* Angina: 50–200 mg PO bid max 400 mg/d; ER form dose qd. *HTN:* 50–200 mg PO bid max 450 mg/d, ER form dose qd. *AMI:* 5 mg IV q2min × 3 doses, then 50 mg PO q6h × 48 h, then 100 mg PO bid. *CHF: (XL form preferred)* 12.5–25 mg/d PO × 2 wk, ↑ 2-wk intervals, target: 200 mg max, use low dose w/ greatest severity; *ECC 2010. AMI:* 5 mg slow IV q5min, total 15 mg; then 50 mg PO, titrate to effect. *Peds 1–17 y.* HTN IR form 1–2 mg/kg/d PO, max 6 mg/kg/d (200 mg/d). ≥ *6 y: HTN* ER form 1 mg/kg/d PO, initial max 50 mg/d, ↑ PRN to 2 mg/kg/d max; ↓ w/ hepatic failure; take w/ meals **W/P:** [C, M] Uncompensated CHF, ↓ HR, heart block, hepatic impair, MyG, PVD, Raynaud, thyrotoxicosis **CI:** For HTN/angina SSS (unless paced), severe PVD, cardiogenic shock, severe PAD, 2nd-, 3rd-H block, pheochromocytoma. For MI sinus brady < 45 BPM, 1st-degree block (PR > 0.24 s), 2nd- and 3rd-degree block, SBP < 100 mm Hg, severe CHF, cardiogenic shock **Disp:** Tabs 25, 50, 100 mg; ER tabs 25, 50, 100, 200 mg; Inj 1 mg/mL **SE:** Drowsiness, insomnia, ED, ↓ HR, bronchospasm **Notes:** IR:ER 1:1 daily dose but ER/XL is qd. OK to split XL tab but do not crush/chew

Metronidazole (Flagyl, Flagyl ER, MetroCream, MetroGel, MetroLotion) BOX: Carcinogenic in rats Uses: *Bone/joint, endocarditis, intra-Abd, meningitis, & skin Infxns; amebiasis & amebic liver abscess; trichomoniasis in pt and partner; bacterial vaginosis; PID; giardiasis; antibiotic associated pseudomembranous colitis (C. difficile), eradicate H. pylori w/ combo Rx, rosacea, prophylactic in postop colorectal surgery* Acts: Interferes w/ DNA synth.

Spectrum: Excellent anaerobic, *C. difficile* **Dose:** *Adults. Anaerobic Infxns:* 500 mg IV q6–8h. *Amebic dysentery:* 500–750 mg/d PO q8h × 5–10 d. *Trichomonas:* 250 mg PO tid for 7 d or 2 g PO × 1 (Rx partner). *C. difficile:* 500 mg PO or IV q8h for 7–10 d (PO preferred; IV only if pt NPO), if no response, change to PO vancomycin. *Vaginosis:* 1 applicator intravag qd or bid × 5 d, or 500 mg PO bid × 7 d or 750 mg PO qd × 7 d. *Acne rosacea/skin:* Apply bid. *Giardia:* 500 mg PO bid × 5–7 d. *H. pylori:* 250–500 mg PO w/ meals & hs × 14 d, combine w/ other antibiotic & a proton pump inhib or H₂ antagonist. *Peds. Anaerobic Infxns:* PO: 15–35 mg/kg/d ÷ q8h *IV:* 30 mg/kg IV/d ÷ q6H, 4 g/d max × dose. *Amebic dysentery:* 35–50 mg/kg/24 h PO in 3 ÷ doses for 5–10 d; *Trichomonas:* 15–30 mg/kg/d PO ÷ q8h × 7 d. *C. difficile:* 30 mg/kg/d PO ÷ q6h × 10 d, max 2 g/d; ↓ w/ severe hepatic/renal impair **W/P:** [B, –] Avoid EtOH, w/ warfarin, CYP3A4 substrates (Table 10, p 319), ↑ Li levels **CI:** 1st tri of PRG **Disp:** Tabs 250, 500 mg; ER tabs 750 mg; caps 375 mg; IV 500 mg/100 mL; lotion 0.75%; gel 0.75, 1%; intravag gel

0.75% (5 g/applicator 37.5 mg in 70-g tube), cream 0.75, 1% **SE:** Disulfiram-like Rxn; dizziness, HA, GI upset, anorexia, urine discoloration, flushing, metallic taste **Notes:** For trichomoniasis, Rx pt's partner; no aerobic bacteria activity; use in combo w/ serious mixed Infxns; wait 24 h after 1st dose to breast-feed or 48 h if extended Rx, take ER on empty stomach

Mexiletine (Generic) **BOX:** Mortality risks noted for flecainide and/or encainide (class I antiarrhythmics). Reserve for use in pts w/ life-threatening ventricular arrhythmias **Uses:** *Suppress symptomatic vent arrhythmias* **DN Acts:** Class Ib antiarrhythmic (Table 9, p 318) **Dose:** *Adults.* 200–300 mg PO q8h. Initial 200 mg q8h, can load w/ 400 mg if needed, ↑ q2–3d, 1200 mg/d max, ↓ dose w/ hepatic impairment or CHF, administer ATC & w/ food **W/P:** [C, +] CHF, may worsen severe arrhythmias; interacts w/ hepatic inducers & suppressors **CI:** Cardiogenic shock or 2nd-/3rd-degree AV block w/o pacemaker **Disp:** Caps 150, 200, 250 mg **SE:** Lightheadedness, dizziness, anxiety, incoordination, ataxia, hepatic damage, blood dyscrasias, PVCs, N/V, tremor **Notes:** ✓ LFTs, CBC, false(+) ANA

Micafungin (Mycamine) **Uses:** *Candidemia, acute dissem and esophageal candidiasis, Candida peritonitis & abscesses; prophylaxis Candida Infxn w/ HSCT* **Acts:** Echinocandin; ↓ fungal cell wall synth **Dose:** *Candidemia, acute disseminated candidiasis, Candida peritonitis & abscesses:* 100 mg IV daily; *Esophageal candidiasis:* 150 mg IV daily; *Prophylaxis of Candida Infxn:* 50 mg IV daily over 1 h **W/P:** [C, ?/–] Sirolimus, nifedipine, itraconazole dosage adj may be necessary **CI:** Component or other echinocandin allergy **Disp:** Inj 50, 100 mg vials **SE:** N/V/D, HA, pyrexia, Abd pain, ↓ K⁺, ↓ plt, histamine Sxs (rash, pruritus, facial swelling, vasodilatation), anaphylaxis, anaphylactoid Rxn, hemolysis, hemolytic anemia, ↑ LFTs, hepatotox, renal impair

Miconazole (Monistat 1 Combo, Monistat 3, Monistat 7) (OTC) (Monistat-Derm) **Uses:** *Candidal Infxns, dermatomycoses (tinea pedis/tinea cruris/tinea corporis/tinea versicolor/candidiasis)* **Acts:** Azole antifungal, alters fungal membrane permeability **Dose:** *Intravag:* 100 mg supp or 2% cream intravag qhs × 7 d or 200 mg supp or 4% cream intravag qhs × 3 d. *Derm:* Apply bid, A.M./P.M. *Tinea versicolor:* Apply qd. Treat tinea pedis and tinea corporis for 1 mo and other Infxns for 2 wk. *Peds ≥12 y.* 100 mg supp or 2% cream intravag qhs × 7 d or 200 mg supp or 4% cream intravag qhs × 3 d. Not for OTC use in children < 2 y **W/P:** [C, ?] Azole sensitivity **Disp:** *Monistat-Derm:* (Rx) Cream 2%; *Monistat 1 combo:* 2% cream w/ 1200 mg supp, *Monistat 3:* Vag cream 4%, supp 200 mg; *Monistat 7:* 2% cream, supp 100 mg; lotion 2%; powder 2%; effervescent tab 2%, oint 2%, spray 2%; Vag supp 100, 200, 1200 mg; Vag cream 2%, 4%; [OTC] **SE:** Vag burning; on skin contact dermatitis, irritation, burning **Notes:** May interfere w/ condom and diaphragm, do not use w/ tampons

Miconazole/Zinc Oxide/Petrolatum (Vusion) **Uses:** *Candidal diaper rash* **Acts:** Combo antifungal **Dose:** *Peds ≤ 4 wk.* Apply at each diaper change × 7 d

W/P: [C, ?] **CI:** None **Disp:** Miconazole/zinc oxide/petrolatum oint 0.25/15/81.35%, 50-, 90-g tube **SE:** None **Notes:** Keep diaper dry, not for prevention

Midazolam (Generic) [C-IV] **BOX:** Associated w/ resp depression and resp arrest especially when used for sedation in noncritical care settings. Reports of airway obst, desaturation, hypoxia, and apnea w/ other CNS depressants. Cont monitoring required; initial doses in elderly & debilitated should be conservative **Uses:** *Preop sedation, conscious sedation for short procedures & mechanically ventilated pts, induction of general anesthesia* **Acts:** Short-acting benzodiazepine **Dose:** **Adults.** 1–5 mg IV or IM or 0.02–0.35 mg/kg based on indication; titrate to effect. **Peds.** *Preop:* > *6 mo:* 0.5–0.75 mg/kg PO, 20 mg max. > *6 mo:* 0.1–0.15 mg/kg IM × 1 max 10 mg. *General anesthesia:* 0.025–0.1 mg/kg IV q2min for 1–3 doses PRN to induce anesthesia (↓ in elderly, w/ narcotics or CNS depressants) **W/P:** [D, M] w/ CYP3A4 substrate (Table 10, p 319), multiple drug interactions **CI:** NAG; w/ fosamprenavir, atazanavir, nelfinavir, ritonavir, intrathecal/epidural Inj of parenteral forms. **Disp:** Inj 1, 5 mg/mL; syrup 2 mg/mL **SE:** Resp depression; ↓ BP w/ conscious sedation, N **Notes:** Reversal w/ flumazenil; monitor for resp depression

Midodrine (Proamatine) **BOX:** Indicated for pts for whom orthohypotension significantly impairs daily life despite standard care **Uses:** *Tx orthostatic hypotension* **Acts:** Vasopressor/antihypotensive; α_1-agonist **Dose:** 10 mg PO tid when pt plans to be upright **W/P:** [C, ?] **CI:** Pheochromocytoma, renal Dz, thyrotoxicosis, severe heart Dz, urinary retention, supine HTN **Disp:** Tabs 2.5, 5, 10 mg **SE:** Supine HTN, paresthesia, urinary retention **Notes:** SBP ≥ 200 mm Hg in ~13% pts given 10 mg

Mifepristone (Korlym) **BOX:** Antiprogestational; can cause termination of PRG. Exclude PRG before use or Rx is interrupted for > 14 d in ♀ of reproductive potential **Uses:** *Control hyperglycemia w/ Cushing synd and type 2 DM in nonsurgical or failed surgical candidates* **Acts:** Antiprogestin; glucocorticoid receptor blocker **Dose:** Start 300 mg PO qd w/ meal, ↑ PRN 1200 mg/d max (20 mg/kg/d); mod renal hepatic impair 600 mg/d max **W/P:** [X, –] Do not use w/ severe hepatic impair or w/ OCP; avoid w/ ↑ QT or drugs that ↑ QT; ✓ for adrenal insufficiency, ✓ K⁺; ✓ Vag bleed or w/ anticoagulants; caution w/ drugs metabolized by CYP3A, CYP2C8/2C9, CYP2B6 (eg, bupropion, efavirenz) **CI:** PRG, w/ simvastatin, lovastatin, CYP3A substrates, long-term steroids, unexplained uterine bleed, endometrial hyperplasia/cancer **Disp:** 300 mg tab **SE:** N/V, fatigue, HA, ↓ K⁺, arthralgia, edema, ↑ BP, dizziness, ↓ appetite, endometrial hypertrophy **Notes:** RU486 discontinued

Miglitol (Glyset) **Uses:** *Type 2 DM* **Acts:** α-Glucosidase inhib; delays carbohydrate digestion **Dose:** Initial 25 mg PO tid; maint 50–100 mg tid (w/ 1st bite of each meal), titrate over 4–8 wk **W/P:** [B, –] w/ Digitalis & digestive enzymes, not rec w/ SCr > 2 mg/dL **CI:** DKA, obstructive/inflammatory GI disorders; colonic ulceration **Disp:** Tabs 25, 50, 100 mg **SE:** Flatulence, D, Abd pain **Notes:** Use alone or w/ sulfonylureas

Milnacipran (Savella) BOX: Antidepressants associated w/ ↑ risk of suicide ideation in children and young adults Uses: *Fibromyalgia* Acts: Antidepressant, SNRI Dose: 50 mg PO bid, max 200 mg/d; ↓ to 25 mg bid w/ CrCl < 30 mL/min W/P: [C, /?] Caution w/ hepatic impair, hepatox, serotonin syndrome, ↑ bleeding risk CI: NAG, w/ recent MAOI Disp: Tabs: 12.5, 25, 50, 100 mg SE: HA, N/V, constipation, dizziness, ↑ HR, ↑ BP Notes: Monitor HR and BP

Milrinone (Primacor) Uses: *CHF acutely decompensated*, Ca antagonist intoxication Acts: Phosphodiesterase inhib, (+) inotrope & vasodilator; little chronotropic activity Dose: 50 mcg/kg, IV over 10 min then 0.375–0.75 mcg/kg/min IV Inf; ↓ w/ renal impair W/P: [C, ?] CI: Allergy to drug; w/ inamrinone Disp: Inj 200 mcg/mL SE: Arrhythmias, ↓ BP, HA Notes: Monitor fluids, lytes, CBC, Mg²⁺, BP, HR; not for long-term use

Mineral Oil [OTC] Uses: *Constipation, bowel irrigation, fecal impaction*
Acts: Lubricant laxative Dose: *Adults. Constipation:* 15–45 mL PO/d PRN. *Fecal impaction or after barium:* 118 mL rectally × 1. *Peds > 6 y. Constipation:* 5–25 mL PO qd. *2–12 y: Fecal impaction:* 59 mL rectally × 1. W/P: [?, ?] w/ N/V, difficulty swallowing, bedridden pts; may ↓ absorption of vits A, D, E, K, warfarin CI: Colostomy/ileostomy, appendicitis, diverticulitis, UC Disp: All [OTC] liq, PO microemulsion 2.5 mL/5 mL, rectal enema 118 mL SE: Lipid pneumonia (aspiration of PO), N/V, temporary anal incontinence Notes: Take PO upright, do not use PO in peds < 6 y

Mineral Oil/Pramoxine HCl/Zinc Oxide (Tucks Ointment [OTC]) Uses: *Temporary relief of anorectal disorders (itching, etc)* Acts: Topical anesthetic Dose: *Adults & Peds ≥ 12 y.* Cleanse, rinse, & dry, apply externally or into anal canal w/ tip 5×/d × 7 d max. W/P: [?, ?] Do not place into rectum CI: None Disp: Oint 1% 30-g tube SE: Local irritation Notes: DC w/ or if rectal bleeding occurs or if condition worsens or does not improve w/in 7 d

Minocycline (Arestin, Dynacin, Minocin, Solodyn, Generic) Uses:
Mod–severe nonnodular acne (Solodyn), anthrax, rickettsiae, skin Infxn, URI, UTI, nongonococcal urethritis, amebic dysentery, asymptomatic meningococcal carrier, Mycobacterium marinum, adjunct to dental scaling for periodontitis (Arestin) Acts: Tetracycline, bacteriostatic, ↓ protein synth Dose: *Adults & Peds > 12 y. Usual:* 200 mg, then 100 mg q12h or 100–200 mg IV or PO, then 50 mg qid. *Gonococcal urethritis, men:* 100 mg q12h × 5 d. *Syphilis:* Usual dose × 10–15 d. *Meningococcal carrier:* 100 mg q12h × 5 d. *M. marinum:* 100 mg q12h × 6–8 wk. *Uncomp urethral, endocervical, or rectal Infxn:* 100 mg q12h × 7 d minimum. *Adults & Peds > 12 y. Acne: (Solodyn)* 1 mg/kg PO qd × 12 wk. *> 8 y:* 4 mg/kg initially then 2 mg/kg q12h w/ food to ↓ irritation, hydrate well, ↓ dose or extend interval w/ renal impair. W/P: [D, –] Associated w/ pseudomembranous colitis, w/ renal impair, may ↓ OCP, or w/ warfarin may ↑ INR CI: Allergy, children < 8 y Disp: Tabs 50, 75, 100 mg; tabs ER (Solodyn) 45, 65, 90, 115, 135 mg, caps (Minocin) 50, 100 mg, susp 50 mg/mL (Arestin) topical power SE: D, HA, fever, rash, joint pain, fatigue, dizziness, photosens, hyperpigmentation, SLE synd,

pseudotumor cerebri **Notes:** Do not cut/crush/chew; keep away from children, tooth discoloration in < 8 y or w/ use last half of PRG

Minoxidil, Oral (Generic) **BOX:** May cause pericardial effusion, occasional tamponade, and angina pectoris may be exacerbated. Only for nonresponders to max doses of 2 other antihypertensives and a diuretic. Administer under supervision w/ a β-blocker and diuretic. Monitor for ↓ BP in those receiving guanethidine w/ malignant HTN **Uses:** *Severe HTN* **Acts:** Peripheral vasodilator **Dose:** *Adults & Peds > 12 y.* 5 mg PO qd, titrate q3d, 100 mg/d max usual range 2.5–80 mg/d in 1–2 ÷ doses. *Peds.* 0.2–1 mg/kg/24 h ÷ PO q12–24h, titrate q3d, max 50 mg/d; ↓ w/ elderly, renal Insuff **W/P:** [C, –] Caution in renal impairment, CHF **CI:** Pheochromocytoma, component allergy **Disp:** Tabs 2.5, 10 mg **SE:** Pericardial effusion & vol overload w/ PO use; hypertrichosis w/ chronic use, edema, ECG changes, Wt gain **Notes:** Avoid for 1 mo after MI

Minoxidil, Topical (Theroxidil, Rogaine) [OTC] **Uses:** *Male & female pattern baldness* **Acts:** Stimulates vertex hair growth **Dose:** Apply 1 mL bid to area, D/C if no growth in 4 mo. **W/P:** [?, ?] **CI:** Component allergy **Disp:** Soln & aerosol foam 2, 5% **SE:** Changes in hair color/texture **Notes:** Requires chronic use to maintain hair

Mipomersen (Kynamro) **BOX:** May ↑ transaminases and/or cause hepatic steatosis. Monitor ALT/AST and bili baseline & regularly; hold if ALT/AST > 3× ULN (see label; D/C w/ significant liver tox; restricted KYNAMRO REMS distribution **Uses:** *Homozygous familial hypercholesterolemia* **Acts:** Oligonucleotide inhib apo B-100 synth **Dose:** *Adults.* 200 mg SQ 1 × wk **W/P:** [B, ?/–] **CI:** Mod–severe hepatic impair, active liver Dz, component allergy **Disp:** Inj 200 mg/mL (1 mL vial/syringe) **SE:** Inj site Rxns, flu-like Sxs; hepatotox, N/V, Abd pain, angina, palpitations, fatigue, pyrexia, edema, musculoskeletal pain, HA, insomnia, HTN

Mirabegron (Myrbetriq) **Uses:** *OAB* **Acts:** β-3 adrenergic agonist; relaxes smooth muscle **Dose:** *Adults.* 25 mg PO daily; ↑ to 50 mg daily after 8 wk PRN; 25 mg max daily w/ severe renal or mod hepatic impair; swallow whole **W/P:** [C, –] w/ Severe uncontrolled HTN; urinary retention w/ BOO & antimuscarinic drugs; w/ drugs metabolized by CYP2D6; do not use w/ ESRD or severe hepatic impair **CI:** None **Disp:** Tabs ER 25, 50 mg **SE:** HTN, HA, UTI, nasopharyngitis, N/D, constipation, Abd pain, dizziness, tachycardia, URI, arthralgia, edema

Mirtazapine (Remeron, Remeron SolTab, Generic) **BOX:** ↑ Risk of suicidal thinking and behavior in children, adolescents, and young adults w/ major depression and other psychological disorders. Not for peds **Uses:** *Depression* **Acts:** α₂-Antagonist antidepressant, ↑ norepinephrine & 5-HT **Dose:** 15 mg PO hs, up to 45 mg/d hs **W/P:** [C, M] Has anticholesterol effects, w/ Sz, clonidine, CNS depressant use, CYP1A2, CYP3A4 inducers/inhib w/ hepatic & renal impairment **CI:** MAOIs w/in 14 d **Disp:** Tabs 7.5, 15, 30, 45 mg; rapid dispersion tabs (SolTab) 15, 30, 45 mg **SE:** Somnolence, ↑ cholesterol, constipation, xerostomia, Wt gain, agranulocytosis, ↓ BP, edema, musculoskeletal pain **Notes:** Do not ↑ dose < q1–2wk;

handle rapid tabs w/ dry hands, do not cut or chew; not FDA approved for Rx of bipolar depression; do not D/C abruptly

Misoprostol (Cytotec, Generic) BOX: Use in PRG can cause Ab, premature birth, or birth defects; do not use to ↓ decrease ulcer risk in women of childbearing age; must comply w/ birth control measures Uses: *Prevent NSAID-induced gastric ulcers; medical termination of PRG < 49 d w/ mifepristone*; induce labor (cervical ripening); incomplete & therapeutic Ab Acts: Prostaglandin (PGE-1); antisecretory & mucosal protection; induces uterine contractions Dose: *Ulcer prevention:* 100–200 mcg PO qid w/ meals; in females, start 2nd/3rd d of next nl period. *Induction of labor (term):* 25–50 mcg intravag. *PRG termination:* 400 mcg PO on day 3 of mifepristone; take w/ food W/P: [X, –] CI: PRG, component allergy Disp: Tabs 100, 200 mcg SE: Miscarriage w/ severe bleeding; HA, D, Abd pain, constipation. Notes: Not used for induction of labor w/ previous C-section or major uterine surgery

Mitomycin (Mitosol [Topical], Generic) BOX: Administer only by physician experienced in chemotherapy; myelosuppressive; can induce hemolytic uremic synd w/ irreversible renal failure Uses: *Stomach, pancreas*, breast, colon CA; squamous cell carcinoma of the anus; NSCLC, head & neck, cervical; bladder CA (intravesically), *Mitosol* for glaucoma surgery Acts: Alkylating agent; generates oxygen-free radicals w/ DNA strand breaks Dose: (Per protocol) 20 mg/m² q6–8wk IV or 10 mg/m² combo w/ other myelosuppressive drugs q6–8wk. *Bladder CA:* 20–40 mg in 40 mL NS via a urethral catheter once/wk; ↓ in renal/hepatic impair W/P: [D, –] w/ Cr > 1.7 mg/dL/ ↑ cardiac tox w/ vinca alkaloids/doxorubicin CI: ↓ Plt, coagulation disorders, ↑ bleeding tendency, PRG Disp: Inj 5, 20, 40 mg; *Mitosol* 0.2 mg/vial SE: ↓ BM (persists for 3–8 wk, may be cumulative; minimize w/ lifetime dose < 50–60 mg/m²), N/V, anorexia, stomatitis, renal tox, microangiopathic hemolytic anemia w/ renal failure (hemolytic–uremic synd), venoocclusive liver Dz, interstitial pneumonia, alopecia, extrav Rxns, contact dermatitis; CHF w/ doses > 30 mg/m²

Mitoxantrone (Generic) BOX: Administer only by physician experienced in chemotherapy; except for acute leukemia, do not use w/ ANC count of < 1500 cells/ mm³; severe neutropenia can result in Infxn, follow CBC; cardiotoxic (CHF), secondary AML reported Uses: *AML (w/ cytarabine), ALL, CML, PCA, MS, lung CA*, breast CA, & NHL Acts: DNA-intercalating agent; ↓ DNA synth by interacting w/ topoisomerase II Dose: Per protocol; ↓ w/ hepatic impair, leukopenia, thrombocytopenia W/P: [D, –] Reports of secondary AML, w/ MS ↑ CV risk, do not treat MS pt w/ low LVEF CI: PRG, sig ↓ in LVEF Disp: Inj 2 mg/mL SE: ↓ BM, N/V, stomatitis, alopecia (infrequent), cardiotox, urine discoloration, secretions & scleras may be blue-green Notes: Maintain hydration; baseline CV evaluation w/ ECG & LVEF; cardiac monitoring prior to each dose; not for intrathecal use

Modafinil (Provigil, Generic) [C-IV] Uses: *Improve wakefulness in pts w/ excess daytime sleepiness (narcolepsy, sleep apnea, shift work sleep disorder)*

Acts: Alters dopamine & norepinephrine release, ↓ GABA-mediated neurotransmission **Dose:** 200 mg PO q A.M.; ↓ dose 50% w/ elderly/hepatic impair **W/P:** [C, M] CV Dz; ↑ effects of warfarin, diazepam, phenytoin; ↓ OCP, cyclosporine, & theophylline effects **CI:** Component allergy **Disp:** Tabs 100, 200 mg **SE:** Serious rash including SJS, HA, N, D, paresthesias, rhinitis, agitation, psychological Sx **Notes:** CV assessment before using

Moexipril (Univasc, Generic) **BOX:** ACE inhib can cause fetal injury/death in 2nd/3rd tri; D/C w/ PRG **Uses:** *HTN, post-MI*, DN **Acts:** ACE inhib **Dose:** 7.5–30 mg in 1–2 ÷ doses 1 h ac ↓ in renal impair **W/P:** [C (1st tri, D 2nd & 3rd tri), ?] **CI:** ACE inhib sensitivity **Disp:** Tabs 7.5, 15 mg; **SE:** ↓ BP, edema, angioedema, HA, dizziness, cough, ↑ K⁺

Mometasone and Formoterol (Dulera) **BOX:** Increased risk of worsening wheezing or asthma-related death in pediatric/adolescent pts w/ long-acting β₂-adrenergic agonists; use only if asthma not controlled on agent such as inhaled steroid **Uses:** *Maint Rx for asthma* **Acts:** Corticosteroid (mometasone) w/ LA bronchodilator β₂ agonist (formoterol) **Dose:** *Adults & Peds > 12 y.* 2 Inh q12h **W/P:** [C, ?/M] w/ P450 3A4 inhib (eg, ritonavir), adrenergic/beta blockers, meds that ↑ QT interval; candida Infxn of mouth/throat, immunosuppression, adrenal suppression, ↓ bone density, w/ glaucoma/cataracts, may ↑ glucose, ↓ K; other LABA should not be used **CI:** Acute asthma attack; component hypersensitivity **Disp:** MDI 120 inhal/canister (mcg mometasone/mcg formoterol) 100/5, 200/5 **SE:** Nasopharyngitis, sinusitis, HA, palpitations, CP, rapid heart rate, tremor or nervousness, oral candidiasis **Notes:** For pts not controlled on other meds (eg, low-medium dose Inh steroids) or whose Dz severity warrants 2 maint therapies

Mometasone, Inhaled (Asmanex Twisthaler) **Uses:** *Maint Rx for asthma* **Acts:** Corticosteroid **Dose:** *Adults & Peds > 11 y. On bronchodilators alone or inhaled steroids:* 220 mcg × 1 q P.M. or in ÷ doses (max 440 mcg/d). *On oral steroids:* 440 mcg bid (max 880 mcg/d) w/ slow oral taper. *Peds 4–11 y.* 110 mcg × 1 q P.M. (max 110 mcg/d) **W/P:** [C, ?/M] Candida Infxn of mouth/throat; hypersens Rxns possible; may worsen certain Infxn (TB, fungal, etc); monitor for ↑ / ↓ cortisol Sxs; ↓ bone density; ↓ growth in peds; monitor for NAG or cataracts; may ↑ glucose **CI:** Acute asthma attack; component hypersens/milk proteins **Disp:** MDI inhal mometasone 110 mcg *Twisthaler* delivers 100 mcg/actuation; 220 mcg *Twisthaler* delivers 200 mcg/actuation **SE:** HA, allergic rhinitis, pharyngitis, URI, sinusitis, oral candidiasis, dysmenorrhea, musculoskeletal/back pain, dyspepsia **Notes:** Rinse mouth after use; treat paradoxical bronchospasm w/ inhaled bronchodilator

Mometasone, Nasal (Nasonex) **Uses:** *Nasal Sx allergic/seasonal rhinitis; prophylaxis of seasonal allergic rhinitis; nasal polyps in adults* **Acts:** Corticosteroid **Dose:** *Adults & Peds ≥ 12 y. Rhinitis:* 2 sprays/each nostril qd. **Adults.** *Nasal polyps:* 2 sprays/each nostril bid *Peds 2–11 y.* 1 spray/each nostril qd **W/P:** [C, M] Monitor for adverse effects on nasal mucosa (bleeding, candidal Infxn, ulceration, perf); may worsen existing Infxns; monitor for NAG, cataracts; monitor for ↑ / ↓ cortisol Sxs; ↓ growth in peds **CI:** Component hypersens **Disp:** 50 mcg mometasone/spray **SE:** Viral Infxn, pharyngitis, epistaxis, HA

Montelukast (Singulair, Generic) Uses: *Prevent/chronic Rx asthma ≥ 12 mo; seasonal allergic rhinitis ≥ 2 y; perennial allergic rhinitis ≥ 6 mo; prevent exercise induced bronchoconstriction (EIB) ≥ 15 y; prophylaxis & Rx of chronic asthma, seasonal allergic rhinitis* **Acts:** Leukotriene receptor antagonist **Dose:** *Asthma: Adults & Peds > 15 y.* 10 mg/d PO in P.M. *6–23 mo:* 4-mg pack granules qd. *2–5 y:* 4 mg/d PO q P.M. *6–14 y:* 5 mg/d PO q P.M. **W/P:** [B, M] **CI:** Component allergy **Disp:** Tabs 10 mg; chew tabs 4, 5 mg; granules 4 mg/pack **SE:** HA, dizziness, fatigue, rash, GI upset, Churg-Strauss synd, flu, cough, neuropsych events (agitation, restlessness, suicidal ideation) **Notes:** Not for acute asthma; use w/in 15 min of opening package

Morphine (Avinza XR, Astramorph/PF, Duramorph, Infumorph, MS Contin, Kadian SR, Oramorph SR, Roxanol) [C-II] **BOX:** Do not crush/chew SR/CR forms; swallow whole or sprinkle on applesauce. 100 and 200 mg for opioid-tolerant pt only for mod–severe pain when pain control needed for an extended period and not PRN. Be aware of misuse, abuse, diversion. No alcoholic beverages while on therapy **Uses:** *Rx severe pain*, AMI, acute pulmonary edema **Acts:** Narcotic analgesic; SR/CR forms for chronic use **Dose:** *Adults.* *Short-term use PO:* 5–30 mg q4h PRN; *IV/IM:* 2.5–15 mg q2–6h; *Supp:* 10–30 mg q4h. SR formulations 15–60 mg q8–12h (do not chew/crush). *IT/epidural* (Duramorph, Infumorph, Astramorph/PF): Per protocol in Inf device. *ECC 2010.* *STEMI:* 2–4 mg IV (over 1–5 min), then give 2–8 mg IV q5–15min as needed. *NSTEMI:* 1–5 mg slow IV if Sxs unrelieved by nitrates or recur; use w/ caution; can be reversed w/ 0.4–2 mg IV naloxone. *Peds > 6 mo.* 0.1–0.2 mg/kg/dose IM/IV q2–4h PRN; 0.15–0.2 mg/kg PO q3–4h PRN **W/P:** [C, +/–] Severe resp depression possible; w/ head injury; chewing delayed release forms can cause severe rapid release of morphine. Administer *Duramorph* in staffed environment d/t cardiopulmonary effects. IT doses 1/10 of epidural dose **CI:** (many product specific) Severe asthma, resp depression, GI obst/ileus; *Oral soln:* CHF d/t lung Dz, head injury, arrhythmias, brain tumor, acute alcoholism, DTs, Sz disorders; *MS Contin and Kadian* CI include hypercarbia. **Disp:** IR tabs 15, 30 mg; soln 10, 20, 100 mg/5 mL; supp 5, 10, 20, 30 mg; Inj 2, 4, 5, 8, 10, 15, 25, 50 mg/mL; *MS Contin CR* tabs 15, 30, 60, 100, 200 mg; *Oramorph SR* tabs 15, 30, 60, 100 mg; *Kadian SR* caps 10, 20, 30, 40, 50, 60, 70, 80, 100, 130, 150, 200 mg; *Avinza XR* caps 30, 60, 90, 120 mg; *Duramorph/Astramorph PF:* Inj 0.5, 1 mg/mL; *Infumorph* 10, 25 mg/mL. **SE:** Narcotic SE (resp depression, sedation, constipation, N/V, pruritus, diaphoresis, urinary retention, biliary colic), granulomas w/ IT **Notes:** May require scheduled dosing to relieve severe chronic pain

Morphine and Naltrexone (Embeda) [C-II] **BOX:** For mod–severe chronic pain; do not use as PRN analgesic; swallow whole or sprinkle contents of cap on applesauce; do not crush/dissolve, chew caps—rapid release & absorption of morphine may be fatal & of naltrexone may lead to withdrawal in opioid-tolerant pts; do not consume EtOH or EtOH-containing products; 100/4 mg caps for opioid-tolerant pts only for use in opioid tolerant pts only, may cause fatal resp. depression; high potential for abuse **Uses:** *Chronic mod–severe pain* **Acts:** Mu-opioid receptor agonist & antagonist **Dose:** *Adult.* Individualize PO q12–24h; if opioid naive start 20/0.8 mg q24h; titrate q48h; ↓ start dose in elderly, w/ hepatic/renal insuff; taper to D/C **W/P:** [C, –] w/ EtOH, CNS depress, muscle relaxants, use w/ in 14 d of D/C of MAOI **CI:** Resp depression, acute/severe asthma/hypercarbia, ileus, hypersens **Disp:** Caps ER (morphine mg/naltrexone mg) 20/0.8, 30/1.2, 50/2, 60/2.4, 80/3.2, 100/4 **SE:** N/V/D, constipation, somnolence, dizziness, HA, ↓ BP, pruritus, insomnia, anxiety, resp depression, Sz, MI, apnea, withdrawal w/ abrupt D/C, anaphylaxis, biliary spasm

Moxifloxacin (Avelox) **BOX:** ↑ Risk of tendon rupture and tendonitis; ↑ risk w/ age > 60, transplant pts; may ↑ Sx of MG **Uses:** *Acute sinusitis & bronchitis, skin/soft-tissue/intra-Abd Infxns, conjunctivitis, CAP* TB, anthrax, endocarditis **Acts:** 4th-gen quinolone; ↓ DNA gyrase. *Spectrum:* Excellent gram(+) except MRSA & *E. faecium;* good gram(–) except *P. aeruginosa, Stenotrophomonas maltophilia, & Acinetobacter* sp; good anaerobic **Dose:** 400 mg/d PO/IV daily; avoid cation products, antacids tid **W/P:** [C, –] Quinolone sensitivity; interactions w/ Mg^{2+}, Ca^{2+}, Al^{2+}, Fe^{2+} -containing products, & class IA & III antiarrhythmic agents (Table 9, p 318) **CI:** Quinolone/component sensitivity **Disp:** Tabs 400 mg, ABC Pak 5 tabs, Inj **SE:** Dizziness, N, QT prolongation, Szs, photosens, peripheral neuropathy risk

Moxifloxacin, Ophthalmic (Moxeza, Vigamox) **Uses:** *Bacterial conjunctivitis* **Acts:** See Moxifloxacin **Dose:** Instill into affected eye/s: *Moxeza* 1 gtt bid × 7 d; *Vigamox* 1 gtt tid × 7 d **W/P:** [C, M] Not well studied in peds < 12 mo **CI:** Quinolone/component sensitivity **Disp:** Ophthal soln 0.5% **SE:** ↓ Visual acuity, ocular pain, itching, tearing, conjunctivitis; prolonged use may result in fungal overgrowth; do not wear contacts w/ conjunctivitis

Multivitamins, Oral [OTC] (See Table 12, p 322)

Mupirocin (Bactroban, Bactroban Nasal) **Uses:** *Impetigo (oint); skin lesion infect w/ S. aureus or S. pyogenes; eradicate MRSA in nasal carriers* **Acts:** ↓ Bacterial protein synth **Dose:** *Topical:* Apply small amount 3x/d × 5–14 d. *Nasal:* Apply 1/2 single-use tube bid in nostrils × 5 d **W/P:** [B, ?/M] **CI:** Do not use w/ other nasal products **Disp:** Oint 2%; cream 2%; nasal oint 2% 1-g single-use tubes **SE:** Local irritation, rash **Notes:** Pt to contact healthcare provider if no improvement in 3–5 d

Mycophenolic Acid (Myfortic, Generic) **BOX:** ↑ Risk of Infxns, lymphoma, other CAs, progressive multifocal leukoencephalopathy (PML), risk of PRG loss and malformation, female of childbearing potential must use contraception **Uses:** *Prevent rejection after renal transplant* **Acts:** Cytostatic to lymphocytes

Dose: *Adults.* 720 mg PO bid. Doses differ based on transplant *Peds. BSA 1.19–1.58 m²:* 540 mg bid. *BSA > 1.58 m²:* Adult dose; used w/ steroids or tacrolimus. ↓ w/ renal Insuff/neutropenia; take on empty stomach **W/P:** [D, –] **CI:** Component allergy **Disp:** Delayed release tabs 180, 360 mg **SE:** N/V/D, GI bleed, pain, fever, HA, Infxn, HTN, anemia, leukopenia, pure red cell aplasia, edema **Notes:** Cellcept & Myfortic dosage forms should not be used interchangeably

Mycophenolate Mofetil (CellCept, Generic) **BOX:** ↑ Risk of Infxns, lymphoma, other CAs, progressive multifocal leukoencephalopathy (PML); risk of PRG loss and malformation; female of childbearing potential must use contraception **Uses:** *Prevent organ rejection after transplant* **Acts:** Cytostatic to lymphocytes **Dose:** *Adults.* 1 g PO bid, doses differ based on transplant *Peds. BSA 1.2–1.5 m²:* 750 mg PO bid. *BSA > 1.5 m²:* 1 g PO bid; used w/ steroids & cyclosporine or tacrolimus; ↓ in renal Insuff or neutropenia. *IV:* Infuse over > 2 h. *PO:* Take on empty stomach, do not open caps **W/P:** [D, –] **CI:** Component allergy; IV use in polysorbate 80 allergy **Disp:** Caps 250, 500 mg; susp 200 mg/mL, Inj 500 mg **SE:** N/V/D, pain, fever, HA, Infxn, HTN, anemia, leukopenia, edema **Notes:** Cellcept & Myfortic are not interchangeable

Nabilone (Cesamet) [C-II] **Uses:** *Refractory chemotherapy-induced emesis* **Acts:** Synthetic cannabinoid **Dose:** *Adults.* 1–2 mg PO bid 1–3 h before chemotherapy, 6 mg/d max; may continue for 48 h beyond final chemotherapy dose *Peds:* ↑ Per protocol; < 18 kg 0.5 mg bid; 18–30 kg 1 mg bid; > 30 kg 1 mg tid **W/P:** [C, –] Elderly, HTN, heart failure, w/ psychological illness, substance abuse; high protein binding w/ 1st-pass metabolism may lead to drug interactions **Disp:** Caps 1 mg **SE:** Drowsiness, vertigo, xerostomia, euphoria, ataxia, HA, difficulty concentrating, tachycardia, ↓ BP **Notes:** May require initial dose evening before chemotherapy; Rx only quantity for single Tx cycle

Nabumetone (Relafen, Generic) **BOX:** May ↑ risk of CV events & GI bleeding, perforation; CI w/ postop CABG **Uses:** *OA and RA*, pain **Acts:** NSAID; ↓ prostaglandins **Dose:** 1000–2000 mg/d ÷ daily-bid w/ food **W/P:** [C, –] Severe hepatic Dz, peptic ulcer Dz, anaphylaxis w/ "ASA triad" **CI:** NSAID sensitivity, perioperative pain, after CABG surgery **Disp:** Tabs 500, 750 mg **SE:** Dizziness, rash, GI upset, edema, peptic ulcer, ↑ BP, photosens

Nadolol (Corgard) **BOX:** Do not abruptly withdraw **Uses:** *HTN & angina migraine prophylaxis*, prophylaxis of variceal hemorrhage **Acts:** Competitively blocks β-adrenergic receptors (β₁, β₂) **Dose:** 40–80 mg/d; ↑ to 240 mg/d (angina) or 320 mg/d (HTN) at 3- to 7-d intervals; ↓ in renal Insuff & elderly **W/P:** [C +/M] **CI:** Uncompensated CHF, shock, heart block, asthma **Disp:** Tabs 20, 40, 80 mg **SE:** Nightmares, paresthesias, ↓ BP, ↓ HR, fatigue, ↓ sex function

Nafarelin, Metered Spray (SYNAREL) **Uses:** *Endometriosis, CPP* **Acts:** GnRH agonist; ↓ gonadal steroids w/ use > 4 wk **Dose:** *Adults: Endometriosis:* 400 mcg/d (1 spray q A.M./P.M. alternate nostril; if no amenorrhea ↑ 2 sprays bid, start d 2–4 of menstrual cycle *Peds: CPP:* 1600 mcg/d (2 sprays each nostril q A.M./P.M.), can ↑ to 1800 mcg/d **W/P:** [X, –] **CI:** Component hypersens, undiagnosed uterine bleeding, PRG, breast-feeding **Disp:** 0.5-oz bottle 60 sprays (200 mcg/spray) **SE:** ♀: hot flashes, headaches, emotional lability, ↓ libido, vaginal dryness, acne, myalgia, ↓ breast size, ↓ BMD; **Peds:** drug sensitivity Rxn, acne, transient ↑ breast enlargement/pubic hair, Vag bleed, emotional lability, body odor, seborrhea **Notes:** ✓ PRG test before use; for endometriosis only if > 18 y, and no more than 6 mo; no sig effect w/ rhinitis, if needed, use decongestant 2 h before dose

Nafcillin (Nallpen, Generic) Uses: *Infxns d/t susceptible strains of *Staphylococcus & Streptococcus** **Acts:** Bactericidal; antistaphylococcal PCN; ↓ cell wall synth *Spectrum:* Good gram(+) except MRSA & enterococcus, no gram(–), poor anaerobe **Dose:** *Adults.* 1–2 g IV q4–6h. *Peds.* 50–200 mg/kg/d ÷ q4–6h **W/P:** [B, ?] **CI:** PCN allergy, allergy to corn-related products **Disp:** Inj powder l, 2 g **SE:** Interstitial nephritis, N/D, fever, rash, allergic Rxn **Notes:** In setting of both hepatic & renal impairment, modification of dose may be necessary

Naftifine (Naftin) Uses: *Tinea pedis, cruris, & corporis* **Acts:** Allylamine antifungal, ↓ cell membrane ergosterol synth **Dose:** Apply daily (cream) or bid (gel) **W/P:** [B, ?] **CI:** Component sensitivity **Disp:** 1% cream; gel **SE:** Local irritation

Nalbuphine (Generic) Uses: *Mod–severe pain; preop & obstetric analgesia* **Acts:** Narcotic agonist–antagonist; ↓ ascending pain pathways **Dose:** *Adults.* *Pain:* 10 mg/70 kg IV/IM/SQ q3–6h; adjust PRN; 20 mg/dose or 160 mg/d max. *Anesthesia: Induction:* 0.3–3 mg/kg IV over 10–15 min; maint 0.25–0.5 mg/kg IV. *Peds.* 0.2 mg/kg IV or IM, 20 mg/dose or 160 mg/d max; ↓ w/ renal/in hepatic impair **W/P:** [B, M] w/ Opiate use **CI:** Component sensitivity **Disp:** Inj 10, 20 mg/mL **SE:** CNS depression, drowsiness; caution, ↓ BP

Naloxone (Generic) Uses: *Opioid addiction (diagnosis) & OD* **Acts:** Competitive narcotic antagonist **Dose:** *Adults.* 0.4–2 mg IV, IM, or SQ q2min; total dose 10 mg max. *Peds.* 0.01–0.1 mg/kg/dose IV, IM, or SQ; repeat IV q3min × 3 doses PRN; *ECC 2010. Total reversal of narcotic effects:* 0.1 mg/kg q2min PRN; max dose 2 mg; smaller doses (1–5 mcg/kg may be used); cont Inf 2–160 mcg/kg/h **W/P:** [C, ?] May precipitate acute withdrawal in addicts **Disp:** Inj 0.4, 1 mg/mL **SE:** ↓ BP, tachycardia, irritability, GI upset, pulm edema **Notes:** If no response after 10 mg, suspect nonnarcotic cause

Naltrexone (ReVia, Vivitrol, Generic) BOX: Can cause hepatic injury, CI w/ active liver Dz Uses: *EtOH & narcotic addiction* **Acts:** Antagonizes opioid receptors **Dose:** *EtOH/narcotic addiction:* 50 mg/d PO; must be opioid-free for 7–10 d; *EtOH dependence:* 380 mg IM q4wk (*Vivitrol*) **W/P:** [C, M] Monitor for Inj site reactions (*Vivitrol*) **CI:** Acute hep, liver failure, opioid use **Disp:** Tabs 50 mg; Inj 380 mg (*Vivitrol*) **SE:** Hepatotox; insomnia, GI upset, joint pain, HA, fatigue

Naphazoline (Albalon, Naphcon, Generic), Naphazoline, & Pheniramine (Naphcon A, Visine A) Uses: *Relieve ocular redness & itching caused by allergy* **Acts:** Sympathomimetic (α-adrenergic vasoconstrictor) & antihistamine (pheniramine) **Dose:** 1–2 gtt up to q6h, 3 d max **W/P:** [C, +] **CI:**

NAG, in children < 6 y, w/ contact lenses, component allergy **SE:** CV stimulation, dizziness, local irritation **Disp:** Ophthal 0.012, 0.025, 0.1%/15 mL; naphazoline & pheniramine 0.025%/0.3% soln

Naproxen (Aleve [OTC], Anaprox, Anaprox DS, EC-Naprosyn, Naprelan, Naprosyn, Generic) **BOX:** May ↑ risk of CV events & GI bleeding **Uses:** *Arthritis & pain* **Acts:** NSAID; ↓ prostaglandins **Dose:** *Adults & Peds > 12 y.* 200–500 mg bid-tid to 1500 mg/d max. > 2 y: JRA 5 mg/kg/dose bid; ↓ in hepatic impair **W/P:** [C, (D 3rd tri), –] **CI:** NSAID or ASA triad sensitivity, peptic ulcer, post-CABG pain, 3rd-tri PRG **Disp:** Tabs: 250, 375, 500 mg; *DR:* 375, 500, 750 mg; *CR:* 375, 550 mg; susp 25 mg/5 mL (*Aleve*) 200 mg multiple OTC forms **SE:** Dizziness, pruritus, GI upset, peptic ulcer, edema **Notes:** Take w/ food to ↓ GI upset; 220 mg naproxen sodium = 200 mg naproxen base

Naproxen/Esomeprazole (Vimovo) **BOX:** ↑ Risk MI, stroke, PE; CI, CABG surgery pain; ↑ risk GI bleed, gastric ulcer, gastric/duodenal perforation **Uses:** *Pain and/or swelling, RA, OA, ankylosing spondylitis, ↓ risk NSAID-assoc gastric ulcers* **Acts:** NSAID; ↓ prostaglandins & PPI, ↓ gastric acid **Dose:** 375/20 mg (naproxen/esomeprazole) to 500/20 mg PO bid **W/P:** [C 1st, 2nd tri; D 3rd; –] **CI:** PRG 3rd tri; asthma, urticaria from ASA or NSAID; mod–severe hepatic/renal **Disp:** Tabs (naproxen/esomeprazole) DR 375/20 mg; 500/20 mg **SE:** N/D, Abd pain, gastritis, ulcer, ↑ BP, CHF, edema, serious skin rash (eg, Stevens-Johnson synd, etc), ↓ renal Fxn, papillary necrosis **Notes:** Risk of GI adverse events elderly; atrophic gastritis w/ long-term PPI use; possible ↑ risk of fractures w/ all PPI; may ↑ Li levels; may cause MTX tox; may ↑ INR on warfarin; may ↓ effect BP meds; may ↓ absorption drugs requiring acid environment

Naratriptan (Amerge, Generic) **Uses:** *Acute migraine* **Acts:** Serotonin 5-HT$_1$ receptor agonist **Dose:** 1–2.5 mg PO once; repeat PRN in 4 h; 5 mg/24 h max; ↓ in mild renal/hepatic Insuff, take w/ fluids **W/P:** [C, M] **CI:** Severe renal/hepatic impair, avoid w/ angina, ischemic heart Dz, uncontrolled HTN, cerebrovascular synds, & ergot use **Disp:** Tabs 1, 2.5 mg **SE:** Dizziness, sedation, GI upset, paresthesias, ECG changes, coronary vasospasm, arrhythmias

Natalizumab (Tysabri) **BOX:** PML reported **Uses:** *Relapsing MS to delay disability and ↓ recurrences, Crohn Dz* **Acts:** Integrin receptor antagonist **Dose:** *Adults.* 300 mg IV q4wk; 2nd-line Tx only **CI:** PML; immune compromise or w/ immunosuppressant **W/P:** [C, ?/–] Baseline MRI to rule out PML **Disp:** Vial 300 mg **SE:** Infxn, immunosuppression; Inf Rxn precluding subsequent use; HA, fatigue, arthralgia **Notes:** Give slowly to ↓ Rxns; limited distribution (TOUCH Prescribing program); D/C immediately w/ signs of PML (weakness, paralysis, vision loss, impaired speech, cognitive ↓); evaluate at 3 and 6 mo, then q6mo thereafter

Nateglinide (Starlix, Generic) **Uses:** *Type 2 DM* **Acts:** ↑ Pancreatic insulin release **Dose:** 120 mg PO tid 1–30 min ac; ↓ to 60 mg tid if near target HbA$_{1c}$ **W/P:** [C, –] w/ CYP2C9 metabolized drug (Table 10, p 319) **CI:** DKA, type 1 DM **Disp:** Tabs 60, 120 mg **SE:** Hypoglycemia, URI; salicylates, nonselective β-blockers may enhance hypoglycemia **Notes:** If a meal is skipped, the dose should be held

Nebivolol (Bystolic) **Uses:** *HTN* **Acts:** β₁-Selective blocker **Dose:** *Adults.* 5 mg PO daily, ↑ q2wk to 40 mg/d max, ↓ w/ CrCl < 30 mL/min **W/P:** [D, +/–] w/ Bronchospastic Dz, DM, heart failure, pheochromocytoma, w/ CYP2D6 inhib **CI:** ↓ HR, cardiogenic shock, decompensated CHF, severe hepatic impair **Disp:** Tabs 2.5, 5, 10, 20 mg **SE:** HA, fatigue, dizziness

Nefazodone (Generic) **BOX:** Fatal hep & liver failure possible, D/C if LFTs > 3× ULN, do not retreat; closely monitor for worsening depression or suicidality, particularly in ped pts **Uses:** *Depression* **Acts:** ↓ Neuronal uptake of serotonin & norepinephrine **Dose:** Initial 100 mg PO bid; usual 300–600 mg/d in 2 ÷ doses **W/P:** [C, M] **CI:** w/ MAOIs, pimozide, carbamazepine, alprazolam; active liver Dz **Disp:** Tabs 50, 100, 150, 200, 250 mg **SE:** Postural ↓ BP & allergic Rxns; HA, drowsiness, xerostomia, constipation, GI upset, liver failure **Notes:** Monitor LFTs, HR, BP

Nelarabine (Arranon) **BOX:** Fatal neurotox possible **Uses:** *T-cell ALL or T-cell lymphoblastic lymphoma unresponsive > 2 other regimens* **Acts:** Nucleoside (deoxyguanosine) analog **Dose:** *Adults.* 1500 mg/m² IV over 2 h days 1, 3, 5 of 21-d cycle. *Peds.* 650 mg/m² IV over 1 h days 1–5 of 21-d cycle **W/P:** [D, ?/–] **Disp:** Vial 250 mg **SE:** Neuropathy, ataxia, Szs, coma, hematologic tox, GI upset, TLS (Tumor lysis syndrome) HA, blurred vision **Notes:** Prehydration, urinary alkalinization, allopurinol before dose; monitor CBC

Nelfinavir (Viracept) **Uses:** *HIV Infxn, other agents* **Acts:** Protease inhib causes immature, noninfectious virion production **Dose:** *Adults.* 750 mg PO tid or 1250 mg PO bid. *Peds.* 25–35 mg/kg PO tid or 45–55 mg/kg bid; take w/ food **W/P:** [B, –] Many drug interactions; do not use w/salmeterol, colchicine (w/ renal/hepatic failure); adjust dose w/ bosentan, tadalafil for PAH; do not use tid dose w/ PRG **CI:** Phenylketonuria, w/ triazolam/midazolam use or drug dependent on CYP3A4 (Table 10, p 319); w/ alpha 1-adrenoreceptor antagonist (alfuzosin), PDE5 inhibitor sildenafil **Disp:** Tabs 250, 625 mg; powder 50 mg/g; **SE:** Food ↑ absorption; interacts w/ St. John's wort; dyslipidemia, lipodystrophy, D, rash **Notes:** PRG registry; tabs can be dissolved in water; monitor LFTs

Neomycin (Neo-Fradin, Generic) **BOX:** Systemic absorption of oral route may cause neuro-/oto-/nephrotox; resp paralysis possible w/ any route of administration **Uses:** *Hepatic coma, bowel prep* **Acts:** Aminoglycoside, poorly absorbed PO; ↓ GI bacterial flora **Dose:** *Adults.* 3–12 g/24 h PO in 3–4 ÷ doses; 12 g/d max *Peds.* 50–100 mg/kg/24 h PO in 3–4 ÷ doses **W/P:** [C, ?/–] Renal failure, neuromuscular disorders, hearing impair **CI:** Intestinal obst **Disp:** Tabs 500 mg; PO soln 125 mg/5 mL **SE:** Hearing loss w/ long-term use; rash, N/V **Notes:** Do not use parenterally (↑ tox); part of the Condon bowel prep; also topical form

Neomycin, Bacitracin, & Polymyxin B (Neosporin Ointment) (See Bacitracin, Neomycin, & Polymyxin B, Topical, p 61)

Neomycin, Colistin, & Hydrocortisone (Cortisporin-TC Otic Drops); Neomycin, Colistin, Hydrocortisone, & Thonzonium (Cortisporin-TC Otic Susp) Uses: *Otitis externa*, Infxns of mastoid/fenestration cavities **Acts:** Antibiotic w/ anti-inflammatory **Dose:** *Adults.* 5 gtt in ear(s) q6–8h. **Peds.** 3–4 gtt in ear(s) q6–8h **CI:** Component allergy; HSV, vaccinia, varicella **W/P:** [B, ?] **Disp:** Otic gtt & susp **SE:** Local irritation, rash **Notes:** Shake well, limit use to 10 d to minimize ototox

Neomycin, Polymyxin, & Hydrocortisone Ophthalmic (Generic) Uses: *Ocular bacterial Infxns* **Acts:** Antibiotic w/ anti-inflammatory **Dose:** Apply a thin layer to the eye(s) or 1 gtt 1–4×/d **W/P:** [C, ?] **Disp:** Ophthal soln; ophthal oint **SE:** Local irritation **Notes:** Do not wear contacts during Tx

Neomycin, Polymyxin, & Hydrocortisone Otic (Cortisporin Otic Solution, Generic Susp) Uses: *Otitis externa and infected mastoidectomy and fenestration cavities* **Acts:** Antibiotic & anti-inflammatory **Dose:** *Adults.* 3–4 gtt in the ear(s) q6–8 h **Peds > 2 y.** 3 gtt in the ear(s) q6–8 h. **CI:** Viral Infxn, hypersens to components **W/P:** [C, ?] **Disp:** Otic susp (generic); otic soln (Cortisporin) **SE:** Local irritation

Neomycin, Polymyxin B, & Dexamethasone (Maxitrol) Uses: *Steroid-responsive ocular conditions w/ bacterial Infxn* **Acts:** Antibiotic w/ anti-inflammatory corticosteroid **Dose:** 1–2 gtt in eye(s) q3–4h; apply oint in eye(s) q6–8 h **CI:** Component allergy; viral, fungal, TB eye Dz **W/P:** [C, ?] **Disp:** Oint: neomycin sulfate 3.5 mg/polymyxin B sulfate 10,000 units/dexamethasone 0.1%/g; susp: identical/1 mL, 5mL bottle **SE:** Local irritation **Notes:** Use under supervision of ophthalmologist; contacts should not be worn during therapy

Neomycin, Polymyxin B, & Prednisolone (Poly-Pred Ophthalmic) Uses: *Steroid-responsive ocular conditions w/ bacterial Infxn* **Acts:** Antibiotic & anti-inflammatory **Dose:** 1–2 gtt in eye(s) q4–6h; apply oint in eye(s) q6–8 **W/P:** [C, ?] **Disp:** Susp neomycin/polymyxin B/prednisolone 0.5%/mL **SE:** Irritation **Notes:** Use under supervision of ophthalmologist; do not wear contacts during Tx

Neomycin & Dexamethasone (AK-Neo-Dex Ophthalmic, Neo-Decadron Ophthalmic) Uses: *Steroid-responsive inflammatory conditions of the cornea, conjunctiva, lid, & anterior segment* **Acts:** Antibiotic w/ anti-inflammatory corticosteroid **Dose:** 1–2 gtt in eye(s) q3–4h or thin coat q6–8h until response, then ↓ to daily **W/P:** [C, ?] **Disp:** Cream: neomycin 0.5%/dexamethasone 0.1%; oint: neomycin 0.35%/dexamethasone 0.05%; soln: neomycin 0.35%/dexamethasone 0.1% **SE:** Local irritation **Notes:** Use under ophthalmologist's supervision; no contacts w/ use

Neomycin & Polymyxin B (Neosporin Cream) [OTC] Uses: *Infxn in minor cuts, scrapes, & burns* **Acts:** Bactericidal **Dose:** Apply 2–4 × d **W/P:** [C, ?] **CI:** Component allergy **Disp:** Cream: neomycin 3.5 mg/polymyxin B 10,000 units/g **SE:** Local irritation **Notes:** Different from *Neosporin oint*

Neomycin-Polymyxin Bladder Irrigant [Neosporin GU Irrigant]
Uses: *Cont irrigant prevent bacteriuria & gram(–) bacteremia associated w/ indwelling catheter* **Acts:** Bactericidal; not for *Serratia* sp or streptococci **Dose:** 1 mL irrigant in 1 L of 0.9% NaCl; cont bladder irrigation w/ 1 L of soln/24 h 10 d max **W/P:** [D] **CI:** Component allergy **Disp:** Soln neomycin sulfate 40 mg & polymyxin B 200,000 units/mL; amp 1, 20 mL **SE:** Rash, neomycin ototox or nephrotox (rare) **Notes:** Potential for bacterial/fungal super-Infxn; not for Inj; use only 3-way catheter for irrigation

Nepafenac (Nevanac) **Uses:** *Inflammation postcataract surgery* **Acts:** NSAID **Dose:** 1 gtt in eye(s) tid 1 d before, and continue 14 d after surgery **CI:** NSAID/ASA sensitivity **W/P:** [C, ?/–] May ↑ bleeding time, delay healing, causes keratitis **Disp:** Susp 0.1% 3 mL **SE:** Capsular opacity, visual changes, foreign-body sensation, ↑ IOP **Notes:** Prolonged use ↑ risk of corneal damage; shake well before use; separate from other drops by > 5 min

Nesiritide (Natrecor) **Uses:** *Acutely decompensated CHF* **Acts:** Human B-type natriuretic peptide **Dose:** 2 mcg/kg IV bolus, then 0.01 mcg/kg/min IV **W/P:** [C, ?/–] When vasodilators are not appropriate **CI:** SBP < 100 mm Hg, cardiogenic shock **Disp:** Vials 1.5 mg **SE:** ↓ BP, HA, GI upset, arrhythmias, ↑ Cr **Notes:** Requires cont BP monitoring; some studies indicate ↑ in mortality; 175 kg max dose Wt studied

Nevirapine (Viramune, Viramune XR, Generic) **BOX:** Reports of fatal hepatotox even w/ short-term use; severe life-threatening skin Rxns (SJS, toxic epidermal necrolysis, & allergic Rxns); monitor closely during first 18 wk of Rx **Uses:** *HIV Infxn* **Acts:** Nonnucleoside RT inhib **Dose:** *Adults.* Initial 200 mg/d PO × 14 d, then 200 mg bid, 400 mg daily (XR) *Peds > 15.* 150 mg/m² PO daily ×14 d, then 150 mg/m² PO bid (w/o regard to food) **W/P:** [B, –] OCP Disp: Tabs 200 mg; *(Viramune XR)* tab ER 100, 400 mg; susp 50 mg/5 mL **SE:** Life-threatening rash; HA, fever, D, neutropenia, hep **Notes:** HIV resistance when used as monotherapy; use in combo w/ at least 2 additional antiretroviral agents. Restart once daily dosing ×14 d if stopped > 7 d. Not recommended if CD4 > 250 mcL in women or > 400 mcL in men unless benefit > risk of hepatotox; always perform lead-in trial w/ IR formulation

Niacin (Nicotinic Acid) (Niaspan, Slo-Niacin, Niacor, Nicolar) [Some OTC Forms] **Uses:** *Sig hyperlipidemia/hypercholesteremia, nutritional supl* **Acts:** Vit B₃; ↓ lipolysis; ↓ esterification of triglycerides; ↑ lipoprotein lipase **Dose:** *Hypercholesterolemia:* Start 500 mg PO qhs, ↑ 500 mg q4wk, maint 1–2 g/d; 2 g/d max; qhs w/ low fat snack; do not crush/chew; niacin supl 1 ER tab PO qd or 100 mg PO qd; *Pellagra:* Up to 500 mg/d **W/P:** [C, +] **CI:** Liver Dz, peptic ulcer, arterial hemorrhage **Disp:** ER tabs *(Niaspan)* 500, 750, 1000 mg & *(Slo-Niacin)* 250, 500, 750 mg; tab 500 mg *(Niacor)*; many OTC: tab 50, 100, 250, 500 mg, ER caps 125, 250, 400 mg, ER tab 250, 500 mg, elixir 50 mg/5 mL **SE:** Upper body/facial flushing & warmth; hepatox, GI upset, flatulence, exacerbate peptic ulcer, HA, paresthesias, liver damage, gout, altered glucose control in DM **Notes:** ASA/NSAID 30–60 min prior to ↓ flushing; ✓ cholesterol, LFTs, if on statins (eg, Lipitor, etc) also ✓ CPK and K⁺; *RDA adults:* male 16 mg/d, female 14 mg/d

Niacin/Lovastatin (Advicor) Uses: *Hypercholesterolemia* Acts: Combo antilipemic agent, w/ HMG-CoA reductase inhib **Dose:** *Adults.* Niacin 500 mg/ lovastatin 20 mg, titrate q4wk, max niacin 2000 mg/lovastatin 40 mg **W/P:** [X, –] See individual agents, D/C w/ LFTs > 3× ULN **CI:** PRG **Disp:** Niacin mg/lovastatin mg: 500/20, 750/20, 1000/20, 1000/40 tabs **SE:** Flushing, myopathy/rhabdomyolysis, N, Abd pain, ↑ LFTs **Notes:** ↓ Flushing by taking ASA or NSAID 30 min before

Niacin/Simvastatin (Simcor) Uses: *Hypercholesterolemia* Acts: Combo antilipemic agent w/ HMG-CoA reductase inhib **Dose:** *Adults* Niacin 500 mg/simvastatin 20 mg, titrate q4wk not to exceed niacin 2000 mg/simvastatin 40 mg; max 1000 mg/20 mg/d w/ amlodipine and ranolazine **W/P:** [X, –] See individual agents, discontinue Rx if LFTs > 3× ULN **CI:** PRG, active liver Dz, PUD, arterial bleeding, w/ strong CYP3A4 inhib, w/ gemfibrozil, cyclosporine, danazol, verapamil, or diltiazem, hypersens to components **Disp:** Niacin mg/simvastatin mg: 500/20, 500/40, 750/20, 1000/20, 1000/40 tabs **SE:** Flushing, myopathy/rhabdomyolysis, N, Abd pain, ↑ LFTs **Notes:** ↓ Flushing by taking ASA or NSAID 30 min before

Nicardipine (Cardene, Cardene SR, Generic) Uses: *Chronic stable angina & HTN*; prophylaxis of migraine **Acts:** CCB **Dose:** *Adults. PO:* 20–40 mg PO tid. *SR:* 30–60 mg PO bid. *IV:* 5 mg/h IV cont Inf; ↑ by 2.5 mg/h q15min to max 15 mg/h. *Peds.* (Not established) *PO:* 20–30 mg PO q8h. *IV:* 0.5–5 mcg/kg/min; ↓ in renal/hepatic impair **W/P:** [C, ?/–] Heart block, CAD **CI:** Cardiogenic shock, aortic stenosis **Disp:** Caps 20, 30 mg; SR caps 30, 45, 60 mg; Inj 2.5 mg/mL **SE:** Flushing, tachycardia, ↓ BP, edema, HA **Notes:** *PO-to-IV conversion:* 20 mg tid = 0.5 mg/h, 30 mg tid = 1.2 mg/h, 40 mg tid = 2.2 mg/h; take w/ food (not high fat)

Nicotine, Gum (Nicorette, Others) [OTC] Uses: *Aid to smoking cessation, relieve nicotine withdrawal* Acts: Systemic delivery of nicotine **Dose:** Wk 1–6 one piece q1–2h PRN; wk 7–9 one piece q2–4h PRN; wk 10–12 one piece q4–8h PRN; max 24 pieces/d **W/P:** [C, ?] **CI:** Life-threatening arrhythmias, unstable angina **Disp:** 2 mg, 4 mg/piece; mint, orange, original flavors **SE:** Tachycardia, HA, GI upset, hiccups **Notes:** Must stop smoking & perform behavior modification for max effect; use at least 9 pieces first 6 wk; > 25 cigarettes/d use 4 mg; < 25 cigarettes/d use 2 mg

Nicotine, Nasal Spray (Nicotrol NS) Uses: *Aid to smoking cessation, relieve nicotine withdrawal* Acts: Systemic delivery of nicotine **Dose:** 0.5 mg/actuation; 1–2 doses/h, 5 doses/h max; 40 doses/d max **W/P:** [D, M] **CI:** Life-threatening arrhythmias, unstable angina **Disp:** Nasal inhaler 10 mg/mL **SE:** Local irritation, tachycardia, HA, taste perversion **Notes:** Must stop smoking & perform behavior modification for max effect; 1 dose = 1 spray each nostril = 1 mg

Nicotine, Transdermal (Habitrol, NicoDerm CQ [OTC], Others) Uses: *Aid to smoking cessation; relief of nicotine withdrawal* Acts: Systemic delivery of nicotine **Dose:** Individualized; 1 patch (14–21 mg/d) & taper over 6 wk **W/P:** [D, M] **CI:** Life-threatening arrhythmias, unstable angina, adhesive allergy **Disp:** *Habitrol* & *NicoDerm CQ:* 7, 14, 21 mg of nicotine/24 h **SE:** Insomnia, pruritus, erythema, local site Rxn, tachycardia, vivid dreams **Notes:** Wear patch 16–24 h; must stop smoking & perform behavior modification for max effect; > 10 cigarettes/d start w/ 21-mg patch; < 10 cigarettes/d 14-mg patch; do not cut patch; rotate site

Nifedipine (Adalat CC, Afeditab CR, Procardia, Procardia XL, Generic) Uses: *Vasospastic or chronic stable angina & HTN*; tocolytic Acts: CCB Dose: *Adults.* SR tabs 30–90 mg/d. *Tocolysis:* per local protocol. *Peds.* 0.25–0.5 mg/kg/24 h ÷ 3–4×/d W/P: [C, +] Heart block, aortic stenosis, cirrhosis CI: IR preparation for urgent or emergent HTN; acute MI Disp: Caps 10, 20 mg; SR tabs 30, 60, 90 mg SE: HA common on initial Rx; reflex tachycardia may occur w/ regular-release dosage forms; peripheral edema, ↓ BP, flushing, dizziness Notes: Adalat CC & Procardia XL not interchangeable; SL administration not OK

Nilotinib (Tasigna) BOX: May ↑ QT interval; sudden deaths reported, use w/ caution in hepatic failure; administer on empty stomach Uses: *Ph(+) CML, refractory or at 1st diagnosis* Acts: TKI Dose: *Adults.* 300 mg bid—newly diagnosed; 400 mg bid—resistant/intolerant on empty stomach 1 h prior or 2 h post meal. W/P: [D, ?/–] Avoid w/ CYP3A4 inhib/inducers (Table 10, p 319), adjust w/ hepatic impair, heme tox, QT ↑, avoid QT-prolonging agents, w/ Hx pancreatitis, ↓ absorption w/ gastrectomy CI: ↓ K⁺, ↓ Mg²⁺, long QT synd Disp: 200 mg caps SE: ↓ WBC, ↓ plt, anemia, N/V/D, rash, edema, ↑ lipase, tumor lysis synd Notes: Use chemotherapy precautions when handling

Nilutamide (Nilandron) BOX: Interstitial pneumonitis possible; most cases in first 3 mo; check CXR before and during Rx Uses: *Combo w/ surgical castration for metastatic PCa* Acts: Nonsteroidal antiandrogen Dose: 300 mg/d PO × 30 d, then 150 mg/d W/P: [Not used in females] CI: Severe hepatic impair, resp Insuff Disp: Tabs 150 mg SE: Interstitial pneumonitis, hot flashes, ↓ libido, impotence, N/V/D, gynecomastia, hepatic dysfunction Notes: May cause Rxn when taken w/ EtOH, follow LFTs

Nimodipine (Generic) BOX: Do not give IV or by other parenteral routes; can cause death Uses: *Prevent vasospasm following subarachnoid hemorrhage* Acts: CCB Dose: 60 mg PO q4h for 21 d; start w/in 96 h of subarachnoid hemorrhage; ↓ in hepatic failure W/P: [C, ?] CI: Component allergy Disp: Caps 30 mg SE: ↓ BP, HA, constipation, rash Notes: Give via NG tube if caps cannot be swallowed whole

Nisoldipine (Sular, Generic) Uses: *HTN* Acts: CCB Dose: 8.5–34 mg/d PO; take on empty stomach; ↓ start doses w/ elderly or hepatic impair W/P: [C, –] Disp: ER tabs 8.5, 17, 25.5, 34 mg SE: Edema, HA, flushing, ↓ BP Notes: Nisoldipine Geomatrix (Sular) formulation not equivalent to original formulation (ER)

Nitazoxanide (Alinia) Uses: **Cryptosporidium, Giardia lamblia, C. difficile associated D** **Acts:** Antiprotozoal interferes w/ pyruvate ferredoxin oxidoreductase. *Spectrum: Cryptosporidium, Giardia* **Dose: Adults.** 500 mg PO q12h × 3 d; for *C. difficile* × 10 d. **Peds 1–3 y.** 100 mg PO q12h × 3 d. **4–11 y:** 200 mg PO q12h × 3 d. > **12 y:** 500 mg q12h × 3 d; take w/ food **W/P:** [B, ?] Not effective in HIV or immunocompromised **Disp:** 100 mg/5 mL PO susp, 500 tab **SE:** Abd pain **Notes:** Susp contains sucrose, interacts w/ highly protein-bound drugs

Nitrofurantoin (Furadantin, Macrobid, Macrodantin, Generic) Uses: **Prophylaxis & Rx UTI** **Acts:** Interferes w/ metabolism & cell wall synthesis. *Spectrum:* Some gram(+) & (−) bacteria; *Pseudomonas, Serratia,* & most *Proteus* resistant **Dose: Adults.** Prophylaxis: 50–100 mg/d PO. Rx: 50–100 mg PO qid × 7 d; *Macrobid* 100 mg PO bid × 7 d. **Peds.** Prophylaxis: 1–2 mg/kg/d ÷ in 1–2 doses, max 100 mg/d. Rx: 5–7 mg/kg/24 h in 4 ÷ doses (w/ food/milk/antacid) **W/P:** [B, +/not OK if child < 1 mo] Avoid w/ CrCl < 60 mL/min **CI:** Renal failure, infants < 1 mo, PRG at term **Disp:** Caps 25, 50, 100 mg; (*Furadantin*) susp 25 mg/5 mL **SE:** GI effects, dyspnea, various acute/chronic pulm Rxns, peripheral neuropathy, hemolytic anemia w/ G6PD deficiency, rare aplastic anemia **Notes:** Macrocrystals (*Macrodantin*) < N than other forms; not for comp UTI; may turn urine brown; ineffective for pyelonephritis or cystitis

Nitroglycerin (Nitrostat, Nitrolingual, Nitro-Bid Ointment, Nitro-Bid IV, Nitrodisc, Transderm-Nitro, NitroMist, Others) Uses: **Angina pectoris, acute & prophylactic Rx, CHF, BP control** **Acts:** Relaxes vascular smooth muscle, dilates coronary arteries **Dose: Adults.** SL: 1 tab q5min SL PRN for 3 doses. Translingual: 1–2 metered-doses sprayed onto PO mucosa q3–5min, max 3 doses. PO: 2.5–9 mg tid. IV: 5–20 mcg/min, titrated to effect. Topical: Apply 1/2 in oint to chest wall tid, wipe off at night. Transdermal: 0.2–0.4 mg/h/patch daily; Aerosol: 1 spray at 5-min intervals, max 3 doses *ECC 2010.* IV bolus. 12.5–25 mcg (if no spray or SL dose given); Inf: Start 10 mcg/min, ↑ by 10 mcg/min q3–5min until desired effect; ceiling dose typically 200 mcg/min. SL: 0.3–0.4 mg, repeat q5min. Aerosol spray: Spray 0.5–1 s at 5-min intervals. **Peds.** 0.25–0.5 mcg/kg/min IV, titrate; *ECC 2010.* Heart failure, HTN emergency, pulm HTN: Cont Inf 0.25–0.5 mcg/kg/min initial, titrate 1 mcg/kg/min q15–20min (typical dose 1–5 mcg/kg/min) **W/P:** [B, ?] Restrictive cardiomyopathy **CI:** w/ Sildenafil, tadalafil, vardenafil, head trauma, NAG, pericardial tamponade, constrictive pericarditis. **Disp:** SL tabs 0.3, 0.4, 0.6 mg; translingual spray 0.4 mg/dose; SR caps 2.5, 6.5, 9 mg; Inj 0.1, 0.2, 0.4 mg/mL (premixed); 5 mg/mL Inj soln; oint 2%; transdermal patches 0.1, 0.2, 0.4, 0.6 mg/h; aerosol (*NitroMist*) 0.4 mg/spray; (*Rectiv*) intra-anal 0.4% **SE:** HA, ↓ BP, lightheadedness, GI upset **Notes:** Nitrate tolerance w/ chronic use after 1–2 wk; minimize by providing 10–12 h nitrate-free period daily, using shorter-acting nitrates tid, & removing LA patches & oint before sleep to ↓ tolerance

Nitroprusside (Nitropress) **BOX:** Warning: Cyanide tox & excessive hypotension **Uses:** *Hypertensive crisis, acute decompensated heart failure, controlled ↓ BP periop (↓ bleeding)*, aortic dissection, pulm edema **Acts:** ↓ Systemic vascular resistance **Dose:** *Adults & Peds.* 0.25–10 mcg/kg/min IV Inf, titrate; usual dose 3 mcg/kg/min. *ECC 2010.* 0.1 mcg/kg/min start, titrate (max dose 5–10 mcg/kg/min). *Peds. ECC 2010. Cardiogenic shock, severe HTN:* 0.3–1 mcg/kg/min, then titrate to 8 mcg/kg/min PRN **W/P:** [C, ?] ↓ Cerebral perfusion **CI:** High output failure, compensatory HTN **Disp:** Inj 25 mg/mL **SE:** Excessive hypotensive effects, palpitations, HA **Notes:** Thiocyanate (metabolite w/ renal excretion) w/ tox at 5–10 mg/dL, more likely if used for > 2–3 d; w/ aortic dissection use w/ β-blocker; continuous BP monitoring essential

Nizatidine (Axid, Axid AR [OTC], Generic) **Uses:** *Duodenal ulcers, GERD, heartburn* **Acts:** H₂-receptor antagonist **Dose:** *Adults.* Active ulcer: 150 mg PO bid or 300 mg PO hs; maint 150 mg PO hs. *GERD:* 150 mg PO bid. *Heartburn:* 75 mg PO bid. *Peds. GERD:* 10 mg/kg PO bid, 150 mg bid max; ↓ in renal impair **W/P:** [B, ?] **CI:** H₂-receptor antagonist sensitivity **Disp:** Tab 75 mg [OTC]; caps 150, 300 mg; soln 15 mg/mL **SE:** Dizziness, HA, constipation, D **Notes:** Contains bisulfites

Norepinephrine (Levophed) **Uses:** *Acute ↓ BP, cardiac arrest (adjunct)* **Acts:** Peripheral vasoconstrictor of arterial/venous beds **Dose:** *Adults.* 8–30 mcg/min IV, titrate. *Peds.* 0.05–0.1 mcg/kg/min IV, titrate **W/P:** [C, ?] **CI:** ↓ BP d/t hypovolemia, vascular thrombosis, do not use w/ cyclopropane/halothane anesthetics **Disp:** Inj 1 mg/mL **SE:** ↓ HR, arrhythmia **Notes:** Correct vol depletion as much as possible before vasopressors; interaction w/ TCAs leads to severe HTN; use large vein to avoid extrav; phentolamine 5–10 mg/10 mL NS injected locally for extrav

Norethindrone Acetate/Ethinyl Estradiol Tablets (FemHRT) (See Estradiol/Norethindrone Acetate)

Norfloxacin (Noroxin, Chibroxin Ophthalmic) **BOX:** Use associated w/ tendon rupture, tendonitis, & myasthenia gravis exacerbation **Uses:** *Comp & uncomp UTI d/t gram(−) bacteria, prostatitis, gonorrhea*, infectious D, conjunctivitis **Acts:** Quinolone, ↓ DNA gyrase, bactericidal *Spectrum:* Broad gram(+) and (−) *E. faecalis, E. coli, K. pneumoniae, P. mirabilis, P. aeruginosa, S. epidermidis, S. saprophyticus* **Dose:** *Uncomp UTI (E. coli, K. pneumoniae, P. mirabilis):* 400 mg PO bid × 3 d; other uncomp UTI Rx × 7–10 d. *Comp UTI:* 400 mg PO q12h for 10–21 d. *Gonorrhea:* 800 mg × 1 dose. *Prostatitis:* 400 mg PO bid × 28 d. *Gastroenteritis, traveler's D:* 400 mg PO bid × 1–3 d; take 1 h ac or 2 h pc. *Adults & Peds > 1 y.* Ophthal: 1 gtt each eye qid for 7 d; CrCl < 30 mL/min use 400 mg qd **W/P:** [C, −] Quinolone sensitivity, w/ some antiarrhythmics ↑ QT **CI:** Hx allergy or tendon problems **Disp:** Tabs 400 mg; ophthal 3 mg/mL **SE:** Photosens, HA, dizziness, asthenia, GI upset, pseudomembranous colitis; ocular burning w/ ophthal, peripheral neuropathy risk w/PO only **Notes:** Interactions w/ antacids, theophylline, caffeine; good conc in the kidney & urine, poor blood levels; not for urosepsis; CDC suggests do not use for GC

Nortriptyline (Aventyl, Pamelor) BOX: ↑ Suicide risk in pts < 24 y w/ major depressive/other psychological disorders especially during 1st month of Tx; risk ↓ pts > 65 y; observe all pts for clinical Sxs; not for ped use Uses: *Endogenous depression* Acts: TCA; ↑ synaptic CNS levels of serotonin &/or norepinephrine Dose: Adults. 25 mg PO tid-qid; > 150 mg/d not OK. Elderly: 10–25 mg hs. Peds 6–7 y. 10 mg/d. 8–11 y: 10–20 mg/d. > 11 y: 25–35 mg/d, ↓ w/ hepatic Insuff W/P: [D, –] NAG, CV Dz CI: TCA allergy, use w/ MAOI Disp: Caps 10, 25, 50, 75 mg; (Aventyl) soln 10 mg/5 mL SE: Anticholinergic (blurred vision, retention, xerostomia, sedation) Notes: Max effect may take > 2–3 wk

Nystatin (Mycostatin, Nilstat, Nystop) Uses: *Mucocutaneous Candida Infxns (oral, skin, Vag)* Acts: Alters membrane permeability. Spectrum: Susceptible Candida sp Dose: Adults & Peds. PO: 400,000–600,000 units PO "swish & swallow" qid. Vag: 1 tab Vag hs × 2 wk. Topical: Apply bid-tid to area. Peds Infants. 200,000 units PO q6h. W/P: [B (C PO), +] Disp: PO susp 100,000 units/mL; PO tabs 500,000 units; troches 200,000 units; Vag tabs 100,000 units; topical cream/oint 100,000 units/g, powder 100,000 units/g SE: GI upset, SJS Notes: Not absorbed through mucus membranes/intact skin, poorly absorbed through GI; not for systemic Infxns; see also Triamcinolone/Nystatin

Octreotide (Sandostatin, Sandostatin LAR, Generic) Uses: *↓ Severe D associated w/ carcinoid & neuroendocrine GI tumors (eg, vasoactive intestinal peptide-secreting tumor [VIPoma], ZE synd), acromegaly*; bleeding esophageal varices Acts: LA peptide; mimics natural somatostatin Dose: Adults. 100–600 mcg/d SQ/IV in 2–4 ÷ doses; start 50 mcg daily-bid. Sandostatin LAR (depot): 10–30 mg IM q4wk. Peds. 1–10 mcg/kg/24 h SQ in 2–4 ÷ doses W/P: [B, +] Hepatic/renal impair Disp: Inj 0.05, 0.1, 0.2, 0.5, 1 mg/mL; 10, 20, 30 mg/5 mL LAR depot SE: N/V, Abd discomfort, flushing, edema, fatigue, cholelithiasis, hyper-/hypoglycemia, hep, hypothyroidism Notes: Stabilize for at least 2 wk before changing to LAR form

Ofatumumab (Arzerra) Uses: *Rx refractory CLL* Acts: MoAb, binds CD20 molecule on nl & abnormal B-lymphocytes w/ cell lysis Dose: Adults. 300 mg (0.3 mg/mL) IV week 1, then 2000 mg (2 mg/mL) weekly × 7 doses, then 2000 mg q4wks × 4 doses. Titrate Inf: start 12 mL/h × 30 min, ↑ 25 mL/h for 30 min, ↑ to 50 mL/h × 30 min, ↑ to 100 mL/h × 30 min, then titrate to max Inf 200 mL/h. W/P: [C, ?] ✓ WBC, screen high risk for hep B, can reactivate, D/C immediately Disp: Inj 20 mg/mL (5 mL) SE: Infusion Rxns (bronchospasm, pulmonary edema, ↑ / ↓ BP, syncope, cardiac ischemia, angioedema), ↓ WBC, anemia, fever, fatigue, rash, N/D, pneumonia, Infxns, PML Notes: Premed w/ acetaminophen, antihistamine, and IV steroid

Ofloxacin (Floxin) BOX: Use associated w/ tendon rupture and tendonitis Uses: *Lower resp tract, skin, & skin structure, & UTI, prostatitis, uncomp gonorrhea, & Chlamydia Infxns* Acts: Bactericidal; ↓ DNA gyrase. Broad spectrum gram(+) & (–): S. pneumoniae, S. aureus, S. pyogenes, H. influenzae, P. mirabilis, N. gonorrhoeae, C. trachomatis, E. coli Dose: Adults. 200–400 mg PO bid or

IV q12h. ↓ in renal impair, take on empty stomach **W/P:** [C, –] ↓ Absorption w/ antacids, sucralfate, Al^{2+}, Ca^{2+}, Mg^{2+}, Fe^{2+}, Zn^+-containing drugs, Hx Szs **CI:** Quinolone allergy **Disp:** Tabs 200, 300, 400 mg; Inj 20, 40 mg/mL; ophthal & otic 0.3% **SE:** N/V/D, photosens, insomnia, HA, local irritation, ↑ QTc interval, peripheral neuropathy risk *Notes: Floxin* brand D/C

Ofloxacin, Ophthalmic (Ocuflox Ophthalmic) Uses: *Bacterial conjunctivitis, corneal ulcer* **Acts:** See Ofloxacin **Dose:** *Adults & Peds > 1 y.* 1–2 gtt in eye(s) q2–4h × 2 d, then qid × 5 more d **W/P:** [C, +/–] **CI:** Quinolone allergy **Disp:** Ophthal 0.3% soln **SE:** Burning, hyperemia, bitter taste, chemosis, photophobia

Ofloxacin, Otic (Floxin Otic, Floxin Otic Singles) Uses: *Otitis externa; chronic suppurative otitis media w/ perf drums; otitis media in peds w/ tubes* **Acts:** See Ofloxacin **Dose:** *Adults & Peds > 13 y. Otitis externa:* 10 gtt in ear(s) daily × 7 d. *Peds 1–12 y. Otitis media* 5 gtt in ear(s) bid × 10 d **W/P:** [C, –] **CI:** Quinolone allergy **Disp:** Otic 0.3% soln 5/10 mL bottles; singles 0.25 mL foil pack **SE:** Local irritation **Notes:** OK w/ tubes/perforated drums; 10 gtt = 0.5 mL

Olanzapine (Zyprexa, Zydis) BOX: ↑ Mortality in elderly w/ dementia-related psychosis Uses: *Bipolar mania, schizophrenia*, psychotic disorders, acute agitation in schizophrenia **Acts:** Dopamine & serotonin antagonist; atypical antipsychotic. **Dose:** *Bipolar/schizophrenia:* 5–10 mg/d, weekly PRN, 20 mg/d max. *Agitation;* atypical antipsychotic 5–10 mg IM q2–4h PRN, 30 mg d/max **W/P:** [C, –] **Disp:** Tabs 2.5, 5, 7.5, 10, 15, 20 mg; ODT (*Zyprexa Zydis*) 5, 10, 15, 20 mg; Inj 10 mg **SE:** HA, somnolence, orthostatic ↓ BP, tachycardia, dystonia, xerostomia, constipation, hyperglycemia; ↑ Wt, ↑ prolactin levels; and sedation may be ↑ in peds **Notes:** Takes wk to titrate dose; smoking ↓ levels; may be confused w/ *Zyrtec* or *Zyprexa Relprevv*

Olanzapine, LA Parenteral (Zyprexa Relprevv) BOX: ↑ Risk for severe sedation/coma following parenteral Inj, observe closely for 3 h in appropriate facility; restricted distribution; ↑ mortality in elderly w/ dementia-related psychosis; not approved for dementia-related psychosis Uses: *Schizophrenia* Acts: See Olanzapine **Dose:** IM: 150 mg/q2 wk, 300 mg/q4wk, 210 mg/q2wk, 405 mg/q4 wk, or 300 mg/q2wk **W/P:** [C, –] IM only, do not confuse w/ *Zyprexa* IM; can cause neuroleptic malignant synd, ↑ glucose/lipids/prolactin, ↓ BP, tardive dyskinesia, cognitive impair, ↓ CBC **CI:** None **Disp:** Vials, 210, 300, 405 mg **SE:** HA, sedation, ↑ Wt, cough, N/V/D, ↑ appetite, dry mouth, nasopharyngitis, somnolence **Notes:** ✓ Glucose/lipids/CBC baseline and periodically: establish PO tolerance before Δ to IM

Olmesartan, Olmesartan, & Hydrochlorothiazide (Benicar, Benicar HCT) BOX: Use in PRG 2nd/3rd tri can harm fetus; D/C when PRG detected Uses: *Hypertension, alone or in combo* **Acts:** *Benicar* angiotensin II receptor blocker (ARB); *Benicar HCT* ARB w/ diuretic HCTZ **Dose:** *Adults. Benicar* 20–40 mg qd; *Benicar HCT 20–40 mg* olmesartan *w/ 12.5–25 mg HCTZ based on effect Peds 6–16 y. Benicar:* < 35 kg start 10 mg PO, range 10–20 mg qd; ≥ 35 kg start 20 mg PO qd, target 20–40 mg qd **W/P:** [C 1st tri, D 2nd, 3rd, ?/–] *Benicar HCT* not rec w/ CrCl < 30 mL/min; follow closely if volume depleted w/ start of med **CI:** Component allergy **Disp:** (*Benicar*) Tabs 5, 20, 40 mg; (*Benicar HCT*) mg olmesartan/mg HCTZ: 20/12.5, 40/12.5, 40/25 **SE:** Dizziness, ↓ K⁺ w/ HCTZ product (may require replacement) **Notes:** If *Benicar* does not control BP a diuretic can be added or *Benicar HCT* used; ? ↑ sprue-like enteropathy

Olmesartan/Amlodipine/Hydrochlorothiazide (Tribenzor) Uses: *Hypertension* **Acts:** Combo angiotensin II receptor blocker, CCB, thiazide diuretic **Dose:** Begin w/ 20/5/12.5 olmesartan/amlodipine/HCTZ, ↑ to max 40/10/25 mg **W/P:** [C 1st tri, D 2nd, 3rd; –] **CI:** Anuria; sulfa allergy; PRG, neonate exposure, CrCl < 30 mg/min, age > 75 y, severe liver Dz **Disp:** Tabs: (olmesartan mg/amlodipine mg/HCTZ mg) 20/5/12.5, 40/5/12.5, 40/5/25, 40/10/12.5, 40/10/25 **SE:** Edema, HA, fatigue, N/D, muscle spasms, jt swelling, URI, syncope **Notes:** Avoid w/ vol depletion; thiazide diuretics may exacerbate SLE, associated NA glaucoma; ? ↑ sprue-like enteropathy

Olopatadine, Nasal (Patanase) Uses: *Seasonal allergic rhinitis* **Acts:** H₁-receptor antagonist **Dose:** 2 sprays each nostril bid **W/P:** [C, ?] **Disp:** 0.6% 240-Spray bottle **SE:** Epistaxis, bitter taste somnolence, HA, rhinitis

Olopatadine, Ophthalmic (Patanol, Pataday) Uses: *Allergic conjunctivitis* **Acts:** H₁-receptor antagonist **Dose:** *Patanol:* 1 gtt in eye(s) bid; *Pataday:* 1 gtt in eye(s) qd **W/P:** [C, ?] **Disp:** *Patanol:* soln 0.1% 5 mL *Pataday:* 0.2% 2.5 mL **SE:** Local irritation, HA, rhinitis **Notes:** Wait 10 min after to insert contacts

Olsalazine (Dipentum) Uses: *Maintain remission in UC* **Acts:** Topical anti-inflammatory **Dose:** 500 mg PO bid (w/ food) **W/P:** [C, –] **CI:** Salicylate sensitivity **Disp:** Caps 250 mg **SE:** D, HA, blood dyscrasias, rash

Omacetaxine (Synribo) Uses: *CML w/ resist &/or intol to ≥ 2 TKI* **Acts:** Inhib protein synthesis **Dose:** *Adults.* Induct: 1.25 mg/m² SQ bid × 14 consecutive d 28 d cycle, repeat until hematologic response achieved; Maint: 1.25 mg/m² SQ twice daily × 7 consecutive d 28-d cycle, continue as long as beneficial; adjust based on toxicity (see label) **W/P:** [D, –] Severe myelosuppression (✓ CBC q 1–2 wk); severe bleeding (✓ plt); glucose intol (✓ glucose); embryo-fetal tox **CI:** None **Disp:** Inj powder 3.5 mg/vial **SE:** Anemia, neutropenia, ↓ plts/WBC, N/V/D, fatigue, asthenia, Inj site Rxn, pyrexia, Infxn, bleeding, ↑ glucose, constipation, Abd pain, edema, HA, arthralgia, insomnia, cough, epistaxis, alopecia, rash

Omalizumab (Xolair) BOX: Reports of anaphylaxis 2–24 h after administration, even in previously treated pts Uses: *Mod–severe asthma in ≥ 12 y w/ reactivity to an allergen & when Sxs inadequately controlled w/ inhaled steroids* **Acts:** Anti-IgE Ab **Dose:** 150–375 mg SQ q2–4wk (dose/frequency based on serum IgE level & body Wt; see PI) **W/P:** [B, ?/–] **CI:** Component allergy, acute bronchospasm **Disp:** 150-mg single-use 5-mL vial **SE:** Site Rxn, sinusitis, HA, anaphylaxis reported in 3 pts **Notes:** Continue other asthma meds as indicated

Omega-3 Fatty Acid [Fish Oil] (Lovaza) Uses: *Rx hypertriglyceridemia* Acts: Omega-3 acid ethyl esters, ↓ thrombus inflammation & triglycerides Dose: *Hypertriglyceridemia:* 4 g/d ÷ in 1–2 doses W/P: [C, –], Fish hypersens; PRG, risk factor w/ anticoagulant use; w/ bleeding risk CI: Hypersens to components Disp: 1000-mg gel caps SE: Dyspepsia, N, GI pain, rash, flu-like synd Notes: Only FDA-approved fish oil supl; not for exogenous hypertriglyceridemia (type 1 hyperchylomicronemia); many OTC products. D/C after 2 mo if triglyceride levels do not ↓ ; previously called "Omacor"

Omeprazole (Prilosec, Prilosec [OTC]) Uses: *Duodenal/gastric ulcers (adults), GERD, and erosive gastritis (adults and children)*, prevent NSAID ulcers, ZE synd, *H. pylori* Infxns Acts: PPI Dose: *Adults.* 20–40 mg PO daily-bid × 4–8 wk; *H. pylori* 20 mg PO bid × 10 d w/ amoxicillin & clarithromycin or 40 mg PO × 14 d w/ clarithromycin; pathologic hypersecretory cond 60 mg/d (varies); 80 mg/d max. *Peds (1–16 y) 5–<10 kg:* 5 mg/d; *10–20 kg:* 10 mg PO qd. *> 20 kg:* 20 mg PO qd; 40 mg/d max W/P: [C, –/+] w/ Drugs that rely on gastric acid (eg, ampicillin); avoid w/ atazanavir and nelfinavir; caution w/ warfarin, diazepam, phenytoin; do not use w/ clopidogrel (controversial ↓ effect); response does not R/O malignancy Disp: OTC tabs 20 mg; *Prilosec* DR caps 10, 20, 40 mg; *Prilosec* DR susp 2.5, 10 mg SE: HA, Abd pain, N/V/D, flatulence Notes: Combo w/ antibiotic Rx for *H. pylori*; ? ↑ risk of fractures, *C. difficile*, CAP w/ all PPI; risk of hypomagnesemia w/ long-term use

Omeprazole, Sodium Bicarbonate (Zegerid, Zegerid OTC) Uses: *Duodenal/gastric ulcers, GERD and erosive gastritis (↓ GI bleed in critically ill pts)*, prevent NSAID ulcers, ZE synd, *H. pylori* Infxns Acts: PPI w/ sodium bicarb Dose: *Duodenal ulcer:* 20 PO daily-bid × 4–8 wk; *Gastric ulcer:* 40 PO daily-bid × 4–8 wk; *GERD no erosions* 20 mg PO daily × 4 wk, w/ *erosions* treat 4–6 wk; *UGI bleed prevention:* 40 mg q6–8h then 40 mg/d × 14 d W/P: [C, –/+] w/ drugs that rely on gastric acid (eg, ampicillin); avoid w/ atazanavir and nelfinavir; w/ warfarin, diazepam, phenytoin; do not use w/ clopidogrel (controversial ↓ effect); response does not R/O malignancy Disp: Omeprazole mg/sodium bicarb mg: *Zegerid OTC* caps 20/1100; *Zegerid* 20/1100, mg 40/1100; *Zegerid powder packet* for oral susp 20/1680, 40/1680 SE: HA, Abd pain, N/V/D, flatulence Notes: Not approved in peds; take 1 h ac; mix powder in small cup w/ 2 tbsp water (not food or other liq) refill and drink; do not open caps; possible ↑ risk of fractures, *C. difficile*, CAP w/ all PPI; risk of hypomagnesemia w/ long-term use, monitor

Omeprazole, Sodium Bicarbonate, Magnesium Hydroxide (Zegerid w/ Magnesium Hydroxide) Uses: *Duodenal or gastric ulcer, GERD, maintenance esophagitis* Acts: PPI w/ acid buffering; Dose: 20–40 mg omeprazole daily, empty stomach 1 h pc; *Duodenal ulcer, GERD:* 20 mg 4–8 wk; *Gastric ulcer:* 40 mg 4–8 wk; *Esophagitis maint:* 20 mg W/P: [C, ?/–] w/ Resp alkalosis, ↓ K^+, ↓ Ca^{+2}; ↑ drug levels metabolized by cytochrome P450; may ↑ INR w/ warfarin; may ↓ absorption drugs requiring acid environment CI: ↓ Renal Fxn;

Disp: Chew tabs, 20, 40 mg omeprazole; w/ 600 mg $NaHCO_3$; 700 mg $MgOH_2$ **SE:** N, V, D, Abd pain, HA **Notes:** Atrophic gastritis w/ long-term PPI; ? ↑ risk of fractures, *C. difficile*, CAP w/ all PPI; long-term use + Ca^{2+} → milk-alkali syndrome

Ondansetron (Zofran, Zofran ODT, Generic) **Uses:** *Prevent chemotherapy-associated & postop N/V* **Acts:** Serotonin receptor (5-HT_3) antagonist **Dose:** *Adults & Peds.* *Chemotherapy:* 0.15 mg/kg/dose IV prior to chemotherapy, then 4 & 8 h after 1st dose or 4–8 mg PO tid; 1st dose 30 min prior to chemotherapy & give on schedule, not PRN. *Adults.* *Postoperation:* 4 mg IV immediately preanesthesia or postoperation. *Peds.* *Postoperation:* < *40 kg:* 0.1 mg/kg. > *40 kg:* 4 mg IV; ↓ w/ hepatic impair **W/P:** [B, +/–] Arrhythmia risk, may ↑ QT interval **Disp:** Tabs 4, 8, 24 mg, soln 4 mg/5 mL, Inj 2 mg/mL; *Zofran* ODT tabs 4, 8 mg; **SE:** D, HA, constipation, dizziness **Notes:** ODT contains phenylalanine. No single IV dose > 16 mg

Ondansetron, Oral Soluble Film (Zuplenz) **Uses:** *Prevent chemotherapy/RT-associated & postop N/V* **Acts:** Serotonin receptor (5-HT_3) antagonist **Dose:** *Adults.* *Highly emetogenic chemo:* 24 mg (8 mg film × 3) 30 min pre-chemo; *RT N & V:* 8 mg film tid. *Adults & Peds > 12 y.* *Mod emetogenic chemo:* 8 mg film 30 min pre-chemo, then 8 mg in 8 h; 8 mg film bid × 1–2 d after chemo. *Adults.* *Postop:* 16 mg (8 mg film × 2) 1 h preop; ↓ w/ hepatic impair **W/P:** [B, +/–] **CI:** w/ Apomorphine (↓ *BP, LOC*). **Disp:** Oral soluble film 4, 8 mg **SE:** HA, malaise/fatigue, constipation, D **Notes:** Use w/ dry hands, do not chew/swallow; place on tongue, dissolves in 4–20 s; peppermint flavored

Oprelvekin (Neumega) BOX: Allergic Rxn w/ anaphylaxis reported; D/C w/ any allergic Rxn **Uses:** *Prevent ↓ plt w/ chemotherapy* **Acts:** ↑ Proliferation & maturation of megakaryocytes (IL-11) **Dose:** *Adults.* 50 mcg/kg/d SQ for 10–21 d. *Peds > 12 y.* 75–100 mcg/kg/d SQ for 10–21 d. < *12 y.* Use only in clinical trials; ↓ w/ CrCl < 30 mL/min 25 mcg/kg. **W/P:** [C, ?/–] **Disp:** 5 mg powder for Inj **SE:** Tachycardia, palpitations, arrhythmias, edema, HA, dizziness, visual disturbances, papilledema, insomnia, fatigue, fever, N, anemia, dyspnea, allergic Rxns including anaphylaxis **Notes:** D/C 48 h before chemo

Oral Contraceptives (See Table 5, p 306) BOX: Cigarette smoking ↑ risk of serious CV SEs; ↑ risk w/ > 15 cigarettes/d, > 35 y; strongly advise women on OCP to not smoke. Pt should be counseled that these products do not protect against HIV and other STD **Uses:** *Birth control; regulation of anovulatory bleeding; dysmenorrhea; endometriosis; polycystic ovaries; acne* (Note: FDA approvals vary widely, see PI) **Acts:** *Birth control:* Suppresses LH surge, prevents ovulation; progestins thicken cervical mucus, ↓ fallopian tubule cilia, ↑ endometrial thickness to ↓ chances of fertilization. *Anovulatory bleeding:* Cyclic hormones mimic body's natural cycle & regulate endometrial lining, results in regular bleeding q28d; may ↓ uterine bleeding & dysmenorrhea **Dose:** Start day 1 menstrual cycle or 1st Sunday after onset of menses; 28-d cycle pills take daily; 21-d cycle pills take daily, no pills during last 7 d of cycle (during menses); some available as transdermal patch; Intrauterine ring **W/P:** [X, +] Migraine, HTN, DM, sickle cell Dz, gallbladder Dz; monitor for breast Dz; w/ drospirenone containing OCP ✓ K⁺ if taking drugs w/ ↑ K⁺ risk; drospirenone implicated in ↑ VTE risk. **CI:** AUB, PRG, estrogen-dependent malignancy, ↑ hypercoagulation/liver Dz, hemiplegic migraine, smokers > 35 y; drospirenone has mineralocorticoid effect; do not use w/ renal/liver/adrenal problems. **Disp:** See Table 5, p 306. 28-d cycle pills (21 active pills + 7 placebo or Fe or folate supl); 21-d cycle pills (21 active pills) **SE:** Intramenstrual bleeding, oligomenorrhea, amenorrhea, ↑ appetite/Wt gain, ↓ libido, fatigue, depression, mood swings, mastalgia, HA, melasma, ↑ Vag discharge, acne/greasy skin, corneal edema, N; drospirenone containing pills have ↑ blood clots compared to other progestins **Notes:** Taken correctly, up to 99.9% effective for contraception; no STDs prevention instruct in use of condoms to reduce STD use additional barrier contraceptive; long-term, can ↓ risk of ectopic PRG, benign breast Dz, ovarian & uterine CA. Suggestions for OCP prescribing and/or regimen changes are noted below. Listing of other forms of Rx birth control on p 26.

- *Rx menstrual cycle control:* Start w/ monophasic × 3 mo before switching to another brand; w/ continued bleeding change to pill w/ ↑ estrogen
- *Rx birth control:* Choose pill w/ lowest SE profile for particular pt; SEs numerous; d/t estrogenic excess or progesterone deficiency; each pill's SE profile can be unique (see PI); newer extended-cycle combos have shorter/fewer hormone-free intervals, ? ↓ PRG risk; OCP troubleshooting SE w/ suggested OCP.
  - *Absent menstrual flow:* ↑ Estrogen, ↓ progestin: Brevicon, Necon 1/35, Norinyl 1/35, Modicon, Necon 1/50, Norinyl 1/50, Ortho-Cyclen, Ortho-Novum 1/50, Ortho-Novum 1/35, Ovcon 35
  - *Acne:* Use ↑ estrogen, ↓ androgenic: Brevicon, Ortho-Cyclen, Demulen 1/50, Estrostep, Ortho Tri-Cyclen, Mircette, Modicon, Necon, Ortho Evra, Yasmin, Yaz
  - *Break-through bleed:* ↑ Estrogen, ↑ progestin, ↓ androgenic: Demulen 1/50, Desogen, Estrostep, Loestrin 1/20, Ortho-Cept, Ovcon 50, Yasmin, Zovia 1/50
  - *Breast tenderness or ↑ Wt:* ↓ Estrogen, ↓ progestin: Use ↓ estrogen pill rather than current; Alesse, Levlite, Loestrin 1/20 Fe, Ortho Evra, Yasmin, Yaz
  - *Depression:* ↓ Progestin: Alesse, Brevicon, Levlite, Modicon, Necon, Ortho Evra, Ovcon 35, Ortho-Cyclen, Ortho Tri-Cyclen Tri-Levlen, Triphasil, Trivora
  - *Endometriosis:* ↓ Estrogen, ↑ progestin: Demulen 1/35, Loestrin 1.5/30, Loestrin 1/20 Fe, Lo Ovral, Levlen, Levora, Nordette, Zovia 1/35; cont w/o placebo pills or w/ 4 d of placebo pills
  - *HA:* ↓ Estrogen, ↓ progestin: Alesse, Levlite, Ortho Evra
  - *Moodiness &/or irritability:* ↓ Progestin: Alesse, Brevicon, Levlite, Modicon, Necon 1/35, Ortho Evra, Ortho-Cyclen, Ortho Tri-Cyclen, Ovcon 35, Tri-Levlen, Triphasil, Trivora
  - *Severe menstrual cramping:* ↑ Progestin: Demulen 1/50, Desogen, Loestrin 1.5/30, Mircette, Ortho-Cept, Yasmin, Yaz, Zovia 1/50E, Zovia 1/35E

Orphenadrine (Norflex, Generic) Uses: *Discomfort associated w/ painful musculoskeletal conditions* Acts: Central atropine-like effect; indirect skeletal muscle relaxation, euphoria, analgesia Dose: 100 mg PO bid, 60 mg IM/IV q12h W/P: [C, +/–] CI: NAG, GI/ or bladder obst, cardiospasm, MyG Disp: SR tabs 100 mg; Inj 30 mg/mL SE: Drowsiness, dizziness, blurred vision, flushing, tachycardia, constipation

Oseltamivir (Tamiflu) Uses: *Prevention & Rx influenza A & B* Acts: ↓ Viral neuraminidase Dose: *Adults. Tx:* 75 mg PO bid for 5 d w/in 48 h of Sx onset; *Prophylaxis:* 75 mg PO daily × 10 d w/in 48 h of contact *Peds. Tx: Dose bid × 5 d: < 15 kg:* 30 mg. *15–23 kg:* 45 mg. *23–40 kg:* 60 mg. *> 40 kg:* Adult dose. *Prophylaxis:* Same dosing but once daily for 10 d ↓ w/ renal impair W/P: [C, ?/–] CI: Component allergy Disp: Caps 30, 45, 75 mg, powder 6 mg/mL for suspension (Note. 12 mg/mL dose is being phased out due to dosing concerns) SE: N/V, insomnia, reports of neuropsychological events in children (self-injury, confusion, delirium) Notes: Start w/in 48 h of Sx onset or exposure; 2009 H1N1 strains susceptible; ✓ CDC updates http://www.cdc.gov/h1n1flu/guidance/

Oxacillin (Generic) Uses: *Infxns d/t susceptible S. aureus, Streptococcus & other organisms* Acts: Bactericidal; ↓ cell wall synth. *Spectrum:* Excellent gram(+), poor gram(–) Dose: *Adults.* 250–500 mg (2 g severe) IM/IV q4–6h. *Peds.* 150–200 mg/kg/d IV ÷ q4–6h W/P: [B, M] CI: PCN sensitivity Disp: Powder for Inj 500 mg, 1, 2, 10 g SE: GI upset, interstitial nephritis, blood dyscrasias, may ↓ OCP effectiveness

Oxaliplatin (Eloxatin) BOX: Administer w/ supervision of physician experienced in chemotherapy. Appropriate management is possible only w/ adequate diagnostic & Rx facilities. Anaphylactic-like Rxns reported Uses: *Adjuvant Rx stage III colon CA (primary resected) & metastatic colon CA w/ 5-FU* Acts: Metabolized to platinum derivatives, crosslinks DNA Dose: Per protocol; see PI. *Premedicate:* Antiemetic w/ or w/o dexamethasone W/P: [D, –] See Box CI: Allergy to components or platinum Disp: Inj 50, 100 mg SE: Anaphylaxis, granulocytopenia, paresthesia, N/V/D, stomatitis, fatigue, neuropathy, hepatotox, pulm tox Notes: 5-FU & leucovorin are given in combo; epi, corticosteroids, & antihistamines alleviate severe Rxns

Oxandrolone (Oxandrin, Generic) [C-III] BOX: Risk of peliosis hepatis, liver cell tumors, may ↑ risk atherosclerosis Uses: *Wt ↑ after Wt ↓ from severe trauma, extensive surgery* Acts: Anabolic steroid; ↑ lean body mass Dose: *Adults.* 2.5–20 mg/d PO ÷ bid-qid *Peds.* ≤ 0.1 mg/kg/d ÷ bid-qid W/P: [X, ?/–] ↑ INR w/ warfarin CI: PRG, prostate CA, breast CA, breast CA w/ hypercalcemia, nephrosis Disp: Tabs 2.5, 10 mg SE: Acne, hepatotox, dyslipidemia Notes: ✓ lipids & LFTs; Use intermittently, 2–4 wk typical

Oxaprozin (Daypro, Generic) BOX: May ↑ risk of cardiovascular CV events & GI bleeding Uses: *Arthritis & pain* Acts: NSAID; ↓ prostaglandin synth Dose: *Adults.* 600–1200 mg/daily (÷ dose helps GI tolerance); ↓ w/ renal/hepatic impair **Peds. JRA (Daypro):** 22–31 kg: 600 mg/d. 32–54 kg: 900 mg/d **W/P:** [C (D 3rd tri), ?] Peptic ulcer, bleeding disorders **CI:** ASA/NSAID sensitivity, perioperative pain w/ CABG **Disp:** Tabs 600 mg **SE:** CNS inhibition, sleep disturbance, rash, GI upset, peptic ulcer, edema, renal failure, anaphylactoid Rxn w/ "ASA triad" (asthmatic w/ rhinitis, nasal polyps and bronchospasm w/ NSAID use)

Oxazepam (Generic) [C-IV] Uses: *Anxiety, acute EtOH withdrawal*, anxiety w/ depressive Sxs **Acts:** Benzodiazepine; diazepam metabolite **Dose: Adults.** 10–15 mg PO tid-qid ÷ doses **Peds > 6 y.** 1 mg/kg/d ÷ doses **W/P:** [D, ?/–] **CI:** Component allergy, NAG **Disp:** Caps 10, 15, 30 mg; tabs 15 mg **SE:** Sedation, ataxia, dizziness, rash, blood dyscrasias, dependence **Notes:** Avoid abrupt D/C

Oxcarbazepine (Oxtellar XR, Trileptal, Generic) Uses: *Partial Szs*, bipolar disorders **Acts:** Blocks voltage-sensitive Na$^+$ channels, stabilization of hyperexcited neural membranes **Dose: Adults.** 300 mg PO bid, ↑ weekly to target maint 1200–2400 mg/d. **Peds.** 8–10 mg/kg bid, 600 mg/d max, ↑ weekly to target maint dose; ↓ w/ renal Insuff **W/P:** [C, –] Carbamazepine sensitivity **CI:** Component sensitivity **Disp:** Tabs 150, 300, 600 mg; (*Oxtellar XR*) ER tabs 150, 300, 600 mg; susp 300 mg/5 mL **SE:** ↓ Na$^+$, HA, dizziness, fatigue, somnolence, GI upset, diplopia, concentration difficulties, fatal skin/multiorgan hypersens Rxns **Notes:** Do not abruptly D/C, ✓ Na$^+$ if fatigued; advise about SJS and topic epidermal necrolysis

Oxiconazole (Oxistat) Uses: *Tinea cruris, tinea corporis, tinea pedis, tinea versicolor* **Acts:** ? ↓ Ergosterols in fungal cell membrane. **Spectrum:** Most *Epidermophyton floccosum, Trichophyton mentagrophytes, Trichophyton rubrum, Malassezia furfur* **Dose:** Apply thin layer daily-bid **W/P:** [B, M] **CI:** Component allergy **Disp:** Cream, lotion 1% **SE:** Local irritation

Oxybutynin (Ditropan, Ditropan XL, Generic) Uses: *Symptomatic relief of urgency, nocturia, incontinence w/ neurogenic or reflex neurogenic bladder* **Acts:** Anticholinergic, relaxes bladder smooth muscle, ↑ bladder capacity **Dose: Adults.** 5 mg bid-tid, 5 mg 4×/d max. XL 5–10 mg/d, 30 mg/d max. **Peds > 5 y.** 5 mg PO bid-tid; 15 mg/d max. **Peds 1–5 y.** 0.2 mg/kg/dose 2–4×/d (syrup 5 mg/5 mL); 15 mg/d max; ↓ in elderly; periodic drug holidays OK **W/P:** [B, ?] **CI:** NAG, MyG, GI/GU obst, UC, megacolon **Disp:** Tabs 5 mg; XL tabs 5, 10, 15 mg; syrup 5 mg/5 mL **SE:** Anticholinergic (drowsiness, xerostomia, constipation, tachycardia); ↑ QT interval, memory impair; ER form empty shell expelled in stool

Oxybutynin, Topical (Gelnique) Uses: *OAB* **Acts:** Anticholinergic, relaxes bladder smooth muscle, ↑ bladder capacity **Dose:** 1 g sachet qd to dry skin (Abd/shoulders/thighs/upper arms) **W/P:** [B, ?/–] **CI:** Gastric or urinary retention; NAG **Disp:** Gel 10%, 1-g sachets (100 mg oxybutynin) **SE:** Anticholinergic (lethargy, xerostomia, constipation, blurred vision, ↑ HR); rash, pruritus, redness, pain at site; UTI **Notes:** Cover w/ clothing, skin-to-skin transfer can occur; gel is flammable; after applying wait 1 h before showering

Oxybutynin Transdermal System (Oxytrol)   Uses: *Rx OAB* Acts: Anticholinergic, relaxes bladder smooth muscle, ↑ bladder capacity Dose: One 3.9 mg/d system apply 2×/wk (q3–4d) to Abd, hip, or buttock W/P: [B, ?/–] CI: GI/GU obst, NAG gluc SE: Anticholinergic, itching/ redness at site Notes: Do not apply to same site w/in 7 d

Oxycodone (OxyContin, Roxicodone, Generic) [C-II]   BOX: High abuse potential; controlled release only for extended chronic pain, not for PRN use; 60-, 80-mg tab for opioid-tolerant pts; do not crush, break, or chew Uses: *Mod-severe pain, usually in combo w/ nonnarcotic analgesics* Acts: Narcotic analgesic Dose: *Adults.* 5 mg PO q6h PRN (IR). *Mod–severe chronic pain:* 10–160 mg PO q12h (ER), can give ER q8h if effect does not last 12 h. *Peds 6–12 y,* 1.25 mg PO q6h PRN. *> 12 y:* 2.5 mg PO q6h PRN; ↓ w/ severe liver/renal Dz, elderly; w/ food W/P: [B (D if prolonged use/near term), M] CI: Allergy, resp depression, acute asthma, ileus w/ microsomal morphine Disp: IR caps (OxyIR) 5 mg; CR Roxicodone tabs 15, 30 mg; ER (OxyContin) 10, 15, 20, 30, 40, 60, 80 mg; liq 5 mg/5 mL; soln conc 20 mg/mL SE: ↓ BP, sedation, resp depression, dizziness, GI upset, constipation, risk of abuse Notes: *OxyContin* for chronic CA pain; do not crush/chew/ cut ER product; sought after as drug of abuse; reformulated *OxyContin* is intended to prevent the opioid medication from being cut, broken, chewed, crushed, or dissolved to release more medication

Oxycodone/Acetaminophen (Percocet, Tylox) [C-II]   Uses: *Mod-severe pain* Acts: Narcotic analgesic Dose: *Adults.* 1–2 tabs/caps PO q4–6h PRN (acetaminophen max dose 4 g/d). *Peds.* Oxycodone 0.05–0.15 mg/kg/dose q4–6h PRN, 5 mg/dose max W/P: [C (D prolonged use or near term), M] CI: Allergy, paralytic ileus, resp depression Disp: Percocet tabs, mg oxycodone/mg APAP: 2.5/325, 5/325, 7.5/325, 10/325, 7.5/500, 10/650; Tylox caps 5 mg oxycodone, 500 mg APAP; soln 5 mg oxycodone & 325 mg APAP/5 mL SE: ↓ BP, sedation, dizziness, GI upset, constipation Notes: See Acetaminophen note p 36

Oxycodone/Aspirin (Percodan) [C-II]   Uses: *Mod–severe pain* Acts: Narcotic analgesic w/ NSAID Dose: *Adults.* 1–2 tabs/caps PO q4–6h PRN. *Peds.* Oxycodone 0.05–0.15 mg/kg/dose q4–6h PRN, up to 5 mg/dose; ↓ in severe hepatic failure W/P: [D, –] w/ Peptic ulcer, CNS depression, elderly, Hx Szs CI: Component allergy, children (< 16 y) w/ viral Infxn (Reyes synd), resp depression, ileus, hemophilia Disp: *Generics:* 4.83 mg oxycodone hydrochloride, 0.38 mg oxycodone terephthalate, 325 mg ASA; *Percodan* 4.83 mg oxycodone hydrochloride, 325 mg ASA SE: Sedation, dizziness, GI upset/ulcer, constipation, allergy Notes: Monitor for possible drug abuse; max 4 g ASA/d

Oxycodone/Ibuprofen (Combunox) [C-II]   BOX: May ↑ risk of serious CV events; CI in perioperative CABG pain; ↑ risk of GI events such as bleeding Uses: *Short-term (not > 7 d) management of acute mod–severe pain* Acts: Narcotic w/ NSAID Dose: 1 tab q6h PRN 4 tab max/24 h; 7 d max W/P: [C, –] w/ Impaired renal/hepatic Fxn; COPD, CNS depression, avoid in PRG CI: Paralytic ileus, 3rd-tri PRG, allergy to ASA or NSAIDs, where opioids are CI **Disp:** Tabs 5 mg oxycodone/400 mg ibuprofen **SE:** N/V, somnolence, dizziness, sweating, flatulence, ↑ LFTs **Notes:** ✓ Renal Fxn; abuse potential w/ oxycodone

Oxymorphone (Opana, Opana ER) [C-II] **BOX:** *(Opana ER)* Abuse potential, controlled release only for chronic pain; do not consume EtOH-containing beverages, may cause fatal OD **Uses:** *Mod–severe pain, sedative* **Acts:** Narcotic analgesic **Dose:** 10–20 mg PO q4–6h PRN if opioid-naïve or 1–1.5 mg SQ/IM q4–6h PRN or 0.5 mg IV q4–6h PRN; starting 20 mg/dose max PO; *Chronic pain:* ER 5 mg PO q12h; if opioid-naïve ↑ PRN 5–10 mg PO q12h q3–7d; take 1 h pc or 2 h ac; ↓ dose w/ elderly, renal/hepatic impair **W/P:** [B, ?] **CI:** ↑ ICP, severe resp depression, w/ EtOH or liposomal morphine, severe hepatic impair **Disp:** Tabs 5, 10 mg; ER 5, 10, 20, 30, 40 mg **SE:** ↓ BP, sedation, GI upset, constipation, histamine release **Notes:** Related to hydromorphone

Oxytocin (Pitocin, Generic) **BOX:** Not rec for elective induction of labor **Uses:** *Induce labor, control postpartum hemorrhage* **Acts:** Stimulate muscular contractions of the uterus **Dose:** 0.0005–0.001 units/min IV Inf; titrate 0.001–0.002 units/min q30–60min **W/P:** [Uncategorized, +/–] **CI:** Where Vag delivery not favorable, fetal distress **Disp:** Inj 10 units/mL **SE:** Uterine rupture, fetal death; arrhythmias, anaphylaxis, H_2O intoxication **Notes:** Monitor vital signs; nasal form for breast-feeding only; postpartum bleeding 10–40 units in 1000 mL @ sufficient rate to stop bleeding

Paclitaxel (Abraxane, Taxol, Generic) **BOX:** Administration only by physician experienced in chemotherapy; fatal anaphylaxis and hypersens possible; severe myelosuppression possible **Uses:** *Ovarian & breast CA, PCa*, Kaposi sarcoma, NSCLC **Acts:** Mitotic spindle poison; promotes microtubule assembly & stabilization against depolymerization **Dose:** Per protocols; use glass or polyolefin containers (eg, nitroglycerin tubing set); PVC sets leach plasticizer; ↓ in hepatic failure **W/P:** [D, –] **CI:** Neutropenia ANC < 1500 cells/mm^3, < 1000 cells/mm^3 in w/ AIDS related karposis syndrome; solid tumors, component allergy **Disp:** Inj 6 mg/mL, vial 5, 16.7, 25, 50 mL; *(Abraxane)* 100 mg/vial **SE:** ↓ BM, peripheral neuropathy, transient ileus, myalgia, ↓ HR, ↓ BP, mucositis, N/V/D, fever, rash, HA, phlebitis; hematologic tox schedule-dependent; leukopenia dose-limiting by 24-h Inf; neurotox limited w/ short (1–3 h) Inf; allergic Rxns (dyspnea, ↓ BP, urticaria, rash) **Notes:** Maintain hydration; allergic Rxn usually w/in 10 min of Inf; minimize w/ corticosteroid, antihistamine pretreatment

Palifermin (Kepivance) **Uses:** *Oral mucositis w/ BMT* **Acts:** Synthetic keratinocyte GF **Dose:** *Phase 1:* 60 mcg/kg IV daily × 3, 3rd dose 24–48 h before chemotherapy. *Phase 2:* 60 mcg/kg IV daily × 3, after stem cell Inf (at least 4 d from last dose) **W/P:** [C, ?/–] **CI:** Hypersensitivity to palifermin, *E. coli*–derived proteins, or any component & formulation **Disp:** Inj 6.25 mg **SE:** Unusual mouth sensations, tongue thickening, rash, ↑ amylase & lipase **Notes:** *E. coli*–derived; separate phases by 4 d; safety unknown w/ nonhematologic malignancies

Paliperidone (Invega, Invega Sustenna) BOX: Not for dementia-related psychosis Uses: *Schizophrenia* Acts: Risperidone metabolite, antagonizes dopamine, and serotonin receptors Dose: *Invega:* 6 mg PO q A.M., 12 mg/d max; CrCl 50–79 mL/min: 6 mg/d max; CrCl 10–49 mL/min: 3 mg/d max. *Invega Sustenna:* 234 mg day 1, 156 mg 1 week later IM (deltoid), then 117 mg monthly (deltoid or gluteal); range 39–234 mg/mo W/P: [C, ?/–] w/ ↓ HR, ↓ K⁺/Mg²⁺, renal/hepatic impair; w/ phenothiazines, ranolazine, ziprasidone, prolonged QT, Hx arrhythmia CI: Risperidone/paliperidone hypersens Disp: *Invega:* ER tabs 1.5, 3, 6, 9 mg; *Invega Sustenna:* Prefilled syringes 39, 78, 117, 156, 234 mg SE: Impaired temp regulation, ↑ QT & HR, HA, anxiety, dizziness, N, dry mouth, fatigue, EPS Notes: Do not chew/cut/crush pill; determine tolerability to oral risperidone or paliperidone before using injectable

Palivizumab (Synagis) Uses: *Prevent RSV Infxn* Acts: MoAb Dose: *Peds.* 15 mg/kg IM monthly, typically Nov–Apr; AAP rec max 3 doses for those born 32–34 6/7 wk w/o significant congenital heart/lung Dz W/P: [C, ?] Renal/hepatic dysfunction CI: Component allergy Disp: Vials 50, 100 mg SE: Hypersens Rxn, URI, rhinitis, cough, ↑ LFTs, local irritation

Palonosetron (Aloxi) BOX: May ↑ QTc interval Uses: *Prevent acute & delayed N/V w/ emetogenic chemotherapy; prevent postoperative N/V* Acts: 5-HT₃-receptor antagonist Dose: *Chemotherapy:* 0.25 mg IV 30 min prior to chemotherapy. *Postoperative N/V:* 0.075 mg immediately before induction W/P: [B, ?] CI: Component allergy Disp: 0.05 mg/mL (1.5 & 5 mL vials) SE: HA, constipation, dizziness, Abd pain, anxiety

Pamidronate (Generic) Uses: *Hypercalcemia of malignancy, Paget Dz, palliate symptomatic bone metastases* Acts: Bisphosphonate; ↓ nl & abnormal bone resorption Dose: *Hypercalcemia:* 60–90 mg IV over 2–24 h or 90 mg IV over 24 h if severe; may repeat in 7 d. *Paget Dz:* 30 mg/d IV slow Inf over 4 h × 3 d. *Osteolytic bone mets in myeloma:* 90 mg IV over 4 h qmo. *Osteolytic bone mets breast CA:* 90 mg IV over 2 h q3–4wk; 90 mg/max single dose. W/P: [D, ?/–] Avoid invasive dental procedures w/ use CI: PRG, bisphosphonate sensitivity Disp: Inj 30, 60, 90 mg SE: Fever, malaise, convulsions, Inj site Rxn, uveitis, fluid overload, HTN, Abd pain, N/V, constipation, UTI, bone pain, ↓ K⁺, ↓ Ca²⁺, ↓ Mg²⁺, hypophosphatemia; jaw osteonecrosis (mostly CA pts; avoid dental work), renal tox Notes: Perform dental exam pretherapy; follow Cr, hold dose if Cr ↑ by 0.5 mg/dL w/ nl baseline or by 1 mg/dL w/ abnormal baseline; restart when Cr returns w/in 10% of baseline; may ↑ atypical subtrochanteric femur fractures

Pancrelipase (Creon, Pancreaze, Panakare Plus, Pertzye, Ultresa, Voikace, Zenpep, Generic) Uses: *Exocrine pancreatic secretion deficiency (eg, CF, chronic pancreatitis, pancreatic Insuff), steatorrhea of malabsorption* Acts: Pancreatic enzyme supl; amylase, lipase, protease Dose: 1–3 caps (tabs) w/ meals & snacks; ↑ to 8 caps (tabs); do not crush or chew EC products; dose dependent on digestive requirements of pt; avoid antacids W/P: [C, ?/–] CI: Pork product allergy, acute pancreatitis **Disp:** Caps, tabs **SE:** N/V, Abd cramps **Notes:** Individualize Rx; dosing based on lipase component

Pancuronium (Generic)   **BOX:** Should only be administered by adequately trained individuals **Uses:** *Paralysis w/ mechanical ventilation* **Acts:** Nondepolarizing neuromuscular blocker **Dose:** *Adults & Peds > 1 mo.* Initial 0.06–0.1 mg/kg; maint 0.01 mg/kg 60–100 min after, then 0.01 mg/kg q25–60min PRN; ↓ w/ renal/hepatic impair; intubate pt & keep on controlled ventilation; use adequate sedation and analgesia **W/P:** [C, ?/–] **CI:** Component or bromide sensitivity **Disp:** Inj 1, 2 mg/mL **SE:** Tachycardia, HTN, pruritus, other histamine/hypersens Rxns **Notes:** Cross-reactivity w/ other neuromuscular blocker possible

Panitumumab (Vectibix)   **BOX:** Derm tox common (89%) and severe in 12%; can be associated w/ Infxn (sepsis, abscesses requiring I&D; w/ severe derm tox, hold or D/C and monitor for Infxn; severe Inf Rxns (anaphylactic Rxn, bronchospasm, fever, chills, hypotension) in 1%; w/ severe Rxns, immediately D/C Inf and possibly permanent D/C **Uses:** *Rx EGFR-expressing metastatic colon CA* **Acts:** Anti-EGFR MoAb **Dose:** 6 mg/kg IV Inf over 60 min over 60 min q14d; doses > 1000 mg over 90 min ↓ Inf rate by 50% w/ grade 1–2 Inf Rxn, D/C permanently w/ grade 3–4 Rxn. For derm tox, hold until < grade 2 tox. If improves < 1 mo, restart 50% original dose. If tox recurs or resolution > 1 mo permanently D/C. If ↓ dose tolerated, ↑ dose by 25% **W/P:** [C, –] D/C nursing during, 2 mo after **Disp:** 20 mg/mL vial (5, 10 mL) **SE:** Rash, acneiform dermatitis, pruritus, paronychia, ↓ Mg²⁺, Abd pain, N/V/D, constipation, fatigue, dehydration, photosens, conjunctivitis, ocular hyperemia, ↑ lacrimation, stomatitis, mucositis, palm fibrosis, severe derm tox, Inf Rxns **Notes:** May impair female fertility; ✓ lytes; wear sunscreen/hats, limit sun exposure

Pantoprazole (Protonix, Generic)   **Uses:** *GERD, erosive gastritis*, ZE synd, PUD **Acts:** Proton pump inhib **Dose:** *Adult:* 40 mg/d PO; do not crush/chew tabs; 40 mg IV/d (not > 3 mg/min) **Peds:** 0.5–1 mg/kg/d ages 6–13 y limited data **W/P:** [B, ?/–] Do not use w/ clopidogrel (↓ effect) **Disp:** Tabs, DR 20, 40 mg; 40 mg powder for oral susp (mix in applesauce or juice, give immediately); Inj 40 mg **SE:** CP, anxiety, GI upset, ↑ LFTs **Notes:** ? ↑ Risk of fractures w/ all PPI; risk of hypomagnesemia w/ long-term use, monitor; ↑ *C. difficile* risk

Paregoric [Camphorated Tincture of Opium] [C-III]   **Uses:** *D*, pain & neonatal opiate withdrawal synd **Acts:** Narcotic **Dose:** *Adults.* 5–10 mL PO 1–4×/d PRN. *Peds.* 0.25–0.5 mL/kg 1–4×/d. **W/P:** [B (D w/ prolonged use/high dose near term, +] **CI:** Toxic D; convulsive disorder, morphine sensitivity **Disp:** Liq 2 mg morphine = 20 mg opium/5 mL **SE:** ↓ BP, sedation, constipation **Notes:** Contains anhydrous morphine from opium; do not confuse w/ opium tincture; short-term use only; contains benzoic acid (benzyl alcohol metabolite)

Paroxetine (Brisdelle)   **BOX:** Potential for suicidal thinking/behavior; monitor closely **Uses:** *Mod–severe menopause vasomotor Sx (not for psych use)* **Acts:** SSRI, nonhormonal Rx for condition **Dose:** 7.5 mg PO qhs **W/P:** [X, ?/M] Serotonin synd, bleed/ w NSAID, ↓ Na⁺, ↓ tamoxifen effect, fractures, mania/hypomania activation, Szs, akathisia, NAG, cognitive/motor impair, w/ strong CYP2D6 inhib **CI:** w/ or w/in 14 d of MAOI, w/ thioridazine/pimozide/PRG **Disp:** Caps 7.5 mg **SE:** HA, fatigue, N/V **Notes:** See other paroxetine listings

Paroxetine (Paxil, Paxil CR, Pexeva, Generic) **BOX:** Closely monitor for worsening depression or emergence of suicidality, particularly in children, adolescents, and young adults; not for use in peds **Uses:** *Depression, OCD, panic disorder, social anxiety disorder*, PMDD **Acts:** SSRI **Dose:** 10–60 mg PO single daily dose in A.M.; CR 25 mg/d PO; ↑ 12.5 mg/wk (max range 26–62.5 mg/d) **W/P:** [D, ?/] ↑ Bleeding risk **CI:** w/ MAOI, thioridazine, pimozide, linezolid, methylthioninium chloride (methylene blue) **Disp:** Tabs 10, 20, 30, 40 mg; susp 10 mg/5 mL; CR 12.5, 25, 37.5 mg **SE:** HA, somnolence, dizziness, GI upset, N/D, ↓ appetite, sweating, xerostomia, tachycardia, ↓ libido, ED, anorgasmia

Pasireotide (Signifor) **Uses:** *Cushing Dz* **Acts:** Somatostatin analogue inhib ACTH secretion **Dose:** *Adults.* 0.6–0.9 mg SQ 2×/d; titrate on response/tolerability; hepatic impair (Child-Pugh B): 0.3–0.6 mg SQ twice daily, (Child-Pugh C): avoid **W/P:** [C, –] w/ Risk for ↓ HR or ↑ QT; w/ drugs that ↓ HR, ↑ QT, cyclosporine, bromocriptine **CI:** None **Disp:** Inj single-dose 0.3, 0.6, 0.9 mg/mL **SE:** N/V/D, hyperglycemia, HA, Abd pain, cholelithiasis, fatigue, DM, hypocortisolism, ↓ HR, QT prolongation, ↑ glucose, ↑ LFTs, ↓ pituitary hormones, Inj site Rxn, edema, alopecia, asthenia, myalgia, arthralgia **Notes:** Prior to and periodically (see label), ✓ FPG, HbA1c, LFTs, ECG, gallbladder US

Pazopanib (Votrient) **BOX:** Administer only by physician experienced in chemotherapy. Severe and fatal hepatotox observed. **Uses:** *Rx advanced RCC* metastatic soft-tissue sarcoma after chemotherapy **Acts:** TKI **Dose:** *Adults.* 800 mg PO once daily, ↓ to 200 mg daily if moderate hepatic impair, not rec in severe hepatic Dz (bili > 3× ULN) **W/P:** [D, –] Avoid w/ CYP3A4 inducers/inhib and QTc prolonging drugs, all SSRI. **CI:** Severe hepatic Dz **Disp:** 200-mg tablet **SE:** ↑ BP, N/V/D, GI perf, anorexia, hair depigmentation, ↓ WBC, ↓ plt, ↑ bleeding, ↑ AST/ALT/bili, ↓ Na, CP, ↑ QT **Notes:** Hold for surgical procedures. Take 1 h ac or 2 h pc

Pegfilgrastim (Neulasta) **Uses:** *↓ Frequency of Infxn in pts w/ nonmyeloid malignancies receiving myelosuppressive anti-CA drugs that cause febrile neutropenia* **Acts:** Granulocyte and macrophage-stimulating factor **Dose:** *Adults.* 6 mg SQ × 1/chemotherapy cycle **W/P:** [C, M] w/ Sickle cell **CI:** Allergy to *E. coli*-derived proteins or filgrastim **Disp:** *Syringes:* 6 mg/0.6 mL **SE:** Splenic rupture, HA, fever, weakness, fatigue, dizziness, insomnia, edema, N/V/D, stomatitis, anorexia, constipation, taste perversion, dyspepsia, Abd pain, granulocytopenia, neutropenic fever, ↑ LFTs & uric acid, arthralgia, myalgia, bone pain, ARDS, alopecia, worsen sickle cell Dz **Notes:** Never give between 14 d before & 24 h after dose of cytotoxic chemotherapy

Peginterferon Alfa-2a [Pegylated Interferon] (Pegasys) **BOX:** Can cause or aggravate fatal or life-threatening neuropsychological, autoimmune, ischemic, and infectious disorders. Monitor pts closely **Uses:** *Chronic hep C w/ compensated liver Dz* **Acts:** Immune modulator **Dose:** 180 mcg (1 mL) SQ see package insert; SQ dosing; ↓ in renal impair **W/P:** [C, /?–] **CI:** Autoimmune hep, decompensated liver Dz **Disp:** 180 mcg/mL Inj **SE:** Depression, insomnia, suicidal behavior, GI upset, ↓ WBC and plt, alopecia, pruritus; do not confuse w/ peginterferon alfa-2b

Peginterferon Alfa-2b [Pegylated Interferon] (PegIntron) BOX: Can cause or aggravate fatal or life-threatening neuropsychological, autoimmune, ischemic, and infectious disorders; monitor pts closely **Uses:** *Rx hep C* **Acts:** Immune modulator **Dose:** Typical dose (see package insert) 1 mcg/kg/wk SQ; 1.5 mcg/kg/wk combo w/ ribavirin **W/P:** [C, ?/–] w/ Psychological disorder Hx **CI:** Autoimmune hep, decompensated liver Dz, hemoglobinopathy **Disp:** Vials 50, 80, 120, 150 mcg/0.5 mL; Redipen 50, 80, 120, 150 mcg/5 mL; reconstitute w/ 0.7 mL w/ sterile water **SE:** Depression, insomnia, suicidal behavior, GI upset, neutropenia, thrombocytopenia, alopecia, pruritus **Notes:** Give hs or w/ APAP to ↓ flu-like Sxs; monitor CBC/plt; use immediately or store in refrigerator × 24 h; do not freeze

Pegloticase (Krystexxa) BOX: Anaphylaxis/Inf Rxn reported; admin in settings prepared to manage these Rxns; premed w/ antihistamines and cortico-steroids **Uses:** *Refractory gout* **Acts:** PEGylated recombinant urate-oxidase enzyme **Dose:** 8 mg IV q2wk (in 250 mL NS/½NS over 120 min) premed w/ antihistamines and corticosteroids **W/P:** [C, –] **CI:** G6PD deficiency **Disp:** Inj 8 mg/mL in 1 mL vial **SE:** Inf Rxn (anaphylaxis, urticaria, pruritis, erythema, CP, dyspnea); may cause gout flare, N **Notes:** ✓ uric acid level before each Inf, consider D/C if 2 consecutive levels > 6 mg/dL; do not IV push

Pemetrexed (Alimta) **Uses:** *w/ Cisplatin in nonresectable mesothelioma*, NSCLC **Acts:** Antifolate antineoplastic **Dose:** 500 mg/m² IV over 10 min q3wk; hold if CrCl < 45 mL/min; give w/ vit B₁₂ (1000 mcg IM q9wk) & folic acid (350– 1000 mcg PO daily); start 1 wk before; dexamethasone 4 mg PO bid × 3, start 1 d before on Rx **W/P:** [D, –] w/ Renal/hepatic/BM impair **CI:** Component sensitivity **Disp:** 500-mg vial **SE:** Neutropenia, thrombocytopenia, N/V/D, anorexia, stomatitis, renal failure, neuropathy, fever, fatigue, mood changes, dyspnea, anaphylactic Rxns **Notes:** Avoid NSAIDs, follow CBC/plt; ↓ dose w/ grade 3–4 mucositis

Pemirolast (Alamast) **Uses:** *Allergic conjunctivitis* **Acts:** Mast cell stabilizer **Dose:** 1–2 gtt in each eye qid **W/P:** [C, ?/–] **Disp:** 0.1% (1 mg/mL) in 10-mL bottles **SE:** HA, rhinitis, cold/flu Sxs, local irritation **Notes:** Wait 10 min before inserting contacts

Penbutolol (Levatol) **Uses:** *HTN* **Acts:** β-Adrenergic receptor blocker, β₁, β₂ **Dose:** 20–40 mg/d; ↓ in hepatic Insuff **W/P:** [C 1st tri; D if 2nd/3rd tri, M] **CI:** Asthma, cardiogenic shock, cardiac failure, heart block, ↓ HR, COPD, pulm edema **Disp:** Tabs 20 mg **SE:** Flushing, ↓ BP, fatigue, hyperglycemia, GI upset, sexual dysfunction, bronchospasm **Notes:** ISA

Penciclovir (Denavir) Uses: *Herpes simplex (herpes labialis/cold sores)* Acts: Competitive inhib of DNA polymerase Dose: Apply at 1st sign of lesions, then q2h while awake × 4 d W/P: [B, ?/–] CI: Allergy, previous Rxn to famciclovir Disp: Cream 1% SE: Erythema, HA Notes: Do not apply to mucous membranes

Penicillin G, Aqueous (Potassium or Sodium) (Pfizerpen, Pentids) Uses: *Bacteremia, endocarditis, pericarditis, resp tract Infxns, meningitis, neurosyphilis, skin/skin structure Infxns* Acts: Bactericidal; ↓ cell wall synth. *Spectrum:* Most gram(+) (not staphylococci), streptococci, *N. meningitidis*, syphilis, clostridia, & anaerobes (not *Bacteroides*) Dose: *Adults.* Based on indication range 0.6–24 mill units/d in ÷ doses q4h. *Peds Newborns < 1 wk.* 25,000–50,000 units/kg/dose IV q12h. *Infants 1 wk–< 1 mo:* 25,000–50,000 units/kg/dose IV q8h. *Children:* 100,000–400,000 units/kg/24h IV ÷ q4h; ↓ in renal impair W/P: [B, M] CI: Allergy Disp: Powder for Inj SE: Allergic Rxns; interstitial nephritis, D, Szs Notes: Contains 1.7 mEq of K+/mill units

Penicillin V (Pen-Vee K, Veetids, Others) Uses: Susceptible streptococcal Infxns, otitis media, URIs, skin/soft-tissue Infxns (PCN-sensitive staphylococci) Acts: Bactericidal; ↓ cell wall synth. *Spectrum:* Most gram(+), including streptococci Dose: *Adults.* 250–500 mg PO q6h, q8h, q12h. *Peds.* 25–50 mg/kg/24 h PO in 3–4 ÷ dose above the age of 12 y, dose can be standardized vs Wt based; ↓ in renal impair; take on empty stomach W/P: [B, M] CI: Allergy Disp: Tabs 125, 250, 500 mg; susp 125, 250 mg/5 mL SE: GI upset, interstitial nephritis, anaphylaxis, convulsions Notes: Well-tolerated PO PCN; 250 mg = 400,000 units of PCN G

Penicillin G Benzathine (Bicillin) Uses: *Single-dose regimen for streptococcal pharyngitis, rheumatic fever, glomerulonephritis prophylaxis, & syphilis* Acts: Bactericidal; ↓ cell wall synth. *Spectrum:* See Penicillin G Dose: *Adults.* 1.2–2.4 mill units deep IM Inj q2–4wk. *Peds.* 50,000 units/kg/dose, 2.4 mill units/ dose max; deep IM Inj q2–4 wk W/P: [B, M] CI: Allergy Disp: Inj 300,000, 600,000 units/mL; Bicillin L-A benzathine salt only; Bicillin C-R combo of benzathine & procaine (300,000 units procaine w/ 300,000 units benzathine/mL or 900,000 units benzathine w/ 300,000 units procaine/2 mL) SE: Inj site pain, acute interstitial nephritis, anaphylaxis Notes: IM use only; sustained action, w/ levels up to 4 wk; drug of choice for noncongenital syphilis

Penicillin G Procaine (Wycillin, Others) Uses: *Infxns of resp tract, skin/soft tissue, scarlet fever, syphilis* Acts: Bactericidal; ↓ cell wall synth. *Spectrum:* PCN G-sensitive organisms that respond to low, persistent serum levels Dose: *Adults.* 0.6–4.8 mill units/d in ÷ doses q12–24h; give probenecid at least 30 min prior to PCN to prolong action. *Peds.* 25,000–50,000 units/kg/d IM ÷ dailybid W/P: [B, M] CI: Allergy Disp: Inj 300,000, 500,000, 600,000 units/mL SE: Pain at Inj site, interstitial nephritis, anaphylaxis Notes: LA parenteral PCN; levels up to 15 h

Pentamidine (Pentam 300, NebuPent) Uses: *Rx & prevention of PCP* Acts: ↓ DNA, RNA, phospholipid, & protein synth Dose: *Rx: Adults &*

Peds. 4 mg/kg/24 h IV daily × 14–21 d. *Prevention: Adults & Peds > 5 y.* 300 mg once q4wk, give via Respirgard II nebulizer; ↓ IV w/ renal impair **W/P:** [C, ?] **CI:** Component allergy, use w/ didanosine **Disp:** Inj 300 mg/vial; aerosol 300 mg **SE:** Pancreatic cell necrosis w/ hyperglycemia; pancreatitis, CP, fatigue, dizziness, rash, GI upset, renal impair, blood dyscrasias (leukopenia, thrombocytopenia) **Notes:** Follow CBC, glucose, pancreatic Fxn monthly for first 3 mo; monitor for ↓ BP following IV dose; prolonged use may ↑ Infxn risk

Pentazocine (Talwin, Talwin Compound, Talwin NX) [C-IV] BOX: Oral use only; severe and potentially lethal Rxns from misuse by Inj **Uses:** *Mod–severe pain* **Acts:** Partial narcotic agonist–antagonist **Dose:** *Adults.* 30 mg IM or IV; 50–100 mg PO q3–4h PRN. *Peds 5–8 y.* 15 mg IM q4h PRN. *9–14 y:* 30 mg IM q4h PRN; ↓ in renal/hepatic impair **W/P:** [C (1st tri, D w/ prolonged use/high dose near term), +/–] **CI:** Allergy, ↑ ICP (unless ventilated) **Disp:** Talwin Compound tab 12.5 mg + 325 mg ASA; Talwin NX 50 mg + 0.5 mg naloxone; Inj 30 mg/mL **SE:** Considerable dysphoria; drowsiness, GI upset, xerostomia, rash **Notes:** 30–60 mg IM = 10 mg of morphine IM; Talwin NX has naloxone to curb abuse by nonoral route

Pentobarbital (Nembutal) [C-II] **Uses:** *Insomnia (short-term), convulsions*, sedation, induce coma w/ severe head injury **Acts:** Barbiturate **Dose:** *Adults. Sedative:* 150–200 mg IM, 100 mg IV, may repeat up to 500 mg max. *Hypnotic:* 100–200 mg PO or PR hs PRN. *Induced coma:* Load 5–10 mg/kg IV, w/ maint 1–3 mg/kg/h IV. *Peds. Induced coma:* As adult **W/P:** [D, +/–] Severe hepatic impair **CI:** Allergy **Disp:** Caps 50, 100 mg; elixir 18.2 mg/5 mL (= 20 mg pentobarbital); supp 30, 60, 120, 200 mg; Inj 50 mg/mL **SE:** Resp depression, ↓ BP w/ aggressive IV use for cerebral edema; ↓ HR, ↓ BP, sedation, lethargy, resp ↓, hangover, rash, SJS, blood dyscrasias **Notes:** Tolerance to sedative–hypnotic effect w/in 1–2 wk

Pentosan Polysulfate Sodium (Elmiron) **Uses:** *Relieve pain/discomfort w/ interstitial cystitis* **Acts:** Bladder wall buffer **Dose:** 100 mg PO tid; on empty stomach w/ H_2O 1 h ac or 2 h pc **W/P:** [B, ?/–] **CI:** Hypersensitivity to pentosan or related compounds (LMWH, heparin) **Disp:** Caps 100 mg **SE:** Alopecia, N/D, HA, ↑ LFTs, anticoagulant effects, ↓ plts, rectal bleed **Notes:** Reassess after 3 mo; related to LMWH, heparin

Pentoxifylline (Trental, Generic) **Uses:** *Rx Sxs of peripheral vascular Dz* **Acts:** ↓ Blood cell viscosity, restores RBC flexibility **Dose:** *Adults.* 400 mg PO tid pc; Rx min 8 wk for effect; ↓ to bid w/ GI/CNS SEs **W/P:** [C, +/–] **CI:** Cerebral/retinal hemorrhage, methylxanthine (caffeine) intolerance **Disp:** Tabs CR 400 mg; Tabs ER 400 mg **SE:** Dizziness, HA, GI upset

Perampanel (Fycompa) BOX: Serious/life-threatening psychiatric & behavioral Rxns (aggression, hostility, irritability, anger, homicidal threats/idea-tion) reported; monitor; ↓ dose or D/C if Sxs are severe/worsen **Uses:** *Adjunct in partial-onset Sz w/ or w/o secondarily generalized Szs* **Acts:** Noncompetitive AMPA glutamate receptor antag **Dose:** *Adults & Peds ≥ 12 y.* 2 mg PO qhs if not on enzyme-inducing AEDs; 4 mg PO qhs if on enzyme-inducing AEDs; ↑ 2 mg qhs weekly; 12 mg qhs max; elderly, ↑ at 2-wk intervals; mild–mod hepatic impair 6 mg max & 4 mg w/ ↑ dose q 2wk; severe hepatic/renal impair or dialysis: avoid **W/P:** [C, –] √ For suicidal behavior; avoid strong CYP3A inducers; monitor/ dose adjust w/ CYP450 inducers; 12-mg daily dose may ↓ effect of OCP w/ levonorgestrel **CI:** None **Disp:** Tabs 2, 4, 6, 8, 10, 12 mg **SE:** N, dizziness, vertigo, ataxia, gait balance/disturb, falls, somnolence, fatigue, irritability, ↑ Wt, anxiety, aggression, anger, blurred vision

Perindopril Erbumine (Aceon, Generic) BOX: ACE inhib can cause death to developing fetus; D/C immediately w/ PRG Uses: *HTN*, CHF, DN, post-MI **Acts:** ACE inhib **Dose:** 2–8 mg/d ÷ dose; 16 mg/d max; avoid w/ food; ↓ w/ elderly/renal impair **W/P:** [C (1st tri, D 2nd & 3rd tri), ?/–] ACE inhib-induced angioedema **CI:** Bilateral RAS, primary hyperaldosteronism **Disp:** Tabs 2, 4, 8 mg **SE:** Weakness, HA, ↓ BP, dizziness, GI upset, cough **Notes:** OK w/ diuretics

Permethrin (Elimite, Nix, Generic [OTC]) Uses: *Rx lice/scabies* **Acts:** Pediculicide **Dose:** *Adults & Peds > 2 y. Lice:* Saturate hair & scalp; allow 10 min before rinsing. *Scabies:* Apply cream head to toe; leave for 8–14 h, wash w/ H_2O **W/P:** [B, ?/–] **CI:** Allergy > 2 mo **Disp:** Topical lotion 1%; cream 5% **SE:** Local irritation **Notes:** Sprays available (*Rid, A200, Nix*) to disinfect clothing, bedding, combs, & brushes; lotion not OK in peds < 2 mo; may repeat after 7 d

Perphenazine (Generic) Uses: *Psychotic disorders, severe N* **Acts:** Phenothiazine, blocks brain dopaminergic receptors **Dose:** *Adults. Antipsychotic:* 4–16 mg PO tid; max 64 mg/d. **Notes:** Starting doses for schizophrenia lower in nonhospitalized pts N/V: 8–16 mg/d in ÷ doses. *Peds 1–6 y.* 4–6 mg/d PO in ÷ doses. *6–12 y:* 6 mg/d PO in ÷ doses. *> 12 y:* 4–16 mg PO 2–4×/d; ↓ in hepatic Insuff **W/P:** [C, ?/–] NAG, severe ↑/↓ BP **CI:** Phenothiazine sensitivity, BM depression, severe liver or cardiac Dz **Disp:** Tabs 2, 4, 8, 16 mg **SE:** ↓ BP, ↑/↓ HR, EPS, drowsiness, Szs, photosens, skin discoloration, blood dyscrasias, constipation

Pertuzumab (Perjeta) BOX: Embryo-fetal death & birth defects. Animal studies: oligohydramnios, delayed renal development, & death. Advise pt of risk & need for effective contraception Uses: *HER2-pos metastatic breast CA w/ trastuzumab & docetaxel in pts who have not received prior anti-HER2 therapy or chemo* **Acts:** HER2 dimerization inhib **Dose:** *Adults.* 840 mg 60 min IV Inf × 1; then 420 mg 30–60 min IV Inf q3wk; see label tox dose adjust **W/P:** [D, –] LV dysfxn (monitor LVEF); Inf Rxn **CI:** None **Disp:** Inj vial 420 mg/14 mL **SE:** N/V/D, alopecia, ↓ RBC/WBC, fatigue, rash, peripheral neuropathy, hypersens, anaphylaxis, pyrexia, asthenia, stomatitis, pruritus, dry skin, paronychia, HA, dysgeusia, dizziness, myalgia, arthralgia, URI, insomnia

Phenazopyridine (Pyridium, Azo-Standard, Urogesic, Many Others) [OTC] Uses: *Lower urinary tract irritation* **Acts:** Anesthetic on urinary tract mucosa **Dose:** *Adults.* 100–200 mg PO tid; 2 d max w/ antibiotics for UTI; ↓ w/ renal Insuff **W/P:** [B, ?] Hepatic Dz **CI:** Renal failure, CrCl < 50 mL/min **Disp:** Tabs (Pyridium) 100, 200 mg [OTC] 45, 97.2, 97.5 mg **SE:** GI disturbances, red-orange urine color (can stain clothing, contacts), HA, dizziness, acute renal failure, methemoglobinemia, tinting of sclera/skin **Notes:** Take w/ food

Phenelzine (Nardil) **BOX:** Antidepressants ↑ risk of suicidal thinking and behavior in children and adolescents w/ major depressive disorder and other psychological disorders; not for peds use **Uses:** *Depression*, bulimia **Acts:** MAOI **Dose:** *Adults.* 15 mg PO tid, ↑ to 60–90 mg/d ÷ doses. *Elderly:* 17.5–60 mg/d ÷ doses **W/P:** [C, –] Interacts w/ SSRI, ergots, triptans **CI:** CHF, Hx liver Dz, pheochromocytoma **Disp:** Tabs 15 mg **SE:** Postural ↓ BP; edema, dizziness, sedation, rash, sexual dysfunction, xerostomia, constipation, urinary retention **Notes:** 2–4 wk for effect; avoid tyramine-containing foods (eg, cheeses)

Phenobarbital (Generic) [C-IV] **Uses:** *Sz disorders*, insomnia, anxiety **Acts:** Barbiturate **Dose:** *Adults. Sedative–hypnotic:* 30–120 mg/d PO or IM PRN. *Anticonvulsant:* Load 10–20 mg/kg × 1 IV then 1–3 mg/kg/24 h PO or IV. *Peds. Sedative–hypnotic:* 2–3 mg/kg/24 h PO or IM hs PRN. *Anticonvulsant:* Load 15–20 mg/kg × 1 IV then 3–5 mg/kg/24 h PO ÷ in 2–3 doses; ↓ w/ CrCl < 10 mL/min **W/P:** [D, M] **CI:** Porphyria, hepatic impair, dyspnea, airway obst **Disp:** Tabs 15, 30, 60, 100 mg; elixir 20 mg/5 mL; Inj 60, 65, 130 mg/mL **SE:** ↓ HR, ↓ BP, hangover, SJS, blood dyscrasias, resp depression **Notes:** Tolerance develops to sedation; paradoxical hyperactivity seen in ped pts; long half-life allows single daily dosing. Levels: *Trough:* Just before next dose. *Therapeutic: Trough:* 15–40 mcg/mL; *Toxic: Trough:* > 40 mcg/mL *half-life:* 40–120 h

Phentermine (Adipex-P, Suprenza, Generic) **Uses:** *Wt loss in exogenous obesity* **Acts:** Anorectic/sympathomimetic amine **Dose:** *Adults.* 1 daily in A.M., lowest dose possible; place on tongue, allow to dissolve, then swallow **W/P:** [X, –] **CI:** CV Dz, hyperthyroidism, glaucoma, PRG, nursing, w/in 14 d of MOAI **Disp:** Tabs 15, 30, 37.5 mg; (*Suprenza*) ODT 15, 30, 37.5 mg **SE:** Pulm hypertension; aortic/mitral/tricuspid regurg valve Dz; dependence, ↑ HR, ↑ BP, palpitations, insomnia, HA, psychosis, restlessness, mood change, impotence, dry mouth, taste disturbance **Notes:** Avoid use at night

Phentermine/Topiramate (Qsymia) [C-IV] **Uses:** *Wt management w/ BMI ≥ 30 kg/m^2 or ≥ 27 kg/m^2 w/ Wt-related comorbidity* **Acts:** Anorectic (sympathomimetic amine w/ anticonvulsant) **Dose:** *Adults.* 3.75/23 mg PO daily × 14 d, then 7.5/46 mg PO daily; max dose 15/92 mg daily or 7.5/46 mg w/ mod/severe renal impair or mod hepatic impair; D/C if not > 3% Wt loss on 7.5/46 mg dose or 5% Wt loss on 15/92 mg dose by week 12; D/C max dose gradually to prevent Szs **W/P:** [X, –] **CI:** PRG, glaucoma, hyperthyroidism, use w/ or w/in 14 d of MAOI **Disp:** Caps (phentermine/topiramate ER) 3.75/23, 7.5/46, 11.25/69, 15/92 mg **SE:** Paresthesia, dizziness, dysgeusia, insomnia, constipation, dry mouth, ↑ HR, ↑ BP, palpitations, HA, restlessness, mood change, memory impair, metabolic acidosis, kidney stones, ↑ Cr, acute myopia, glaucoma, depression, suicidal behavior/ideation **Notes:** √ PRG baseline & qmo; effective contraception necessary, √ HR/BP/electrolytes REMS restricted distribution

Phenylephrine, Nasal (Neo-Synephrine Nasal [OTC]) BOX: Not for use in peds < 2 y Uses: *Nasal congestion* Acts: α-Adrenergic agonist Dose: *Adults.* 0.25–1% 2–3 sprays/drops in each nostril 94 h PRN. *Peds 2–6 y.* 0.125% 1 drop/nostril q2–4h. *6–12 y:* 1–2 sprays/nostril q4h 0.25% 2–3 drops W/P: [C, +/–] HTN, acute pancreatitis, hep, coronary Dz, NAG, hyperthyroidism CI: ↓ HR, arrhythmias Disp: Nasal spray 0.25, 0.5, 1%; drops: 0.125, 0.25 mg/mL SE: Arrhythmias, HTN, nasal irritation, dryness, sneezing, rebound congestion w/ prolonged use, HA Notes: Do not use > 3 d

Phenylephrine, Ophthalmic (Neo-Synephrine Ophthalmic, AK-Dilate, Zincfrin [OTC]) Uses: *Mydriasis, ocular redness [OTC], perioperative mydriasis, posterior synechiae, uveitis w/ posterior synechiae* Acts: α-Adrenergic agonist Dose: *Adults. Redness:* 1 gtt 0.12% q3–4h PRN up to qid. *Exam mydriasis:* 1 gtt 2.5% (15 min–1 h for effect). *Preop:* 1 gtt 2.5–10% 30–60 min preop. *Peds.* As adult, only use 2.5% for exam, preop, and ocular conditions W/P: [C, May cause late-term fetal anoxia/↓ HR, +/–] HTN, w/ elderly w/ CAD CI: NAG Disp: Ophthal soln 0.12% (Zincfrin OTC), 2.5, 10% SE: Tearing, HA, irritation, eye pain, photophobia, arrhythmia, tremor

Phenylephrine, Oral (Sudafed, Others [OTC]) BOX: Not for use in peds < 2 y Uses: *Nasal congestion* Acts: α-Adrenergic agonist Dose: *Adults.* 10–20 mg PO q4h PRN, max 60 mg/d. *Peds.* 4 5 y: 2.5 mg q4h max 6 doses/d, > 6–12: 5 mg q4h, max 30 mg/d ≥ 12: adult dosing W/P: [C, +/–] HTN, acute pancreatitis, hep, coronary Dz, NAG, hyperthyroidism CI: MAOI w/in 14 d, NAG, severe ↑ BP or CAD, urinary retention Disp: Liq 7.5 mg/5 mL; drops: 1.25/0.8 mL, 2.5 mg/5 mL; tabs 5, 10 mg; chew tabs 10 mg; tabs once daily 10 mg; strips: 1.25, 2.5, 10 mg; many combo OTC products SE: Arrhythmias, HTN, HA, agitation, anxiety, tremor, palpitations; can be chemically processed into methamphetamine; products now sold behind pharmacy counter w/o prescription

Phenylephrine, Systemic (Generic) BOX: Prescribers should be aware of full prescribing information before use Uses: *Vascular failure in shock, allergy, or drug-induced ↓ BP* Acts: α-Adrenergic agonist Dose: *Adults. Mild–mod ↓ BP:* 2–5 mg IM or SQ ↑ BP for 2 h; 0.1–0.5 mg IV elevates BP for 15 min. *Severe ↓ BP/ shock:* Cont Inf at 100–180 mcg/min; after BP stable *Peds.* ↓ *BP:* 5–20 mcg/kg/ dose IV q10–15min or 0.1–0.5 mcg/kg/min IV Inf, titrate to effect W/P: [C, +/–] HTN, acute pancreatitis, hep, coronary Dz, NAG, hyperthyroidism CI: ↓ HR, arrhythmias Disp: Inj 10 mg/mL SE: Arrhythmias, HTN, peripheral vasoconstriction ↑ w/ oxytocin, MAOIs, & TCAs; HA, weakness, necrosis, ↓ renal perfusion Notes: Restore blood vol if loss has occurred; use large veins to avoid extrav; phentolamine 10 mg in 10–15 mL of NS for local Inj to Rx extrav

Phenytoin (Dilantin, Generic) Uses: *Sz disorders* Acts: ↓ Sz spread in the motor cortex Dose: *Adults & Peds. Load:* 15–20 mg/kg IV, 50 mg/min max or PO in 400-mg doses at 4-h intervals; *Adults. Maint:* Initial 200 mg PO or IV bid or 300 mg hs then follow levels; alternatively 5–7 mg/kg/d based on IBW ÷

daily-tid, *Peds. Maint:* 4–7 mg/kg/24h PO or IV ÷ daily-bid; avoid PO susp (erratic absorption) **W/P:** [D, +] **CI:** Heart block, sinus bradycardia **Disp:** *Dilantin Infatab:* chew 50 mg. *Dilantin/Phenytek:* caps 100 mg; caps, ER 30, 100, 200, 300 mg; susp 125 mg/5 mL; Inj 50 mg/mL **SE:** Nystagmus/ataxia early signs of tox; gum hyperplasia w/ long-term use. *IV:* ↓ BP, ↓ HR, arrhythmias, phlebitis; peripheral neuropathy, rash, blood dyscrasias, SJS **Notes:** Levels: *Trough:* Just before next dose. *Therapeutic:* 10–20 mcg/mL *Toxic:* > 20 mcg/mL Phenytoin albumin bound, levels = bound & free phenytoin; w/ ↓ albumin & azotemia, low levels may be therapeutic (nl free levels); do not change dosage at intervals < 7–10 d; hold tube feeds 1 h before and after dose if using oral susp; avoid large dose ↑

Physostigmine (Generic) Uses: *Reverse toxic CNS effects of atropine & scopolamine OD* **Acts:** Reversible cholinesterase inhib **Dose:** *Adults.* 0.5–2 mg IV or IM q20 min *Peds.* 0.01–0.03 mg/kg/dose IV q5–10 min up to 2 mg total PRN **W/P:** [C, ?] **CI:** GI/GU obst, CV Dz, asthma **Disp:** Inj 1 mg/mL **SE:** Rapid IV administration associated w/ Szs; cholinergic SEs; sweating, salivation, lacrimation, GI upset, asystole, changes in HR **Notes:** Excessive readministration can result in cholinergic crisis; crisis reversed w/ atropine; contains bisulfite (allergy possible)

Phytonadione [Vitamin K₁] (Mephyton, Generic) BOX: Hypersens Rxns associated w/ or immediately following Inf Uses: *Coagulation disorders d/t faulty formation of factors II, VII, IX, X*; hyperalimentation **Acts:** Cofactor for production of factors II, VII, IX, & X **Dose:** *Adults & Peds. Anticoagulant-induced prothrombin deficiency:* 1–10 mg PO or IV slowly. *Hyperalimentation:* 10 mg IM or IV qwk. *Infants:* 0.5–1 mg/dose; IM w/in 1 h of brith, or PO **W/P:** [C, +] **CI:** Allergy **Disp:** Tabs 5 mg; Inj 2, 10 mg/mL **SE:** Anaphylaxis from IV dosage; give IV slowly; GI upset (PO), Inj site Rxns **Notes:** w/ Parenteral Rx, 1st change in PT/INR usually seen in 12–24 h; use makes rewarfarinization more difficult; see label for dosing algorithm based on INR of S/Sx of bleeding

Pimecrolimus (Elidel) BOX: Associated w/ rare skin malignancies and lymphoma, limit to area, not for age < 2 y Uses: *Atopic dermatitis* refractory, severe perianal itching **Acts:** Inhibits T lymphocytes **Dose:** *Adults & Peds > 2 y.* Apply bid **W/P:** [C, ?/–] w/ Local Infxn, lymphadenopathy; immunocompromised; avoid in pts < 2 y **CI:** Allergy component, < 2 y **Disp:** Cream 1% **SE:** Phototox, local irritation/burning, flu-like Sxs, may ↑ malignancy **Notes:** Use on dry skin only; wash hands after; 2nd-line/short-term use only

Pimozide (Orap) BOX: ↑ Mortality in elderly w/ dementia-related psychosis Uses: * Tourette Dz* agitation, psychosis **Acts:** Typical antipsychotic, dopamine antagonist **Dose:** Inital 1–2 mg/d to max of 10 mg/d or 0.2 mg/kg/d (whichever is less); ↓ hepatic impair **W/P:** [C/–] NAG, elderly, hepatic impair, neurologic Dz, **CI:** compound hypersens, CNS depression, coma, dysrhythmia, ↑ QT syndrome, w/ QT prolonging drugs, ↓ K, ↓ Mg, w/ CYP3A4 inhib (Table 10, p 319) **Disp:** Tabs 1, 2 mg **SE:** CNS (somnolence, agitation, others), rash, xerostomia, weakness, rigidity, visual changes, constipation, ↑ salivation, akathisia, tardive dyskinesia, neuroleptic malignant syndrome, ↑ QT **Notes:** ✓ ECG

Pindolol (Generic) Uses: *HTN* Acts: β-Adrenergic receptor blocker, β$_1$, β$_2$, ISA Dose: 5–10 mg bid, 60 mg/d max; ↓ in hepatic/renal failure W/P: [B (1st tri; D 2nd/3rd tri), +/–] CI: Uncompensated CHF, cardiogenic shock, ↓ HR, heart block, asthma, COPD Disp: Tabs 5, 10 mg SE: Insomnia, dizziness, fatigue, edema, GI upset, dyspnea; fluid retention may exacerbate CHF

Pioglitazone (Actos, Generic) BOX: May cause or worsen CHF Uses: *Type 2 DM* Acts: ↑ Insulin sensitivity, a thiazolidinedione Dose: 15–45 mg/d PO W/P: [C, –] w/ Hx bladder CA; do not use w/ active bladder CA CI: CHF, hepatic impair Disp: Tabs 15, 30, 45 mg SE: Wt gain, myalgia, URI, HA, hypoglycemia, edema, ↑ fracture risk in women; may ↑ bladder CA risk Notes: Not 1st-line agent

Pioglitazone/Metformin (ACTOplus Met, ACTOplus MET XR, Generic) BOX: Metformin can cause lactic acidosis, fatal in 50% of cases; pioglitazone may cause or worsen CHF Uses: *Type 2 DM as adjunct to diet and exercise* Acts: Combined ↑ insulin sensitivity w/ ↓ hepatic glucose release Dose: Initial 1 tab PO daily or bid, titrate; max daily pioglitazone 45 mg & metformin 2550 mg; XR: 1 tab PO daily w/ evening meal; max daily pioglitazone 45 mg & metformin IR 2550 mg, metformin ER 2000 mg; give w/ meals W/P: [C, –] Stop w/ radiologic IV contrast agents; w/ Hx bladder CA; do not use w/ active bladder CA CI: CHF, renal impair, acidosis Disp: Tabs (pioglitazone mg/metformin mg): 15/500, 15/850; Tabs XR (pioglitazone mg/metformin ER mg) 15/1000, 30/1000 mg SE: Lactic acidosis, CHF, ↓ glucose, edema, Wt gain, myalgia, URI, HA, GI upset, liver damage Notes: Follow LFTs; ↑ fracture risk in women receiving pioglitazone; pioglitazone may ↑ bladder CA risk

Piperacillin/Tazobactam (Zosyn, Generic) Uses: *Infxns of skin, bone, resp & urinary tract, Abd, sepsis* Acts: 4th-gen PCN plus β-lactamase inhib; bactericidal; ↓ cell wall synth. *Spectrum:* Good gram(+), excellent gram(–); anaerobes & β-lactamase producers Dose: *Adults.* 3.375–4.5 g IV q6h; ↓ in renal Insuff W/P: [B, M] CI: PCN or β-lactam sensitivity Disp: Frozen and powder for Inj: 2.25, 3.375, 4.5 g SE: D, HA, insomnia, GI upset, serum sickness-like Rxn, pseudomembranous colitis Notes: Often used in combo w/ aminoglycoside

Pirbuterol (Maxair, Autohaler) Uses: *Prevention & Rx reversible bronchospasm* Acts: β$_2$-Adrenergic agonist Dose: 2 Inh q4–6h; max 12 Inh/d W/P: [C, ?/–] Disp: Aerosol 0.2 mg/actuation (contains ozone-depleting CFCs; will be gradually removed from US market) SE: Nervousness, restlessness, trembling, HA, taste changes, tachycardia Notes: Teach pt proper inhaler technique

Piroxicam (Feldene, Generic) BOX: May ↑ risk of cardiovascular CV events & GI bleeding Uses: *Arthritis & pain* Acts: NSAID; ↓ prostaglandins Dose: 10–20 mg/d W/P: [C/D if 3rd tri, –] GI bleeding CI: ASA/NSAID sensitivity Disp: Caps 10, 20 mg SE: Dizziness, rash, GI upset, edema, acute renal failure, peptic ulcer

Pitavastatin (Livalo) Uses: *Reduce elevated total cholesterol* Acts: Statin, inhibits HMG-CoA reductase Dose: 1–4 mg once/d w/o regard to meals; CrCl < 60 mL/min start 1 mg w/ 2 mg max W/P: [X, /–] May cause myopathy and rhabdomyolysis CI: Active liver Dz, w/ lopinavir/ritonavir/cyclosporine, severe renal impair not on dialysis Disp: Tabs 1, 2, 4 mg SE: Muscle pain, back pain, jt pain, and constipation, ↑ LFTs Notes: ✓ LFTs; OK w/ grapefruit

Plasma Protein Fraction (Plasmanate) Uses: *Shock & ↓ BP* Acts: Plasma vol expander Dose: *Adults.* *Initial:* 250–500 mL IV (not > 10 mL/min); subsequent Inf based on response. *Peds.* 10–15 mL/kg/dose IV; subsequent Inf based on response; safety & efficacy in children not established W/P: [C, +] CI: Renal Insuff, CHF, cardiopulmonary bypass Disp: Inj 5% SE: ↓ BP w/ rapid Inf; hypocoagulability, metabolic acidosis, PE Notes: 0.25 mEq K/L & 145 mEq Na/L; not substitute for RBC

Plerixafor (Mozobil) Uses: *Mobilize stem cells for ABMT in lymphoma and myeloma in combo w/ G-CSF* Acts: Hematopoietic stem cell mobilizer Dose: 0.24 mg/kg SQ daily; max 40 mg/d); CrCl < 50 mL/min: 0.16 mg/kg, max 27 mg/d) W/P: [D, /?] CI: Disp: IV: 20 mg/mL (1.2 mL) SE: HA, N/V/D, Inj site Rxns, ↑ WBC, ↓ plt Notes: Give w/ filgrastim 10 mcg/kg

Pneumococcal 13-Valent Conjugate Vaccine (Prevnar 13) Uses: *Immunization against pneumococcal Infxns in infants & children* Acts: Active immunization Dose: 0.5 mL IM/dose; series of 4 doses; 1st dose age 2 mo; then 4 mo, 6 mo, and 12–15 mo; if previous *Prevnar* switch to *Prevnar 13*; if completed *Prevnar* series, supplemental dose *Prevnar 13* at least 8 wk after last *Prevnar* dose W/P: [C, +] w/ ↓ plt CI: Sensitivity to components/diphtheria toxoid, febrile illness Disp: Inj SE: Local Rxns, anorexia, fever, irritability, ↑/↓ sleep, V, D Notes: Keep epi (1:1000) available for Rxns; replaces *Prevnar* (has additional factors); does not replace *Pneumovax-23* in age > 24 mo w/ immunosuppression; inactivated capsular antigens

Pneumococcal Vaccine, Polyvalent (Pneumovax 23) Uses: *Immunization against pneumococcal Infxns in pts at high risk (all pts > 65 y, also asplenia, sickle cell Dz, HIV, and other immunocompromised and w/ chronic illnesses)* Acts: Active immunization Dose: 0.5 mL IM or SQ W/P: [C, ?] CI: Do not vaccinate during immunosuppressive Rx Disp: Inj 0.5 mL SE: Fever, Inj site Rxn also hemolytic anemia w/ other heme conditions, ↓ plt w/ stable ITP, anaphylaxis, Guillain-Barré synd Notes: Keep epi (1:1000) available for Rxns. Revaccinate q3–5 y if very high risk (eg, asplenia, nephrotic synd), consider revaccination if > 6 y since initial or if previously vaccinated w/ 14-valent vaccine; inactivated capsular antigens

Podophyllin (Podocon-25, Condylox Gel 0.5%, Condylox) Uses: *Topical Rx of benign growths (genital & perianal warts [condylomata acuminata]*, papillomas, fibromas) Acts: Direct antimitotic effect; exact mechanism unknown Dose: *Condylox gel & Condylox:* Apply bid for 3 consecutive d/wk then hold for 4 d may repeat 4 × 0.5 mL/d max; *Podocon-25:* Use sparingly on the lesion, leave on for only 30–40 min for 1st application, then 1–4 h on subsequent applications, thoroughly wash off; limit < 5 mL or < 10 cm²/Rx **W/P:** [X, ?] Immunosuppression **CI:** DM, bleeding lesions **Disp:** *Podocon-25* (w/ benzoin) 15-mL bottles; *Condylox gel* 0.5% 3.5-g clear gel; *Condylox soln* 0.5% 3.5-g clear **SE:** Local Rxns, sig absorption; anemias, tachycardia, paresthesias, GI upset, renal/hepatic damage **Notes:** *Podocon-25* applied by the clinician; do not dispense directly to pt

Polyethylene Glycol [PEG]-Electrolyte Soln (GoLYTELY, Colyte)
Uses: *Bowel prep prior to examination or surgery* **Acts:** Osmotic cathartic **Dose:** *Adults.* Following 3- to 4-h fast, drink 240 mL of soln q10min until 4 L consumed or until BMs are clear. *Peds.* 25–40 mL/kg/h for 4–10 h until BM clear; max dose 4L? **W/P:** [C, ?] **CI:** GI obst, bowel perforation, megacolon, UC **Disp:** Powder for recons to 4 L **SE:** Cramping or N, bloating **Notes:** 1st BM should occur in approximately 1 h; chilled soln more palatable; flavor packets available

Polyethylene Glycol [PEG] 3350 (MiraLAX [OTC]) **Uses:** *Occasional constipation* **Acts:** Osmotic laxative **Dose:** 17-g powder (1 heaping tsp) in 8 oz (1 cup) of H_2O & drink; max 14 d **W/P:** [C, ?] Rule out bowel obst before use **CI:** GI obst, allergy to PEG **Disp:** Powder for reconstitution; bottle cap holds 17 g **SE:** Upset stomach, bloating, cramping, gas, severe D, hives **Notes:** Can add to H_2O, juice, soda, coffee, or tea

Pomalidomide (Pomalyst) **BOX:** CI in PRG. A thalidomide analogue: a teratogen that causes life-threatening birth defects. Obtain 2 negative PRG tests prior to use; use 2 methods of contraception or abstain from sex during & for 4 wk after stopping. Only available through POMALYST REMS Program. Risk for VTE **Uses:** *Multiple myeloma w/ 2 prior therapies including lenalidomide & bortezomib & w/ Dz prog on or w/in 60 d of therapy* **Acts:** Immunomodulatory w/ antineoplastic activity **Dose:** *Adults.* 4 mg PO daily d 1–21 of 28-d cycle; repeat until Dz prog; on empty stomach, swallow whole; see label for tox dose adjustments; avoid w/ SCr > 3 mg/dL, bili > 2 mg/dL, AST/ALT > 3 × ULN **W/P:** [X, –] √ for hematologic tox; avoid w/ strong inhib/induc CYP1A2, CYP3A, or P-glycoprotein; smoking ↓ efficacy **CI:** PRG **Disp:** Caps 1, 2, 3, 4 mg **SE:** Fatigue, asthenia, ↓ WBC/HGB/plts, N/V/D, constipation, dyspnea, URI, back pain, pyrexia, VTE, dizziness, confusion, neuropathy, hypersens Rxn, rash **Notes:** Do not donate blood during Tx & × 1 mo after; males must use condom during sex w/ Tx & × 28 d after; do not donate sperm

Posaconazole (Noxafil) **Uses:** *Prevent Aspergillus and Candida Infxns in severely immunocompromised; Rx oropharyngeal candida* **Acts:** ↓ Cell membrane ergosterol synth **Dose:** *Adults. Invasive fungal prophylaxis:* 200 mg PO tid. *Oropharyngeal candidiasis:* 100 mg bid on day 1, then 100 mg daily × 13 d *Peds > 13 y.* See adult dose **W/P:** [C, ?] Multiple drug interactions; ↑ QT, cardiac Dzs, severe renal/liver impair **CI:** Component hypersens; w/ many drugs including alfuzosin, astemizole, alprazolam, phenothiazines, terfenadine, triazolam, others **Disp:** Soln 40 mg/mL **SE:** ↑ QT, ↑ LFTs, hepatic failure, fever, N/V/D, HA, Abd pain, anemia, ↓ plt, ↓ K+ rash, dyspnea, cough, anorexia, fatigue **Notes:** Monitor LFTs, CBC, lytes; administer w/ meal or nutritional supplement

Potassium Citrate (Urocit-K, Generic) Uses: *Alkalinize urine, prevention of urinary stones (uric acid, calcium stones if hypocitraturic)* Acts: Urinary alkalinizer Dose: 30–60 mEq/d based on severity of hypocitraturia. Max 100 mEq/d W/P: [A, +] CI: Severe renal impair, dehydration, ↑ K+, peptic ulcer; w/ K+-sparing diuretics, salt substitutes Disp: Tabs 5, 10, 15 mEq/d SE: GI upset, ↓ Ca2+, ↑ K+, metabolic alkalosis

Potassium Iodide [Lugol Soln] (Iosat, SSKI, Thyro-Block, ThyroSafe, ThyroShield) [OTC] Uses: *Thyroid storm*, ↓ vascularity before thyroid surgery, block thyroid uptake of radioactive iodine (nuclear scans or nuclear emergency), thin bronchial secretions Acts: Iodine supl Dose: *Adults & Peds > 2 y. Preop thyroidectomy:* 50–100 mg PO tid (1–2 gtts or 0.05–0.1 mL SSKI); give 10 d preop. *Protection:* 130 mg/d. *Peds. Protection: < 1 y:* 16.25 mg qd. *1 mo–3y:* 32.5 mg qd. *3–18 y:* 65 mg once daily W/P: [D, +] ↑ K+, TB, PE, bronchitis, renal impair CI: Iodine sensitivity Disp: Tabs 65, 130 mg; soln (saturated soln of potassium iodide [SSKI]) 1 g/mL; Lugol soln, strong iodine 100 mg/mL; syrup 325 mg/5 mL SE: Fever, HA, urticaria, angioedema, goiter, GI upset, eosinophilia Notes: w/ Nuclear radiation emergency, give until radiation exposure no longer exists

Potassium Supplements (Kaon, Kaochlor, K-Lor, Slow-K, Micro-K, Klorvess, Generic) Uses: *Prevention or Rx of ↓ K+* (eg, diuretic use) Acts: K+ supl Dose: *Adults.* 20–100 mEq/d PO ÷ 1–4×/d; IV 10–20 mEq/h, max 40 mEq/h & 150 mEq/d (monitor K+ levels frequently and in presence of continuous ECG monitoring w/ high-dose IV). *Peds.* Calculate K+ deficit; 1–3 mEq/kg/d PO ÷ 1-4× /d; IV max dose 0.5–1 mEq/kg/× 1–2 h W/P: [A, +] Renal Insuff, use w/ NSAIDs & ACE inhib CI: ↑ K+ Disp: PO forms (Table 6, p 314) Inj SE: GI irritation; ↓ HR, ↑ K+, heart block Notes: Mix powder & liq w/ beverage (unsalted tomato juice, etc); swallow SR tabs must be swallowed whole; follow monitor K+; Cl− salt OK w/ alkalosis; w/ acidosis use acetate, bicarbonate, citrate, or gluconate salt; do not administer IV K+ undiluted

Pralatrexate (Folotyn) Uses: *Tx refractory T-cell lymphoma* Acts: Folate analogue metabolic inhib; ↓ dihydrofolate reductase Dose: *Adults.* IV push over 3–5 min: 30 mg/m2 once weekly for 6 wk W/P: [D, −] Disp: Inj 20 mg/mL (1 mL, 2 mL) SE: ↓ Plt, anemia, ↓ WBC, mucositis, N/V/D, edema, fever, fatigue, rash Notes: Give folic acid supplements prior to and after; ANC should be ≥ 1000/mm3

Pramipexole (Mirapex, Mirapex ER, Generic) Uses: *Parkinson Dz (Mirapex, Mirapex ER),* restless leg synd *(Mirapex)* Acts: Dopamine agonist Dose: *Mirapex:* 1.5–4.5 mg PO, initial 0.375 mg/d in 3 ÷ doses; titrate slowly; *RLS:* 0.125–0.5 mg PO 2–3 h before bedtime. *Mirapex ER:* Start 0.375 PO daily, ↑ dose every 5–7 d to 0.75, then by 0.75 mg to max 4.5 mg/d W/P: [C, ?/−] Daytime falling asleep, ↓ BP CI: None Disp: *Mirapex:* Tabs 0.125, 0.25, 0.5, 0.75, 1, 1.5 mg; *Mirapex*

ER: 0.375, 0.75, 1.5, 2.25, 3, 3.75, 4.5 mg **SE:** Somnolence, N, constipation, dizziness, fatigue, hallucinations, dry mouth, muscle spasms, edema

Pramoxine (Anusol Ointment, ProctoFoam-NS, Others) Uses: *Relief of pain & itching from hemorrhoids, anorectal surgery*; topical for burns & dermatosis **Acts:** Topical anesthetic **Dose:** Apply freely to anal area 3–5x/d **W/P:** [C, ?] **Disp:** [OTC] All 1%; foam (*ProctoFoam-NS*), cream, oint, lotion, gel, pads, spray **SE:** Contact dermatitis, mucosal thinning w/ chronic use

Pramoxine/Hydrocortisone (ProctoFoam-HC) Uses: *Relief of pain & itching from hemorrhoids* **Acts:** Topical anesthetic, anti-inflammatory **Dose:** Apply freely to anal area tid-qid **W/P:** [C, ?/–] **Disp:** *Cream:* pramoxine 1% acetate 1/2.5/2.35%, *foam:* pramoxine 1% hydrocortisone 1%; *lotion;* pramoxine 1% hydrocortisone 1/2.5%; *ointment* pramoxine 1% & hydrocortisone 1/2.5% **SE:** Contact dermatitis, mucosal thinning w/ chronic use

Prasugrel (Effient) BOX: Can cause significant, sometimes fatal, bleeding; do not use w/ planned CABG, w/ active bleeding, Hx TIA / stroke or pts > 75 y **Uses:** *↓ Thrombotic CV events (eg, stent thrombosis) post-PCI*, administer ASAP in ECC setting w/ high-risk ST depression or T-wave inversion w/ planned PCI **Acts:** ↓ Plt aggregation **Dose:** 10 mg/d; Wt < 60 kg, consider 5 mg/d; 60 mg PO loading dose in ECC; use at least 12 mo w/ cardiac stent (bare or drug eluting); consider > 15 mo w/ drug eluting stent **W/P:** [B, ?] Active bleeding; ↑ bleed risk; w/ CYP3A4 substrates **CI:** Active bleed, Hx TIA/stroke risk factors: > 75 y, propensity to bleed, Wt < 60 kg, CABG, meds that ↑ bleeding **Disp:** Tabs 5, 10 mg **SE:** ↑ Bleeding time, ↑ BP, GI intolerance, HA, dizziness, rash, ↓ WBC **Notes:** Plt aggregation to baseline ~ 7 d after D/C, plt transfusion reverses acutely

Pravastatin (Pravachol, Generic) Uses: *↓ Cholesterol* **Acts:** HMG-CoA reductase inhib **Dose:** 10–80 mg PO hs; ↓ in sig renal/hepatic impair **W/P:** [X, –] w/ Gemfibrozil **CI:** Liver Dz or persistent LFTs ↑ **Disp:** Tabs 10, 20, 40, 80 mg **SE:** Use caution w/ concurrent gemfibrozil; HA, GI upset, hep, myopathy, renal failure **Notes:** OK w/ grapefruit juice

Prazosin (Minipress, Generic) Uses: *HTN* **Acts:** Peripherally acting α-adrenergic blocker **Dose:** *Adults.* 1 mg PO tid; can ↑ to 20 mg/d max PRN. *Peds.* 0.05–0.1 mg/kg/d in 3 ÷ doses; max 0.5 mg/kg/d **W/P:** [C, ?] Use w/ phosphodiesterase-5 (PDE5) inhib (eg, sildenafil) can cause ↓ BP **CI:** Component allergy, concurrent use of PDE5 inhib **Disp:** Caps 1, 2, 5 mg; tabs ER 2.5, 5 mg **SE:** Dizziness, edema, palpitations, fatigue, GI upset **Notes:** Can cause orthostatic ↓ BP, take the 1st dose hs; tolerance develops to this effect; tachyphylaxis may result

Prednisolone (Flo-Pred, Omnipred, Orapred, Pediapred, Generic) (See Steroids, p 259 & Table 2, p 301)

Prednisone (Generic)(See Steroids, p 259 & Table 2, p 301)

Pregabalin (Lyrica, Generic) Uses: *DM peripheral neuropathy pain; postherpetic neuralgia; fibromyalgia; adjunct w/ adult partial onset Szs* **Acts:** Nerve transmission modulator, antinociceptive, antiseizure effect; mechanism ?; related to gabapentin **Dose:** *Neuropathic pain:* 50 mg PO tid, ↑ to 300 mg/d w/in 1 wk based on response, 300 mg/d max *Postherpetic neuralgia:* 75–150 mg bid or 50–100 mg tid; start 75 mg bid or 50 mg tid; ↑ to 300 mg/d w/in 1 wk PRN; if pain persists after 2–4 wk, ↑ to 600 mg/d. *Partial onset Sz:* start 150 mg/d (75 mg bid or 50 mg tid) may ↑ to max 600 mg/d; ↓ w/ CrCl < 60; w/ or w/o food **W/P:** [C, –] w/ Sig renal impair (see PI), w/ elderly & severe CHF avoid abrupt D/C **CI:** Hypersensitivity **Disp:** Caps 25, 50, 75, 100, 150, 200, 225, 300 mg; soln 20 mg/mL **SE:** Dizziness, drowsiness, xerostomia, edema, blurred vision, Wt gain, difficulty concentrating; suicidal ideation **Notes:** w/ D/C, taper over at least 1 wk

Probenecid (Probalan, Generic) Uses: *Prevent gout & hyperuricemia; extends levels of PCNs & cephalosporins* **Acts:** Uricosuric, renal tubular blocker of weak organic anions **Dose:** *Adults. Gout:* 250 mg bid × 1 wk, then 500 mg PO bid; can ↑ by 500 mg/mo up to 2–3 g/d. *Antibiotic effect:* 1–2 g PO 30 min before dose. *Peds > 2 y.* 25 mg/kg, then 40 mg/kg/d PO qid **W/P:** [B, ?] **CI:** Uric acid kidney stones, initiations during accute gout attack, coadministration of salicylates, age < 2 y, MDD, renal impair **Disp:** Tabs 500 mg **SE:** HA, GI upset, rash, pruritus, dizziness, blood dyscrasias

Procainamide (Generic) **BOX:** Positive ANA titer or SLE w/ prolonged use; only use in life-threatening arrhythmias; hematologic tox can be severe, follow CBC **Uses:** *Supraventricular/ventricular arrhythmias* **Acts:** Class 1a antiarrhythmic (Table 9, p 318) **Dose:** *Adults. Recurrent VF/VT:* 20–50 mg/min IV (total 17 mg/kg max). *Maint:* 1–4 mg/min. *Stable wide-complex tachycardia of unknown origin, AF w/ rapid rate in WPW:* 20 mg/min IV until arrhythmia suppression, ↓ BP, or QRS widens > 50%, then 1–4 mg/min. *Recurrent VF/VT:* 20–50 mg/min IV; max total 17 mg/kg. *ECC 2010. Stable monomorphic VT, refractory reentry SVT, stable wide-complex tachycardia, AFib w/ WPW:* 20 mg/ min IV until one of these: arrhythmia stopped, hypotension, QRS widens > 50%, total 17 mg/kg; then maint IV inf 1–4 mg/min. *Peds. ECC 2010. SVT, aflutter, VT (w/ pulses):* 15 mg/kg IV/IO over 30–60 min **W/P:** [C, +] In renal/hepatic impair **CI:** Complete heart block, 2nd-/3rd-degree heart block w/o pacemaker, torsades de pointes, SLE **Disp:** Inj 100, 500 mg/mL **SE:** ↓ BP, lupus-like synd, GI upset, taste perversion, arrhythmias, tachycardia, heart block, angioneurotic edema, blood dyscrasias **Notes:** Levels: *Trough:* Just before next dose. *Therapeutic:* 4–10 mcg/mL; *N*-acetyl procainamide (NAPA) + procaine 10–30 mcg/mL *Toxic* (procainamide only): > 10 mcg/mL; NAPA + procaine > 30 mcg/mL *half-life:* procaine 3–5 h, NAPA 6–10 h

Procarbazine (Matulane) **BOX:** Highly toxic; handle w/ care; should be administard under the supervision of an experienced CA chemotherapy physician **Uses:** *Hodgkin Dz*, NHL, brain & lung tumors **Acts:** Alkylating agent; ↓ DNA & RNA synth **Dose:** Per protocol **W/P:** [D, ?] w/ EtOH ingestion **CI:** Inadequate BM reserve **Disp:** Caps 50 mg **SE:** ↓ BM, hemolytic Rxns (w/ G6PD deficiency),

N/V/D; disulfiram-like Rxn; cutaneous & constitutional Sxs; myalgia, arthralgia, CNS effects, azoospermia, cessation of menses

Prochlorperazine (Compro, Procomp, Generic) BOX: ↑ Mortality in elderly pts w/ dementia related psychosis Uses: *N/V, agitation, & psychotic disorders* Acts: Phenothiazine; blocks postsynaptic dopaminergic CNS receptors Dose: *Adults.* Antiemetic: 5–10 mg PO 3–4×/d or 25 mg PR bid or 5–10 mg deep IM q4–6h. Antipsychotic: 10–20 mg IM acutely or 5–10 mg PO 3–4×/d for maint; ↑ doses may be required for antipsychotic effect. *Peds.* 0.1–0.15 mg/kg/dose IM q4–6h or 0.4 mg/kg/24 h PO/PR ÷ 3–4×/d W/P: [C, +/−] NAG, severe liver/cardiac Dz CI: Phenothiazine sensitivity, BM suppression; age < 2 y or Wt < 9 kg Disp: Tabs 5, 10 mg; syrup 5 mg/5 mL; supp 25 mg; Inj 5 mg/mL SE: EPS common; Rx w/ diphenhydramine or benztropine

Promethazine (Promethegan, Generic) BOX: Do not use in pts < 2 y; resp depression risk; tissue damage, including gangrene w/ extravasation Uses: *N/V, motion sickness, adjunct to postop analgesics, sedation, rhinitis* Acts: Phenothiazine; blocks CNS postsynaptic mesolimbic dopaminergic receptors Dose: *Adults.* 12.5–50 mg PO, PR, or IM 2–4×/d PRN. *Peds > 2 y* 0.1–0.5 mg/kg/dose PO/ or IM 4–6h PRN W/P: [C, +/−] Use w/ agents w/ resp depressant effects CI: Component allergy, NAG, age < 2 y Disp: Tabs 12.5, 25, 50 mg; syrup 6.25 mg/5 mL; supp 12.5, 25, 50 mg; Inj 25, 50 mg/mL SE: Drowsiness, tardive dyskinesia, EPS, lowered Sz threshold, ↓ BP, GI upset, blood dyscrasias, photosens, resp depression in children Notes: IM/PO preferred route; not SQ or intra-arterial

Propafenone (Rythmol, Rhythmol SR, Generic) BOX: Excess mortality or nonfatal cardiac arrest rate possible; avoid use w/ asymptomatic and symptomatic non–life-threatening ventricular arrhythmias Uses: *Life-threatening ventricular arrhythmias, AF* Acts: Class Ic antiarrhythmic (Table 9, p 318) Dose: *Adults.* 150–300 mg PO q8h. *Peds.* 8–10 mg/kg/d ÷ in 3–4 doses; may ↑ 2 mg/kg/d, 20 mg/kg/d max W/P: [C, ?] w/ Ritonavir, MI w/in 2 y, w/ liver/renal impair, safety in peds not established CI: Uncontrolled CHF, bronchospasm, cardiogenic shock, AV block w/o pacer Disp: Tabs 150, 225, 300 mg; SR caps 225, 325, 425 mg SE: Dizziness, unusual taste, 1st degree heart block, arrhythmias, prolongs QRS & QT intervals; fatigue, GI upset, blood dyscrasias

Propantheline (Pro-Banthine, Generic) Uses: *PUD*, symptomatic Rx of small intestine hypermotility, spastic colon, ureteral spasm, bladder spasm, pylorospasm Acts: Antimuscarinic Dose: *Adults.* 15 mg PO ac & 30 mg PO hs; ↓ in elderly. *Peds.* 2–3 mg/kg/24 h PO ÷ 3–4×/d W/P: [C, ?] CI: NAG, UC, toxic megacolon, GI atony in elderly, MG, GI/GU obst Disp: 15 mg SE: Anticholinergic (eg, xerostomia, blurred vision)

Propofol (Diprivan, Generic) Uses: *Induction & maint of anesthesia; sedation in intubated pts* Acts: Sedative–hypnotic; mechanism unknown; acts in 40 s Dose: *Adults.* Anesthesia: 2–2.5 mg/kg (also *ECC 2005*), then 100–200 mcg/kg/min Inf. ICU sedation: 5 mcg/kg/min IV, ↑ PRN 5–10 mcg/kg/min q5–10 min,

5–50 mcg/kg/min cont Inf. *Peds. Anesthesia:* 2.5–3.5 mg/kg induction; then 125–300 mcg/kg/min; ↓ in elderly, debilitated, ASA II/IV pts **W/P:** [B, –] **CI:** If general anesthesia CI, sensitivity to egg, egg products, soybeans, soybean products **Disp:** Inj 10 mg/mL **SE:** May ↑ triglycerides w/ extended dosing; ↓ BP, pain at site, apnea, anaphylaxis **Notes:** 1 mL has 0.1-g fat; monitor during Inf for "propofol Inf synd" (eg, heart failure, rhabdomyolysis, renal failure) mostly peds

Propoxyphene (Darvon-N); Propoxyphene/Acetaminophen (Generic); Propoxyphene/Aspirin (Generic) [C-IV] Notes: In November 2010 the FDA banned all products containing propoxyphene due to the increased risk of abnormal and potentially fatal heart rhythm disturbances

Propranolol (Inderal LA, Innopran XL, Generic) Uses: *HTN, angina, MI, hyperthyroidism, essential tremor, hypertrophic subaortic stenosis, pheochromocytoma; prevents migraines & atrial arrhythmias*, thyrotoxicosis **Acts:** ß-Adrenergic receptor blocker, β_1, β_2; only β-blocker to block conversion of T_4 to T_3 **Dose: *Adults.*** *Angina:* 80–320 mg/d PO ÷ 2–4×/d or 80–320 mg/d SR. *Arrhythmia:* 10–30 mg/dose PO q6–8h or 1 mg IV slowly, repeat q5min, 5 mg max. *HTN:* 40 mg PO bid or 60–80 mg/d SR, weekly to max 640 mg/d. *Hypertrophic subaortic stenosis:* 20–40 mg PO 3–4×/d. *MI:* 180–240 mg PO 3–4×/d. *Migraine prophylaxis:* 80 mg/d ÷ 3–4×/d, ↑ weekly 160–240 mg/d ÷ 3–4 ×/d max; wean if no response in 6 wk. *Pheochromocytoma:* 30–60 mg/d ÷ 3–4×/d. *Thyrotoxicosis:* 1–3 mg IV × 1; 10–40 mg PO q6h. *Tremor:* 40 mg PO bid, ↑ PRN 320 mg/d max *ECC 2010: SVT:* 0.5–1 mg IV given over 1 min; repeat PRN up to 0.1 mg/kg. ***Peds.*** *Arrhythmia:* 0.5–1.0 mg/kg/d ÷ 3–4×/d, ↑ PRN q3–7d to 8 mg/kg max; 0.01–0.1 mg/kg IV over 10 min, 1 mg max infants, 3 mg max children. *HTN:* 0.5–1.0 mg/kg ÷ 3–4×/day, PRN q3–7d to 8 mg/kg/d max; ↓ in renal impair **W/P:** [C (1st tri, D if 2nd or 3rd tri), +] **CI:** Uncompensated CHF, cardiogenic shock, HR, heart block, PE, severe resp Dz **Disp:** Tabs 10, 20, 40, 80 mg; SR caps 60, 80, 120, 160 mg; oral soln 4, 8, mg/mL; Inj 1 mg/mL **SE:** ↓ HR, ↓ BP, fatigue, GI upset, ED

Propylthiouracil (Generic) **BOX:** Severe liver failure reported; use only if pt cannot tolerate methimazole; d/t fetal anomalies w/ methimazole, PTU may be DOC in 1st tri Uses: *Hyperthyroidism* **Acts:** ↓ Production of T_3 & T_4 & conversion of T_4 to T_3 **Dose: *Adults.*** *Initial:* 100 mg PO q8h (may need up to 1200 mg/d); after pt euthyroid (6–8 wk), taper dose by 1/2 q4–6wk to maint, 50–150 mg/24 h; can usually D/C in 2–3 y; ↓ in elderly. ***Peds.*** *Initial:* 5–7 mg/kg/24 h PO ÷ q8h. *Maint:* 1/3–2/3 of initial dose **W/P:** [D, –] See Box **CI:** Allergy **Disp:** Tabs 50 mg **SE:** Fever, rash, leukopenia, dizziness, GI upset, taste perversion, SLE-like synd, ↑ LFT, liver failure **Notes:** Monitor pt clinically; report any S/Sx of hepatic dysfunction, ✓ TFT and LFT

Protamine (Generic) **BOX:** Severe ↓ BP, CV collapse, noncardiogenic pulm edema, pulm vasoconstriction, and pulm HTN can occur; risk factors: high dose/ overdose, repeat doses, prior protamine use, current or use of prior protamine-containing product (eg, NPH or protamine zinc insulin, some beta-blockers), fish allergy, prior vasectomy, severe LV dysfunction, abnormal pulm testing; weigh risk/benefit in pts w/ 1 or more risk factors; resuscitation equipment must be available **Uses:** *Reverse heparin effect* **Acts:** Neutralize heparin by forming a stable complex **Dose:** Based on degree of heparin reversal; give IV slowly; 1 mg reverses ~ 100 units of heparin given in the preceding 30 min; 50 mg max **W/P:** [C, ?] **CI:** Allergy **Disp:** Inj 10 mg/mL **SE:** Follow coagulation markers; anticoagulant effect if given w/o heparin; ↓ BP, ↓ HR, dyspnea, hemorrhage **Notes:** ✓ aPTT ~ 15 min after use to assess response

Prothrombin Complex Concentrate (Human) (Kcentra) **BOX:** Risk of fatal & nonfatal arterial & venous TE. Weigh risk of TE vs benefit of reversing VKA. May not be suitable for pts w/ Hx of TE w/in the past 3 mo **Uses:** *Urgent reversal of VKA (vitamin K antagonist) induced coag factor deficiency in pts w/ acute major bleed* **Acts:** Nonactivated 4F-PCC containing 4F K-dep factors II, VII, IX, X & antithrombotic proteins C & S **Dose:** *INR 2–< 4:* 25 units of factor IX/kg (max 2500 units); *INR 4–6:* 35 units of factor IX/kg (max 3500 units); *INR > 6:* 50 units of factor IX/kg (max 5000 units); IV only @ 0.12 mL/kg/min (max 8.4 mL/min); give w/ vit K **W/P:** [C, ?/–] Hypersens Rxn; ✓ S/Sxs of thrombosis; from human plasma, infectious agent risk **CI:** Hx anaphylactic/severe Rxn to factors II, VII, IX, X, protein C & S, heparin, antithrombin III, human albumin; DIC; Hx HIT **Disp:** Inj 500 units/vial (20–31 factor IX units/mL, potency on each carton) **SE:** N/V, HA, arthralgia, ↓ BP, stroke, PE, DVT

Pseudoephedrine (Many OTC Mono and Combination Brands) **Uses:** *Decongestant* **Acts:** Stimulates α-adrenergic receptors w/ vasoconstriction **Dose:** *Adults. IR:* 60 mg PO q4–6h PRN; *ER:* 120 mg PO q12h, 240 mg/d max. *Peds 2–5 y.* 15 mg q4–6h, 60 mg/24 h max. *6–12 y:* 30 mg q4–6h, 120 mg/24 h max; ↓ w/ renal Insuff **W/P:** [C, +] Not rec for use in peds < 2 y **CI:** Poorly controlled HTN or CAD, w/ MAOIs w/in 14 d, urinary retention **Disp:** IR tabs 30, 60 mg; ER caplets 60, 120 mg; ER tabs 120, 240 mg; liq 15, 30 mg/5 mL; syrup 15, 30 mg/5mL; multiple combo OTC products **SE:** HTN, insomnia, tachycardia, arrhythmias, nervousness, tremor **Notes:** Found in many OTC cough/cold preparations; OTC restricted distribution by state (illicit ingredient in methamphetamine production)

Psyllium (Konsyl, Metamucil, Generic) **Uses:** *Constipation & colonic diverticular Dz* **Acts:** Bulk laxative **Dose:** 1.25–30 g/d varies w/ specific product **W/P:** [B, ?] *Effer-Syllium* (effervescent psyllium) usually contains K+, caution w/ renal failure; phenylketonuria (in products w/ aspartame) **CI:** Suspected bowel obst **Disp:** Large variety available: granules; powder, caps, wafers **SE:** D, Abd cramps, bowel obst, constipation, bronchospasm **Notes:** Maintain adequate hydration

Pyrazinamide (Generic) **Uses:** *Active TB in combo w/ other agents* **Acts:** Bacteriostatic; unknown mechanism **Dose:** *Adults.* Dose varies based on Tx option chosen daily 1 × 2 wk–3 × wk; dosing based on lean body Wt; ↓ dose in renal/hepatic impair. *Peds.* 20–40 mg/kg/d PO ÷ daily-bid; ↓ w/ renal/hepatic impair **W/P:** [C, +/–] **CI:** Severe hepatic damage, acute gout **Disp:** Tabs 500 mg **SE:** Hepatotox, malaise, GI upset, arthralgia, myalgia, gout, photosens **Notes:** Use in combo w/ other anti-TB drugs; consult http://www.cdc.gov/tb/ for latest TB recommendations; dosage regimen differs for "directly observed" Rx

Pyridoxine [Vitamin B₆] (Generic) Uses: *Rx & prevention of vit B₆ deficiency* **Acts:** Vit B₆ supl **Dose:** *Adults. Deficiency:* 10–20 mg/d PO. *Drug-induced neuritis:* 100–200 mg/d; 25–100 mg/d prophylaxis. *Peds.* 5–25 mg/d × 3 wk **W/P:** [A (C if doses exceed RDA), +] **CI:** Component allergy tabs 25, 50, 100, 250, 500 mg; tab SR 500 mg; liquid 200 mg, 15 mg; Inj: 100 mg/mL; caps: 50, 250

Quetiapine (Seroquel, Seroquel XR, Generic) **BOX:** Closely monitor pts for worsening depression or emergence of suicidality, particularly in ped pts; not for use in peds; ↑ mortality in elderly w/ dementia-related psychosis **Uses:** *Acute exacerbations of schizophreniab, bipolar Dz* **Acts:** Serotonin & dopamine antagonism **Dose:** 150–750 mg/d; initiate at 25–100 mg bid-tid; slowly ↑ dose; *XR:* 400–800 mg PO q P.M.; start ↑ 300 mg/d, 800 mg/d max ↓ dose w/ hepatic & geriatric pts **W/P:** [C, –] **CI:** Component allergy **Disp:** Tabs 25, 50, 100, 200, 300, 400 mg; tabs XR: 50, 150, 200, 300, 400 mg **SE:** Confusion w/ nefazodone; HA, somnolence, ↑ Wt, ↓ BP, dizziness, cataracts, neuroleptic malignant synd, tardive dyskinesia, ↑ QT interval

Quinapril (Accupril, Generic) **BOX:** ACE inhib used during PRG can cause fetal injury & death **Uses:** *HTN, CHF, DN, post-MI* **Acts:** ACE inhib **Dose:** 10–80 mg PO daily; ↓ in renal impair **W/P:** [D, +] w/ RAS, vol depletion **CI:** ACE inhib sensitivity, angioedema, PRG **Disp:** Tabs 5, 10, 20, 40 mg **SE:** Dizziness, HA, ↓ BP, impaired renal Fxn, taste perversion, cough

Quinidine (Generic) **BOX:** Mortality rates when used to treat non–life-threatening arrhythmias **Uses:** *Prevention of tachydysrhythmias, malaria* **Acts:** Class IA antiarrhythmic **Dose:** *Adults.* Antiarrhythmic IR: 200–400 mg/dose q6h; ER: 300 mg q8–12h (sulfate) 324 mg q8–12h (gluconate) *Peds.* 15–60 mg/kg/24 h PO in 4–5 ÷ doses; ↓ in renal impair **W/P:** [C, +] **CI:** TTP, thrombocytopenia, medications that prolong QT interval, digitalis tox & AV block; conduction disorders **Disp:** *Sulfate:* Tabs 200, 300 mg; SR tabs 300 mg. *Gluconate:* SR tabs 324 mg; Inj 80 mg/mL **SE:** Extreme ↓ BP w/ IV use; syncope, QT prolongation, GI upset, arrhythmias, fatigue, cinchonism (tinnitus, hearing loss, delirium, visual changes), fever, hemolytic anemia, thrombocytopenia, rash **Levels:** *Trough:* just before next dose. *Therapeutic:* 2–5 mcg/mL, some pts require higher levels *Toxic:* > 10 mcg/mL *half-life:* 6–8h; sulfate salt 83% quinidine; gluconate salt 62% quinidine; use w/ drug that slows AV conduction (eg, digoxin, diltiazem, β-blocker) 267 mg of quinidine gluconate = 200 mg of quinidine sulfate

Quinupristin/Dalfopristin (Synercid) **Uses:** *Vancomycin-resistant Infxns d/t E. faecium & other gram(+)* **Acts:** ↓ Ribosomal protein synth. *Spectrum:* Vancomycin-resistant *E. faecium*, methicillin-susceptible *S. aureus, S. pyogenes*; not against *E. faecalis* **Dose:** *Adults & Peds.* 7.5 mg/kg IV q12h (central line preferred); incompatible w/ NS or heparin; flush IV w/ dextrose; ↓ w/ hepatic failure **W/P:** [B, M] Multiple drug interactions w/ drugs metabolized by CYP3A4 (eg, cyclosporine)

CI: Component allergy **Disp:** Inj 500 mg (150 mg quinupristin/350 mg dalfopristin) **SE:** Hyperbilirubinemia, Inf site Rxns & pain, arthralgia, myalgia

Rabeprazole (AcipHex) Uses: *PUD, GERD, ZE* H. pylori **Acts:** Proton pump inhib **Dose:** 20 mg/d; may ↑ to 60 mg/d; H. pylori 20 mg PO bid × 7 d (w/ amoxicillin and clarithromycin); do not crush/chew tabs; do not use clopidogrel **W/P:** [B, ?/–] Do not use w/ clopidogrel, possible ↓ effect (controversial) **Disp:** Tabs 20 mg ER **SE:** HA, fatigue, GI upset **Notes:** ? ↑ Risk of fractures, C. difficile, CAP w/ all PPI; risk of hypomagnesemia w/ long-term use, monitor

Raloxifene (Evista) BOX: Increased risk of venous thrombocmbolism and death from stroke Uses: *Prevent osteoporosis, breast CA prevention* **Acts:** Partial antagonist of estrogen, behaves like estrogen **Dose:** 60 mg/d **W/P:** [X, –] **CI:** Thromboembolism, PRG **Disp:** Tabs 60 mg **SE:** CP, insomnia, rash, hot flashes, GI upset, hepatic dysfunction, leg cramps

Raltegravir (Isentress) Uses: *HIV in combo w/ other antiretroviral agents* **Acts:** HIV-integrase strand transfer inhib **Dose:** 400 mg PO bid, 800 mg PO bid if w/ rifampin; w/ or w/o food **W/P:** [C, –] **CI:** None **Disp:** Tabs 400 mg **SE:** Development of immune reconstitution synd: ↑ CK, myopathy, and rhabdomyolysis, insomnia, N/D, HA, fever, ↑ cholesterol, paranoia, and anxiety **Notes:** Monitor lipid profile; initial therapy may cause immune reconstitution synd (inflammatory response to residual opportunistic Infxns (eg, M. avium, Pneumocystis jiroveci)

Ramelteon (Rozerem) Uses: *Insomnia* **Acts:** Melatonin receptor agonist **Dose:** 8 mg PO 30 min before bedtime **W/P:** [C, ?/–] w/ CYP1A2 inhib **CI:** w/ Fluvoxamine; hypersens **Disp:** Tabs 8 mg **SE:** Somnolence, dizziness **Notes:** Avoid w/ high-fat meal, do not break

Ramipril (Altace, Generic) BOX: ACE inhib used during PRG can cause fetal injury & death Uses: *HTN, CHF, DN, post-MI* **Acts:** ACE inhib **Dose:** 1.25–20 mg/d PO ÷ daily-bid; ↓ in renal failure **W/P:** [C-1st tri/D-2nd & 3rd, +] **CI:** ACE inhib-induced angioedema **Disp:** Caps 1.25, 2.5, 5, 10 mg **SE:** Cough, HA, dizziness, ↓ BP, renal impair, angioedema **Notes:** OK in combo w/ diuretics

Ranibizumab (Lucentis) Uses: *Neovascular "wet" macular degeneration* **Acts:** VEGF inhib **Dose:** 0.5 mg intravitreal Inj qmo **W/P:** [C, ?] Hx thromboembolism **CI:** Periocular Infxn **Disp:** Inj 10 mg/mL **SE:** Endophthalmitis, retinal detachment/hemorrhage, cataract, intraocular inflammation, conjunctival hemorrhage, eye pain, floaters

Ranitidine (Zantac, Zantac EFFERDose [OTC], Generic) Uses: *Duodenal ulcer, active benign ulcers, hypersecretory conditions, & GERD* **Acts:** H_2-receptor antagonist **Dose:** *Adults.* *Ulcer:* 150 mg PO bid, 300 mg hs, or 50 mg IV q6–8h; or 400 mg IV/d cont Inf, then maint of 150 mg PO hs. *Hypersecretion:* 150 mg PO bid, up to 600 mg/d. *GERD:* 300 mg PO bid; maint 300 mg PO hs. *Dyspepsia:* 75 mg PO daily. *Peds.* 1.5–2 mg/kg/dose IV q6–8h or 2 mg/kg/dose PO q12h; ↓ in renal Insuff/failure **W/P:** [B, +] **CI:** Component allergy **Disp:** Tabs 75, 150 mg [OTC], 150, 300 mg; caps 150, 300 mg;

effervescent tabs 25 mg (contains phenylalanine); syrup 15 mg/mL; Inj 25 mg/mL **SE:** Dizziness, sedation, rash, GI upset **Notes:** PO & parenteral doses differ

Ranolazine (Ranexa) **Uses:** *Chronic angina* **Acts:** ↓ Ischemia-related Na$^+$ entry into myocardium **Dose:** *Adults.* 500 mg bid–1000 mg PO bid **CI:** w/ Cirrhosis, CYP3A inhib/inducers (Table 10, p 319) **W/P:** [C, ?/–] HTN may develop w/ renal impair, agents that ↑ QTc, ↓ K$^+$ **Disp:** SR tabs 500, 1000 mg **SE:** Dizziness, HA, constipation, arrhythmias **Notes:** Not 1st line; use w/ amlodipine, nitrates, or β-blockers

Rasagiline Mesylate (Azilect) **Uses:** *Early Parkinson Dz monotherapy; levodopa adjunct w/ advanced Dz* **Acts:** MAO B inhib **Dose:** *Adults. Early Dz:* 1 mg PO daily, start 0.5 mg PO daily w/ levodopa; ↓ w/ CYP1A2 inhib or hepatic impair **CI:** MAOIs, sympathomimetic amines, meperidine, methadone, tramadol, propoxyphene, dextromethorphan, mirtazapine, cyclobenzaprine, St. John's wort, sympathomimetic vasoconstrictors, SSRIs **W/P:** [C, ?] Avoid tyramine-containing foods; mod–severe hepatic impair **Disp:** Tabs 0.5, 1 mg **SE:** Arthralgia, indigestion, dyskinesia, hallucinations, ↓ Wt, postural ↓ BP, N/V, constipation, xerostomia, rash, sedation, CV conduction disturbances **Notes:** Rare melanoma reported; periodic skin exams (skin CA risk); D/C 14 d prior to elective surgery; initial ↓ levodopa dose OK

Rasburicase (Elitek) **BOX:** Anaphylaxis possible; do not use in G6PD deficiency and hemolysis; can cause methemoglobinemia; can interfere w/ uric acid assays; collect blood samples and store on ice **Uses:** *Reduce ↑ uric acid d/t tumor lysis* **Acts:** Catalyzes uric acid **Dose:** *Adult & Peds.* 0.20 mg/kg IV over 30 min, daily × 5; do not bolus, redosing based uric acid levels **W/P:** [C, ?/–] Falsely ↓ uric acid values **CI:** Anaphylaxis, screen for G6PD deficiency to avoid hemolysis, methemoglobinemia **Disp:** 1.5, 7.5 mg powder Inj **SE:** Fever, neutropenia, GI upset, HA, rash **Notes:** Place blood test tube for uric acid level on ice to stop enzymatic Rxn; removed by dialysis; doses as low as 0.05 mg/kg have been used effectively in clinical trials

Regorafenib (Stivarga) **BOX:** May cause severe/fatal hepatotox. Monitor LFTs & dose adjust or D/C for ↑ LFTs or hepatocellular necrosis **Uses:** *Metastatic colorectal CA & GIST (see labeling/institution protocol)* **Acts:** Kinase inhibitor **Dose:** *Adults.* 160 mg PO q A.M. on d 1–21 of 28-d cycle; w/ low-fat food, swallow whole; see label for toxicity dose adjust **W/P:** [D, –] Fetal tox; avoid w/ strong CYP3A4 inhib/induc **CI:** None **Disp:** Tabs 40 mg **SE:** Fatigue, asthenia, N/V/D, Abd pain, ↓ appetite, ↓ Wt, HTN, HFSR, mucositis, dysphonia, Infxn, pain, rash, fever, hemorrhage, wound healing complications, RPLS, cardiac ischemia/infarction, derm tox, GI perforation/fistula

Repaglinide (Prandin) **Uses:** *Type 2 DM* **Acts:** ↑ Pancreatic insulin release **Dose:** 0.5–4 mg ac, PO start 1–2 mg, ↑ to 16 mg/d max; take pc **W/P:** [C, ?/–] **CI:** DKA, type 1 DM **Disp:** Tabs 0.5, 1, 2 mg **SE:** HA, hyper-/hypoglycemia, GI upset

Repaglinide/Metformin (PrandiMet) **BOX:** Associated w/ lactic acidosis, risk ↑ w/ sepsis, dehydration, renal/hepatic impair, ↑ alcohol, acute CHF; Sxs include myalgias, malaise, resp distress, Abd pain, somnolence; Labs: ↓ pH, ↑

anion gap, ↑ blood lactate; D/C immediately & hospitalize if suspected **Uses:** *Type ? DM* **Acts:** Meglitinide & biguanide (see metformin) **Dose:** *Adults.* 1/500 mg bid w/in 15 min pc (skip dose w/ skipped meal); max 10/2500 mg/d or 4/1000 mg/meal **W/P:** [C, –] suspend use w/ iodinated contrast, do not use w/ NPH insulin, use w/ cationic drugs or CYP2C8 & CYP3A4 inhib **CI:** SCr > 1.4 mg/dL (females) or > 1.5 mg/dL (males); metabolic acidosis; w/ gemfibrozil **Disp:** Tabs (repaglinide/metformin mg) 1/500, 2/500 **SE:** Hypoglycemia, HA, N/V/D, anorexia, weakness, myalgia, rash, ↓ vit B_{12}

Retapamulin (Altabax) **Uses:** *Topical Rx impetigo in pts > 9 mo* **Acts:** Pleuromutilin antibiotic, bacteriostatic, ↓ bacteria protein synth; *Spectrum:* S. *aureus* (not MRSA), S. *pyogenes* **Dose:** Apply bid × 5 d **W/P:** [B, ?] **Disp:** 1% ointment **SE:** Local irritation **Notes:** Rx should not exceed 2% BSA in peds or 100 cm² BSA in adults

Reteplase (Retavase) **Uses:** *Post-AMI* **Acts:** Thrombolytic **Dose:** 10 units IV over 2 min, 2nd dose in 30 min, 10 units IV over 2 min; *ECC 2010.* 10 units IV bolus over 2 min; 30 min later, 10 units IV bolus over 2 min w/ NS flush before and after each dose. **W/P:** [C, ?/–] **CI:** Internal bleeding, spinal surgery/trauma, Hx CNS AVM/CVA, bleeding diathesis, severe uncontrolled ↑ BP, sensitivity to thrombolytics **Disp:** IC it: 10.4 units **SE:** Bleeding including CNS, allergic Rxns

Ribavirin (Copegus, Rebetol, Virazole, Generic) **BOX:** Monotherapy for chronic hep C ineffective; hemolytic anemia possible, teratogenic and embryocidal; use 2 forms of birth control for up to 6 mo after D/C drug; decrease in resp Fxn when used in infants as Inh **Uses:** *RSV Infxn in infants [Virazole];* hep C (in combo w/ peg-interferon α-2b)* **Acts:** Unknown **Dose:** *RSV:* 6 g in 300 mL sterile H_2O, Inh over 12–18 h. *Hep C:* See individual product labeling for dosing based on Wt & genotype **W/P:** [X, ?] May accumulate on soft contacts lenses **CI:** PRG, autoimmune hep, CrCl < 50 mL/min **Disp:** Powder for aerosol 6 g; tabs 200, 400, 600 mg, caps 200 mg, soln 40 mg/mL **SE:** Fatigue, HA, GI upset, anemia, myalgia, alopecia, bronchospasm, ↓ HCT; pancytopenia reported **Notes:** Virazole aerosolized by a SPAG, monitor resp Fxn closely; ✓ Hgb/Hct; PRG test monthly; 2 forms birth control, hep C viral genotyping may modify dose

Rifabutin (Mycobutin) **Uses:** *Prevent MAC Infxn in AIDS pts w/ CD4 count < 100 mcL* **Acts:** ↓ DNA-dependent RNA polymerase activity **Dose:** *Adults.* 150–300 mg/d PO. *Peds ≤ 1 y.* 15–25 mg/kg/d PO *Others:* 5 mg/kg/d, max 800 mg/d **W/P:** [B, ?/–] WBC < 1000 cells/mm³ or plts < 50,000 cells/mm³; ritonavir **CI:** Allergy **Disp:** Caps 150 mg **SE:** Discolored urine, rash, neutropenia, leukopenia, myalgia, ↑ LFTs **Notes:** SE/interactions similar to rifampin

Rifampin (Rifadin, Rimactane, Generic) **Uses:** *TB & Rx & prophylaxis of N. meningitidis, H. influenzae, or S. aureus carriers*; adjunct w/ severe S. *aureus* **Acts:** ↓ DNA-dependent RNA polymerase activity **Dose:** *Adults.* N. meningitidis & H. influenzae carrier: 600 mg/d PO for 4 d. *TB:* 600 mg PO or IV daily or 2×/wk w/ combo regimen. **Peds.** 10–20 mg/kg/dose PO or IV daily-bid; ↓ in hepatic failure **W/P:** [C, +] w/ Fosamprenavir, multiple drug interactions **CI:** Allergy, active *N. meningitidis* Infxn, w/ saquinavir/ritonavir **Disp:** Caps 150, 300 mg; Inj 600 mg **SE:** Red-orange–colored bodily fluids, ↑ LFTs, flushing, HA **Notes:** Never use as single agent w/ active TB

Rifapentine (Priftin) Uses: *Pulm TB* **Acts:** ↓ DNA-dependent RNA polymerase. *Spectrum: Mycobacterium tuberculosis* **Dose:** *Intensive phase:* 600 mg PO 2×/wk for 2 mo; separate doses by > 3 d. *Continuation phase:* 600 mg/wk for 4 mo; part of 3–4 drug regimen **W/P:** [C, +/– red-orange breast milk] Strong CYP450 inducer, ↓ protease inhib efficacy, antiepileptics, β-blockers, CCBs **CI:** Rifamycins allergy **Disp:** 150-mg tabs **SE:** Neutropenia, hyperuricemia, HTN, HA, dizziness, rash, GI upset, blood dyscrasias, ↑ LFTs, hematuria, discolored secretions **Notes:** Monitor LFTs

Rifaximin (Xifaxan) Uses: *Traveler's D (noninvasive strains of *E. coli* in pts > 12 y (*Xifaxan*); hepatic encephalopathy (*Xifaxan 550*) > 18 y* **Acts:** Not absorbed, derivative of rifamycin. *Spectrum: E. coli* **Dose:** Diarrhea (*Xifaxan*): 1 tab PO, tid daily × 3 d; encephalopathy (*Xifaxan 550*) > 550 mg PO bid **W/P:** [C, ?/–] Hx allergy; pseudomembranous colitis; w/ severe (Child-Pugh C) hepatic impair **CI:** Allergy to rifamycins **Disp:** Tabs: *Xifaxan:* 200 mg; *Xifaxan 550:* 550 mg **SE:** *Xifaxan:* Flatulence, HA, Abd pain, rectal tenesmus and urgency; N; *Xifaxan 550:* Edema, N, dizziness, fatigue, ascites, flatulence, HA **Notes:** D/C if D Sx worsen or persist > 24–48 h, or w/ fever or blood in stool

Rilpivirine (Edurant) Uses: *HIV in combo w/ other antiretroviral agents* **Acts:** NRTI **Dose:** *Adults.* 25 mg daily **W/P:** [B, –] **CI:** None **Disp:** Tab 25 mg **SE:** HA, depression, insomnia, rash, ↑ AST/ALT, ↑ cholesterol, ↑ SCr **Notes:** Take w/ food; metabolized via CYP3A; CYP3A inducers may ↓ virologic response, CYP3A inhib may ↑ levels; ↑ gastric pH ↓ absorption

Rimantadine (Flumadine, Generic) Uses: *Prophylaxis & Rx of influenza A viral Infxns* **Acts:** Antiviral **Dose:** *Adults & Peds > 9 y.* 100 mg PO bid. *Peds 1–9 y.* 5 mg/kg/d PO, 150 mg/d max; daily w/ severe renal/hepatic impair & elderly; initiate w/in 48 h of Sx onset **W/P:** [C, –] w/ Cimetidine; avoid w/ PRG, breast-feeding **CI:** Component & amantadine allergy **Disp:** Tabs 100 mg **SE:** Orthostatic ↓ BP, edema, dizziness, GI upset, ↓ Sz threshold **Notes:** See CDC (*MMWR*) for current influenza A guidelines

Rimexolone (Vexol Ophthalmic) Uses: *Postop inflammation & uveitis* **Acts:** Steroid **Dose:** *Adults & Peds > 2 y. Uveitis:* 1–2 gtt/h daytime & q2h at night, taper to 1 gtt q6h. *Postop:* 1–2 gtt qid × 2 wk **W/P:** [C, ?/–] Ocular Infxns **Disp:** Susp 1% **SE:** Blurred vision, local irritation **Notes:** Taper dose

Risedronate (Actonel, Actonel W/ Calcium, Generic) Uses: *Paget Dz; Rx/prevention glucocorticoid-induced/postmenopausal osteoporosis, ↑ bone mass in osteoporotic men; w/ calcium only FDA approved for female osteoporosis* **Acts:** Bisphosphonate; ↓ osteoclast-mediated bone resorption **Dose:** *Paget Dz:*

30 mg/d PO for 2 mo. *Osteoporosis Rx/prevention:* 5 mg daily or 35 mg qwk or 150 mg qmo; 30 min before 1st food/drink of the d; stay upright for at least 30 min after dose **W/P:** [C, ?/–] Ca^{2+} supls & antacids ↓ absorption; jaw osteonecrosis, avoid dental work **CI:** Component allergy, ↓ Ca^{2+}, esophageal abnormalities, unable to stand/sit for 30 min, CrCl < 30 mL/min **Disp:** Tabs 5, 30, 35, 150 mg; Risedronate 35 mg (4 tabs)/calcium carbonate 1250 mg (24 tabs) **SE:** Back pain, HA, Abd pain, dyspepsia, arthralgia; flu-like Sxs, hypersensitivity (rash, etc), esophagitis, bone pain, eye inflammation **Notes:** Monitor LFTs, Ca^{2+}, $PO3^{+}$, K^{+}; may ↑ atypical subtrochanteric femur fractures

Risedronate, Delayed-Release (Atelvia) Uses: *Postmenopausal osteoporosis* **Acts:** See Risedronate **Dose:** One 35 mg tab 1 × wk; in ʌ м following breakfast w/ 4-oz water; do not lie down for 30 min **W/P:** [C, ?/–] Ca^{2+} & Fe^{2+} supls/antacids ↓ absorption; do not use w/ Actonel or CrCl < 30 mL/min; jaw osteonecrosis reported, avoid dental work; may ↑ subtrochanteric femur fractures; severe bone/jt pain **CI:** Component allergy, ↓ Ca^{2+}, esophageal abnormalities, unable to stand/sit for 30 min **Disp:** DR Tabs 35 mg **SE:** D, influenza, arthralgia, back/Abd pain; rare hypersens, eye inflam **Notes:** Correct ↓ Ca^{2+} before use; ✓ Ca^{2+}

Risperidone, Oral (Risperdal, Risperdal M-Tab, Generic) BOX: ↑ Mortality in elderly w/ dementia-related psychosis Uses: *Psychotic disorders (schizophrenia)*, dementia of the elderly, bipolar disorder, mania, Tourette disorder, autism **Acts:** Benzisoxazole antipsychotic **Dose:** *Adults & Peds.* See PI for Dz specific dosing, ↓ dose w/ elderly, renal/hepatic impair **W/P:** [C, –], ↑ BP w/ antihypertensives, clozapine **CI:** Component allergy **Disp:** Tabs 0.25, 0.5, 1, 2, 3, 4 mg; soln 1 mg/mL, *M-Tab* (ODT) tabs 0.5, 1, 2, 3, 4 mg **SE:** Orthostatic ↓ BP, EPS w/ high dose, tachycardia, arrhythmias, sedation, dystonias, neuroleptic malignant synd, sexual dysfunction, constipation, xerostomia, ↓ WBC, neutropenia and agranulocytosis, cholestatic jaundice **Notes:** Several weeks for effect

Risperidone, Parenteral (Risperdal Consta) BOX: Not approved for dementia-related psychosis; ↑ mortality risk in elderly dementia pts on atypical antipsychotics; most deaths d/t CV or infectious events Uses: Schizophrenia **Acts:** Benzisoxazole antipsychotic **Dose:** 25 mg q2wk IM may ↑ to max 50 mg q2wk; w/ renal/hepatic impair start PO Risperdal 0.5 mg PO bid × 1 wk titrate weekly **W/P:** [C, –], ↑ BP w/ antihypertensives, clozapine **CI:** Component allergy **Disp:** Inj 25, 37.5, 50 mg/vial **SE:** See Risperidone, oral **Notes:** Long-acting Inj; give PO dose w/ initial Inj & continue × 3 wk

Ritonavir (Norvir) BOX: Life-threatening adverse events when used w/ certain nonsedating antihistamines, sedative hypnotics, antiarrhythmics, or ergot alkaloids d/t inhibited drug metabolism Uses: *HIV* combo w/ other antiretrovirals **Actions:** Protease inhib; ↓ maturation of immature noninfectious virions to mature infectious virus **Dose:** *Adults.* Initial 300 mg PO bid, titrate over 1 wk to 600 mg PO bid (titration will ↓ GI SE). *Peds > 1 mo.* Initiate @ 250 mg/m² titrate by 50 mg/m² q 2–3d, goal 350–400 mg/m², max 600 mg bid; adjust w/ fosamprenavir, indinavir, nelfinavir, & saquinavir; take w/ food **W/P:** [B, +] w/ Ergotamine, amiodarone, bepridil, bosentan, colchicine, PDE inhib, flecainide, propafenone, quinidine, pimozide, midazolam, triazolam **CI:** Component allergy **Disp:** Caps & tabs 100 mg; soln 80 mg/mL **SE:** ↑ Triglycerides, ↑ LFTs, N/V/D/C, Abd pain, taste perversion, anemia, weakness, HA, fever, malaise, rash, paresthesias **Notes:** Refrigerate

Rivaroxaban (Xarelto) **BOX:** May ↑ risk of spinal/epidural hematoma w/ paralysis & increase risk of stroke w/ premature D/C, monitor closely **Uses:** *Prevention DVT in knee/hip replacement surgery & prevention of stroke and systemic embolism in pts w/ nonvalvular Afib * **Acts:** Factor Xa inhib **Dose:** 10 mg PO qd × 35 d (hip) or 12 d (knee), stroke 20 mg daily; w or w/o food **W/P:** [C, −] w/ CYP3A4 inhib/inducers, other anticoagulants or plt inhib; avoid w/CrCl < 30 mL/min or mod/severe hepatic impair **CI:** Active bleeding; component hypersens **Disp:** Tabs 10 mg **SE:** Bleeding **Notes:** See PI for information about timing of stopping or starting dosage in relation to other anticoagulants

Rivastigmine (Exelon, Generic) **Uses:** *Mild–mod dementia in Alzheimer Dz* **Acts:** Enhances cholinergic activity **Dose:** 1.5 mg bid; ↑ to 6 mg bid, w/ ↑ at 2-wk intervals (take w/ food) **W/P:** [B, ?] w/ β-Blockers, CCBs, smoking, neuromuscular blockade, digoxin **CI:** Rivastigmine or carbamate allergy **Disp:** Caps 1.5, 3, 4.5, 6 mg; soln 2 mg/mL **SE:** Dose-related GI effects, N/V/D, dizziness, insomnia, fatigue, tremor, diaphoresis, HA, Wt loss (in 18–26%) **Notes:** Swallow caps whole, do not break/chew/crush; avoid EtOH

Rivastigmine, Transdermal (Exelon Patch, Generic) **Uses:** *Mild–mod Alzheimer and Parkinson Dz dementia* **Acts:** Acetylcholinesterase inhib **Dose:** *Initial:* 4.6-mg patch/d applied to back, chest, upper arm, ↑ 9.5 mg after 4 wk if tolerated **W/P:** [?, ?] Sick sinus synd, conduction defects, asthma, COPD, urinary obst, Szs; death from multiple patches at same time reported **CI:** Hypersens to rivastigmine, other carbamates **Disp:** Transdermal patch 5 cm² (4.6 mg/24 h), 10 cm² (9.5 mg/24 h) **SE:** N/V/D

Rizatriptan (Maxalt, Maxalt MLT, Generic) **Uses:** *Rx acute migraine* **Acts:** Vascular serotonin receptor agonist **Dose:** 5–10 mg PO, repeat in 2 h, PRN, 30 mg/d max **W/P:** [C, M] **CI:** Angina, ischemic heart Dz, ischemic bowel Dz, hemiplegic/basilar migraine, uncontrolled HTN, ergot or serotonin 5-HT₁ agonist use w/in 24 h, MAOI use w/in 14 d **Disp:** Tab 5, 10 mg; *Maxalt MLT:* OD tabs 5, 10 mg. **SE:** CP, palpitations, N, V, asthenia, dizziness, somnolence, fatigue

Rocuronium (Zemuron, Generic) **Uses:** *Skeletal muscle relaxation during rapid-sequence intubation, surgery, or mechanical ventilation* **Acts:** Nondepolarizing neuromuscular blocker **Dose:** *Rapid sequence intubation:* 0.6–1.2 mg/kg IV. *Continuous Inf:* 8–12 mcg/kg/min IV; adjust/titrate based on *train of four* monitoring; ↓ in hepatic impair **W/P:** [C, ?] Anaphylactoid reactions can occur. Concomitant use of corticosteroids has been associated w/ myopathy **CI:** Component or omer neuromuscular blocker allergy **Disp:** Inj preservative-free 10 mg/mL **SE:** BP changes, tachycardia **Notes:** Cross-reactivity w/ other neuromuscular blocker possible

Roflumilast (Daliresp) Uses: *↓ Exacerbations severe COPD* **Acts:** Selective phosphodiesterase -4 inhib (PDE4), ↑ cAMP w/ ↓ inflammation **Dose:** *Adults.* 500 mcg daily **W/P:** [C, –] Metabolized by CYP3A4 and 1A2; CYP3A4 and 1A2 inhib (cimetidine, erythromycin) increase levels, inducers (rifampin, carbamazepine) can decrease blood levels **CI:** Mod–severe liver impair **Disp:** Tabs 500 mcg **SE:** Worsening depression/suicidal behavior/ideation; N/D, ↓ Wt, HA, insomnia, anxiety **Notes:** Not a bronchodilator, not for acute exacerbations

Romidepsin (Istodax) Uses: *Rx cutaneous T-cell lymphoma in pts who have received at least one prior systemic therapy* **Acts:** Histone deacetylase (HDAC) inhib **Dose:** 14 mg/m^2 IV over 4 h days 1, 8, and 15 of a 28-d cycle; repeat cycles every 28 d if tolerated; Tx D/C or interruption w/ or w/o dose reduction to 10 mg/m^2 to manage adverse drug reactions **W/P:** [D, ?] Risk of ↑QT, hematologic tox; strong CYP3A4 inhibs may ↑ conc **Disp:** Inj 10 mg **SE:** N, V, fatigue, Infxn, anorexia, ↓ plt **Notes:** Hazardous agent, precautions for handling and disposal

Romiplostim (Nplate) **BOX:** ↑ Risk for heme malignancies and thromboembolism. D/C may worsen ↓ plt Uses: *Rx ↓ plt d/t ITP w/ poor response to other therapies* **Acts:** Thrombopoietic, thrombopoietin receptor agonist **Dose:** *Adults.* 1 mcg/kg SQ weekly, adjust 1 mcg/kg/wk to plt count > 50,000/mm^3; max 10 mcg/kg/wk **W/P:** [C, /?] **CI:** None **Disp:** 500 mcg/mL (250-mcg vial) **SE:** HA, fatigue, dizziness, N/V/D, myalgia, epistaxis **Notes:** ✓ CBC/diff/plt weekly; plt ↑ 4–9 d, peak 12–16 d; D/C if no ↑ plt after 4 wk max dose; ↓ dose w/ plt count > 200,000/mm^3 for 2 wk

Ropinirole (Requip, Requip XL, Generic) Uses: *Rx of Parkinson Dz, restless leg synd (RLS)* **Acts:** Dopamine agonist **Dose:** *Parkinson Dz:* IR initial 0.25 mg PO tid, weekly ↑ 0.25 mg/dose, to 1 mg PO tid (may continue to titrate weekly to max dose of 24 mg/d); ER: 2 mg PO daily, titrate qwk by 2 mg/d to max 24 mg/d *RLS:* initial 0.25 mg PO 1–3 h before bedtime **W/P:** [C, ?/–] Severe CV/renal/hepatic impair **CI:** Component allergy **Disp:** Tabs IR 0.25, 0.5, 1, 2, 3, 4, 5 mg; tabs ER 2, 4, 6, 8, 12 mg **SE:** Syncope, postural ↓ BP, N/V, HA, somnolence, dose-related hallucinations, dyskinesias, dizziness **Notes:** D/C w/ 7-d taper

Rosiglitazone (Avandia) **BOX:** May cause or worsen CHF; may increase myocardial ischemia Uses: *Type 2 DM* **Acts:** Thiazolidinedione; ↑ insulin sensitivity **Dose:** 4–8 mg/d PO or in 2 ÷ doses (w/o regard to meals) **W/P:** [C, –] w/ ESRD, CHF, edema, ↑? CA risk; severe CHF (NYHA class III IV) **Disp:** Tabs 2, 4, 8 mg **SE:** May ↑ CV, CHF & ? CA risk; Wt gain, hyperlipidemia, HA, edema, fluid retention, worsen CHF, hyper/hypoglycemia, hepatic damage w/ ↑ LFTs **Notes:** Increased MI risk now requires REMS restricted distribution program

Rosuvastatin (Crestor) Uses: *Rx primary hypercholesterolemia & mixed dyslipidemia* **Acts:** HMG-CoA reductase inhib **Dose:** 5–40 mg PO daily; max 5 mg/d w/ cyclosporine, 10 mg/d w/ gemfibrozil or CrCl < 30 mL/min (avoid Al-Mg-based antacids for 2 h after) **W/P:** [X, ?/–] **CI:** Active liver Dz, unexplained ↑ LFTs **Disp:** Tabs 5, 10, 20, 40 mg **SE:** Myalgia, constipation, asthenia, Abd pain, N, myopathy, rarely rhabdomyolysis **Notes:** May ↑ warfarin effect; monitor LFTs at baseline, 12 wk, then q6mo; ↓ dose in Asian pts; OK w/ grapefruit

Rotavirus Vaccine, Live, Oral, Monovalent (Rotarix) Uses: *Prevent rotavirus gastroenteritis in peds* Acts: Active immunization w/ live attenuated rotavirus Dose: *Peds 6–24 wk.* 1st dose PO at 6 wk of age, wait at least 4 wk then a 2nd dose by 24 wk of age. W/P: [C, ?] CI: Component sensitivity, uncorrected congenital GI malformation, severe combined immunodeficiency (SCID), intussusception Disp: Single-dose vial SE: Irritability, cough, runny nose, fever, anaphylactic Rxn, D, ↓ appetite, otitis media, V Notes: Conclude by age 24 wk; can be given to infant in house w/ immunosuppressed fam member or mother who is breast-feeding. Safety and effectiveness not studied in immunocompromised infants

Rotavirus Vaccine, Live, Oral, Pentavalent (RotaTeq) Uses: *Prevent rotavirus gastroenteritis* Acts: Active immunization w/ live attenuated rotavirus Dose: *Peds 6–24 wk.* Single dose PO at 2, 4, & 6 mo W/P: [?, ?] CI: Component sensitivity, uncorrected congenital GI malformation, severe combined immunodeficiency (SCID), intussusception Disp: Oral susp 2-mL single-use tubes SE: Irritability, cough, runny nose, fever, anaphylactic Rxn, D, ↓ appetite, otitis media, V Notes: Begin series by age 12 wk and conclude by age 32 wk; can be given to infant in house w/ immunosuppressed fam member or mother who is breast-feeding. Safety and effectiveness not studied in immunocompromised infants

Rotigotine (Neupro) Uses: *Parkinson Dz, RLS* Acts: Dopamine agonist Dose: *Adults. Parkinson Dz:* 2 mg/24 h (early Dz) or 4 mg/24 h (advanced Dz); ↑ by 2 mg/24 h qwk PRN to max of 6 mg/24 h (early Dz) or 8 mg/24 h (advanced Dz); *RLS:* 1 mg/24 h; ↑ by 1 mg/24 h qwk PRN to max 3 mg/24 h; apply patch 1×/d to dry, intact skin; ↓ gradually w/ D/C W/P: [C, ?/–] Allergic Rxns w/ sulfite sens CI: Hypersens Disp: Transdermal sys 1, 2, 3, 4, 6, 8 mg/24 h SE: N/V, site Rxn, somnolence, dizziness, anorexia, hyperhidrosis, insomnia, peripheral edema, dyskinesia, HA, postural hypotension, syncope, ↑ HR, ↑ BP, hallucinations, psychotic-like/compulsive behavior Notes: Do not use same site more than once q14 d

Rufinamide (Banzel) Uses: *Adjunct Lennox-Gastaut Szs* Acts: Anticonvulsant Dose: *Adults. Initial:* 400–800 mg/d ÷ bid (max 3200 mg/d ÷ bid) *Peds ≥ 4 y. Initial:* 10 mg/kg/d ÷ bid, target 45 mg/kg/d ÷ bid; 3200 mg/d max W/P: [C, –/–] Familial short QT synd CI: Tab: 200, 400 mg; susp 40 mg/mL (460 mL) SE: ↓ QT, HA, somnolence, N/V, ataxia, rash Notes: Monitor for rash; use w/ OCP may lead to contraceptive failure; dose adjust w/ valproate; initial dose not > 400 mg

Ruxolitinib (Jakafi) Uses: *Myelofibrosis* Acts: Inhib Janus-associated kinases, mediators of hematologic and immunologic cytokines and growth factors Dose: 20 mg bid if plt > 200,000 × 10^9/L; 15 mg bid if plt 100,000–200,000 × 10^9/L; ↑ based on response, 25 mg bid max; stop Tx if plt < 50,0000 × 10^9/L; restart when > 50,000 × 10^9/L; 20 mg bid if plt > 125,000 × 10^9/L; 15 mg bid if plt 100–125,000 × 10^9/L; 10 mg bid if plt 75–100,000 × 10^9/L × 2 wk, if stable ↑ to 15 mg bid; if plt 50–75,000 × 10^9/L, 5 mg bid × 2 wk, if stable ↑ to 10 mg bid if no ↓ in spleen size or symptoms D/C after 6 mo **W/P:** [C, –] **Do not** use if ESRD **and not** on dialysis; ↓ dose w/ strong CYP3A4 inhib **CI:** None **Disp:** Tabs 5, 10, 15, 20, 25 mg **SE:** ↓ Plt, ↓ WBC, anemia, bruising, HA, dizziness, serious Infxns including zoster **Notes:** w/ D/C for reason other than ↓ plt, taper 5 mg bid each wk

Salmeterol (Serevent Diskus) **BOX:** Long-acting β₂-agonists, such as salmeterol, may ↑ risk of asthma-related death. Do not use alone, only as additional Rx for pts not controlled on other asthma meds; LABAs may ↑ risk of asthma-related hospitalization in pediatric and adolescent pts **Uses:** *Asthma, exercise-induced asthma, COPD* **Acts:** Sympathomimetic bronchodilator, long acting β₂-agonist **Dose:** *Adults & Peds > 12 y.* 1 Diskus-dose inhaled bid **W/P:** [C, ?/–] **CI:** Acute asthma; monotherapy concomitant use of inhaled steroid, status asthticus **Disp:** 50 mcg/dose, dry powder discus, **SE:** HA, pharyngitis, tachycardia, arrhythmias, nervousness, GI upset, tremors **Notes:** Not for acute attacks; must use w/ steroid or short-acting β-agonist

Saquinavir (Invirase) **BOX:** Invirase and Fortovase not bioequivalent/ interchangeable; must use Invirase in combo w/ ritonavir, which provides saquinavir plasma levels = those w/ Fortovase **Uses:** *HIV Infxn* **Acts:** HIV protease inhib **Dose:** 1000 mg PO bid w/in 2 h of a full meal (dose w/ ritonavir 100 mg PO bid) w/in 2 h pc (dose adjust w/ delavirdine, lopinavir, & nelfinavir) **W/P:** [B, ?] **CI:** Complete AV block w/o implanted pacemaker; concomitant use antiarrhythmics, ergot derivatives, sedatives/hypnotics, trazodone, sildenafil, statins, rifamins, congenital ↑ QT synd; severe hepatic impair; refractory ↓ K⁺/↓ Mg²⁺; anaphylaxis to component **Disp:** Caps 200 mg, tabs 500 mg **SE:** Dyslipidemia, lipodystrophy, rash, hyperglycemia, GI upset, weakness **Notes:** Take w/in 2 h of a meal, avoid direct sunlight

Sargramostim [GM-CSF] (Leukine) **Uses:** *Myeloid recovery following BMT or chemotherapy* **Acts:** Recombinant GF, activates mature granulocytes & macrophages **Dose:** *Adults & Peds.* 250 mcg/m²/d IV cont until ANC > 1500 cells/m² for 3 consecutive days **W/P:** [C, ?/–] Li, corticosteroids > 10% blasts, allergy to yeast, concurrent chemotherapy/RT **Disp:** Inj 250, 500 mcg **SE:** Bone pain, fever, ↑ BP, tachycardia, flushing, GI upset, myalgia **Notes:** Rotate Inj sites; use APAP PRN for pain

Saxagliptin (Onglyza) **Uses:** *Monotherapy/combo type 2 DM* **Acts:** DDP-4 inhib, ↑ insulin synth/release **Dose:** 2.5 or 5 mg 1×/d w/o regard to meals; 2.5 mg once/d w/ CrCl < 50 mL/min or w/ strong CYP3A4/5 inhib (eg, atazanavir, clarithromycin, indinavir, itraconazole, ketoconazole, nefazodone, nelfinavir, ritonavir, saquinavir, telithromycin) **W/P:** [B, ?] May ↓ glucose when used w/ insulin secretagogues (eg, sulfonylureas); w/ pancreatitis **CI:** Hypersens Rxn **Disp:** Tabs 2.5, 5 mg **SE:** Peripheral edema, hypoglycemia, UTI, HA, Abd pain

Saxagliptin/Metformin (Kombiglyze XR) **BOX:** Lactic acidosis can occur w/ metformin accumulation; ↑ risk w/ sepsis, vol depletion, CHF, renal/ hepatic impair, excess alcohol; if lactic acidosis suspected D/C med and hospitalize

Uses: *Type 2 DM* **Acts:** Dipeptidyl peptidase-4 (DDP-4) inhib, ↑ insulin synth/release & biguanide; ↓ hepatic glucose production & intestinal absorption of glucose; ↑ insulin sens **Dose:** 5/500 mg–5/2000 mg saxagliptin/metformin HCl XR PO daily w/ evening meal **W/P:** [B, ?/–] w/ 10 diagonsed contrast studies **CI:** SCr > 1.4 mg/dL (females) or > 1.5 mg/dL (males); met acidosis **Disp:** Tabs mg saxagliptin/mg metformin XR 5/500, 5/1000, 2.5/1000 **SE:** Lactic acidosis; ↓ vit B₁₂ levels; ↓ glucose w/ insulin secretagogue; N/V/D, anorexia, HA, URI, UTI, urticaria, myalgia **Notes:** Do not exceed 5 mg/2000 mg saxagliptin/metformin HCl XR; do not crush or chew; w/ strong CYP3A4/5 inhib do not exceed 2.5 mg saxagliptin/d

Scopolamine, Transdermal (Transderm-Scop) **Uses:** *Prevent N/V associated w/ motion sickness, anesthesia, opiates* **Acts:** Anticholinergic, antiemetic **Dose:** 1 mg/72 h, 1 patch behind ear q3d; apply > 4 h before exposure **W/P:** [C, +] w/ APAP, levodopa, ketoconazole, digitalis, KCl **CI:** NAG, GI or GU obst, thyrotoxicosis, paralytic ileus **Disp:** Patch 1.5 mg, (releases 1 mg over 72 h) **SE:** Xerostomia, drowsiness, blurred vision, tachycardia, constipation **Notes:** Do not blink excessively after dose, wait 5 min before dosing other eye; antiemetic activity w/ patch requires several hours

Secobarbital (Seconal) [C-II] **Uses:** *Insomnia, short-term use*, preanesthetic agent **Acts:** Rapid-acting barbiturate **Dose:** *Adults.* 100–200 mg hs, 100–300 mg preop. *Peds.* 2–6 mg/kg/dose, 100 mg/max; ↓ in elderly **W/P:** [D, +] w/ CYP2C9, 3A3/4, 3A5/7 inducer (Table 10, p 319); ↑ tox w/ other CNS depressants **CI:** Hypersensitivity to barbiturates, marked hepatic impairment dyspnea or airway obstruction, porphyria, PRG **Disp:** Caps 100 mg **SE:** Tolerance in 1–2 wk; resp depression, porphyria, porphyria, dyspnea

Selegiline, Oral (Eldepryl, Zelapar, Generic) **BOX:** Closely monitor for worsening depression or emergence of suicidality, particularly in ped pts **Uses:** *Parkinson Dz* **Acts:** MAOI **Dose:** 5 mg PO bid; 1.25–2.5 once daily ODT tabs PO q A.M. (before breakfast w/o liq) 2.5 mg/d max; ↓ in elderly **W/P:** [C, ?] w/ Drugs that induce CYP3A4 (Table 10, p 319) (eg, phenytoin, carbamazepine, nafcillin, phenobarbital, & rifampin); avoid w/ antidepressants **CI:** w/ Meperidine, MAOI, dextromethorphan, tramadol, methadone, general anesthesia w/in 10 d, pheochromocytoma **Disp:** Tabs/caps 5 mg; once-daily tabs 1.25 mg **SE:** N, dizziness, orthostatic ↓ BP, arrhythmias, tachycardia, edema, confusion, xerostomia **Notes:** ↓ Carbidopa/levodopa if used in combo; see transdermal form

Selegiline, Transdermal (Emsam) **BOX:** May ↑ risk of suicidal thinking and behavior in children and adolescents w/ MDD **Uses:** *Depression* **Acts:** MAOI **Dose:** *Adults.* Apply patch daily to upper torso, upper thigh, or outer upper arm **CI:** Tyramine-containing foods w/ 9- or 12-mg doses; serotonin-sparing agents **W/P:** [C, –] ↑ Carbamazepine and oxcarbazepine levels **Disp:** ER Patches 9, 12 mg **SE:** Local Rxns requiring topical steroids; HA, insomnia, orthostatic, ↓ BP, serotonin synd, suicide risk **Notes:** Rotate site; see oral form

Selenium Sulfide (Exsel Shampoo, Selsun Blue Shampoo, Selsun Shampoo) Uses: *Scalp seborrheic dermatitis*, scalp itching & flaking d/t *dandruff*; tinea versicolor Acts: Antiseborrheic Dose: *Dandruff, seborrhea:* Massage 5–10 mL into wet scalp, leave on 2–3 min, rinse, repeat; use 2× wk, then once q1–4wk PRN. *Tinea versicolor:* Apply 2.5% daily on area & lather w/ small amounts of water; leave on 10 min, then rinse W/P: [C, ?] Avoid contact w/ open wounds or mucus membranes CI: Component allergy Disp: Shampoo [OTC]; 2.5% lotion SE: Dry or oily scalp, lethargy, hair discoloration, local irritation Notes: Do not use more than 2×/wk

Sertaconazole (Ertaczo) Uses: *Topical Rx interdigital tinea pedis* Acts: Imidazole antifungal. *Spectrum: Trichophyton rubrum, Trichophyton mentagrophytes, Epidermophyton floccosum* Dose: *Adults & Peds > 12.* Apply between toes & immediate surrounding healthy skin bid × 4 wk W/P: [C, ?] Avoid occlusive dressing CI: Component allergy Disp: 2% Cream SE: Contact dermatitis, dry/burning skin, tenderness Notes: Use in immunocompetent pts; not for oral, intravag, ophthal use

Sertraline (Zoloft, Generic) BOX: Closely monitor pts for worsening depression or emergence of suicidality, particularly in ped pts Uses: *Depression, panic disorders, PMDD, OCD, PTSD*, social anxiety disorder, eating disorders, premenstrual disorders Acts: ↓ Neuronal uptake of serotonin Dose: *Adults. Depression:* 50–200 mg/d PO. *PTSD:* 25 mg PO daily × 1 wk, then 50 mg PO daily, 200 mg/d max. *Peds 6–12 y.* 25 mg PO daily. *13–17 y:* 50 mg PO daily W/P: [C, ?/–] Serotonin syndrome: ↑ risk w/ concomitant use of serotonin antagonists (haloperidol, etc), hepatic impair CI: MAOI use w/in 14 d; concomitant pimozide Disp: Tabs 25, 50, 100 mg; 20 mg/mL oral SE: Activate manic/hypomanic state, ↑/↓ Wt, insomnia, somnolence, fatigue, tremor, xerostomia, N/D, dyspepsia, ejaculatory dysfunction, ↓ libido, hepatotox

Sevelamer Carbonate (Renvela) Uses: *Control ↑ PO_4^{3-} in ESRD* Acts: Intestinal phosphate binder Dose: Start 0.8 or 1.6 g PO tid w/ meals; titrate 0.8 g/meal for target PO_4 3.5–5.5 mg/dL; switch g/g among sevelamer forms, titrate PRN W/P: [C, ?] w/ Swallow disorders, bowel problems, may ↓ absorption of vits D, E, K, ↓ ciprofloxacin & other medicine levels CI: Bowel obst Disp: Tab 800 mg, powder 0.8/2.4 g SE: N/V/D, dyspepsia, Abd pain, flatulence, constipation Notes: Separate other meds 1 h before or 3 h after

Sevelamer HCl (Renagel) Uses: *↓ PO_4^{3-} in ESRD* Acts: Binds intestinal PO_4^{3-} Dose: *Initial:* PO_4^{3-} > 5.5 and < 7.5 mg/dL: 800 mg PO tid; ≥ 7.5 mg/dL: 1200–1600 mg PO tid. *Switching from sevelamer carbonate:* per-g basis; titrate ↑/↓ 1 tab/meal 2-wk intervals PRN; take w/ food 2–4 caps PO tid w/ meals; adjust based on PO_4^{3-}; max 4 g/dose W/P: [C, ?] May ↓ absorption of vits D, E, K, ↓ ciprofloxacin & other medicine levels CI: ↓ PO_4^{3-}, bowel obst Disp: Tab 400, 800 mg SE: N/V/D, dyspepsia, ↑ Ca^{2+} Notes: Do not open/chew caps; separate other meds 1 h before or 3 h after; 800 mg sevelamer = 667 mg Ca acetate

Sildenafil (Viagra, Revatio) Uses: *Viagra:* *ED*; *Revatio:* *Pulm artery HTN (adult only)* Acts: ↓ Phosphodiesterase type 5 (PDE5) (responsible for cGMP breakdown); ↑ cGMP activity to relax smooth muscles & ↑ flow to corpus cavernosum and pulm vasculature; ? antiproliferative on pulm artery smooth muscle **Dose:** *ED:* 25–100 mg PO 1 h before sexual activity, max 1/d; ↓ if > 65 y *Revatio: Pulm HTN:* 20 mg PO tid or 10 mg IV tid **W/P:** [B, ?] w/ CYP3A4 inhib (Table 10, p 319), retinitis pigmentosa; hepatic/severe renal impair; w/ sig hypo-/hypertension **CI:** w/ Nitrates or if sex not advised; w/ protease inhib **Disp:** Tabs *Viagra:* 25, 50, 100 mg, tabs *Revatio:* Tabs 20 mg; Inj 5–10 mg/vial **SE:** HA; flushing; dizziness; blue haze visual change, hearing loss, priapism **Notes:** Cardiac events in absence of nitrates debatable; transient global amnesia reports; avoid fatty food w/ dose; not for peds use

Silodosin (Rapaflo) **Uses:** *BPH* **Acts:** α-blockers of prostatic $α_{1a}$ **Dose:** 8 mg/d; 4 mg/d w/ CrCl 30–50 mL/min; take w/ food **W/P:** [B, ?] Not for use in females; do not use w/ other α-blockers or glycoprotein inhib (ie, cyclosporine); R/O PCa before use; IFIS possible w/ cataract surgery **CI:** Severe hepatic/renal impair (CrCl < 30 mL/min), w/ CYP3A4 inhib (eg, ketoconazole, clarithromycin, itraconazole, ritonavir) **Disp:** Caps 4, 8 mg **SE:** Retrograde ejaculation, dizziness, D, syncope, somnolence, orthostatic ↓ BP, nasopharyngitis, nasal congestion, intraoperative floppy iris syndrome during contract surgery **Notes:** Not for use as antihypertensive; no effect on QT interval

Silver Nitrate (Generic) **Uses:** *Removal of granulation tissue & warts; prophylaxis in burns* **Acts:** Caustic antiseptic & astringent **Dose:** *Adults & Peds.* Apply to moist surface 2–3 × wk for 2–3 wk or until effect **W/P:** [C, ?] Do not use on broken skin **Disp:** Topical impregnated applicator sticks, soln 0.5, 10, 25, 50%; topical ointment 10% **SE:** May stain tissue black, usually resolves; local irritation, methemoglobinemia **Notes:** D/C if redness or irritation develops; no longer used in US for newborn prevention of gonococcus conjunctivitis

Silver Sulfadiazine (Silvadene, Generic) **Uses:** *Prevention & Rx of Infxn in 2nd- & 3rd-degree burns* **Acts:** Bactericidal **Dose:** *Adults & Peds.* Aseptically cover the area w/ 1/16-in coating bid **W/P:** [B unless near term, ?/–] **CI:** Infants < mo, PRG near term **Disp:** Cream 1% **SE:** Itching, rash, skin discoloration, blood dyscrasias, hep, allergy **Notes:** Systemic absorption w/ extensive application

Simethicone (Generic [OTC]) **Uses:** Flatulence **Acts:** Defoaming, alters gas bubble surface tension action **Dose:** *Adults & Peds > 12 y.* 40–360 mg PO after meals and at bedtime PRN; 500 mg/d max. *Peds < 2 y.* 20 mg PO qid PRN. *2–12 y:* 40 mg PO qid PRN **W/P:** [C, ?] **CI:** GI perforation or obst **Disp:** [OTC] Tabs 80, 125 mg; caps 125 mg; susp 40 mg/0.6 mL; chew tabs 80, 125 mg; caps: 125, 180 mg; ODT strip: 40, 62.5 mg **SE:** N/D **Notes:** Available in combo products OTC

Simvastatin (Zocor) **Uses:** ↓ Cholesterol **Acts:** HMG-CoA reductase inhib **Dose:** *Adults.* 5–40 mg PO q P.M.; w/ meals; ↓ in renal Insuff; w/o grapefruit. *Peds 10–17 y.* 10 mg, 40 mg max **W/P:** [X, –] Max 10 mg daily w/ verapamil, diltiazem; max 20 mg daily w/ amlodipine, ranolazine, amiodarone; 80 mg dose restricted to those taking > 12 mo w/o muscle tox; w/ Chinese pt on lipid modifying meds **CI:** PRG, liver Dz, strong CYP3A4 inhib **Disp:** Tabs 5, 10, 20, 40, 80 mg **SE:** HA, GI upset, myalgia, myopathy (pain, tenderness, weakness w/ creatine kinase 10 × ULN) and rhabdomyolysis, hep **Notes:** Combo w/ ezetimibe/simvastatin; follow LFTs; ↑ blood glucose w/ DM

Sipuleucel-T (Provenge) Uses: *Asymptomatic/minimally symptomatic metastatic castrate resistant PCa* **Acts:** Autologous (pt specific) cellular immunotherapy **Dose:** 3 doses over 1 mo @ 2-wk intervals; premed w/ APAP & diphenhydramine **W/P:** [N/A, N/A] Confirm identity/expir date before Inf; acute transfusion Rxn possible; not tested for transmissible Dz **CI:** None **Disp:** 50 mill units autologous CD54+ cells activated w/ PAP GM-CSF in 250 mL LR **SE:** Chills, fatigue, fever, back pain, N, jt ache, HA **Notes:** Pt must undergo leukopheresis, and shipping and autologous cell processing at manufacturing facility before each Inf

Sirolimus [Rapamycin] (Rapamune) **BOX:** Use only by physicians experienced in immunosuppression; immunosuppression associated w/ lymphoma, ↑ Infxn risk; do not use in lung transplant (fatal bronchial anastomotic dehiscence); do not use in liver transplant: ↑ risk hepatic arterythrombosis, graft failure, and mortality (w/ evidence of Infxn) Uses: *Prevent organ rejection in new renal Tx pts* **Acts:** ↓ T-lymphocyte activation and proliferation **Dose:** *Adults > 40 kg:* 6 mg PO on day 1, then 2 mg/d PO. *Peds < 40 kg & ≥13 y:* 3 mg/m² load, then 1 mg/m²/d (in H₂O/orange juice; no grapefruit juice w/ sirolimus); take 4 h after cyclosporine; ↓ in hepatic impair **W/P:** [C, ?/–] Impaired wound healing & angioedema; grapefruit juice, ketoconazole **CI:** Component allergy **Disp:** Soln 1 mg/mL, tab 0.5, 1, 2 mg **SE:** HTN, edema, CP, fever, HA, insomnia, acne, rash, ↑ cholesterol, GI upset, ↑/↓ K⁺, Infxns, blood dyscrasias, arthralgia, tachycardia, renal impair, graft loss & death in liver transplant (hepatic artery thrombosis), ascites **Notes:** Levels: *Trough:* 4–20 ng/mL; varies w/ assay method and indication

Sitagliptin (Januvia) Uses: *Monotherapy or combo for type 2 DM* **Acts:** Dipeptidyl peptidase-4 (DDP-4) inhib, ↑ insulin synth/release **Dose:** 100 mg PO daily; CrCl 30–50: 50 mg PO daily; CrCl < 30 mL/min: 25 mg PO daily **W/P:** [B/?] May cause ↓ blood sugar when used w/ insulin secretagogues such as sulfonylureas **CI:** Component hypersens **Disp:** Tabs 25, 50, 100 mg **SE:** URI; peripheral edema, asopharyngitis **Notes:** No evidence for ↑ CV risk

Sitagliptin/Metformin (Janumet) **BOX:** See metformin, p 189 Uses: *Adjunct to diet and exercise in type 2 DM* **Acts:** See individual agents **Dose:** 1 tab PO bid, titrate; 100 mg sitagliptin & 2000 mg metformin/d max; take w/ meals **W/P:** [B, ?/–] **CI:** Type 1 DM, DKA, male Cr > 1.5; female Cr > 1.4 mg/dL **Disp:** Tabs 50/500, 50/1000 mg **SE:** Nasopharyngitis, N/V/D, flatulence, Abd discomfort, dyspepsia, asthenia, HA **Notes:** Hold w/ contrast study; ✓ Cr, CBC

Sitagliptin/Simvastatin (Juvisync) Uses: *DM2 w/ hyperlipidemia* **Acts:** ↑ Insulin synth/release and ↓ chol, ↓ VLDL, ↓ triglycerides, ↑ HDL; dipeptidyl peptidase-4 (DPP-4) inhib w/ HMG-CoA reductase inhib **Dose:** Start 100/40 mg or maintain simvastatin dose **W/P:** [X, –] ↑ AST/ALT; myopathy (↑ risk of myopathy w/ age > 65 y, female, renal impair, meds (eg, niacin, amiodarone, CCBs, fibrates, colchicine); renal failure, hypoglycemia w/ sulfonylureas, or insulin; pancreatitis, anaphylaxis **CI:** Hx hypersens Rxn; w/ CYP3A4 inhib, gemfibrozil, cyclosporine, danazol, ketoconazole, itraconazole, erythromycin, clarithromycin, HIV protease inhib; liver Dx; PRG or women who may get PRG; nursing **Disp:** Tabs mg sitagliptin/mg simvastatin: 100/10, 100/20, 100/40, 50/10, 50/20, 50/40 **SE:** *Simvastatin:* HA, GI upset, myalgia, myopathy (pain, tenderness, weakness w/ creatine kinase 10× ULN) and rhabdomyolysis, hep; sitagliptin: URI, nasopharyngitis, UTI, HA **Notes:** ↑ Myopathy w/ coadministration of CYP3A4 inhib; risk of myopathy dose related

Smallpox Vaccine (ACAM2000) BOX: Acute myocarditis and other infectious complications possible; CI in immunocompromised, eczema or exfoliative skin conditions, infants < 1 y Uses: Immunization against smallpox (variola virus) **Acts:** Active immunization (live attenuated cowpox virus) **Dose:** *Adults. Primary and revaccination:* 15 punctures w/ bifurcated needle dipped in vaccine into deltoid, ✓ site for Rxn in 6–8 d; if major Rxn, site scabs, & heals, leaving scar **W/P:** [D, ?] **CI:** *Nonemergency use:* febrile illness, immunosuppression, Hx eczema & in household contacts. *Emergency:* No absolute CI **Disp:** Vial for reconstitution: 100 mill pock-forming units/mL **SE:** Malaise, fever, regional lymphadenopathy, encephalopathy, rashes, spread of inoculation to other sites; SJS, eczema vaccinatum w/ severe disability **Notes:** Avoid infants for 14 d; intradermal use only; restricted distribution; Dryvax discontinued

Sodium Bicarbonate [NaHCO₃] (Generic) Uses: *Alkalinization of urine, RTA, metabolic acidosis, ↑ K⁺, TCA OD* **Acts:** Alkalinizing agent **Dose:** *Adults. ECC 2010.* Cardiac arrest w/ good ventilation, hyperkalemia, OD of TCAs, ASA, cocaine, diphenhydramine: 1 mEq/kg IV bolus; repeat 1/2 dose q10min PRN. *Metabolic acidosis:* 2–5 mEq/kg IV over 8 h & PRN based on acid–base status. ↑ K⁺: 50 mEq IV over 5 min. *Alkalize urine:* 4 g (48 mEq) PO, then 12–24 mEq q4h; adjust based on urine pH; 2 amp (100 mEq)/1 L D₅W at 100–250 mL/h IV, monitor urine pH & serum bicarbonate. *Chronic renal failure:* 1–3 mEq/kg/d. *Distal RTA:* 0.5–2 mEq/kg/d in 4–5 ÷ doses. *Peds.* Sodium bicarbonate *ECC 2010. Severe metabolic acidosis, hyperkalemia:* 1 mEq/kg IV slow bolus; 4.2% conc in infants <1 mo. *Chronic renal failure:* See Adults dosage. *Distal RTA:* 2–3 mEq/kg/d PO. *Proximal RTA:* 5–10 mEq/kg/d; titrate based on serum bicarbonate. *Urine alkalinization:* 84–840 mg/kg/d (1–10 mEq/kg/d) in ÷ doses; adjust based on urine pH **W/P:** [C, ?] **CI:** Alkalosis, ↑ Na⁺, severe pulm edema, ↓ Ca²⁺ **Disp:** Powder, tabs; 325 mg = 3.8 mEq; 650 mg = 7.6 mEq; Inj 1 mEq/mL, 4.2% (5 mEq/10 mL), 7.5% (8.92 mEq/mL), 8.4% (10 mEq/10 mL) vial or amp **SE:** Belching, edema, flatulence, ↑ Na⁺, metabolic alkalosis **Notes:** 1 g neutralizes 12 mEq of acid; 50 mEq bicarbonate = 50 mEq Na; can make 3 amps in 1 L D₅W = D₅NS w/ 150 mEq bicarbonate

Sodium Citrate/Citric Acid (Bicitra, Oracit) Uses: *Chronic metabolic acidosis, alkalinize urine; dissolve uric acid & cysteine stones* **Acts:** Urinary

alkalinizer **Dose:** *Adults.* 10–30 mL in 1- to 3- oz H_2O pc & hs. *Peds.* 5–15 mL in 1- to 3- oz H_2O pc & hs; best after meals **W/P:** [?, ?] **CI:** Severe renal impair or Na-restricted diets **Disp:** 15- or 30-mL unit dose: 16 (473 mL) or 4 fl oz **SE:** Tetany, metabolic alkalosis, ↑ K^+, GI upset; avoid w/ multiple 50-mL amps; can cause ↑ Na^+/hyperosmolality **Notes:** 1 mL = 1 mEq Na & 1 mEq bicarbonate

Sodium Oxybate/Gamma Hydroxybutyrate/GHB (Xyrem) [C-III]
BOX: Known drug of abuse even at recommended doses; confusion, depression, resp depression may occur **Uses:** *Narcolepsy-associated cataplexy* **Acts:** Inhibitory neurotransmitter **Dose:** *Adults & Peds > 16 y.* 2.25 g PO qhs, 2nd dose 2.5–4 h later; may ↑ 9 g/d max **W/P:** [C, ?/–] **CI:** Succinic semialdehyde dehydrogenase deficiency; potentiates EtOH & other CNS depressants **Disp:** 500 mg/mL (180-mL) PO soln **SE:** Confusion, depression, ↓ diminished level of consciousness, incontinence, sig V, resp depression, psychological Sxs **Notes:** May lead to dependence; GHB abused as a "date rape drug"; controlled distribution (prescriber & pt registration); must be administered when pt in bed

Sodium Phosphate (Osmoprep, Visicol)
BOX: Acute phosphate nephropathy reported w/ permanent renal impair risk; w/ ↑ age, hypovolemia, bowel obstr or colitis, baseline kidney Dz, w/ meds that affect renal perf/Fxn (diuretics, ACE inhib, ARB, NSAIDs) **Uses:** *Bowel prep prior to colonoscopy*, short-term constipation **Acts:** Hyperosmotic laxative **Dose:** 3 tabs PO w/ at least 8-oz clear llq q15min for 6 doses, then 2 additional tabs in 15 min, 3–5 h prior to colonoscopy; 3 tabs q15 min for 6 doses, then 2 additional tabs in 15 min **W/P:** [C, ?] Renal impair, electrolyte disturbances **CI:** Megacolon, bowel obst **Disp:** Tabs 0.398, 1.102 g (32/bottle) **SE:** ↑ QT, ↑ PO_4^{3-}, ↓ calcium, D, flatulence, cramps, Abd bloating/pain

Sodium Polystyrene Sulfonate (Kayexalate, Kionex, Generic)
Uses: *Rx of ↑ K^+* **Acts:** Na^+/K^+ ion-exchange resin **Dose:** *Adults.* 15–60 g PO or 30–50 g PR q6h based on serum K^+. *Peds.* 1 g/kg/dose PO or PR q6h based on serum K^+ **W/P:** [C, ?] Obstructive bowel Dz; ↑ neonates w/ ↓ gut motility **Disp:** Powder; susp 15 g/60 mL sorbitol **SE:** ↑ Na^+, ↓ K^+, GI upset, fecal impaction **Notes:** Enema acts more quickly than PO; PO most effective, onset action > 2 h

Solifenacin (Vesicare)
Uses: *OAB* **Acts:** Antimuscarinic, ↓ detrusor contractions **Dose:** 5 mg PO daily, 10 mg/d max; w/ renal/hepatic impair **W/P:** [C, ?/–] BOO or GI obst, UC, MyG, renal/hepatic impair, QT prolongation risk **CI:** NAG, urinary/gastric retention **Disp:** Tabs 5, 10 mg **SE:** Constipation, xerostomia, dyspepsia, blurred vision, drowsiness **Notes:** CYP3A4 substrate; azole antifungals ↑ levels; recent concern over cognitive effects

Somatropin (Genotropin, Nutropin AQ, Omnitrope, Saizen, Serostim, Zorbtive)
Uses: *HIV-assoc wasting/cachexia* **Acts:** Anabolic peptide hormone **Dose:** 0.1 mg/kg SQ hs; max 6 mg/d **W/P:** [B, ?] Lipodystrophy (rotate sites) **CI:** Active neoplasm; acute critical illness postop; benzyl alcohol sens; hypersens **Disp:** 4, 5, 6 mg powder for Inj **SE:** Arthralgia, edema, ↑ blood glucose

Sorafenib (Nexavar)   Uses: *Advanced RCC*, metastatic liver CA Acts: Tyrosine kinase inhib Dose: *Adults.* 400 mg PO bid on empty stomach W/P: [D, –] w/ Irinotecan, doxorubicin, warfarin; avoid conception (male/female); avoid inducers Disp: Tabs 200 mg SE: Hand–foot syndr; Tx-emergent hypertension; bleeding, ↑ INR, cardiac infarction/ischemia; ↑ pancreatic enzymes, hypophosphatemia, lymphopenia, anemia, fatigue, alopecia, pruritus, D, GI upset, HA, neuropathy Notes: Monitor BP first 6 wk; may require ↓ dose (daily or q other day); impaired metabolism w/ Asian descent; may effect wound healing, D/C before major surgery

Sorbitol (Generic)   Uses: *Constipation* Acts: Osmotic laxative Dose: 30–150 mL PO of a 20–70% soln PRN W/P: [C, ?] CI: Anuria Disp: Liq 70% SE: Edema, lyte loss, lactic acidosis, GI upset, xerostomia Notes: Vehicle for many liq formulations (eg, zinc, Kayexalate)

Sotalol (Betapace, Sorine, Generic)   BOX: To minimize risk of induced arrhythmia, pts initiated/reinitiated on *Betapace AF* should be placed for a minimum of 3 d (on their maint) in a facility that can provide cardiac resuscitation, cont ECG monitoring, & calculations of CrCl. *Betapace* should not be substituted for *Betapace AF* because of labeling; adjust dose base on Crcl. Can cause life-threatening ventricular tachycardia w/ prolonged QT. Do not initiate if QT > 450 ms. If QTc > 500 ms during Tx, ↓ dose. Uses: *Ventricular arrhythmias, AF* Acts: β-Adrenergic-blocking agent Dose: *Adults. CrCl > 60 mL/min:* 80 mg PO bid, may ↑ to 240–320 mg/d. CrCl 30–60 mL/min: 80 mg q24h. CrCl 10–30 mL/min: Dose 80 mg q36–48h. *ECC 2010. SVT and ventricular arrhythmias:* 1–1.5 mg/kg IV over 5 min. *Peds < 2 y.* Dosing dependent on age, renal Fxn, heart rate, QT interval; ≥ 2 y: 30 mg/m² tid; to max dose of 60 mg/m² tid; ↓ w/ renal impair W/P: [B, + (monitor child)] CI: Asthma, ↓ HR, ↑ prolonged QT interval, 2nd/3rd-degree heart block w/o pacemaker, cardiogenic shock, uncontrolled CHF Disp: Tabs 80, 120, 160, 240 mg SE: ↓ HR, CP, palpitations, fatigue, dizziness, weakness, dyspnea

Sotalol (Betapace AF)   BOX: See sotalol (*Betapace*) Uses: *Maintain sinus rhythm for symptomatic AF/a flutter* Acts: β-Adrenergic-blocking agent Dose: *Adults. CrCl > 60 mL/min:* 80 mg PO q12h, max 320 mg/d. *CrCl 40–60 mL/min:* 80 mg PO q24h; ↑ to 120 mg bid during hospitalization; monitor QT interval 2–4 h after each dose, dose reduction or D/C if QT interval ≥ 500 ms. *Peds. < 2 y:* Dose adjusted based on logarithmic scale (refer to pkg insert): *> 2 y:* 9 mg/m²/d ÷ tid, may ↑ to 180 mg/m²/d W/P: [B, +] When converting from other antiarrhythmic CI: Asthma, ↓ HR, ↑ QT interval, 2nd/3rd-degree heart block w/o pacemaker, cardiogenic shock, K⁺ < 4, sick sinus synd, baseline QT > 450 ms uncontrolled CHF, CrCl < 40 mL/min Disp: Tabs 80, 120, 160 mg SE: ↓ HR, CP, palpitations, fatigue, dizziness, weakness, dyspnea Notes: Follow renal Fxn & QT interval; Betapace should not be substituted for Betapace AF because of differences in labeling

Spinosad (Natroba)   Uses: *Head lice* Acts: Neuronal excitation of lice, w/ paralysis & death Dose: Cover dry scalp w/ suspension, then apply to dry hair; rinse off in 10 min, may repeat after 7 d; unlabeled to use < 4 y W/P: [B, ?/–]

Disp: 0.9% topical susp **SE:** Scalp/ocular erythema **Notes:** Shake well before use; use w/ overall lice management program; in benzyl alcohol, serious Rxns in neonates, in breast milk, pump and discard milk for 8 h after use

Spironolactone (Aldactone, Generic) BOX: Tumorogenic in anmial studies; avoid unnecessary use **Uses:** *Hyperaldosteronism, HTN, class III/IV CHF, ascites from cirrhosis* **Acts:** Aldosterone antagonist; K^+-sparing diuretic **Dose:** *Adults. CHF* (NYHA class III–IV) 12.5–25 mg/d (w/ ACE and loop diuretic); *HTN* 25–50 mg/d; *Ascites:* 100–400 mg q A.M w/ 40–160 mg of furosemide, start w/ 100 mg/40 mg, wait at least 3 d before ↑ dose *Peds.* 1–3.3 mg/kg/24 h PO ÷ bid q12–24h, take w/ food **W/P:** [C, + (D/C w/ breast-feeding)] **CI:** ↑ K^+, acute renal failure, anuria **Disp:** Tabs 25, 50, 100 mg **SE:** ↑ K^+ & gynecomastia, arrhythmia, sexual dysfunction, confusion, dizziness, D/N/V, abnormal menstruation

Starch, Topical, Rectal (Tucks Suppositories [OTC]) **Uses:** *Temporary relief of anorectal disorders (itching, etc)* **Acts:** Topical protectant **Dose:** *Adults & Peds ≥ 12 y.* Cleanse, rinse, and dry, insert 1 supp rectally 6×/d × 7 d max. **W/P:** [?, ?] **CI:** None **Disp:** Supp **SE:** D/C w/ or if rectal bleeding occurs or if condition worsens or docs not improve w/in 7 d

Stavudine (Zerit, Generic) BOX: Lactic acidosis & severe hepatomegaly w/ steatosis & pancreatitis reported w/ didanosine **Uses:** *HIV in combo w/ other antiretrovirals* **Acts:** NRTI **Dose:** *Adults > 60 kg.* 40 mg bid. *< 60 kg.* 30 mg bid. *Peds Birth–13 d.* 0.5 mg/kg q12h. *> 14 d & < 30 kg.* 1 mg/kg q12h. *≥ 30 kg.* Adult dose; ↓ w/ renal Insuff **W/P:** [C, –] **CI:** Allergy **Disp:** Caps 15, 20, 30, 40 mg; soln 1 mg/mL **SE:** Peripheral neuropathy, HA, chills, rash, GI upset, anemias, lactic acidosis, ↑ LFTs, pancreatitis **Notes:** Take w/ plenty of H_2O

Steroids, Systemic (See Table 2, p 301) The following relates only to the commonly used systemic glucocorticoids **Uses:** *Endocrine disorders (adrenal Insuff), rheumatoid disorders, collagen–vascular Dzs, derm Dzs, allergic states, cerebral edema*, nephritis, nephrotic synd, immunosuppression for transplantation, ↑ Ca^{2+}, malignancies (breast, lymphomas), preop (pt who has been on steroids in past year, known hypoadrenalism), preop for adrenalectomy); Inj into jts/tissue **Acts:** Glucocorticoid **Dose:** Varies w/ use & institutional protocols.

- *Adrenal Insuff, acute: Adults. Hydrocortisone:* 100 mg IV; then 300 mg/d ÷ q8h for 48 h then convert to 50 mg PO q8h × 6 doses, taper to 30–50 mg/d ÷ bid. *Peds. Hydrocortisone:* 1–2 mg/kg IV, then 150–250 mg/d ÷ q6h–q8h.
- *Adrenal Insuff, chronic (physiologic replacement):* May need mineralocorticoid supl such as Florinef. *Adults. Hydrocortisone:* 20 mg PO q A.M., 10 mg PO q P.M.; *cortisone:* 25–35 mg PO daily. *Dexamethasone:* 0.03–0.15 mg/kg/d or 0.6–0.75 mg/m^2/d ÷ q6–12h PO, IM, IV. *Peds. Hydrocortisone:* 8–10 mg/m^2/d ÷ q8h; some may require up to 12 mg/m^2/d. *Hydrocortisone succinate:* 0.25–0.35 mg/kg/d IM.
- *Asthma, acute: Adults. Methylprednisolone* 40–80 mg in 1–2 ÷ dose PO/ IV or *dexamethasone* 12 mg IV q6h. *Peds. Prednisolone* 1–2 mg/kg/d or

prednisone 1–2 mg/kg/d ÷ daily-bid for up to 5 d; *methylprednisolone* 12 mg/kg/d IV ÷ bid; *dexamethasone* 0.1–0.3 mg/kg/d ÷ q6h.

- *Congenital adrenal hyperplasia: Peds.* Initial *hydrocortisone* 10–20 mg/m²/d in 3 ÷ doses
- *Extubation/airway edema: Adults.* Dexamethasone: 0.5–2 mg/kg/d IM/IV ÷ q6h (start 24 h prior to extubation; continue × 4 more doses). *Peds.* Dexamethasone: 0.5–2 mg/kg/d ÷ q6h (start 24 h before & cont for 4–6 doses after extubation)
- *Immunosuppressive/anti-inflammatory: Adults & Older Peds.* Hydrocortisone: 15–240 mg PO, IM, IV q12h. *Methylprednisolone:* 2–60 mg/d PO in 1–4 ÷ doses, taper to lowest effective dose. *Methylprednisolone Na succinate:* 10–80 mg/d IM or 10–40 mg/d IV. *Adults.* Prednisone or prednisolone: 5–60 mg/d PO ÷ daily-qid. *Infants & Younger Children.* Hydrocortisone: 2.5–10 mg/kg/d PO ÷ q6–8h; 1–5 mg/kg/d IM/IV ÷ bid-daily.
- *Nephrotic synd: Peds.* Prednisolone or prednisone: 2 mg/kg/d PO tid-qid until urine is protein-free for 5 d, use up to 28 d; for persistent proteinuria, 4 mg/kg/dose PO q other day max, 120 mg/d for an additional 28 d; maint 2 mg/kg/dose q other day for 28 d; taper over 4–6 wk (max 80 mg/d).
- *Septic shock (controversial): Adults.* Hydrocortisone: 50 mg IV q6h; max 300 mg/d; some suggest 200 mg/d cont Inf *Peds.* Hydrocortisone: 1–2 mg/kg/d intermittent or continuous Inf; may titrate up to 50 mg/kg/d.
- *Status asthmaticus: Adults & Peds.* Hydrocortisone: 1–2 mg/kg/dose IV q6h for 24h; then ↓ by 0.5–1 mg/kg q6h.
- *Rheumatic Dz: Adults. Intra-articular: Hydrocortisone acetate:* 25–37.5 large jt, 10–25 mg small jt. *Methylprednisolone acetate:* 20–80 mg large jt, 4–10 mg small jt. *Intrabursal: Hydrocortisone acetate:* 25–37.5 mg. *Intra-ganglial: Hydrocortisone acetate:* 25–37.5 mg. *Tendon sheath: Hydrocortisone acetate:* 5–12.5 mg.
- *Perioperative steroid coverage: Hydrocortisone:* 100 mg IV night before surgery, 1 h preop, intraoperative, & 4, 8, & 12 h postp; postop day No. 1 100 mg IV q6h; postop day No. 2 100 mg IV q8h; postop day No. 3 100 mg IV q12h; postop day No. 4 50 mg IV q12h; postop day No. 5 25 mg IV q12h; resume prior PO dosing if chronic use or D/C if only perioperative coverage required.
- *Cerebral edema: Dexamethasone:* 10 mg IV; then 4 mg IV q4–6h

W/P: [C/D, ?] **CI:** Active varicella Infxn, serious Infxn except TB, fungal Infxns **Disp:** Table 2, p 301 **SE:** ↑ Appetite, hyperglycemia, ↓ K⁺, osteoporosis, nervousness, insomnia, "steroid psychosis", adrenal suppression **Notes:** Hydrocortisone succinate for systemic, acetate for intraarticular; never abruptly D/C steroids, taper dose; also used for bacterial and TB meningitis

Steroids, Topical (See Table 3, p 302) **Uses:** *Steroid-responsive dermatoses (seborrheic/atopic dermatitis, neurodermatitis, anogenital pruritus, psoriasis)* **Acts:** Glucocorticoid; ↓ capillary permeability, stabilizes lysosomes to

control inflammation; controls protein synthesis; ↓ migration of leukocytes, fibroblasts **Dose:** Use lowest potency produce for shortest period for effect (see Table 3, p 302) **W/P:** [C, +] Do not use occlusive dressings; high potency topical products not for rosacea, perioral dermatitis; not for use on face, groin, axillae; none for use in a diapered area. **CI:** Component hypersens **Disp:** See Table 3, p 302 **SE:** Skin atrophy w/ chronic use; chronic administration or application over large area may cause adrenal suppression or hyperglycemia

Streptokinase (Generic) **Uses:** *Coronary artery thrombosis, acute massive PE, DVT, & some occluded vascular grafts* **Acts:** Activates plasminogen to plasmin that degrades fibrin **Dose:** *Adults. PE:* Load 250,000 units peripheral IV over 30 min, then 100,000 units/h IV for 24–72 h. *Coronary artery thrombosis:* 1.5 mill units IV over 60 min. *DVT or arterial embolism:* Load as w/ PE, then 100,000 units/h for 24 h; *ECC 2010. AMI:* 1.5 mill units over 1 h. *Peds.* 1000–2000 units/kg over 30 min, then 1000 units/kg/h for up to 24 h. *Occluded catheter (controversial):* 10,000–25,000 units in NS to final vol of catheter (leave in for 1 h, aspirate & flush w/ NS) **W/P:** [C, +] **CI:** Streptococcal Infxn or streptokinase in last 6 mo, active bleeding, CVA, TIA, spinal surgery/trauma in last mo, vascular anomalies, severe hepatic/renal Dz, severe uncontrolled HTN **Disp:** Powder for Inj 250,000, 750,000, 1,500,000 units **SE:** Bleeding, ↓ BP, fever, bruising, rash, GI upset, hemorrhage, anaphylaxis **Notes:** If Inf inadequate to keep clotting time 2–5 × control, see PI for adjustments; antibodies remain 3–6 mo following dose

Streptomycin (Generic) **BOX:** Neuro/oto/renal tox possible; neuromuscular blockage w/ resp paralysis possible **Uses:** *TB combo Rx therapy* streptococcal or enterococcal endocarditis **Acts:** Aminoglycoside; ↓ protein synth **Dose:** *Adults.* IM route. *Endocarditis:* 1 g q12h 1–2 wk, then 500 mg q12h 1–4 wk in combination w/ PCN; *TB:* 15 mg/kg/d (up to 1 g), directly observed therapy (DOT) 2 × wk 20–30 mg/kg/dose (max 1.5 g), DOT 3 × wk 25–30 mg/kg/dose (max 1.5 g). *Peds.* 20–40 mg/kg/d, 1 g/d max; DOT 2 × wk 25–30 mg/kg/d (max 1.5 g/d) dose (max 1g); DOT 3× wk 25–30 mg/kg/dose (max 1.5 g/d); ↓ w/ renal Insuff, either IM (preferred) or IV over 30–60 min **W/P:** [D, –] **CI:** PRG **Disp:** Inj 400 mg/mL (1-g vial) **SE:** ↑ Incidence of vestibular & auditory tox, ↑ neurotox risk in pts w/ impaired renal Fxn **Notes:** Monitor levels: *Peak:* 20–30 mcg/mL, *Trough:* < 5 mcg/mL; *Toxic peak:* > 50 mcg/mL, *Trough:* > 10 mcg/mL

Streptozocin (Zanosar) **BOX:** Administer under the supervision of a physician experienced in the use of chemotherapy. Renal tox dose-related/cumulative and may be severe or fatal. Other major toxicities: N/V, and may be Tx-limiting; liver dysfunction, D, hematologic changes possible. Streptozocin is mutagenic. **Uses:** *Pancreatic islet cell tumors* & carcinoid tumors **Acts:** DNA–DNA (intrastrand) cross-linking; DNA, RNA, & protein synth inhib **Dose:** Per protocol; ↓ in renal failure **W/P:** w/ Renal failure [D, –] **CI:** w/ PRG **Disp:** Inj 1 g **SE:** N/V/D, duodenal ulcers, depression, ↓ BM rare (20%) & mild; nephrotox (proteinuria & azotemia dose related), ↑ LFT hypophosphatemia dose limiting; hypoglycemia; Inj site Rxns **Notes:** ✓ SCr

Succimer (Chemet) Uses: *Lead poisoning (levels > 50 mcg/dL w/ significant symptoms)* Acts: Heavy metal-chelating agent Dose: *Adults & Peds.* 10 mg/kg/dose q8h × 5 d, then 10 mg/kg/dose q12h for 14 d W/P: [C, ?] w/ Hepatic/renal Insuff CI: Allergy Disp: Caps 100 mg SE: Rash, fever, GI upset, hemorrhoids, metallic taste, drowsiness, ↑ LFTs Notes: Monitor lead levels, maintain hydration, may open caps

Succinylcholine (Anectine, Generic) BOX: Acute rhabdomyolysis w/ hyperkalemia followed by ventricular dysrhythmias, cardiac arrest, and death. Seen in children w/ skeletal muscle myopathy (Duchenne muscular dystrophy) Uses: *Adjunct to general anesthesia, facilitates ET intubation; induce skeletal muscle relaxation during surgery or mechanical ventilation* Acts: Depolarizing neuromuscular blocker; rapid onset, short duration (3–5 min) Dose: *Adults.* Rapid sequence intubation 1–1.5 mg/kg IV over 10–30 s or 3–4 mg/kg IM (up to 150 mg) (ECC 2010). *Peds.* 1–2 mg/kg/dose IV, then by 0.3–0.6 mg/kg/dose q5min; ↓ w/ severe renal/hepatic impair W/P: See Box [C, ?] CI: w/ Malignant hyperthermia risk, myopathy, recent major burn, multiple trauma, extensive skeletal muscle denervation Disp: Inj 20, 100 mg/mL SE: Fasciculations, ↑ IOP, ↑ ICP, intragastric pressure, salivation, myoglobinuria, malignant hyperthermia, resp depression, prolonged apnea; multiple drugs potentiate CV effects (arrhythmias, ↓ BP, brady/tachycardia) Notes: May be given IV push/Inf/IM deltoid

Sucralfate (Carafate, Generic) Uses: *Duodenal ulcers*, gastric ulcers, stomatitis, GERD, preventing stress ulcers, esophagitis Acts: Forms ulcer-adherent complex that protects against acid, pepsin, & bile acid Dose: *Adults.* 1 g PO qid, 1 h prior to meals & hs. *Peds.* 40–80 mg/kg/d ÷ q6h; continue 4–8 wk unless healing demonstrated by x-ray or endoscopy; separate from other drugs by 2 h; take on empty stomach ac W/P: [B, ?] CI: Component allergy Disp: Tabs 1 g; susp 1 g/10 mL SE: Constipation; D, dizziness, xerostomia Notes: May accumulate in renal failure

Sulfacetamide (Bleph-10, Cetamide, Klaron, Generic) Uses: *Conjunctival Infxns*, topical acne, seborrheic dermatitis Acts: Sulfonamide antibiotic Dose: Ophthal soln: 1–2 gtt q2–3 h while awake for 7–10 d; 10% oint apply qid & hs; soln for keratitis apply q2–3h based on severity W/P: [C, M] CI: Sulfonamide sensitivity; age < 2 mo Disp: Opthal: Oint soln 10%; topical cream 10%; foam, gel, lotion, pad all 10% SE: Irritation, burning, blurred vision, brow ache, SJS, photosens

Sulfacetamide/Prednisolone (Blephamide) Uses: *Steroid-responsive inflammatory ocular conditions w/ Infxn or a risk of Infxn* Acts: Antibiotic & anti-inflammatory Dose: *Adults & Peds > 2 y.* Apply oint lower conjunctival sac daily-qid; soln 1–3 gtt q4h while awake W/P: [C, ?/–] Sulfonamide sensitivity; age < 2 mo Disp: *Oint:* sulfacetamide 10%/prednisolone 0.2%. *Susp:* sulfacetamide 10%/prednisolone 0.2% SE: Irritation, burning, blurred vision, brow ache, SJS, photosens Notes: OK ophthal susp use as otic agent

Sulfasalazine (Azulfidine, Azulfidine EN, Generic) Uses: *UC, RA, juvenile RA* Acts: Sulfonamide; actions unclear Dose: *Adults. Ulcerative colitis:* Initial, 1 g PO tid-qid; ↑ to a max of 4–6 g/d in 4 ÷ doses; maint 500 mg PO qid. *RA:*

(EC tab) 0.5–1 g/d, ↑ weekly to maint 2 g ÷ bid. *Peds. Ulcerative colitis:* Initial: 40–60 mg/kg/24 h PO ÷ q4–6h; maint: 30 mg/kg/24 h PO ÷ q6h. *RA > 6 y:* 30–50 mg/kg/d in 2 doses, start w/ 1/4–1/3 maint dose, ↑ weekly until dose reached at 1 mo, 2 g/d max **W/P:** [B, M] Not rec w/ renal or hepatic impair **CI:** Sulfonamide or salicylate sensitivity, porphyria, GI or GU obst **Disp:** Tabs 500 mg; EC DR tabs 500 mg **SE:** GI upset; discolors urine; dizziness, HA, photosens, oligospermia, anemias, SJS **Notes:** May cause yellow-orange skin/contact lens discoloration; avoid sunlight exposure

Sulindac (Clinoril) BOX: May ↑ risk of CV events & GI bleeding; do not use for post-CABG pain control **Uses:** *Arthritis & pain* **Acts:** NSAID; ↓ prostaglandins **Dose:** 150–200 mg bid, 400 mg/d max; w/ food **W/P:** [B (D if 3rd tri or near term), ?] not rec w/ severe renal impair **CI:** Allergy to component, ASA or any NSAID, postop pain in CABG **Disp:** Tabs 150, 200 mg **SE:** Dizziness, rash, pruritus, edema, ↓ renal blood flow, renal failure (? fewer renal effects than other NSAIDs), peptic ulcer, GI bleeding

Sumatriptan (Alsuma, Imitrex, Imitrex Statdose, Imitrex Nasal Spray, Sumavel Dosepro, Generic) **Uses:** *Rx acute migraine and cluster HA* **Acts:** Vascular serotonin receptor agonist **Dose:** *Adults.* SQ: 6 mg SQ as a single-dose PRN; repeat PRN in 1 h to a max of 12 mg/24 h. PO: 25–100 mg, repeat in 2 h, PRN, 200 mg/d max. *Nasal spray:* 1 spray into 1 nostril, repeat in 2 h to 40 mg/24 h max. *Peds. Nasal spray: 6–9 y:* 5–20 mg/d *10–17 y:* 5–20 mg, up to 40 mg/d **W/P:** [C, ?] **CI:** IV use, angina, ischemic heart Dz, CV syndromes, PUD, cerebro vascular Dz, uncontrolled HTN, severe hepatic impair, ergot use, MAOI use w/in 14 d, hemiplegic or basilar migraine **Disp:** *Imitrex Oral:* OD tabs 25, 50, 100 mg; *Imitrex Injection:* 4, 6 mg/0.5 mL; ODTs 25, 50, 100 mg; *Imitrex Nasal Spray:* 5, 20 mg/spray; *Alsuma Auto-Injector:* 6 mg/0.5 mL **SE:** Pain & bruising at Inj site; dizziness, hot flashes, paresthesias, CP, weakness, numbness, coronary vasospasm, HTN

Sumatriptan/Naproxen Sodium (Treximet) BOX: ↑ Risk of serious CV (MI, stroke) serious GI events (bleeding, ulceration, perforation) of the stomach or intestines **Uses:** *Prevent migraines* **Acts:** Anti-inflammatory NSAID w/ 5-HT₁ receptor agonist, constricts CNS vessels **Dose:** *Adults.* 1 tab PO; repeat PRN after 2 h; max 2 tabs/24 h, w/ or w/o food **W/P:** [C, –] **CI:** CV Dz, severe hepatic impair, severe ↑ BP **Disp:** Tab naproxen/sumatriptan 500 mg/85 mg **SE:** Dizziness, somnolence, paresthesia, N, dyspepsia, dry mouth, chest/neck/throat/jaw pain, tightness, pressure **Notes:** Do not split/crush/chew

Sumatriptan Needleless System (Sumavel DosePro) **Uses:** *Rx acute migraine and cluster HA* **Acts:** Vascular serotonin receptor agonist **Dose:** *Adults.* SQ: 6 mg SQ as a single-dose PRN; repeat PRN in 1 h to a max of 12 mg/24 h; administer in abdomen/thigh. **W/P:** [C, M] **CI:** See Sumatriptan **Disp:** Needle-free SQ injector 6 mg/0.5 mL **SE:** Injection site Rxn, tingling, warm/hot/burning sensation, feeling of heaviness/pressure/tightness/numbness, feeling strange, lightheadedness, flushing, tightness in chest, discomfort in nasal cavity/sinuses/jaw, changes/vertigo, drowsiness/sedation, HA

Sunitinib (Sutent) **BOX:** Hepatotox that may be severe and/or result in fatal liver failure **Uses:** *Advanced GI stromal tumor (GIST) refractory/intolerant of imatinib; advanced RCC; well-differentiated pancreatic neuroendocrine tumors unresectable, locally advanced, metastatic* **Acts:** TKI; VEGF inhib **Dose:** *Adults.* 50 mg PO daily × 4 wk, followed by 2 wk holiday = 1 cycle; ↓ to 37.5 mg w/ CYP3A4 inhib (Table 10, p 319), to ↑ 87.5 mg or 62.5 mg/d w/ CYP3A4 inducers **CI:** None **W/P:** [D, –] Multiple interactions require dose modification (eg, St. John's wort) **Disp:** Caps 12.5, 25, 50 mg **SE:** ↓ WBC & plt, bleeding, ↑ BP, ↓ ejection fraction, ↑ QT interval, pancreatitis, DVT, Szs, adrenal insufficiency, N/V/D, skin discoloration, oral ulcers, taste perversion, hypothyroidism **Notes:** Monitor left ventricular ejection fraction, ECG, CBC/plts, chemistries (K+/Mg2+/phosphate), TFT & LFTs periodically; ↓ dose in 12.5-mg increments if not tolerated

Tacrolimus (Prograf, Generic) **BOX:** ↑ Risk of Infxn and lymphoma. Only physicians experienced in immunosuppression should prescribe **Uses:** *Prevent organ rejection (kidney/liver/heart)* **Acts:** Calcineurin inhib/immunosuppressant **Dose:** *Adults.* IV: 0.03–0.05 mg/kg/d in kidney and liver, 0.01 mg/kg/d in heart IV Inf *Peds.* IV: 0.03–0.05 mg/kg/d as cont Inf. *PO:* 0.15–0.2 mg/kg/d PO ÷ q12h. *Adults & Peds. Eczema:* Take on empty stomach; ↓ w/ hepatic/renal impair **W/P:** [C, –] w/ Cyclosporine; avoid topical if < 2 y; Neuro & nephrotox, ↑ risk opportunistic Infxns; avoid grapefruit juice **CI:** Component allergy, castor oil allergy w/ IV form **Disp:** Caps 0.5, 1, 5 mg; Inj 5 mg/mL **SE:** HTN, edema, HA, insomnia, fever, pruritus, ↑/↓ K+, hyperglycemia, GI upset, anemia, leukocytosis, tremors, paresthesias, pleural effusion, Szs, lymphoma, posterior reversible encephalopathy syndrome (PRES), BK nephropathy, PML **Notes:** Monitor levels; *Trough:* 5–12 ng/mL based on indication and time since transplant

Tacrolimus, Ointment (Protopic) **BOX:** Long-term safety of topical calcineurin inhibs not established. Avoid long-term use. ↑ Risk of Infxn and lymphoma. Not for peds < 2yr **Uses:** *2nd line mod–severe atopic dermatitis* **Acts:** Topical calcineurin inhib/immunosuppressant **Dose:** *Adult & Peds > 15 y.* Apply thin layer (0.03–0.1%) bid; D/C when S/Sxs clear. *Peds 2–15 y.* Apply thin layer (0.03%) bid, D/C when S/Sxs clear **W/P:** [C, –] Reevaluate if no response in 6 wk; not for < 2 y; avoid cont longterm use, ↑ risk opportunistic Infxns **CI:** Component allergy **Disp:** Oint 0.03, 0.1% **SE:** Local irritation **Notes:** Avoid occlusive dressing; only use 0.03% in peds

Tadalafil (Adcirca) **Uses:** *Pulmonary artery hypertension* **Acts:** PDE5 inhib, ↑ cyclic guanosine monophosphate & NO levels; relaxes pulm artery smooth muscles **Dose:** 40 mg 1 × d w/o regard to meals; ↓ w/ renal/hepatic Insuff **W/P:** [B, –] w/ CV Dz, impaired autonomic control of BP, aortic stenosis α-blockers (except tamsulosin); use w/ CYP3A4 inhib/inducers (eg, ritonavir, ketoconazole); monitor for sudden ↓/loss of hearing or vision (NAION), tinnitus, priapism **CI:** w/ Nitrates, component hypersens **Disp:** Tabs 20 mg **SE:** HA **Notes:** See Tadalafil (*Cialis*) for ED

Tadalafil (Cialis) **Uses:** *ED, BPH* **Acts:** PDE5 inhib, ↑ cyclic guanosine monophosphate & NO levels; relaxes smooth muscles, dilates cavernosal arteries

Dose: *Adults. PRN:* 10 mg PO before sexual activity (5–20 mg max based on response) 1 dose/24 h. *Daily dosing:* 2.5 mg qd, may ↑ to 5 mg qd, *BPH;* 5 mg PO qd; w/o regard to meals; ↓ w/ renal/hepatic Insuff **W/P:** [B, –] w/ α-Blockers (except tamsulosin); use w/ CYP3A4 inhib (Table 10, p 319) (eg, ritonavir, ketoconazole, itraconazole) 2.5 mg/daily dose or 5 mg PRN dose; CrCl < 30 mL/min, hemodialysis/severe hepatic impair, do not use daily dosing **CI:** Nitrates **Disp:** Tabs 2.5, 5, 10, 20 mg **SE:** HA, flushing, dyspepsia, back/limb pain, myalgia, nasal congestion, urticaria, SJS, dermatitis, visual field defect, NIAON, sudden ↓/loss of hearing, tinnitus **Notes:** Longest acting of class (36 h); daily dosing may ↑ drug interactions; excessive EtOH may ↑ orthostasis; transient global amnesia reports

Tafluprost (Zioptan) Uses: **Open-angle glaucoma** Acts: ↓ IOP by ↑ uveoscleral outflow, prostaglandin analog **Dose:** 1 gtt evening **W/P:** [C, ?/–] **CI:** None **Disp:** Soln 0.0015% **SE:** Periorbital/iris pigmentation, eyelash darkening thickening; ↑ number eye redness **Notes:** Pigmentation maybe permanent

Talc [Sterile Talc Powder] (Sclerosol, Generic) Uses: **↓ Recurrence of malignant pleural effusions (pleurodesis)** Acts: Sclerosing agent **Dose:** Mix slurry: 50 mL NS w/ 5-g vial, mix, distribute 25 mL into two 60-mL syringes, vol to 50 mL/syringe w/ NS. Infuse each into chest tube, flush w/ 25 mL NS. Keep tube clamped; have pt change positions q15min for 2 h, unclamp tube; aerosol 4–8 g intrapleurally **W/P:** [B, ?] **CI:** Planned further surgery on site **Disp:** 5 g powder; (*Sclerosol*) 400 mg/spray **SE:** Pain, Infxn **Notes:** May add 10–20 mL 1% lidocaine/syringe; must have chest tube placed, monitor closely while tube clamped (tension pneumothorax), not antineoplastic

Taliglucerase Alfa (Elelyso) Uses: **Long-term enzyme replacement for type 1 Gaucher Dz** Acts: Catalyzes hydrolysis of glucocerebroside to glucose & ceramide **Dose:** *Adults.* 60 units/kg IV every other wk; Inf over 1–2 h **W/P:** [B, ?/–] **CI:** None **Disp:** Inj 200 units/vial **SE:** Inf Rxns (allergic, HA, CP, asthenia, fatigue, urticaria, erythema, ↑ BP, back pain, arthralgia, flushing), anaphylaxis, URI, pharyngitis, influenza, UTI, extremity pain **Notes:** For Rxns: ↓ Inf rate, give antihistamines/antipyretics or D/C

Tamoxifen (Generic) BOX: CA of the uterus or endometrium; stroke, and blood clots can occur Uses: **Breast CA [postmenopausal, estrogen receptor(+)], ↓ risk of breast CA in high-risk, met male breast CA**, ovulation induction Acts: Nonsteroidal antiestrogen; mixed agonist–antagonist effect **Dose:** 20–40 mg/d; doses > 20 mg ÷ bid. *Prevention:* 20 mg PO/d × 5 y **W/P:** [D, –] w/ ↓ WBC, ↓ plts, hyperlipidemia **CI:** PRG, w/ warfarin, Hx thromboembolism **Disp:** Tabs 10, 20 mg **SE:** Uterine malignancy & thrombosis events seen in breast CA prevention trials; menopausal Sxs (hot flashes, N/V) in premenopausal pts; Vag bleeding & menstrual irregularities; skin rash, pruritus vulvae, dizziness, HA, peripheral edema; acute flare of bone metastasis pain & ↑ Ca^{2+}; retinopathy reported (high dose)

Tamsulosin (Flomax, Generic) Uses: **BPH** Acts: Antagonist of prostatic α-receptors **Dose:** 0.4 mg/d, may ↑ to 0.8 mg PO daily **W/P:** [B, ?] Floppy iris syndrome w/ cataract surgery **Disp:** Caps 0.4 mg **SE:** HA, dizziness, syncope, somnolence, ↓ libido, GI upset, retrograde ejaculation, rhinitis, rash, angioedema, IFIS **Notes:** Not for use as antihypertensive; do not open/crush/chew; approved for use w/ dutasteride for BPH

Tapentadol (Nucynta) [C-II] **Box:** Provider should be alert to problems of abuse, misuse, & diversion. Avoid use w/ alcohol. **Uses:** *Mod–severe acute pain* **Acts:** Mu-opioid agonist and norepinephrine reuptake inhib **Dose:** 50–100 mg PO q4–6h PRN (max 600 mg/d); w/ mod hepatic impair: 50 mg q8h PRN (max 3 doses/24 h) ER dosing: initial 50 mg PO bid (max daily dose 500 mg) **W/P:** [C, –] Hx of Szs, CNS depression; ↑ ICP, severe renal impair, biliary tract Dz, elderly, serotonin synd w/ concomitant serotonergic agents **CI:** ↓ Pulm Fxn, use w/ or w/in 14 d of MAOI, Ileus **Disp:** Tabs 50, 75, 100 mg, ER: 50, 100, 150, 200, 250 mg **SE:** N/V, dizziness, somnolence, HA, constipation **Notes:** Taper dose w/ D/C

Tazarotene (Avage, Fabior, Tazorac) **Uses:** *Facial acne vulgaris; stable plaque psoriasis up to 20% BSA* **Acts:** Keratolytic **Dose:** *Adults & Peds > 12 y. Acne:* Cleanse face, dry, apply thin film qhs lesions. *Psoriasis:* Apply qhs **W/P:** [X, ?/–] **CI:** Retinoid sensitivity, PRG, use in women of childbearing age unable to comply w/ birth control requirements **Disp:** Gel 0.05, 0.1%; cream 0.05, 0.1%; foam 0.1% **SE:** Burning, erythema, irritation, rash, photosens, desquamation, bleeding, skin discoloration **Notes:** D/C w/ excessive pruritus, burning, skin redness, or peeling until Sxs resolve; external use only, not for broken or sunburned skin

Teduglutide [rDNA Origin] (Gattex) **Uses:** *Short bowel synd dependent on parenteral support* **Acts:** GLP-2 analog ↑ intest & portal blood flow & ↓ gastric acid secretion **Dose:** *Adults.* 0.05 mg/kg SQ daily; ↓ 50% w/ mod–severe renal impair; alt Inj site between Abd, thighs, arms **W/P:** [B, ?/–] Acceleration neoplastic growth (colonoscopy baseline, 1 y, & q5y); D/C w/ intestinal obstr; biliary/ pancreatic Dz (baseline & q6mo bili, alk phos, lipase, amylase); may ↑ absorption oral meds **CI:** None **Disp:** Inj vial 5 mg **SE:** N/V, Abd pain, Abd distention, Inj site Rxn, HA, URI, fluid overload

Telaprevir (Incivek) **Uses:** *Hep C virus, genotype 1, w/ compensated liver Dz including naive to Tx, nonresponders, partial responders, relapsers; w/ peginterferon and ribavirin* **Acts:** Hep C antiviral; NS3/4A protease inhib **Dose:** *Adults.* 750 mg tid, w/ food, must be used w/ peginterferon and ribavirin × 12 wk, then peginterferon and ribavirin × 12 wk (if hep C undetectable at 4 and 12 wk) or 36 wk (if hep C detectable at 4 and/or 12 wk) **W/P:** [X, –] **CI:** All CIs to peginterferon and ribavirin; men if PRG female partner; w/ CYP3A metabolized drugs (eg, alfuzosin, sildenafil, tadalafil, lovastatin, simvastatin, ergotamines, cisapride, midazolam, rifampin, St. John's wort) **Disp:** Tabs 375 mg **SE:** Rash > 50% of pts, include SJS, drug rash w/ eosinophilia (DRESS); pruritus, anemia, N, V, D, fatigue, anorectal pain, dysgeusia, hemorrhoids **Notes:** Must not be used as monotherapy

Telavancin (Vibativ) **BOX:** Fetal risk; must have PRG test prior to use in childbearing age **Uses:** *Complicated skin/skin structure Infxns d/t susceptible

Gram-positive bacteria* **Acts:** Lipoglycopeptide antibacterial; *Spectrum:* Good gram(+) aerobic and anaerobic include MRSA, MSSA, some VRE; poor gram(−) **Dose:** 10 mg/kg IV q24h; 7.5 mg/kg q24h w/CrCl 30–50 mL/min; 10 mg/kg q48h w/CrCl 10–30 mL/min; **W/P:** [C, ?] Nephrotox, *C. difficile*-associated diarrhea, insomnia, HA Dz, ↑ QTc, interferes w/ some coag tests **CI:** None **Disp:** Inj 250, 750 mg **SE:** Insomnia, psychiatric disorder, taste disturbance, HA, N, V, foamy urine **Notes:** Contains cyclodextrin, which can accumulate in renal dysfunction

Telbivudine (Tyzeka) **BOX:** May cause lactic acidosis and severe hepatomegaly w/ steatosis when used alone or w/ antiretrovirals; D/C of the drug may lead to exacerbations of hep B; monitor LFTs **Uses:** *Rx chronic hep B* **Acts:** Nucleoside RT inhib **Dose:** *CrCl > 50 mL/min:* 600 mg PO daily; *CrCl 30–49 ml /min:* 600 mg q 48h; *CrCl < 30 mL/min:* 600 mg q72h; *ESRD:* 600 mg q96h; dose after hemodialysis **W/P:** [B, ?/–] May cause myopathy; follow closely w/ other myopathy causing drugs **Disp:** Tabs 600 mg **SE:** Fatigue, Abd pain, N/V/D, HA, URI, nasopharyngitis, ↑ LFTs, CPK, myalgia/myopathy, flu-like Sxs, dizziness, insomnia, dyspepsia **Notes:** Use w/ PEG-interferon may ↑ peripheral neuropathy risk

Telithromycin (Ketek) **BOX:** CI in MyG; life-threatening RF occured in PF w/ MyG **Uses:** *Mild–mod CAP* **Acts:** Unique macrolide, blocks ↓ protein synth; bactericidal. *Spectrum: S. aureus, S. pneumoniae, H. influenzae, M. catarrhalis, C. pneumoniae, M. pneumoniae* **Dose:** *CAP:* 800 mg (2 tabs) PO daily × 7–10 d **W/P:** [C, ?] Pseudomembranous colitis, ↑ QTc interval, visual disturbances, hepatic dysfunction; dosing in renal impair unknown **CI:** Macrolide allergy, w/ pimozide or cisapride, Hx of hep or jaundice, w/ macrolide abx, w/ MyG **Disp:** Tabs 300, 400 mg **SE:** N/V/D, dizziness, blurred vision **Notes:** A CYP450 inhib; multiple drug interactions; hold statins d/t ↑ risk of myopathy

Telmisartan (Micardis) **BOX:** Use of renin-angiotensin agents in PRG can cause fetal injury and death, D/C immediately when PRG detected **Uses:** *HTN, CHF* **Acts:** Angiotensin II receptor antagonist **Dose:** 40–80 mg/d **W/P:** [C (1st tri; D 2nd & 3rd tri), ?/–] ↑ K+ **CI:** Angiotensin II receptor antagonist sensitivity **Disp:** Tabs 20, 40, 80 mg **SE:** Edema, GI upset, HA, angioedema, renal impair, orthostatic ↓ BP

Telmisartan/Amlodipine (Twynsta) **BOX:** Use of renin-angiotensin agents in PRG can cause fetal injury and death, D/C immediately when PRG detected **Uses:** *Hypertension* **Acts:** CCB; relaxes coronary vascular smooth muscle & angiotensin II receptor antagonist **Dose:** Start 40/5 mg telmisartan/amlodipine; max 80/10 mg PO/d; ↑ dose after 2 wk **W/P:** [C 1st tri; D 2nd, 3rd; ?/–] ↑ K+ **CI:** PRG **Disp:** Tabs mg telmisartan/mg amlodipine 40/5; 40/10; 80/5; 80/10 **SE:** HA, edema, dizziness, N, ↓ BP **Notes:** Titrate w/ hepatic/renal impair; avoid w/ ACE/other ARBs; correct hypovolemia before; w/ CHF monitor

Temazepam (Restoril, Generic) [C-IV] **Uses:** *Insomnia*, anxiety, depression, panic attacks **Acts:** Benzodiazepine **Dose:** 15–30 mg PO hs PRN; ↓ in elderly **W/P:** [X, ?/–] Potentiates CNS depressive effects of opioids, barbs, EtOH, antihistamines, MAOIs, TCAs **CI:** NAG, PRG **Disp:** Caps 7.5, 15, 22.5,

30 mg **SE:** Confusion, dizziness, drowsiness, hangover **Notes:** Abrupt D/C after > 10 d use may cause withdrawal

Temozolomide (Temodar) **Uses:** *Glioblastoma multiforme (GBM), refractory anaplastic astrocytoma* **Acts:** Alkylating agent **Dose:** *GBM, new:* 75 mg/m^2 PO/IV/d × 42 d w/ RT, maint 150 mg/m^2/d days 1–5 of 28-d cycle × 6 cycles; may ↑ to 200 mg/m^2/d × 5 d every 28 d in cycle 2; *Refractory astrocytoma:* 150 mg/m^2 PO/IV/d × 5 d per 28-d cycle; Adjust dose based on ANC and plt count (per PI and local protocols). **W/P:** [D, ?/–] w/ Severe renal/hepatic impair, myelosuppression (monitor ANC & plt), myelodysplastic synd, secondary malignancies, PCP pneumonia (PCP prophylaxis required) **CI:** Hypersens to components or dacarbazine **Disp:** Caps 5, 20, 100, 140, 180, & 250 mg; powder for Inj 100 mg **SE:** N/V/D, fatigue, HA, asthenia, Sz, hemiparesis, fever, dizziness, coordination abnormality, alopecia, rash, constipation, anorexia, amnesia, insomnia, viral Infxn, ↓ WBC, plt **Notes:** Infuse over 90 min; swallow caps whole; if caps open avoid inhalation and contact w/ skin/mucous membranes

Temsirolimus (Torisel) **Uses:** *Advanced RCC* **Acts:** Multikinase inhib, ↓ mTOR (mammalian target of rapamycin), ↓ hypoxic-induced factors, ↓ VEGF **Dose:** 25 mg IV 30–60 min 1×/wk. Hold w/ ANC < 1000 cells/mcL, plt < 75,000 cells/mcL, or NCI grade 3 tox. Resume when tox grade 2 or less, restart w/ dose ↓ 5 mg/wk not < 15 mg/wk. w/ CYP3A4 inhib: ↓ 12.5 mg/wk. w/ CYP3A4 inducers ↑ 50 mg/wk **W/P:** [D, –] Avoid live vaccines, ↓ wound healing, avoid periop **CI:** Bili > 1.5 × ULN **Disp:** Inj 25 mg/mL w/ 250 mL diluent **SE:** Rash, asthenia, mucositis, N, bowel perforation, angioedema, impaired wound healing, interstitial lung Dz anorexia, edema, ↑ lipids, ↑ glucose, ↑ triglycerides, ↑ LFTs, ↑ Cr, ↓ WBC, ↓ HCT, ↓ plt, ↓ PO$_4$ **Notes:** Premedicate w/ antihistamine; ✓ lipids, CBC, plt, Cr, glucose; w/ sunitinib dose-limiting tox likely; females use w/ contraception

Tenecteplase (TNKase) **Uses:** *Restore perfusion & ↓ mortality w/ AMI* **Acts:** Thrombolytic; TPA **Dose:** 30–50 mg; see table below **W/P:** [C, ?], ↑ Bleeding w/ NSAIDs, ticlopidine, clopidogrel, GPIIb/IIIa antagonists **CI:** Bleeding, AVM aneurysm, CVA, CNS neoplasm, uncontrolled ↑ BP, major surgery (intracranial, intraspinal) or trauma w/in 2 mo **Disp:** Inj 50 mg, reconstitute w/ 10 mL sterile H$_2$O only **SE:** Bleeding, allergy **Notes:** Do not shake w/ reconstitution; start ASA ASAP, IV heparin ASAP w/ aPTT 1.5–2 × UL of control

Tenecteplase Dosing (From 1 vial of reconstituted TNKase)

Weight (kg)	TNKase (mg)	TNKase Volume (mL)
< 60	30	6
60–69	35	7
70–79	40	8
80–89	45	9
≥ 90	50	10

Tenofovir (Viread) **BOX:** Lactic acidosis/hepatomegaly w/ steatosis (some fatal) reported w/ the use of NRTI. Exacerbations of hepatitis reported w/ HBV patients who D/C hep B Rx, including VIREAD. ✓ LFT in these patients and may need to resume hep B Rx **Uses:** *HIV and chronic hep B Infxn* **Acts:** NRTI **Dose:** 300 mg PO daily w/ or w/o meal; CrCl 30–49 mL/min q48h, CrCl 10–29 mL/min 2×/wk **W/P:** [B, –] Didanosine, lopinavir, ritonavir w/ known risk factors for liver Dz **CI:** Hypersens **Disp:** Tabs 300 mg **SE:** GI upset, metabolic synd, hepatotox; insomnia, rash, ↑ CK, Fanconi synd **Notes:** Combo product w/ emtricitabine is *Truvada*

Tenofovir/Emtricitabine (Truvada) **BOX:** Lactic acidosis/hepatomegaly w/ steatosis (some fatal) reported w/ the use of NRTI. Not approved for chronic hep B. Exacerbations of hepatitis reported w/ HBV pts who D/C *Truvada*. May need to resume hep B Rx. If used for PrEP, confirm (–) HIV before and q3mo. Drug-resistant HIV-1 variants have been identified **Uses:** *HIV Infxn pre-exposure prophylaxis (PrEP) for HIV-1* **Acts:** Dual nucleotide RT inhib **Dose:** 1 tab PO daily w/ or w/o a meal; adjust w/ renal impair **W/P:** [B, ?/–] w/ Known risk factors for liver Dz **CI:** None **Disp:** Tabs: 200 mg emtricitabine/300 mg tenofovir **SE:** GI upset, rash, metabolic synd, hepatotox, Fanconi synd; OK peds > 12 y

Terazosin (Hytrin, Generic) **Uses:** *BPH & HTN* **Acts:** α_1-Blocker (blood vessel & bladder neck/prostate) **Dose:** Initial, 1 mg PO hs; ↑ 20 mg/d max; may ↓ w/ diuretic or other BP medicine **W/P:** [C, ?] w/ β-Blocker, CCB, ACE inhib; use w/ phosphodiesterase-5 (PDE5) inhib (eg, sildenafil) can cause ↓ BP, intra op floppy iris synd w/ cataract surgery **CI:** α-Antagonist sensitivity **Disp:** Tabs 1, 2, 5, 10 mg; caps 1, 2, 5, 10 mg angina **SE:** Angina, ↓ BP, & syncope following 1st dose or w/ PDE5 inhib; dizziness, weakness, nasal congestion, peripheral edema, palpitations, GI upset **Notes:** Caution w/ 1st dose syncope; if for HTN, combine w/ thiazide diuretic

Terbinafine (Lamisil, Lamisil AT, Generic [OTC]) **Uses:** *Onychomycosis, athlete's foot, jock itch, ringworm*, cutaneous candidiasis, pityriasis versicolor **Acts:** ↓ Squalene epoxidase resulting in fungal death **Dose:** *PO:* 250 mg/d PO for 6–12 wk. *Topical:* Apply to area tinea pedis bid, tinea cruris & corporus daily-bid, tinea versicolor soln bid; ↓ PO w/ renal/hepatic impair **W/P:** [B, –] PO ↑ effects of drug metabolism by CYP2D6, w/ liver/renal impair **CI:** CrCl < 50 mL/min, WBC < 1000/mm³, severe liver Dz **Disp:** Tabs 250 mg; oral granules 125 mg/pkt, 187.5 mg/pkt *Lamisil AT* [OTC] cream, gel, soln 1% **SE:** HA, DIV/N dizziness, rash, pruritus, alopecia, GI upset, taste perversion, neutropenia, retinal damage, SJS, ↑ LFTs **Notes:** Effect may take months d/t need for new nail growth; topical not for nails; do not use occlusive dressings; PO follow CBC/LFTs

Terbutaline (Generic) **BOX:** Not approved and should not be used > 48–72h for tocolysis. Serious adverse Rxns possible, including death. **Uses:** *Reversible bronchospasm (asthma, COPD); inhib labor* **Acts:** Sympathomimetic; tocolytic **Dose:** *Adults. Bronchodilator:* 2.5–5 mg PO qid or 0.25 mg SQ; repeat in 15 min PRN; max 0.5 mg SQ in 4 h. Max 15 mg/24 h PO. *Metered-dose inhaler:* 1 puff PRN, repeat after 5 min PRN; 6 inhal/24 h max. *Premature labor:* 0.25 mg

SQ every 1–4 h × 24 h, 5 mg max/24 h; 2.5–5 mcg/min IV, ↑ 5 mcg/min q10min as tolerated, 25 mcg/min max. When controlled ↓ to lowest effective dose; SQ pump: basal 0.05–0.10 mg/h, bolus over 25 mg PRN *Peds. PO:* 0.05–0.15 mcg/kg/dose PO tid; max 5 mg/24 h; ↓ in renal failure **W/P:** [C, +] ↑ Tox w/ MAOIs, TCAs; DM, HTN, hyperthyroidism, CV Dz, convulsive disorders, K⁺ **CI:** Component allergy, prolonged tocolysis **Disp:** Tabs 2.5, 5 mg; Inj 1 mg/mL; metered-dose inhaler **SE:** HTN, hyperthyroidism, β₁-adrenergic effects w/ high dose, nervousness, trembling, tachycardia, arrhythmia, HTN, dizziness, ↑ glucose **Notes:** Tocolysis requires close monitoring of mother and fetus

Terconazole (Terazol 3, Terazol 7, Generic) Uses: *Vag fungal Infxns* **Acts:** Topical triazole antifungal **Dose:** 1 applicator-full or 1 supp intravag hs × 3–7 d **W/P:** [C, ?] **CI:** Component allergy **Disp:** Vag cream (Terzol 7) 0.4, (Terzol 3), 0.8%, (Terzol 3) Vag supp 80 mg **SE:** Vulvar/Vag burning **Notes:** Insert high into vagina

Teriflunomide (Aubagio) BOX: Hepatotox; ✓ LFT baseline & ALT qmo × 6 mo. D/C w/ liver injury & begin accelerated elimination procedure; CI in PRG & women of childbearing potential w/o reliable contraception Uses: *Relapsing MS* **Acts:** Pyrimidine synth inhib **Dose:** *Adults.* 7 or 14 mg PO daily **W/P:** [X, –] w/ CYP2C8, CYP1A2 metab drugs, warfarin, ethinylestradiol, levonorgestrel; ↑ elimin w/ cholestyramine or activated charcoal × 11 d; w/ hepatic impair; w/ leflunomide **Disp:** Tabs 7, 14 mg **SE:** ↑ ALT, alopecia, N/D, influenza, paresthesia, ↓ WBC, neuropathy, ↑ BP, SJS, TEN, ARF, ↑ K⁺ **Notes:** ✓ CBC & TB screen prior to Rx; ✓ BP, S/Sxs of Infxn; do not give w/ live vaccines

Teriparatide (Forteo) BOX: ↑ Osteosarcoma risk in animals, use only where potential benefits outweigh risks Uses: *Severe/refractory osteoporosis* **Acts:** PTH (recombinant) **Dose:** 20 mcg SQ daily in thigh or Abd **W/P:** [C, –]; Caution in urolithiasis **Disp:** 250 mcg/mL in 2.4-mL prefilled syringe **SE:** Orthostatic ↓ BP on administration, N/D, ↑ Ca²⁺; leg cramps, ↑ uric acid **Notes:** 2 y max use

Tesamorelin (Egrifta) Uses: *↓ Excess Abd fat in HIV-infected patients w/ lipodystrophy* **Acts:** Binds/stimulates growth hormone-releasing factor receptors **Dose:** 2 mg SQ/d; **W/P:** [X; HIV-infected mothers should not breast-feed] **CI:** Hypothalamic-pituitary axis disorders; hypersensitivity to tesamorelin, mannitol, or any component; head radiation/trauma; malignancy; PRG; child w/ open epiphyses **Disp:** Vial 1 mg **SE:** Arthralgias, Inj site Rxn, edema, myalgia, ↑ glucose, N, V **Notes:** ✓ Gluc, ? ↑ mortality w/ acute critical illness; ↑ IGF

Testosterone (AndroGel 1%, AndroGel 1.62% Androderm, Axiron, Fortesta, Striant, Testim, Testopel) [C-III] BOX: Virilization reported in children exposed to topical testosterone products. Children to avoid contact w/ unwashed or unclothed application sites Uses: *Male hypogonadism (congenital/acquired)* **Acts:** Testosterone replacement; ↑ lean body mass, libido **Dose:** All daily applications *AndroGel 1%:* 50 mg (4 pumps). *AndroGel 1.62%:* 40.5 mg (2 pumps); apply to clean skin on upper body only. *Androderm:* Two 2.5-mg or one 5-mg patch daily. *Axiron:* 60 mg (1 pump = 30 mg each axilla) q A.M. *Fortesta:* 40 mg (4 pumps) on clean, dry thighs; adjust form 1–7 pumps based on blood test 2 h after (days 14 and 35). *Striant:* 30-mg buccal tabs bid. *Testim:* One 5-g gel tube. *Testopel:* 150–450 mg (2–6 pellets) SQ implant q3–6mo (implant two 75-mg pellets for each 25 mg testosterone required weekly; eg: For 75 mg/wk, implant 450 mg (6 pellets). **W/P:** [X, –] May cause polycythemia, worsening of BPH Sx **CI:** PCa, male breast CA, women **Disp:** *AndroGel 1%: 12.5 mg/pump; AndroGel 1.62%: 20.25 mg/pump; Androderm:* 2.5-, 5-mg patches; *Axiron:* Metered-dose pump 30 mg/pump; *Fortesta:* Metered-dose gel pump 10 mg/pump; *Striant:* 30-mg buccal tab. *Testopel:* 75 mg/implant **SE:** Site Rxns, acne, edema, Wt gain, gynecomastia, HTN, ↑ sleep apnea, prostate enlargement, ↑ PSA **Notes:** IM testosterone enanthate (*Delatestryl; Testro-L.A.*) & cypionate (*Depo-Testosterone*) dose q14–28d w/ variable serum levels; PO agents (*methyltestosterone & oxandrolone*) associated w/ hepatic tumors; transdermal/mucosal forms preferred; wash hands immediately after topical applications *AndroGel* formulations not equivalent; ✓ levels and adjust PRN (300–1000 ng/dL testosterone range)

Tetanus Immune Globulin **Uses:** Prophylaxis *passive tetanus immunization* (suspected contaminated wound w/ unknown immunization status, see Table 7, p 315), or Tx of tetanus **Acts:** Passive immunization **Dose:** *Adults & Peds. Prophylaxis:* 250 mg units IM × 1; Tx: 500–6000 (30–300 units/kg) units IM **W/P:** [C, ?] Anaphylaxis Rxn **CI:** Thimerosal sensitivity **Disp:** Inj 250-unit vial/syringe **SE:** Pain, tenderness, erythema at site; fever, angioedema **Notes:** May begin active immunization series at different Inj site if required

Tetanus Toxoid (TT) (Generic) **Uses:** *Tetanus prophylaxis* **Acts:** Active immunization **Dose:** Based on previous immunization, Table 7, p 315 **W/P:** [C, ?/–] **CI:** Thimersal hypersensitivity neurologic Sxs w/ previous use, active Infxn w/ routine primary immunization **Disp:** Inj tetanus toxoid fluid, 5 Lf units/0.5 mL; tetanus toxoid adsorbed, 5 units/0.5 mL **SE:** Inj site erythema, induration, sterile abscess; arthralgias, fever, malaise, neurologic disturbances **Notes:** DTaP rather than TT or Td all adults 19–64 y who have not previously received 1 dose of DTaP (protection adult pertussis); also use DT or Td instead of TT to maintain diphtheria immunity; if IM, use only preservative-free Inj; do not confuse Td (for adults) w/ DT (for children)

Tetrabenazine (Xenazine) **BOX:** ↑ Risk of depression, suicide w/ Huntington Dz **Uses:** *Rx chorea in Huntington Dz* **Acts:** Monoamine depleter **Dose:** Divide 25–100 mg/d ÷ doses; 12.5 mg PO/d × 1 wk, ↑ to 12.5 mg bid, may ↑ to 12.5 mg TID if > 37.5 mg/d tid after 1 wk; if > 50 mg needed, ✓ for CYP2D6 gene; if poor metabolizer, 25 mg/dose, 50 mg/d max; extensive/indeterminate metabolizer 37.5 mg/dose max, 100 mg/d max **W/P:** [C, ?/–] 1/2 dose w/ strong CYP2D6 inhib 50 mg/d max (paroxetine, fluoxetine) **CI:** Wait 20 d after reserpine D/C before use, suicidality, untreated or inadequately treated depression; hepatic impair; w/ MOAI or reserpine **Disp:** Tabs 12.5, 25 mg **SE:** Sedation, insomnia, depression, anxiety, irritability, akathisia, Parkinsonism, balance difficulties, neuroleptic malignant syndrome, fatigue, N, V, dysphagia, ↑ QT, EPS Szs, falls

Tetracycline (Generic) Uses: *Broad-spectrum antibiotic* **Acts:** Bacteriostatic; ↓ protein synth. *Spectrum:* Gram(+): *Staphylococcus, Streptococcus.* Gram(−): *H. pylori.* Atypicals: *Chlamydia, Rickettsia, & Mycoplasma* **Dose:** *Adults.* 250–500 mg PO bid-qid. *Peds > 8 y.* 25–50 mg/kg/24 h PO q6–12h; ↓ w/ renal/hepatic impair, w/o food preferred **W/P:** [D, −] **CI:** PRG, children < 8 y **Disp:** Caps 100, 250, 500 mg; tabs 250, 500 mg; PO susp 250 mg/5 mL **SE:** Photosens, GI upset, renal failure, pseudotumor cerebri, hepatic impair **Notes:** Can stain tooth enamel & depress bone formation in children; do not administer w/ antacids or milk products

Thalidomide (Thalomid) **BOX:** Restricted use; use associated w/ severe birth defects and ↑ risk of venous thromboembolism **Uses:** *Erythema nodosum leprosum (ENL)*, GVHD, aphthous ulceration in HIV(+) **Acts:** ↓ Neutrophil chemotaxis, ↓ monocyte phagocytosis **Dose:** *GVHD:* 50–100 tid, max 600–1200 mg/d. *Stomatitis:* 200 mg bid for 5 d, then 200 mg daily up to 8 wk. *Erythema nodosum leprosum:* 100–300 mg PO qhs **W/P:** [X, −] May ↑ HIV viral load; Hx Szs **CI:** PRG or females not using 2 forms of contraception **Disp:** 50, 100, 150, 200 mg caps **SE:** Dizziness, drowsiness, rash, fever, orthostasis, SJS, thrombosis, fatigue, peripheral neuropathy, Szs **Notes:** MD must register w/ STEPS risk-management program; informed consent necessary; immediately D/C if rash develops

Theophylline (Theo24, Theochron, Theolair, Generic) Uses: *Asthma, bronchospasm* **Acts:** Relaxes smooth muscle of the bronchi & pulm blood vessels **Dose:** *Adults.* 900 mg PO ÷ q6h; SR products may be ÷ q8–12h (maint). *Peds.* 16–22 mg/kg/24 h PO ÷ q6h; SR products may be ÷ q8–12h (maint); ↓ in hepatic failure **W/P:** [C, +] Multiple interactions (eg, caffeine, smoking, carbamazepine, barbiturates, β-blockers, ciprofloxacin, E-mycin, INH, loop diuretics), arrhythmia, hyperthyroidism, uncontrolled Szs **CI:** Corn allergy **Disp:** Elixir 80 mg/15 mL; soln 80 mg/15 mL; ER 12 h caps: 300 mg; ER 12 h tabs: 200, 100, 300, 480 mg; ER 24 h caps: 100, 200, 300, 400 mg; ER 24 h tabs: 400, 600 mg **SE:** N/V, tachycardia, Szs, nervousness, arrhythmias **Notes:** IV levels: Sample 12–24 h after Inf started; *Therapeutic:* 5–15 mcg/mL; *Toxic:* > 20 mcg/mL. PO levels: *Trough:* just before next dose; *Therapeutic:* 5–15 mcg/mL

Thiamine [Vitamin B₁] (Generic) Uses: *Thiamine deficiency (beriberi), alcoholic neuritis, Wernicke encephalopathy* **Acts:** Dietary supl **Dose:** *Adults.* *Deficiency:* 5–30 mg IM or IV TID then 5–30 mg/d for 1 mo. *Wernicke encephalopathy:* 100 mg IV single dose, then 100 mg/d IM for 2 wk. *Peds.* 10–25 mg/d IM for 2 wk, then 5–10 mg/24 h PO for 1 mo **W/P:** [A, +] **CI:** Component allergy **Disp:** Tabs 50, 100, 250, 500 mg; Inj 100 mg/mL **SE:** Angioedema, paresthesias, rash, anaphylaxis w/ rapid IV **Notes:** IV use associated w/ anaphylactic Rxn; give IV slowly

Thioguanine (Tabloid) Uses: *AML, ALL, CML* **Acts:** Purine-based antimetabolite (substitutes for natural purines interfering w/ nucleotide synth) **Dose:** Adult: 2–3 mg/kg/d **Peds:** 60 mg/m²/d for 14 d no renal adjustment in peds; D/C if pt develops jaundice, VOD, portal hypertension; ↓ in severe renal/hepatic impair **W/P:** [D, –] **CI:** Resistance to mercaptopurine **Disp:** Tabs 40 mg **SE:** ↓ BM (leukopenia/thrombocytopenia), N/V/D, anorexia, stomatitis, rash, hyperuricemia, rare hepatotox

Thioridazine **BOX:** Dose-related QT prolongation elderly pts w/ dementia-related psychosis Tx w/ antipsychosis are at an ↑ risk of death **Uses:** *Schizophrenia*, psychosis **Acts:** Phenothiazine antipsychotic **Dose:** *Adults.* Initial, 50–100 mg PO tid; maint 200–800 mg/24 h PO in 2–4 ÷ doses. *Peds > 2 y.* 0.5–3 mg/kg/24 h PO in 2–3 ÷ doses **W/P:** [C, ?] Phenothiazines, QTc-prolonging agents, Al **CI:** Phenothiazine sensitivity, severe CNS depression, severe ↑/↓ BP, heart DZ, coma, combo w/ drugs that prolong QTc or CYPZD6 inhib; pt w/ congenital prolonoged QTc or Hx cardiac arrhythmia **Disp:** Tabs 10, 15, 25, 50, 100 mg **SE:** Low incidence of EPS; ventricular arrhythmias; ↓ BP, dizziness, drowsiness, neuroleptic malignant synd, Szs, skin discoloration, photosens, constipation, sexual dysfunction, blood dyscrasias, pigmentary retinopathy, hepatic impair **Notes:** Avoid EtOH

Thiothixene (Generic) **BOX:** Not for dementia-related psychosis; increased mortality risk in elderly on antipsychotics **Uses:** *Psychosis* **Acts:** ? May antagonize dopamine receptors **Dose:** *Adults & Peds > 12 y. Mild–mod psychosis:* 2 mg PO tid, up to 20–30 mg/d. Rapid tranquilization for agitated pts: 5–10 mg q30–60 min; Avg: 15–30 mg total *Severe psychosis:* 5 mg PO bid; ↑ to max of 60 mg/24 h PRN. *IM use:* 16–20 mg/24 h ÷ bid qid; max 30 mg/d. *Peds < 12 y.* 0.25 mg/kg/24 h PO ÷ q6–12h **W/P:** [C, ?] Avoid w/ ↑ QT interval or meds that can ↑ QT **CI:** Severe CNS depression; circulatory collapse; blood dyscrasias, phenothiazine sensitivity **Disp:** Caps 1, 2, 5, 10 mg **SE:** Drowsiness, EPS most common; ↓ BP, dizziness, drowsiness, neuroleptic malignant synd, Szs, skin discoloration, photosens, constipation, sexual dysfunction, leukopenia, neutropenia and agranulocytosis, pigmented retinopathy, hepatic impair

Tiagabine (Gabitril) **Uses:** *Adjunct in partial Szs*, bipolar disorder **Acts:** Antiepileptic, enhances activity of GABA **Dose:** *Adults & Peds ≥ 12 y.* (*Dose if already on enzyme-inducing AED; use lower dose if not on AED*) Initial 4 mg/d PO, ↑ by 4 mg during 2nd wk; ↑ PRN by 4–8 mg/d based on response, 56 mg/d max; take w/ food **W/P:** [C, –] May ↑ suicidal risk **CI:** Component allergy **Disp:** Tabs 2, 4, 12, 16 mg **SE:** Dizziness, HA, somnolence, memory impair, tremors, N **Notes:** Use gradual withdrawal; used in combo w/ other anticonvulsants

Ticagrelor (Brilinta) **BOX:** ↑ Bleeding risk; can be fatal; daily aspirin > 100 mg may ↓ effectiveness; do not start w/ active bleeding, Hx intracranial bleed, planned CABG; if hypotensive and recent procedure, suspect bleeding; manage any bleed w/o D/C of ticagrelor **Uses:** *↓ CV death and heart attack in ACS* **Acts:** Oral antiplatelet; reversibly binding ADP receptor antagonist inhib **Dose:** Initial 180 mg PO w/ ASA 325 mg, then 90 mg bid w/ ASA 75–100 mg/d **W/P:** [C, –]w/ Mod hepatic impair; w/ strong CYP3A inhib or CYP3A inducers **CI:** Hx intracranial bleed, active pathologic bleeding, severe hepatic impair **Disp:** Tabs 90 mg **SE:** Bleeding, SOB **Notes:** REMS; D/C 5 days preop

Ticarcillin/Potassium Clavulanate (Timentin) Uses: *Infxns of the skin, bone, resp & urinary tract, Abd, sepsis* Acts: Carboxy-PCN; bactericidal; ↓ cell wall synth; clavulanic acid blocks β-lactamase. *Spectrum:* Good gram(+), not MRSA; good gram(−) & anaerobes Dose: *Adults.* 3.1 g IV q4–6h max 24 g ticarcillin component/d *Peds. ≤60 kg* (if ≥ 60 kg, adult dose). 200–300 mg/kg/d IV ÷ q4–6h; ↓ in renal failure W/P: [B, +/−] PCN sensitivity Disp: Inj ticarcillin/clavulanate acid 3.1/0.1-g vial SE: Hemolytic anemia, false(+) proteinuria Notes: Often used in combo w/ aminoglycosides; penetrates CNS w/ meningeal irritation

Ticlopidine (Ticlid) BOX: Neutropenia/agranulocytosis, TTP, aplastic anemia reported Uses: *↓ Risk of thrombotic stroke*, protect grafts status post-CABG, diabetic microangiopathy, ischemic heart Dz, Acts: Plt aggregation inhib Dose: 250 mg PO bid w/ food W/P: [B, ?/−], ↑ Tox of ASA, anticoagulation, NSAIDs, theophylline; do not use w/ clopidogrel (↓ effect) CI: Bleeding, hepatic impair, neutropenia, ↓ plt Disp: Tabs 250 mg SE: Bleeding, GI upset, rash, ↑ LFTs Notes: ✓ CBC first 3 mo

Tigecycline (Tygacil) Uses: *Rx complicated skin & soft-tissue Infxns, & complicated intra-Abd Infxns* Acts: A glycycycline; binds 30 S ribosomal subunits, ↓ protein synthesis; *Spectrum:* Broad gram(+), gram(−), anaerobic, some mycobacterial; *E. coli, E. faecalis* (vancomycin-susceptible isolates), *S. aureus* (methicillin-susceptible/resistant), *Streptococcus* (agalactiae, anginosus grp, pyogenes), *Citrobacter freundii, Enterobacter cloacae, B. fragilis* group, *C. perfringens, Peptostreptococcus* Dose:100 mg, then 50 mg q12h IV over 30–60 min W/P: [D, ?] Hepatic impair, monotherapy w/ intestinal perforation, not OK in peds, w/ tetracycline allergy CI: Component sensitivity Disp: Inj 50-mg vial SE: N/V, Inj site Rxn, anaphylaxis Notes: Not indicated for HAP, VAP (↑ mortality for VAP), bacteremia

Timolol (Generic) BOX: Exacerbation of ischemic heart Dz w/ abrupt D/C Uses: *HTN & MI* Acts: β-Adrenergic receptor blocker, β₁, β₂ Dose: HTN: 10–20 mg bid, up to 60 mg/d. *MI:* 10 mg bid PO W/P: [C (1st tri; D if 2nd or 3rd tri), +] CI: CHF, cardiogenic shock, ↓ HR, heart block, COPD, asthma Disp: Tabs 5, 10, 20 mg SE: Sexual dysfunction, arrhythmia, dizziness, fatigue, CHF

Timolol, Ophthalmic (Betimol, Timoptic, Timoptic XE, Generic) Uses: *Glaucoma* Acts: β-Blocker Dose: 0.25% 1 gt bid; ↓ to daily when controlled; use 0.5% if needed; 1-gtt/d gel W/P: [C, ?/+] Disp: Soln 0.25/0.5%; *Timoptic XE* (0.25) gel-forming soln SE: Local irritation

Tinidazole (Tindamax, Generic) BOX: Off-label use discouraged (animal carcinogenicity w/ other drugs in class) Uses: *Adults/children > 3 y: *Trichomoniasis & giardiasis; intestinal amebiasis or amebic liver abscess* Acts: Antiprotozoal nitroimidazole; *Spectrum: Trichomonas vaginalis, Giardia duodenalis, Entamoeba histolytica* Dose: *Adults.* Trichomoniasis: 2 g PO; Rx partner. *Giardiasis:* 2 g PO. *Amebiasis:* 2 g PO daily × 3 d. *Amebic liver abscess:* 2 g PO daily × 3–5 d. *Peds.* Trichomoniasis: 50 mg/kg PO, 2 g/d max. *Giardiasis:* 50 mg/kg PO, 2 g max. *Amebiasis:* 50 mg/kg PO daily × 3 d, 2 g/d max. *Amebic liver abscess:* 50 mg/kg PO daily × 3–5 d, 2 g/d max; take w/ food W/P: [C, D in 1st tri, −] May be cross-resistant w/ metronidazole; Sz/peripheral neuropathy may require D/C; w/ CNS/hepatic impair **CI:** Metronidazole allergy, 1st-tri PRG, breast-feeding **Disp:** Tabs 250, 500 mg **SE:** CNS disturbances; blood dyscrasias, taste disturbances, N/V, darkens urine **Notes:** D/C EtOH during & 3 d after Rx; potentiates warfarin & Li; clearance ↓ w/ other drugs; crush & disperse in cherry syrup for peds; removed by HD

Tioconazole (Generic [OTC]) **Uses:** *Vag fungal Infxns* **Acts:** Topical antifungal **Dose:** 1 applicator-full intravag hs (single dose) **W/P:** [C, ?] **CI:** Component allergy **Disp:** Vag oint 6.5% **SE:** Local burning, itching, soreness, polyuria **Notes:** Insert high into vagina; may damage condom or diaphragm

Tiotropium (Spiriva) **Uses:** Bronchospasm w/ COPD, bronchitis, emphysema **Acts:** Synthetic anticholinergic-like atropine **Dose:** 1 caps/d inhaled using HandiHaler, **do not** use w/ spacer **W/P:** [C, ?/–] BPH, NAG, MyG, renal impair **CI:** Acute bronchospasm **Disp:** Inh caps 18 mcg **SE:** URI, xerostomia **Notes:** Monitor FEV1 or peak flow

Tirofiban (Aggrastat) **Uses:** *Acute coronary synd* **Acts:** Glycoprotein IIB/IIIa inhib **Dose:** Initial 0.4 mcg/kg/min for 30 min, followed by 0.1 mcg/kg/min 12–24 h; use in combo w/ heparin; *ECC 2010. ACS or PCI:* 0.4 mcg/kg/min IV for 30 min, then 0.1 mcg/kg/min for 18–24 h post PCI; ↓ in renal Insuff **W/P:** [B, ?/–] **CI:** Bleeding, intracranial neoplasm, vascular malformation, stroke/surgery/trauma w/in last 30 d, severe HTN, acute pericarditis **Disp:** Inj 50 mcg/mL **SE:** Bleeding, ↓ HR, coronary dissection, pelvic pain, rash

Tizanidine (Zanaflex, Generic) **Uses:** *Rx spasticity* **Acts:** α₂-Adrenergic agonist **Dose:** *Adults.* 4 mg q6–8h, ↑ 2–4 mg PRN max 12 mg/dose or 36 mg/d; ↓ w/ CrCl < 25 mL/min. *Peds.* Not rec **W/P:** [C, ?/–] Do not use w/ potent CYP1A2 inhib or other α₂-adrenergic agonists **CI:** w/ Fluvoxamine, ciprofloxacin; hypersens **Disp:** Caps 2, 4, 6 mg; tabs 2, 4 mg **SE:** ↓ BP, ↓ HR, somnolence, hepatotox **Notes:** ✓ LFT & BP; do not abruptly D/C, taper dose; take consistently w/ or w/o food

Tobramycin (Nebcin) **Uses:** *Serious gram(–) Infxns* **Acts:** Aminoglycoside; ↓ protein synth. *Spectrum:* Gram(–) bacteria (including *Pseudomonas*) **Dose:** *Adults.* Conventional dosing: 1–2.5 mg/kg/dose IV q8–12h. *Once-daily dosing:* 5–7 mg/kg/dose q24h. *Peds.* 2.5 mg/kg/dose IV q8h; ↓ w/ renal Insuff **W/P:** [D, –] **CI:** PRGlt; aminoglycoside sensitivity **Disp:** Inj 10, 40 mg/mL **SE:** Nephro/ototox **Notes:** Follow CrCl & levels. Levels: *Peak:* 30 min after Inf; *Trough:* < 0.5 before next dose; *Therapeutic Conventional: Peak:* 5–10 mcg/mL, *Trough:* < 2 mcg/mL

Tobramycin, Inhalation (TOBI, TOBI Podhaler) **Uses:** *CF pts w/ P. aeruginosa* **Acts:** Aminoglycoside; ↓ protein synth. *Spectrum:* Gram (–) bacteria **Dose:** *Adults/Peds > 6 y.* 300 mg inhal q12h by nebulizer, cycle 28 d on 28 d off **W/P:** [D, –] w/ Renal/auditory/vestibular/neuromusc dysfxn; avoid w/ other neuro/nephro/ototoxic drugs **CI:** Aminoglycoside sens **Disp:** 300 mg vials for nebulizer; *TOBI Podhaler:* 4-wk supply (56 blister caps w/ inhaler device plus reserve) **SE:** Cough, productive cough, lung disorders, dyspnea, pyrexia, oropharyngeal pain, dysphonia, hemoptysis, ↓ hearing **Notes:** Do not mix w/ dornase alfa in nebulizer; safety not established in peds < 6 y, or w/ FEV1 < 25% or > 80%, or if colonized w/ *Burkholderia cepacia*

Tobramycin Ophthalmic (AKTob, Tobrex, Generic) Uses: *Ocular bacterial Infxns* Acts: Aminoglycoside Dose: 1–2 gtt q2–4h; oint bid-tid; if severe, use oint q3–4h, or 2 gtt q60 min, then less frequently W/P: [B, –] CI: Aminoglycoside sensitivity Disp: Oint & soln tobramycin 0.3% SE: Ocular irritation

Tobramycin/Dexamethasone Ophthalmic (TobraDex) Uses: *Ocular bacterial Infxns associated w/ sig inflammation* Acts: Antibiotic w/ anti-inflammatory Dose: 0.3% oint apply q6–8h or soln 0.3% apply 1–2 gtt 4–6h (↑ to q2h for first 24–48 h) W/P: [C, M] CI: Aminoglycoside sensitivity viral, fungal, or mycobacterium Infxn of eye Disp: Oint & susp 2.5, 5, & 10 mL tobramycin 0.3% & dexamethasone 0.1% SE: Local irritation/edema Notes: Use under ophthalmologist's direction

Tocilizumab (Actemra) BOX: May cause serious Infxn (TB, bacterial, invasive fungal, viral, opportunistic); w/ serious Infxn stop tocilizumab until Infxn controlled Uses: *Mod–severe RA, SJIA* Acts: IL-6 receptor inhib Dose: RA 4–8 mg/kg q4wk; SJIA if < 30 kg 12 mg/kg q2wk; if > 30 kg 8 mg/kg q2wk W/P: [C, ?/–] ANC < 2000/mm³, plt ct < 100,000, AST/ALT > 1.5 ULN; serious Infxn infection; high-risk bowel perforation CI: Hypersensitivity Disp: Inj 20 mg/mL SE: URI, nasopharyngitis, HA, HTN, ↑ AST, rash, D, ↑ LFTs, ↓ ANC Notes: Do not give live vaccines; ✓ CBC/plt counts, LFTs, lipids; PPD, if + treat before starting, w/ prior Hx retreat unless adequate Tx confirmed, monitor for TB, even if –PPD; ↓ mRNA expression of several CYP450 isoenzymes (CYP3A4)

Tofacitinib (Xeljanz) BOX: Serious Infxns (bacterial, viral, fungal, TB, opportunistic) possible. D/C w/ severe Infxn until controlled; test for TB w/ Tx; lymphoma/other CA possible; possible EBV-associated renal transplant lymphoproliferative disorder Uses: *Mod–severe RA w/ inadequate response/intolerance to MTX* Acts: Janus kinase inhib Dose: Adults. 5 mg PO bid; ↓ 5 mg once daily w/ mod–severe renal & mod hepatic impair, w/ potent inhib CYP3A4, w/ meds w/ both mod inhib CYP3A4 & potent inhib CYP2C19 W/P: [C, –] Do not use w/ active Infxn, w/ severe hepatic impair, w/ biologic DMARDs, immunosuppressants, live vaccines, w/ risk of GI perforation CI: None Disp: Tabs 5 mg SE: D, HA, URI, nasopharyngitis, ↑ LFTs, HTN, anemia Notes: OK w/ MTX or other nonbiologic DMARDs; ✓CBC, LFTs, lipids

Tolazamide (Generic) Uses: *Type 2 DM* Acts: Sulfonylurea; ↑ pancreatic insulin release; ↑ peripheral insulin sensitivity; ↓ hepatic glucose output Dose: 100–500 mg/d (no benefit > 1 g/d) W/P: [C, ?/–] Elderly, hepatic or renal impair; G6PD deficiency = ↑ risk for hemolytic anemia CI: Component hypersens, DM type 1, DKA Disp: Tabs 250, 500 mg SE: HA, dizziness, GI upset, rash, hyperglycemia, photosens, blood dyscrasias

Tolbutamide (Generic) Uses: *Type 2 DM* Acts: Sulfonylurea; ↑ pancreatic insulin release; ↑ peripheral insulin sensitivity; ↓ hepatic glucose output Dose: 500–1000 mg bid; 3 g/d max; ↓ in hepatic failure W/P: [C, –] G6PD deficiency = ↑ risk hemolytic anemia **CI:** Sulfonylurea sensitivity **Disp:** Tabs 500 mg **SE:** HA, dizziness, GI upset, rash, photosens, blood dyscrasias, hypoglycemia, heartburn

Tolcapone (Tasmar)   BOX: Cases of fulminant liver failure resulting in death have occurred **Uses:** *Adjunct to carbidopa/levodopa in Parkinson Dz* **Acts:** Catechol-*O*-methyltransferase inhib slows levodopa metabolism **Dose:** 100 mg PO tid w/ 1st daily levodopa/carbidopa dose, then dose 6 & 12 h later; ↓ /w/ renal Insuff **W/P:** [C, ?] **CI:** Hepatic impair; w/ nonselective MAOI; nontraumatic rhabdomyolysis or hyperpynexia **Disp:** Tabs 100 mg **SE:** Constipation, xerostomia, vivid dreams, hallucinations, anorexia, N/D, orthostasis, liver failure, rhabdomyolysis **Notes:** Do not abruptly D/C or ↓ dose; monitor LFTs

Tolmetin (Generic)   BOX: May ↑ risk of CV events & GI bleeding **Uses:** *Arthritis & pain* **Acts:** NSAID; ↓ prostaglandins **Dose:** 400 mg PO tid titrate up max 1.8 g/d max **W/P:** [C, −] **CI:** NSAID or ASA sensitivity; use for pain CABG **Disp:** Tabs 200, 600 mg; caps 400 mg **SE:** Dizziness, rash, GI upset, edema, GI bleeding, renal failure

Tolnaftate (Tinactin [OTC])   Uses: *Tinea pedis, cruris, corporis, manus, versicolor* **Acts:** Topical antifungal **Dose:** Apply to area bid for 2–4 wk **W/P:** [C, ?] **CI:** Nail & scalp Infxns **Disp:** OTC 1% liq; gel; powder; topical cream; ointment, powder, spray soln **SE:** Local irritation **Notes:** Avoid ocular contact, Infxn should improve in 7–10 d

Tolterodine (Detrol, Detrol LA, Generic)   Uses: *OAB (frequency, urgency, incontinence)* **Acts:** Anticholinergic **Dose:** *Detrol:* 1–2 mg PO bid; *Detrol LA:* 2–4 mg/d **W/P:** [C, −] w/ CYP2D6 & 3A3/4 inhib (Table 10, p 319); w/ QT prolongation **CI:** Urinary retention, gastric retention, or uncontrolled NAG **Disp:** Tabs 1, 2 mg; *Detrol LA* tabs 2, 4 mg **SE:** Xerostomia, blurred vision, HA, constipation **Notes:** LA form may use "intact" pill in stool

Tolvaptan (Samsca)   BOX: Hospital use only w/ close monitoring of Na⁺; too rapid Na⁺ correction can cause severe neurologic symptoms. Correct slowly w/ ↑ risk (malnutrition, alcoholism, liver Dz) **Uses:** *Hypervolemic or euvolemic ↓ Na⁺* **Acts:** Vasopressin V_2-receptor antagonist **Dose:** *Adults.* 15 mg PO daily; after ≥ 24 h, may ↑ to 30 mg × 1 daily; max 60 mg × d; titrate at 24-h intervals to Na⁺ goal **W/P:** [C, −] Monitor Na⁺, volume, neurologic status; GI bleed risk w/ cirrhosis, avoid w/ CYP3A inducers and moderate inhib, ↓ dose w/ P-gp inhib, ↑ K⁺ **CI:** Hypovolemic hyponatremia; urgent need to raise Na⁺; in pts incapable of sensing/reacting to thirst; anuria; w/ strong CYP3A inhib **Disp:** Tabs 15, 30 mg **SE:** N, xerostomia, pollakiuria, polyuria, thirst, weakness, constipation, hyperglycemia **Notes:** Monitor K⁺

Topiramate (Topamax, Generic)   Uses: *Adjunctive Rx for complex partial Szs & tonic–clonic Szs*, bipolar disorder, neuropathic pain, migraine prophylaxis **Acts:** Anticonvulsant **Dose:** *Adults: Seizures:* Total dose 400 mg/d; see PI for 8-wk titration schedule. *Migraine prophylaxis:* titrate 100 m/d total. *Peds 2–9:* See ply PI for dosing & dose titration; ↓ w/ renal impair **W/P:** [D, ?/–] **CI:** Component allergy **Disp:** Tabs 25, 50, 100, 200 mg; caps sprinkles 15, 25 mg **SE:** Somnolence, fatigue,

↓ serum bicarbonate, Wt loss, memory impair, metabolic acidosis, kidney stones, fatigue, dizziness, psychomotor slowing, paresthesias, GI upset, tremor, nystagmus, acute glaucoma requiring D/C **Notes:** Metabolic acidosis responsive to ↓ dose or D/C; D/C w/ taper

Topotecan (Hycamtin, Generic) **BOX:** Chemotherapy precautions, for use by physicians familiar w/ chemotherapeutic agents, BM suppression possible **Uses:** *Ovarian CA (cisplatin-refractory), cervical CA, NSCLC*, sarcoma, ped NSCLC **Acts:** Topoisomerase I inhib; ↓ DNA synth **Dose:** 1.5 mg/m²/d as a 1-h IV Inf × 5 d, repeat q3wk; ↓ w/ renal impair **W/P:** [D, –] **CI:** PRG, breast-feeding; severe bone marrow suppression **Disp:** Inj 4-mg vials; caps 0.25, 1.0 mg **SE:** ↑ BM, N/V/D, drug fever, skin rash, interstitial lung Dz

Torsemide (Demadex) **Uses:** *Edema, HTN, CHF, & hepatic cirrhosis* **Acts:** Loop diuretic; ↓ reabsorption of Na⁺ & Cl⁻ in ascending loop of Henle & distal tubule **Dose:** 5–20 mg/d PO or IV; 200 mg/d max **W/P:** [B, ?] **CI:** Sulfonylurea sensitivity, anuria **Disp:** Tabs 5, 10, 20, 100 mg; Inj 10 mg/mL **SE:** Orthostatic ↓ BP, HA, photosens, electrolyte imbalance, blurred vision, renal impair **Notes:** 10–20 mg torsemide = 40 mg furosemide = 1 mg bumetanide

Tramadol (Rybix ODT, Ryzolt ER, Ultram, Ultram ER, Generic) **Uses:** *Mod–severe pain* **Acts:** Centrally acting synthetic opioid analgesic **Dose:** *Adults.* 50–100 mg PO q4–6h PRN, start 25 mg PO q A.M., ↑ q3d to 25 mg PO qid; ↑ 50 mg q3d, 400 mg/d max (300 mg if > 75 y); ER 100–300 mg PO daily; Rybix ODT individualize ↑ 50 mg/d q3d to 200 mg/d or 50 mg qid; after titration 50–100 mg q4–6 PRN, 400 mg/d max. *Peds.* (ER form not rec) 1–2 mg/kg q4–6h (max dose 100 mg); ↓ w/ renal Insuff **W/P:** [C, –] Suicide risk in addiction prone, w/ tranquilizers or antidepressants; ↑ Szs risk w/ MAOI; seratonin syndrome **CI:** Opioid dependency; w/ MAOIs; sensitivity to opioids, acute alcohol intoxication, hynotics, centrally acting analgesics, or w/ psychotropic drugs **Disp:** Tabs 50 mg; ER 100, 200, 300 mg; Rybix ODT 50 mg **SE:** Dizziness, HA, somnolence, GI upset, resp depression, anaphylaxis **Notes:** ↑ Sz resolved; tolerance/dependence may develop; abuse potential d/t mu-opioid agonist activity; Avoid EtOH; do not cut, chew ODT tabs

Tramadol/Acetaminophen (Ultracet) **Uses:** *Short-term Rx acute pain (< 5 d)* **Acts:** Centrally acting opioid analgesic w/ APAP **Dose:** 2 tabs PO q4–6h PRN; 8 tabs/d max. *Elderly/renal impair:* Lowest possible dose; 2 tabs q12h max if CrCl < 30 mL/min **W/P:** [C, –] Szs, hepatic/renal impair, suicide risk in addiction prone, w/ tranquilizers or antidepressants **CI:** Acute intoxication, w/ ethanol, hypnotics, central acting analgesics or psychotropic drugs, hepatic dysfunction **Disp:** Tab 37.5 mg tramadol/325 mg APAP **SE:** SSRIs, TCAs, opioids, MAOIs ↑ risk of Szs; dizziness, somnolence, tremor, HA, N/V/D, constipation, xerostomia, liver tox, rash, pruritus, ↑ sweating, physical dependence **Notes:** Avoid EtOH; abuse potential mu-opioid agonist activity (tramadol); see acetaminophen, p 36

Trandolapril (Mavik, Generic) **BOX:** Use in PRG in 2nd/3rd tri can result in fetal death **Uses:** *HTN*, heart failure, LVD, post-AMI **Acts:** ACE inhib **Dose:** *HTN:* 1–4 mg/d. *Heart failure/LVD:* Start 1 mg/d, titrate to 4 mg/d; ↓ w/ severe renal/hepatic impair **W/P:** [C first, D in 2nd + 3rd, –] ACE inhib sensitivity, angioedema w/ ACE inhib **Disp:** Tabs 1, 2, 4 mg **SE:** ↓ BP, ↓ HR, dizziness, ↑ K⁺, GI upset, renal impair, cough, angioedema **Notes:** African Americans minimum dose is 2 mg vs 1 mg in caucasians

Tranexamic Acid (Lysteda, Generic) **Uses:** *↓ Cyclic heavy menstrual bleeding* **Acts:** ↓ Dissolution of hemostatic fibrin by plasmin **Dose:** 2 tabs tid (3900 mg) 5 d max during monthly menstruation; ↓ w/ renal impair (see label) **W/P:** [B, +/–] ↑ thrombosis risk **CI:** Component sensitivity; active or ↑ thrombosis risk **Disp:** Tabs 650 mg; Inj 100 mg/mL **SE:** HA, sinus and nasal symptoms, Abd pain, back/musculoskeletal/jt pain, cramps, migraine, anemia, fatigue, retinal/ocular occlusion; allergic Rxns **Notes:** Inj used off label trauma associated hemorrage

Tranylcypromine (Parnate) **BOX:** Antidepressants ↑ risk of suicidal thinking and behavior in children and adolescents w/ MDD and other psychiatric disorders **Uses:** *Depression* **Acts:** MAOI **Dose:** 30 mg/d PO ÷ doses, may ↑ 10 mg/d over 1–3 wk to max 60 mg/d **W/P:** [C, +/–] Minimize foods w/ tyramine **CI:** CV Dz, cerebrovascular defects, Pheo, w/ MAOIs, TCAs, SSRIs, SNRIs, sympathomimetics, bupropion, meperidine, dextromethorphan, buspirone **Disp:** Tabs 10 mg **SE:** Orthostatic hypotension, ↑ HR, sex dysfunction, xerostomia **Notes:** False(+) amphetamine drug test

Trastuzumab (Herceptin) **BOX:** Can cause cardiomyopathy and ventricular dysfunction; Inf Rxns and pulm tox reported; use during PRG can lead to pulm hypoplasia, skeletal malformations, & neonatal death **Uses:** *Met breast CA that over express the HER2/neu protein*, breast CA adjuvant, w/ doxorubicin, cyclophosphamide, and paclitaxel pt if HER2/neu(+) **Acts:** MoAb; binds human epidermal growth factor receptor 2 protein (HER2); mediates cellular cytotoxicity **Dose:** Per protocol, typical 2 mg/kg/IV/wk **W/P:** [D, –] CV dysfunction, allergy/Inf Rxns **CI:** None **Disp:** Inj 440 mg **SE:** Anemia, cardiomyopathy, nephrotic synd, pneumonitis, N/V/D, rash, pain, fever, HA, insomnia **Notes:** Inf-related Rxns minimized w/ acetaminophen, diphenhydramine, & meperidine

Trazodone (Oleptro, Generic) **BOX:** Closely monitor for worsening depression or emergence of suicidality, particularly in pts < 24 y. Oleptro not approved in peds **Uses:** *Depression*, hypnotic, augment other antidepressants **Acts:** Antidepressant; ↓ reuptake of serotonin & norepinephrine **Dose:** *Adults & Adolescents. Desyrel:* 50–150 mg PO daily–tid; max 600 mg/d. *Sleep:* 25–50 mg PO, qhs, PRN. *Adults. Oleptro:* Start 150 mg PO daily, may ↑ by 75 mg q3d, max 375 mg/d; take qhs on empty stomach **W/P:** [C, ?/–] Serotonin/neuroleptic malignant syndromes reported; ↑ QTc; may activate manic states; syncope reported; may ↑ bleeding risk; avoid w/in 14 d of MAOI **CI:** Component allergy **Disp:** *Desyrel:* Tabs 50, 100, 150, 300 mg; *Oleptro:* Scored tabs 150, 300 mg **SE:** Dizziness, HA, sedation, N, xerostomia, syncope, confusion, libido, ejaculation dysfunction, tremor, hep, EPS **Notes:** Takes 1–2 wk for Sx improvement; may interact w/ CYP3A4 inhib to ↑ trazodone concentrations, carbamazepine ↓ trazodone concentrations

Treprostinil (Remodulin, Tyvaso) Uses: *NYHA class II–IV pulm arterial HTN* Acts: Vasodilation, ↓ plt aggregation Dose: *Remodulin* 0.625–1.25 ng/kg/min cont Inf/SQ (preferred), titrate to effect; *Tyvaso:* Initial: 18 mcg (3 Inh) q4h 4x/d; if not tolerated, ↓ to 1–2 inhals, then ↑ to 3 inhal; Maint: ↑ additional 3 inhal 1–2 wk intervals; 54 mcg (or 9 inhal) 4x/d max W/P: [B, ?/–] CI: Component allergy Disp: *Remodulin* Inj 1, 2.5, 5, 10 mg/mL; *Tyvaso:* 0.6 mg/mL (2.9 mL) ~6 mcg/inhal SE: Additive effects w/ anticoagulants, antihypertensives; Inf site Rxns; D, N, HA, ↓ BP Notes: Initiate in monitored setting; do not D/C or ↓ dose, abruptly, will cause rebound pulm HTN

Tretinoin, Topical [Retinoic Acid] (Avita, Retin-A, Renova, Retin-A Micro) Uses: *Acne vulgaris, sun-damaged skin, wrinkles* (photo aging), some skin CAs Acts: Exfoliant retinoic acid derivative Dose: *Adults & Peds > 12 y.* Apply daily hs (w/ irritation, ↓ frequency). *Photoaging:* Start w/ 0.025%, ↑ to 0.1% over several mo (apply only q3d if on neck area; dark skin may require bid use) W/P: [C, ?] CI: Retinoid sensitivity Disp: Cream 0.02, 0.025, 0.05, 0.0375, 0.1%; gel 0.01, 0.025, 0.05% micro formulation gel 0.1, 0.04% micro SE: Avoid sunlight; edema; skin dryness, erythema, scaling, changes in pigmentation, stinging, pruritus

Triamcinolone/Nystatin (Generic) Uses: *Cutaneous candidiasis* Acts: Antifungal & anti-inflammatory Dose: Apply lightly to area bid; max 25 mg/d W/P: [C, ?] CI: Varicella; systemic fungal Infxns Disp: Cream & oint: triamcinolone 1 mg/g and 100,000 units nystatin/g SE: Local irritation, hypertrichosis, pigmentation changes Notes: For short-term use (< 7 d)

Triamterene (Dyrenium) Box: Hyperkalemia can occur Uses: *Edema associated w/ CHF, cirrhosis* Acts: K⁺-sparing diuretic Dose: Adults. 100–300 mg/24 h PO ÷ daily-bid. Peds. HTN: 2–4 mg/kg/d in 1–2 ÷ doses; ↓ w/ renal/hepatic impair W/P: [C (Expert opinion), ?] CI: ↑ K⁺, renal impair; caution w/ other K⁺-sparing diuretics Disp: Caps 50, 100 mg SE: ↓ K⁺, ↓ BP, bradycardia, cough, HA

Triazolam (Halcion, Generic) [C-IV] Uses: *Short-term management of insomnia* Acts: Benzodiazepine Dose: 0.125–0.25 mg/d PO hs PRN; ↓ in elderly W/P: [X, ?/–] CI: Concurrent fosamprenavir, ritonavir, nelfinavir, itraconazole, ketoconazole, nefazodone or other moderate/strong CYP3A4 inhib; PRG Disp: Tabs 0.125, 0.25 mg SE: Tachycardia, CP, drowsiness, fatigue, memory impair, GI upset Notes: Additive CNS depression w/ EtOH & other CNS depressants, avoid abrupt D/C

Triethylenethiophosphoramide (Thiotepa, Thioplex, Tespa, TSPA) Uses: *Breast, ovarian CAs, lymphomas* (infrequently used) preparative regimens for allogeneic & ABMT w/ high doses, intravesical for bladder CA, intracavitary effusion control* Acts: Polyfunctional alkylating agent Dose: Per protocol typical 0.3–0.4 mg/kg IV q1–4 wk. *Effusions:* Intracavitary 0.6-0.8 mg/kg; 60 mg into the bladder & retained 2 h q1–4wk; 900–125 mg/m² in ABMT regimens (highest dose w/o ABMT is 180 mg/m²; ↓ in renal failure **W/P:** [D, –] w/ BM suppression, renal and hepatic impair **CI:** Component allergy **Disp:** Inj 15 mg/vial **SE:** ↓ BM, N/V, dizziness, HA, allergy, paresthesias, alopecia **Notes:** Intravesical use in bladder CA infrequent today

Trifluoperazine (Generic) **BOX:** ↑ Mortality in elderly patients w/ dementia-related psychosis **Uses:** *Psychotic disorders* **Acts:** Phenothiazine; blocks postsynaptic CNS dopaminergic receptors **Dose:** *Adults. Schizophrenia/psychosis:* initial 1–2 mg PO bid (out pt) or 2–5 mg PO bid (in pat). Typical 15–20 mg/d, max 40 mg/d. *Nonpsychotic anxiety:* 1–2 mg PO/d, 6 mg/d max. *Peds 6–12 y.* 1 mg PO daily-bid initial, gradually to 15 mg/d; ↓ in elderly/debilitated pts **W/P:** [C, ?/ –] **CI:** Hx blood dyscrasias; phenothiazine sens, severe hepatic Dz **Disp:** Tabs 1, 2, 5, 10 mg **SE:** Orthostatic ↓ BP, EPS, dizziness, neuroleptic malignant synd, skin discoloration, lowered Sz threshold, photosens, blood dyscrasias **Notes:** Several weeks for onset of effects

Trifluridine Ophthalmic (Viroptic) **Uses:** *Herpes simplex keratitis & conjunctivitis* **Acts:** Antiviral **Dose:** 1 gtt q2h, max 9 gtt/d; ↑ to 1 gtt q4h × 7 d after healing begins; Rx up to 21 d **W/P:** [C, ?] **CI:** Component allergy **Disp:** Soln 1% **SE:** Local burning, stinging

Trihexyphenidyl (Generic) **Uses:** *Parkinson Dz, drug-induced EPS* **Acts:** Blocks excess acetylcholine at cerebral synapses **Dose:** *Parkinson.* 1 mg PO daily, ↑ by 2 mg q3–5d to usual dose 6–10 mg/d in 3–4 ÷ doses. *EPS.* 1 mg PO daily, ↑ to 5–15 mg/d in 3–4 ÷ doses **W/P:** [C, –] NAG, GI obst, MyG, BOO **CI:** **Disp:** Tabs 2, 5 mg; elixir 2 mg/5 mL **SE:** Dry skin, constipation, xerostomia, photosens, tachycardia, arrhythmias

Trimethobenzamide (Tigan, Generic) **Uses:** *N/V* **Acts:** ↓ Medullary chemoreceptor trigger zone **Dose:** *Adults.* 300 mg PO or 200 mg IM tid-qid PRN. **W/P:** [C, ?] **CI:** Benzocaine sensitivity; children < 40 kg **Disp:** Caps 300 mg; Inj 100 mg/mL. **SE:** Drowsiness, ↓ BP, dizziness; hepatic impair, blood dyscrasias, Szs, parkinsonian-like synd **Notes:** In the presence of viral Infxns, may mask emesis or mimic CNS effects of Reye synd

Trimethoprim (Primsol, Generic) **Uses:** *UTI d/t susceptible gram(+) & gram(–) organisms; Rx PCP w/ dapsone* suppression of UTI **Acts:** ↓ Dihydrofolate reductase. *Spectrum:* Many gram(+) & (–) except *Bacteroides, Branhamella, Brucella, Chlamydia, Clostridium, Mycobacterium, Mycoplasma, Nocardia, Neisseria, Pseudomonas,* & *Treponema* **Dose:** *Adults.* 100 mg PO bid or 200 mg PO daily; PCP 15 mg/kg ÷ in 3 d w/ dapsone *Peds ≥2 mo:* 4–6 mg/kg/d in 2 ÷ doses; otitis media (> or equal to 6 mo): 10 mg/kg/d in 2 ÷ doses × 10 d; ↓ w/ renal failure **W/P:** [C, +] **CI:** Megaloblastic anemia d/t folate deficiency **Disp:** Tabs 100 mg; *(Primsol)* PO soln 50 mg/5 mL **SE:** Rash, pruritus, megaloblastic anemia, hepatic impair, blood dyscrasias **Notes:** Take w/ plenty of H₂O

Trimethoprim (TMP)/Sulfamethoxazole (SMX) [Co-Trimoxazole], TMP-SMX] (Bactrim, Bactrim DS, Septra DS, Generic) **Uses:** *UTI Rx & prophylaxis, otitis media, sinusitis, bronchitis, prevent PCP pneumonia*

(w/ CD4 count < 200 cells/mm³)* **Acts:** SMX ↓ synth of dihydrofolic acid, TMP ↓ dihydrofolate reductase to impair protein synth. *Spectrum:* Includes *Shigella*, PCP, & *Nocardia* Infxns, *Mycoplasma*, *Enterobacter* sp, *Staphylococcus*, *Streptococcus*, & more **Dose:** All doses based on TMP *Adults.* 1 DS tab PO bid or 8–20 mg/kg/24 h IV in 1–2 ÷ doses. *PCP:* 15–20 mg/kg/d IV or PO (TMP) in 4 ÷ doses. *Nocardia:* 10–15 mg/kg/d IV or PO (TMP) in 4 ÷ doses. PCP prophylaxis: 1 reg tab daily or DS tab 3 × wk. *UTI prophylaxis:* 1 PO bid. *Peds.* 8–10 mg/kg/24 h PO ÷ in 2 doses or 3–4 doses IV; do not use in < 2 mo; ↓ in renal failure; maintain hydration **W/P:** [C (D if near term), –] **CI:** Sulfonamide sensitivity, porphyria, megaloblastic anemia w/ folate deficiency, PRF, breast-feeding Inf < 2 mo, sig hepatic impair **Disp:** Regular tabs 80 mg TMP/400 mg SMX; DS tabs 160 mg TMP/800 mg SMX; PO susp 40 mg TMP/200 mg SMX/5 mL; Inj 80 mg TMP/400 mg SMX/5 mL **SE:** Allergic skin Rxns, photosens, GI upset, SJS, blood dyscrasias, hep **Notes:** Synergistic combo, interacts w/ warfarin

Triptorelin (Trelstar 3.75, Trelstar 11.25, Trelstar 22.5) Uses: *Palliation of advanced PCa* **Acts:** LHRH analog; ↓ GNRH w/ cont dosing; transient ↑ in LH, FSH, testosterone, & estradiol 7–10 d after 1st dose; w/ chronic use (usually 2–4 wk), sustained ↓ LH & FSH w/ ↓ testicular & ovarian steroidogenesis similar to surgical castration **Dose:** 3.75 mg IM q4wk; or 11.25 mg IM q12wk or 22.5 mg q24wk **W/P:** [X, N/A] **CI:** Not indicated in females **Disp:** Inj Depot 3.75 mg; 11.25 mg; 22.5 mg **SE:** Dizziness, emotional lability, fatigue, HA, insomnia, HTN, D, V, ED, retention, UTI, pruritus, anemia, Inj site pain, musculoskeletal pain, osteoporosis, allergic Rxns **Notes:** Only 6-mo formulation; ✓ periodic testosterone levels & PSA

Trospium (Sanctura, Sanctura XR, Generic) Uses: *OAB w/ Sx of urge incontinence, urgency, frequency* **Acts:** Muscarinic antagonist, ↓ bladder smooth muscle tone **Dose:** 20 mg tab PO bid; 60 mg ER caps PO daily A.M., 1 h ac or on empty stomach. ↓ w/ CrCl < 30 mL/min and elderly **W/P:** [C, +/–] w/ EtOH use, in hot environments, UC, MyG, renal/hepatic impair **CI:** Urinary/gastric retention, NAG glaucoma **Disp:** Tab 20 mg; caps ER 60 mg **SE:** Dry mouth, constipation, HA, rash

Ulipristal Acetate (Ella) Uses: *Emergency contraceptive for PRG prevention (unprotected sex/contraceptive failure)* **Acts:** Progesterone agonist/antagonist, delays ovulation **Dose:** 1 tab (30 mg) PO ASAP w/in 5 d of unprotected sex or contraceptive failure **W/P:** [X, –] CYP3A4 inducers ↓ effect **CI:** PRG **Disp:** Tab 30 mg **SE:** HA, N, Abd, dysmenorrhea **Notes:** NOT for routine contraception; fertility after use unchanged, maintain routine contraception; use any day of menstrual cycle

Ustekinumab (Stelara) Uses: *Mod–severe plaque psoriasis* **Acts:** Human IL-12 and -23 antagonist **Dose:** Wt < 100 kg, 45 mg SQ initial and 4 wk later, then 45 mg q12wks. Wt > 100 kg, 90 mg SQ initially and 4 wk later, then 90 mg q 12 wk. **W/P:** [B/?] **Disp:** Prefilled syringe and single-dose vial 45 mg/0.5 mL, 90 mg/1 mL **SE:** Nasopharyngitis, URI, HA, fatigue **Notes:** Do not use w/ live vaccines

Valacyclovir (Valtrex, Generic) Uses: *Herpes zoster; genital herpes; herpes labialis* **Acts:** Prodrug of acyclovir; ↓ viral DNA replication. *Spectrum:*

Herpes simplex I & II **Dose:** *Zoster:* 1 g PO tid × 7 d. *Genital herpes(initial episode):* 1 g bid × 7–10 d, *(recurrent)* 500 mg PO bid × 3 d. *Herpes prophylaxis:* 500–1000 mg/d. *Herpes labialis:* 2 g PO q12h × 1 d ↓ w/ renal failure **W/P:** [B, +] ↑ CNS effects in elderly **Disp:** Caplets 500, 1000 mg; tab 500, 1000 mg **SE:** HA, GI upset, ↑ LFTs, dizziness, pruritus, photophobia

Valganciclovir (Valcyte) **BOX:** Granulocytopenia, anemia, and thrombocytopenia reported. Carcinogenic, teratogenic, and may cause aspermatogenesis **Uses:** *CMV retinitis and CMV prophylaxis in solid-organ transplantation* **Acts:** Ganciclovir prodrug; ↓ viral DNA synth **Dose:** *CMV Retinitis induction:* 900 mg PO bid w/ food × 21 d, then 900 mg PO daily; *CMV prevention:* 900 mg PO daily × 100 d posttransplant, ↓ w/ renal dysfunction **W/P:** [C, ?/–] Use w/ imipenem/cilastatin, nephrotoxic drugs; ANC < 500 cells/mcL, plt < 25,000 cells/mcL; Hgb < 8 g/dL **CI:** Allergy to acyclovir, ganciclovir, valganciclovir **Disp:** Tabs 450 mg; oral solution: 50 mg/mL **SE:** BM suppression, HA, GI upset **Notes:** Monitor CBC & Cr

Valproic Acid (Depakene, Depakote, Stavzor, Generic) **BOX:** Fatal hepatic failure (usually during first 6 mo of Tx, peds < 2 y high risk, monitor LFTs at baseline and frequent intervals), teratogenic effects, and life-threatening pancreatitis reported **Uses:** *Rx epilepsy, mania; prophylaxis of migraines*, Alzheimer behavior disorder **Acts:** Anticonvulsant; ↑ availability of GABA **Dose:** *Adults & Peds. Szs:* 10–15 mg/kg/24 h PO ÷ tid (after initiation by 5–10 mg/kg/d weekly basis until therapetic levels). *Mania:* 750 mg in 3 ÷ doses, ↑ 60 mg/kg/d max. *Migraines:* 250 mg bid, ↑ 1000 mg/d max; ↓ w/ hepatic impair **W/P:** [D, –] Multiple drug interactions **CI:** Severe hepatic impair, urea cycle disorder **Disp:** Caps 250 mg; caps w/ coated particles 125 mg; tabs DR 125, 250, 500 mg; tabs ER 250, 500 mg; caps DR (Stavzor) 125, 250, 500 mg; syrup 250 mg/5 mL; Inj 100 mg/mL **SE:** Somnolence, dizziness, GI upset, diplopia, ataxia, rash, thrombocytopenia, ↓ plt, hep, pancreatitis, ↑ bleeding times, alopecia, ↑ Wt ↑, hyperammonemic encephalopathy in pts w/ urea cycle disorders; if taken during PRG may cause lower IQ tests in children **Notes:** Monitor LFTs & levels: *Trough:* Just before next dose; *Therapeutic: Trough:* 50–100 mcg/mL; *Toxic trough:* > 100 mcg/mL. *Half-life:* 9–16 h; phenobarbital & phenytoin may alter levels

Valsartan (Diovan) **BOX:** Use during 2nd/3rd tri of PRG can cause fetal harm **Uses:** *HTN, CHF, DN* **Acts:** Angiotensin II receptor antagonist **Dose:** 80–160 mg/d, max 320 mg/d **W/P:** [D, ?/–] w/ K⁺-sparing diuretics or K⁺ supls **W/P:** Severe hepatic impair, biliary cirrhosis/obst, primary hyperaldosteronism, bilateral RAS **CI:** None **Disp:** Tabs 40, 80, 160, 320 mg **SE:** ↓ BP, dizziness, HA, viral Infxn, fatigue, Abd pain, D, arthralgia, fatigue, back pain, hyperkalemia, cough, ↑ Cr

Vancomycin (Vancocin, Generic) **Uses:** *Serious MRSA Infxns; enterococcal Infxns; PO Rx of S. aureus and C. difficile pseudomembranous colitis* **Acts:** ↓ Cell wall synth. **Spectrum:** Gram(+) bacteria & some anaerobes (includes MRSA, Staphylococcus, Enterococcus, Streptococcus sp, C. difficile) **Dose:** *Adults.* 15–20 mg/kg IV q8–48h based on CrCl, 15–20 mg/kg/dose; *C. difficile:*

125–500 mg PO q6h × 7 d. *Peds.* 40–60 mg/kg/d IV in ÷ doses q6–12 h; *C. difficile:* 40 mg/kg/d PO in ÷ 3–4 doses × 7–10 d. **W/P:** [B oral + C Inj, –] **CI:** Component allergy; avoid in Hx hearing loss **Disp:** Caps 125, 250 mg; powder for Inj **SE:** Oto-/nephrotoxic, GI upset (PO) **Notes:** Not absorbed PO, effect in gut only; give IV slowly (over 1–3 h) to prevent "red-man synd" (flushing of head/neck/upper torso); IV product used PO for colitis. *Levels: Trough:* < 0.5 h before next dose; *Therapeutic: Trough:* 10–20 mcg/mL; *Trough:* 15–20 mcg/mL. *Half-life:* 6–8 h; peak monitoring is not rec (toxic > 80 mcg/mL)

Vandetanib (Caprelsa) **BOX:** Can ↑ QT interval, Torsades de pointes, sudden death; do not use in pts w/ ↓ K⁺, ↓ Ca²⁺, ↓ Mg²⁺, prolonged QT, avoid drugs that prolong QT, monitor QT baseline, 2–4 wk, 8–12 wk, then q3mo **Uses:** *Advanced medullary thyroid CA* **Acts:** Multi TKI inhib **Dose:** *Adults.* 300 mg/d; ↓ dose w/ ↓ renal Fxn **W/P:** [D, –] Can ↑ QT; avoid w/ CYP3A inducers or drugs that ↑ QT (eg, amiodarone, sotalol, clarithromycin); avoid w/ mod–severe liver impair **CI:** Prolonged QT synd **Disp:** Tabs 100, 300 mg **SE:** Anorexia, Abd pain, N/V, HA, ↑ BP, reversible posterior leukoencephalopathy synd (PRES), fatigue, rash (eg, acne), ↑ QT interval, ILD **Notes:** Half-life 19 d; restricted distribution, providers and pharmacies must be certified; may need ↑ thyroid replacement

Vardenafil (Levitra, Staxyn, Generic) **Uses:** *ED* **Acts:** PDE5 inhib, increases cyclic guanosine monophosphate (cGMP) and NO levels; relaxes smooth muscles, dilates cavernosal arteries **Dose:** *Levitra* 10 mg PO 60 min before sexual activity; titrate; max × 1 = 20 mg; 2.5 mg w/ CYP3A4 inhib (Table 10, p 319); *Staxyn* 1 (10 mg ODT) 60 min before sex, max 1×/d **W/P:** [B, –] w/ CV, hepatic, or renal Dz or if sex activity not advisable; potentiate the hypotensive effects of nitrates, alpha-blockers, and antihypertensives **CI:** w/ Nitrates, **Disp:** *Levitra* Tabs 2.5, 5, 10, 20 mg tabs; *Stayxn* 10 mg ODT (contains phenylalanine) **SE:** ↑ QT interval ↓ BP, HA, dyspepsia, priapism, flushing, rhinitis, sinusitis, flu synd, sudden ↓/loss of hearing, tinnitus, NIAON. **Notes:** Concomitant alpha-blockers may cause ↓ BP; transient global amnesia reports; place Staxyn on tongue to disintegrate w/o liquids; ODT not inter changeable to oral pill; gets higher levels

Varenicline (Chantix) **BOX:** Serious neuropsychiatric events (depression, suicidal ideation/attempt) reported **Uses:** *Smoking cessation* **Acts:** Nicotine receptor partial agonist **Dose:** *Adults.* 0.5 mg PO daily × 3 d, 0.5 mg bid × 4 d, then 1 mg PO bid for 12 wk total; after meal w/ glass of water **W/P:** [C, ?/–] ↓ Dose w/ renal impair, may increase risk of CV events in pts w/ CV Dz **Disp:** Tabs 0.5, 1 mg **SE:** Serious psychological disturbances, N, V, insomnia, flatulence, constipation, unusual dreams **Notes:** Slowly ↑ dose to ↓ N; initiate 1 wk before desired smoking cessation date; monitor for changes in behavior

Varicella Immune Globulin (VarZIG) **BOX:** Prepared from pools of human plasma, which may contain causative agents of hep & other viral Dz; may cause rare hypersensitivity w/ shock; (Investigational, call (800)843-7477) **Uses:** Postexposure prophylaxis for persons w/o immunity, exposure likely to result in

Infxn (household contact > 5 min) and ↑ risk for severe Dz (immunosuppression, PRG) **Acts:** Passive immunization **Dose:** 125 units/10 kg up to 625 units IV (over 3–5 min) or IM (deltoid or proximal thigh); give w/in 4–5 d (best < 72 h) of exposure **W/P:** [?, –] Indicated for PRG women exposed to varicella zoster **CI:** IgA deficiency, Hx, anaphylaxis to immunoglobulins; known immunity to varicella zoster **Disp:** Inj, 125-mg unit vials **SE:** Inj site Rxn, dizziness, fever, HA, N; ARF, thrombosis rare **Notes:** Wait 5 mo before varicella vaccination after varicella immune globulin; may ↓ vaccine effectiveness; observe for varicella for 28 d; if *VariZIG* admin not possible w/in 96 h of exposure consider admin of IGIV (400 mg/kg)

Varicella Virus Vaccine (Varivax) Uses: *Prevent varicella (chickenpox)* **Acts:** Active immunization w/ live attenuated virus **Dose:** *Adults & Peds (> 12 mo).* 0.5 mL SQ, repeat 4–8 wk **W/P:** [C, M] **CI:** Immunosuppression; PRG; fever, untreated TB, neomycin-anaphylactoid Rxn; **Disp:** Powder for Inj, acute febrile Infxn **SE:** Varicella rash, generalized or at Inj site, arthralgias/myalgias, fatigue, fever, HA, irritability, GI upset **Notes:** OK for all children & adults who have not had chickenpox; avoid PRG for 3 mo after; do not give w/in 3 mo of immunoglobulin (IgG) and no IgG w/in 2 mo of vaccination; avoid ASA for 6 wk in peds; avoid high-risk people for 6 wk after vaccination

Vasopressin [Antidiuretic Hormone, ADH] (Pitressin, Generic) Uses: *DI; Rx postop Abd distention*; adjunct Rx of GI bleeding & esophageal varices; asystole, PEA, pulseless VT & VF, adjunct systemic vasopressor (IV drip) **Acts:** Posterior pituitary hormone, potent GI, and peripheral vasoconstrictor **Dose:** *Adults & Peds. DI:* 5–10 units SQ or IM bid-tid. *GI hemorrhage:* 0.2–0.4 units/min; ↓ in cirrhosis; caution in vascular Dz. *VT/VF:* 40 units IV push × 1. *Vasopressor:* 0.01–0.03 units/min *Peds. (ECC 2010). Cardiac arrest:* 0.4–1 unit/kg IV/IO bolus; max dose 40 units. *Hypotension:* 0.2–2 mill units/kg/min cont Inf **W/P:** [C, +] w/ Vascular Dz **CI:** Allergy **Disp:** Inj 20 units/mL **SE:** HTN, arrhythmias, fever, vertigo, GI upset, tremor **Notes:** Addition of vasopressor to concurrent norepinephrine or epi Infs

Vecuronium (Generic) **BOX:** To be administered only by appropriately trained individuals Uses: *Skeletal muscle relaxation* **Acts:** Nondepolarizing neuromuscular blocker; onset 2–3 min **Dose:** *Adults & Peds.* 0.1–0.2 mg/kg IV bolus (also rapid intubation *(ECC 2010)*; maint 0.010–0.015 mg/kg after 25–40 min; additional doses q12–15min PRN; ↓ w/in severe renal/hepatic impair **W/P:** [C, ?] Drug interactions cause ↑ effect (eg, aminoglycosides, tetracycline, succinylcholine) **CI:** Component hypersens **Disp:** Powder for Inj 10, 20 mg **SE:** ↓ HR, ↓ BP, itching, rash, tachycardia, CV collapse, muscle weakness **Notes:** Fewer cardiac effects than succinylcholine

Vemurafenib (Zelboraf) Uses: *Unresectable metastatic melanoma w/ BRAF mutation* **Acts:** BRAF serine-threonine kinase inhib **Dose:** *Adults.* 960 mg bid **W/P:** [D, –] If on warfarin, monitor closely **CI:** None **Disp:** Tab 240 mg **SE:** Rash including SJS; anaphylaxis, pruritus, alopecia, photosens, arthralgias, skin

SCC (> 20%), ↑ QT **Notes:** ✓ Derm exams q2mo for SCC; monitor ECG 15 d and qmo × 3; if QTc > 500 ms, D/C temporarily; mod CYP1A2 inhib, weak CYP2D6 inhib and CYP3A4 inducer

Venlafaxine (Effexor, Effexor XR, Generic)   BOX: Monitor for worsening depression or emergence of suicidality, particularly in ped pts **Uses:** *Depression, generalized anxiety, social anxiety disorder; panic disorder*, OCD, chronic fatigue synd, ADHD, autism **Acts:** Potentiation of CNS neurotransmitter activity **Dose:** 75–225 mg/d ÷ in 2–3 equal doses (IR) or daily (ER); 375 mg IR or 225 mg ER max/d ↓ w/ renal/hepatic impair **W/P:** [C, ?/–] **CI:** MAOIs **Disp:** Tabs IR 25, 37.5, 50, 75, 100 mg; ER caps 37.5, 75, 150 mg; ER tabs 37.5, 75, 150, 225 mg **SE:** HTN, ↑ HR, HA, somnolence, xerostomia, insomnia, GI upset, sexual dysfunction; actuates mania or Szs **Notes:** Avoid EtOH; taper on D/C to avoid withdral Sxs

Verapamil (Calan, Covera HS, Isoptin, Verelan, Generic)   Uses: *Angina, HTN, PSVT, AF, atrial flutter*, migraine prophylaxis, hypertrophic cardiomyopathy, bipolar Dz **Uses:** CCB **Dose:** *Adults. Arrhythmias:* 2nd line for PSVT w/ narrow QRS complex & adequate BP 2.5–10 mg IV over 1–2 min; repeat 5–10 mg in 15–30 min PRN (30 mg max). *Angina:* 80–120 mg PO tid, ↑ 480 mg/24 h max. *HTN:* 80–180 mg PO tid or SR tabs 120–240 mg PO daily to 240 mg bid; *ECC 2010.* Reentry SVT w/ narrow QRS: 2.5–5 mg IV over 2 min (slower in older pts); repeat 5–10 mg in, 15–30 min, PRN max of 20 mg; or 5-mg bolus q15min (max 30 mg). *Peds < 1 y.* 0.1–0.2 mg/kg IV over 2 min (may repeat in 30 min). *1–16 y:* 0.1–0.3 mg/kg IV over 2 min (may repeat in 30 min); 5mg max. *PO:* 3–4 mg/kg/d PO ÷ in 3 doses, max 8 mg/kg/d up to 480 mg/d > *5 y:* 80 mg q6–8h; ↓ in renal/hepatic impair **W/P:** [C, +] Amiodarone/β-blockers/flecainide can cause ↓ HR; statins, midazolam, tacrolimus, theophylline levels may be ↑; use w/ clonidine may cause severe ↓ HR w/ elderly pts **CI:** EF < 30%, severe LV dysfunction, BP < 90 mm Hg, SSS, 2nd-, 3rd-AV block AF/atrial flutter w/ bypass tract **Disp:** *Calan SR:* Caps 120, 180, 240 mg; *Verelan SR:* Caps 120, 180, 240, 360 mg *Verelan PM:* Caps (ER) 100, 200, 300 mg; *Calan:* Tabs 80, 120 mg; *Isoptin SR* 24-h 120, 180, 240 mg; Inj 2.5 mg/mL **SE:** Gingival hyperplasia, constipation, ↓ BP, bronchospasm, HR or conduction disturbances; edema; ↓ BP and bradyarrhythmias taken w/ telithromycin

Vigabatrin (Sabril)   BOX: Vision loss reported D/C w/in 2–4 wk if no effects seen **Uses:** *Refractory complex partial Sz disorder, infantile spasms* **Acts:** ↓ Gamma-aminobutyric acid transaminase (GABA-T) to ↑ levels of brain GABA **Dose:** *Adults.* Initially 500 mg 2×/d, then ↑ daily dose by 500 mg at weekly intervals based on response and tolerability; 1500 mg/d max **Peds.** *Seizures:* 10–15 kg: 0.5–1 g/d ÷ 2×/d; 16–30 kg: 1–1.5 g/d ÷ 2×/d; 31–50 kg: 1.5–3 g/d ÷ 2×/d; > 50 kg: 2–3 g/d ÷ 2×/d; *Infantile spasms:* Initially 50 mg/kg/d ÷ bid, ↑ 25–50 mg/kg/d q3d to 150 mg/kg/d max **W/P:** [C, +/–] ↓ dose by 25% w/ CrCl 50–80 mL/min, ↓ dose 50% w/ CrCl 30–50 mL/min, ↓ dose 75% w/ CrCl 10–30 mL/min; MRI signal changes reported in some infants **Disp:** Tablet 500 mg, powder/oral soln 500 mg/

packet **SE:** Vision loss/blurring, anemia, peripheral neuropathy, fatigue, somnolence, nystagmus, tremor, memory impairment, ↑ Wt, arthralgia, abnormal coordination, confusion **Notes:** ↓ Phenytoin levels reported; taper slowly to avoid withdrawal Szs; restricted distribution; see PI for powder dosing in peds

Vilazodone (Viibryd) **BOX:** ↑ Suicide risk in children/adolescents/young adults on antidepressants for major depressive disorder (MDD) and other psych disorders **Uses:** *MDD* **Acts:** SSRI and 5HT1A receptor partial agonist **Dose:** 40 mg/d; start 10 mg PO/d × 7 d, then 20 mg/d × 7 d, then 40 mg/d; ↓ to 20 mg w/ CYP3A4 inhib **W/P:** [C, ?/–] **CI:** MOAI, < 14 d between D/C MAOI and start **Disp:** Tabs 10, 20, 40 mg **SE:** Serotonin syndrome, neuroleptic malignant syndrome, N/V/D, dry mouth, dizziness, insomnia, restlessness, abnormal dreams, sexual dysfunction **Notes:** NOT approved for peds; w/ D/C, ↓ dose gradually

Vinblastine (Generic) **BOX:** Chemotherapeutic agent; handle w/ caution; only individuals experienced use of vinblastine should administer. **Uses:** *Hodgkin Dz & NHLs, mycosis fungoides, CAs (testis, renal cell, breast, NSCLC), AIDS-related Kaposi sarcoma*, choriocarcinoma, histiocytosis **Acts:** ↓ Microtubule assembly **Dose:** 0.1–0.5 mg/kg/wk (4–20 mg/m^2) (based on specific protocol); ↓ in hepatic failure **W/P:** [D, ?] **CI:** Granulocytopenia, bacterial Infxn **Disp:** Inj 1 mg/mL in 10-mg vial **SE:** ↓ BM (especially leukopenia), N/V, constipation, neurotox, alopecia, rash, myalgia, tumor pain **Notes:** It's use can be fatal

Vincristine (Marqibo, Vincasar, Generic) **BOX:** Chemotherapeutic agent; handle w/ caution, fatal if administered IT; IV only; administration by individuals experienced in use of vincristine only; severe w/ extrav **Uses:** *ALL, breast & small-cell lung CA, sarcoma (eg, Ewing tumor, rhabdomyosarcoma), Wilms tumor, Hodgkin Dz & NHLs, neuroblastoma, multiple myeloma* **Acts:** Promotes disassembly of mitotic spindle, causing metaphase arrest, vinca alkaloid **Dose:** 0.4–1.4 mg/m^2 (single doses 2 mg/max); ↓ in hepatic failure **W/P:** [D, –] **CI:** CharcotMarie-Tooth synd **Disp:** Inj 1 mg/mL **SE:** Neurotox commonly dose limiting, jaw-pain (trigeminal neuralgia), fever, fatigue, anorexia, constipation & paralytic ileus, bladder atony; no sig ↓ BM w/ standard doses; tissue necrosis w/ extrav; myelosuppression ↓

Vinorelbine (Navelbine, Generic) **BOX:** Chemotherapeutic agent; administration by physician experienced in CA chemotherapy only; severe granulocytopenia possible; extravas may cause tissue irritation and necrosis **Uses:** *Breast CA & NSCLC* (alone or w/ cisplatin) **Acts:** ↓ Polymerization of microtubules, impairing mitotic spindle formation; semisynthetic vinca alkaloid **Dose:** 30 mg/m^2/wk; ↓ in hepatic failure **W/P:** [D, –] **CI:** Intrathecal ITuse, granulocytopenia (< 1000/mm^3) **Disp:** Inj 10 mg **SE:** ↓ BM (leukopenia), mild GI, neurotox (6–29%); constipation/paresthesias (rare); tissue damage from extrav, alopecia

Vismodegib (Erivedge) **BOX:** Embryo-fetal death and severe birth defects; verify PRG status before start; advise female and male pts of these risks; advise females on need for contraception and males of potential risk of exposure through semen **Uses:** *Metastatic basal cell carcinoma, postsurgery local recurrence, not surgical candidate* **Acts:** Binds/inhibs transmembrane protein—involved in hedgehog signal transduction **Dose:** 150 mg PO daily **W/P:** [D, –] **CI:** None **Disp:** Caps 150 mg **SE:** N/V/D/C, ↓ Wt, anorexia, dysgeusia, ageusia, arthralgias, muscle spasms, fatigue, alopecia, ↓ Na⁺, ↓ K⁺, azotemia; ↑ SE if coadministered w/ P-gp inhib **Notes:** w/ Missed dose DO NOT make up missed dose, resume w/ next scheduled dose; DO NOT donate blood while on Tx until 7 mo after last Tx; immediately report exposure if PRG

Vitamin B₁ See Thiamine (p 272)
Vitamin B₆ See Pyridoxine (p 242)
Vitamin B₁₂ See Cyanocobalamin (p 93)
Vitamin K See Phytonadione (p 232)
Vitamin, Multi See Multivitamins (Table 12, p 322)

Voriconazole (VFEND, Generic) **Uses:** *Invasive aspergillosis, candidemia, serious fungal Infxns* **Acts:** ↓ Ergosterol synth. *Spectrum: Candida, Aspergillus, Scedosporium, Fusarium* sp **Dose:** *Adults & Peds > 12 y.* IV: 6 mg/kg q2h × 2, then 4 mg/kg bid PO. *< 40 kg:* 100 mg q12h, up to 150 mg. *> 40 kg:* 200 mg q12h, up to 300 mg; w/ mild–mod hepatic impair; IV not rec d/t accumulation of IV diluent; w/ CYP3A4 substrates (Table 10, p 319); do not use w/ clopidogrel (↓ effect) **W/P:** [D, ?/–] SJS, electrolyte disturbances **CI:** w/ Terfenadine, astemizole, cisapride, pimozide, quinidine, sirolimus, rifampin, carbamazepine, longacting barbiturates, ritonavir, rifabutin, ergot alkaloids, St. John's wort; in pt w/ galactose intol; skeletal events w/ long term use; w/ proarrhythmic cond **Disp:** Tabs 50, 200 mg; susp 200 mg/5 mL; Inj 200 mg **SE:** Visual changes, fever, rash, GI upset, ↑ LFTs, edema **Notes:** ✓ for multiple drug interactions (eg, ↓ dose w/ phenytoin); ✓ LFT before and during; ✓ vision w/ use 28 d

Vorinostat (Zolinza) **Uses:** *Rx cutaneous manifestations in cutaneous T-cell lymphoma* **Acts:** Histone deacetylase inhib **Dose:** 400 mg PO daily w/ food; if intolerant. 300 mg PO d × 5 consecutive days each week **W/P:** [D, ?/ –] w/ Warfarin (↑ INR) **CI:** Severe hepatic impair **Disp:** Caps 100 mg **SE:** N/V/D, dehydration, fatigue, anorexia, dysgeusia, DVT, PE, ↓ plt, anemia, ↑ SCr, hyperglycemia, ↑ QTc, edema, muscle spasms **Notes:** Monitor CBC, lytes (K⁺, Mg²⁺, Ca²⁺), glucose, & SCr q2wk × 2 mo then monthly; baseline & periodic ECGs; drink 2 L fluid/d

Warfarin (Coumadin, Jantoven, Generic) **BOX:** Can cause major/fatal bleeding. Monitor INR. Drugs, dietary changes, other factors affect INR. Instruct pts about bleeding risk **Uses:** *Prophylaxis & Rx of PE & DVT, AF w/ embolization*, other postop indications **Acts:** ↓ Vit K-dependent clotting factors in this order: VII-IX-X-II **Dose:** *Adults.* Titrate, INR 2.0–3.0 for most; mechanical valves INR is 2.5–3.5. *American College of Chest Physicians guidelines:* 5 mg initial, may use 7.5–10 mg; ↓ if pt elderly or w/ other bleeding risk factors; maint 2–10 mg/d PO, follow daily INR initial to adjust dosage (Table 8, p 316). *Peds.* 0.05–0.34 mg/kg/24 h PO or IV; follow PT/INR to adjust dosage; monitor vit K intake; ↓ w/ hepatic impair/elderly **W/P:** [X, +] **CI:** Bleeding, peptic ulcer, PRG **Disp:** Tabs 1, 2, 2.5, 3, 4, 5, 6, 7.5, 10 mg; Inj **SE:** Bleeding d/t overanticoagulation or injury & therapeutic INR; bleeding, alopecia, skin necrosis, purple toe synd **Notes:** Monitor vit K intake (↓ effect); INR preferred test; to rapidly correct overanticoagulation w/ vit K, fresh-frozen plasma, or both. Caution on taking w/ other meds that can ↑ risk of bleed. *Common warfarin interactions: Potentiated by:* APAP, EtOH (w/ liver Dz), amiodarone, cimetidine, ciprofloxacin, cotrimoxazole, erythromycin, fluconazole, flu vaccine, isoniazid, itraconazole, metronidazole, omeprazole, phenytoin, propranolol, quinidine, tetracycline. *Inhibited by:* barbiturates, carbamazepine, chlordiazepoxide, cholestyramine, dicloxacillin, nafcillin, rifampin, sucralfate, high–vit K foods. Consider genotyping for VKORC1 & CYP2C9

Witch Hazel (Tucks Pads, Others [OTC]) Uses: After bowel movement, cleansing to decrease local irritation or relieve hemorrhoids; after anorectal surgery, episiotomy, Vag hygiene **Acts:** Astringent; shrinks blood vessels locally **Dose:** Apply PRN **W/P:** [?, ?] External use only **CI:** None **Supplied:** Presoaked pads **SE:** Mild itching or burning

Zafirlukast (Accolate, Generic) Uses: *Adjunctive Rx of asthma* **Acts:** Selective & competitive inhib of leukotrienes *Dose: Adults & Peds > 12 y.* 20 mg bid. *Peds 5–11 y.* 10 mg PO bid (empty stomach) **W/P:** [B,] Interacts w/ warfarin, ↑ INR **CI:** Component allergy, hepatic impair **Disp:** Tabs 10, 20 mg **SE:** Hepatic dysfunction, usually reversible on D/C, HA, dizziness, GI upset; Churg-Strauss synd, neuropsych events (agitation, restlessness, suicidal ideation) **Notes:** Not for acute asthma

Zaleplon (Sonata, Generic) [C-IV] Uses: *Insomnia* **Acts:** A nonbenzodiazepine sedative/hypnotic, a pyrazolopyrimidine **Dose:** 5–20 mg hs PRN; not w/ high-fat meal; ↓ w/ hepatic Insuff, elderly **W/P:** [C, ?/–] Angioedema, anaphylaxis; w/ mental/ psychological conditions **CI:** Component allergy **Disp:** Caps 5, 10 mg **SE:** HA, edema, amnesia, somnolence, photosens **Notes:** Take immediately before desired onset

Zanamivir (Relenza) Uses: *Influenza A & B w/ Sxs < 2 d; prophylaxis for influenza* **Acts:** ↓ Viral neuraminidase **Dose: Adults & Peds > 7 y.** 2 Inh (10 mg) bid × 5d, initiate w/in 48 h of Sxs. *Prophylaxis household:* 10 mg daily × 10 d. *Adults & Peds > 12 y. Prophylaxis community:* 10 mg daily × 28 d **W/P:** [C, ?] Not OK for pt w/ airway Dz, reports of severe bronchospasms **CI:** Component or milk allergy **Disp:** Powder for Inh 5 mg **SE:** Bronchospasm, HA, GI upset, allergic Rxn, abnormal behavior, ear, nose, throat Sx **Notes:** Uses a Diskhaler for administration; dose same time each day; 2009 H1N1 strains susceptible

Ziconotide (Prialt) **BOX:** Psychological, cognitive, neurologic impair may develop over several wk; monitor frequently; may necessitate D/C Uses: *IT Rx of severe, refractory, chronic pain* **Acts:** N-type CCB in spinal cord **Dose:** Max initial dose 2.4 mcg/d IT at 0.1 mcg/h; may ↑ 2.4 mcg/d 2–3×/wk to max 19.2 mcg/d

(0.8 mcg/h) by day 21 **W/P:** [C, ?/–] w/ Neuro-/psychological impair **CI:** Psychosis, bleeding diathesis, spinal canal obst **Disp:** Inj mcg/mL: 100/1, 500/5, 500/20 **SE:** Dizziness, N/V, confusion, psych disturbances, abnormal vision, edema, ↑ SCF, amnesia, ataxia, meningitis; may require dosage adjustment **Notes:** May D/C abruptly; uses specific pumps (eg, Medtronic SynchroMed systems); do not ↑ more frequently than 2–3×/wk

Zidovudine (Retrovir, Generic)   BOX: Neutropenia, anemia, lactic acidosis, myopathy, & hepatomegaly w/ steatosis **Uses:** *HIV Infxn, prevent maternal HIV transmission* **Acts:** NRTI **Dose:** *Adults.* 200 mg PO tid or 300 mg PO bid or 1 mg/kg/dose IV q4h. *PRG:* 100 mg PO 5×/d until labor; during labor 2 mg/kg IV over 1 h then 1 mg/kg/h until cord clamped. *Peds 4 wk–18 y.* 160 mg/m²/dose tid or see table below; ↓ in renal failure **W/P:** [C, ?/–] w/ Ganciclovir, interferon alfa, ribavirin; may alter many other meds (see PI) **CI:** Allergy **Disp:** Caps 100 mg; tab 300 mg; syrup 50 mg/5 mL; Inj 10 mg/mL **SE:** Hematologic tox, HA, fever, rash, GI upset, malaise, myopathy, fat redistribution **Notes:** w/ Severe anemia/ neutropenia dosage interruption may be needed

Recommended Pediatric Dosage of Retrovir

Body Weight (kg)	Total Daily Dose	Dosage Regimen and Dose	
		bid	tid
4 to < 9	24 mg/kg/d	12 mg/kg	8 mg/kg
≥ 9 to < 30	18 mg/kg/d	9 mg/kg	6 mg/kg
≥ 30	600 mg/d	300 mg	200 mg

Zidovudine/Lamivudine (Combivir, Generic)   BOX: Neutropenia, anemia, lactic acidosis, myopathy & hepatomegaly w/ steatosis **Uses:** *HIV Infxn* **Acts:** Combo of RT inhib **Dose:** *Adults & Peds > 12 y.* 1 tab PO bid; ↓ in renal failure **W/P:** [C, ?/–] **CI:** Component allergy **Disp:** Tab zidovudine 300 mg/lamivudine 150 mg **SE:** Hematologic tox, HA, fever, rash, GI upset, malaise, pancreatitis **Notes:** Combo product ↓ daily pill burden; refer to individual component listings

Zileuton (Zyflo, Zyflo CR)   Uses: *Chronic Rx asthma* **Acts:** Leuko-triene inhib (↓ 5-lipoxygenase) **Dose:** *Adults & Peds > 12 y.* 600 mg PO qid; CR 1200 mg bid 1 h after A.M./P.M. meal **W/P:** [C, ?/–] **CI:** Hepatic impair **Disp:** Tabs 600 mg; CR tabs 600 mg **SE:** Hepatic damage, HA, D/N, upper Abd pain, leukopenia, neuropsych events (agitation, restlessness, suicidal ideation) **Notes:** Monitor LFTs qmo × 3, then q2–3mo; take regularly; not for acute asthma; do not chew/crush CR

Ziprasidone (Geodon, Generic)   BOX: ↑ Mortality in elderly w/ dementia-related psychosis **Uses:** *Schizophrenia, acute agitation bipolar disorder* **Acts:** Atypical antipsychotic **Dose:** 20 mg PO bid, may ↑ in 2-d intervals up to 80 mg bid; agitation 10–20 mg IM PRN up to 40 mg/d; separate 10mg doses by 2 h & 20 mg doses by 4 h (w/ food) **W/P:** [C, –] w/ ↓ Mg²⁺, ↓ K⁺ **CI:** QT prolongation, recent MI, uncompensated heart failure, meds that ↑ QT interval **Disp:** Caps 20, 40, 60, 80 mg; susp 10 mg/mL; Inj 20 mg/mL **SE:** ↓ HR; rash, somnolence, resp disorder, EPS, Wt gain, orthostatic ↓ BP **Notes:** ✓ Lytes

Ziv-Aflibercept (Zaltrap) **BOX:** Severe/fatal hemorrhage possible including GI hemorrhage; D/C w/ GI perf; D/C w/ compromised wound healing, suspend Tx 4 wk prior & after surgery & until surgical wound is fully healed **Uses:** *Metastatic colorectal CA (label/institution protocol)* **Acts:** Binds VEGF Λ & PIGF w/ ↓ neovascularization & ↓ vascular permeability **Dose:** 4 mg/kg IV Inf over 1 h q2 wk **W/P:** [C, –] Severe D w/ dehydration; D/C w/ fistula, ATE, hypertensive crisis, RPLS; ✓ urine protein, suspend Tx if proteinuria > 2 g/24 h, D/C w/ nephrotic synd or thrombotic microangiopathy; ✓ neutrophils, delay until ≥ 1.5 × 10⁹/L **CI:** None **Disp:** Inj vial 25 mg/mL (100 mg/4 mL, 200 mg/8 mL) **SE:** D, ↓ WBC, ↓ plts, stomatitis, proteinuria, ↑ ALT/AST, fatigue, epistaxis, Abd pain, ↓ appetite, ↓ Wt, dysphonia, ↑ SCr, HA **Notes:** Males/females: use contraception during Tx & for 3 mo after last dose

Zoledronic Acid (Reclast, Zometa, Generic) **Uses:** *↑ Ca²⁺ of malignancy (HCM), ↓ skeletal-related events in CAP, multiple myeloma, & metastatic bone lesions (Zometa)*; *prevent/Rx of postmenopausal osteoporosis, Paget Dz, ↑ bone mass in men w/ osteoporosis, steroid-induced osteoporosis (Reclast)* **Acts:** Bisphosphonate; ↓ osteoclastic bone resorption **Dose:** Zometa HCM: 4 mg IV over ≥ 15 min; may retreat in 7 d w/ adequate renal Fxn. Zometa bone lesions/ myeloma: 4 mg IV over > 15 min, repeat q3–4wk PRN; extend w/ ↑ Cr. Reclast Rx osteoporosis: 5 mg IV annually. Reclast: Prevent postmenopausal osteoporosis 5 mg IV q2y. Paget: 5 mg IV X 1. **W/P:** [D, ?/–] w/ Diuretics, aminoglycosides; ASA-sensitive asthmatics; avoid invasive dental procedures **CI:** Bisphosphonate allergy; hypocalcemia, angioedema, CrCl < 35 **Disp:** Vial 4 mg, 5 mg **SE:** Fever, flu-like synd, GI upset, insomnia, anemia; electrolyte abnormalities, bone, jt muscle pain, AF, osteonecrosis of jaw, atyp femur Fx **Notes:** Requires vigorous prehydration; do not exceed rec doses/Inf duration to ↓ renal dysfunction; follow Cr; effect prolonged w/ Cr ↑; avoid oral surgery; dental exam recommended prior to Rx; ↓ dose w/ renal dysfunction; give Ca²⁺ and vit D supls; may ↑ atypical subtrochanteric femur fractures

Zolmitriptan (Zomig, Zomig ZMT, Zomig Nasal) **Uses:** *Acute Rx migraine* **Acts:** Selective serotonin agonist; causes vasoconstriction **Dose:** Initial 2.5 mg PO, may repeat after 2 h, 10 mg max in 24 h; nasal 5 mg; if HA returns, repeat after 2 h, 10 mg max 24 h **W/P:** [C, ?/–] **CI:** Ischemic heart Dz, Prinzmetal angina, uncontrolled HTN, accessory conduction pathway disorders, ergots, MAOIs **Disp:** Tabs 2.5, 5 mg; rapid tabs (ZMT) 2.5, 5 mg; nasal 5 mg, **SE:** Dizziness, hot flashes, paresthesias, chest tightness, myalgia, diaphoresis, unusual taste, coronary artery spasm

Zolpidem (Ambien IR, Ambien CR, Edluar, ZolpiMist, Generic) [C-IV] **Uses:** *Short-term Tx of insomnia; *Ambien and Edluar* w/ difficulty of sleep onset; *Ambien CR* w/ difficulty of sleep onset and/or sleep maint* **Acts:** Hypnotic agent **Dose:** *Adults. Ambien:* 5–10 mg or 12.5 mg *CR* PO qhs; *Edluar:* 10 mg SL qhs; *Zolpimist:* 10 mg spray qhs; ↓ dose in elderly, debilitated, & hepatic impair (5 mg or 6.25 mg CR) **W/P:** [C, M] May cause anaphylaxis, angioedema, abnormal thinking, CNS depression, withdrawal; evaluate for other comorbid conditions; next-day psychomotor impairment/impaired driving when Ambien is taken w/ less than a full night of sleep remaining (7–8 h) **CI:** None **Disp:** *Ambien IR:* Tabs 5, 10 mg; *Ambien CR* 6.25, 12.5 mg; *Edluar:* SL tabs 5, 10 mg; *Zolpimist:* Oral soln 5 mg/spray (60 actuations/unit) **SE:** Drowsiness, dizziness, D, drugged feeling, HA, dry mouth, depression **Notes:** Take tabs on empty stomach; be able to sleep 7–8 h; *Zolpimist:* Prime w/ 5 sprays initially, and w/ 1 spray if not used in 14 d; store upright.

Zonegran (Zonegran, Generic) **Uses:** *Adjunct Rx complex partial Szs* **Acts:** Anticonvulsant **Dose:** Initial 100 mg/d PO; may ↑ by 100 mg/d q2wk to 400 mg/d **W/P:** [C, −] ↑ q2wks w/ CYP3A4 inhib; ↓ levels w/ carbamazepine, phenytoin, phenobarbital, valproic acid **CI:** Allergy to sulfonamides **Disp:** Caps 25, 50, 100 mg **SE:** Metabolic acidosis, dizziness, drowsiness, confusion, ataxia, memory impair, paresthesias, psychosis, nystagmus, diplopia, tremor, anemia, leukopenia; GI upset, nephrolithiasis (? d/t metabolic acidosis), SJS; monitor for ↓ sweating & ↑ body temperature **Notes:** Swallow caps whole

Zoster Vaccine, Live (Zostavax) **Uses:** *Prevent varicella zoster in adults > 60 y* **Acts:** Active immunization (live attenuated varicella) virus **Dose:** *Adults.* 0.65 mL SQ × 1 **CI:** Gelatin, neomycin anaphylaxis; fever, untreated TB, immunosuppression, PRG **W/P:** [C, ?/−] **Disp:** Single-dose vial **SE:** Inj site Rxn, HA **Notes:** May be used if previous Hx of zoster; do not use in place of varicella virus vaccine in children; contact precautions not necessary; antivirals and immune globulins may ↓ effectiveness

NATURAL AND HERBAL AGENTS

The following is a guide to some common herbal products. These may be sold separately or in combo with other products. According to the FDA, "Manufacturers of dietary supplements can make claims about how their products affect the structure or function of the body, but they may not claim to prevent, treat, cure, mitigate, or diagnose a disease without prior FDA approval." The table on p 297 summarizes some of the common dangerous aspects of natural and herbal agents.

Black Cohosh Uses: Sx of menopause (eg, hot flashes), PMS, hypercholesterolemia, peripheral arterial Dz; has anti-inflammatory & sedative effects **Efficacy:** May have short-term benefit on menopausal Sx **Dose:** 20–40 mg bid **W/P:** May further ↓ lipids &/or BP w/ prescription meds **CI:** PRG (miscarriage, prematurity reports); lactation **SE:** w/ OD, N/V, dizziness, nervous system & visual changes, ↓ HR, & (possibly) Szs, liver damage/failure

Chamomile Uses: Antispasmodic, sedative, anti-inflammatory, astringent, antibacterial, **Dose:** 10–15 g PO daily (3 g dried flower heads tid-qid between meals; can steep in 250 mL hot H_2O) **W/P:** w/ Allergy to chrysanthemums, ragweed, asters (family *Compositae*) **SE:** Contact dermatitis; allergy, anaphylaxis **Interactions:** w/ Anticoagulants, additive w/ sedatives (benzodiazepines); delayed ↓ gastric absorption of meds if taken together (↓ GI motility)

Cranberry (*Vaccinium macrocarpon*) Uses: Prevention & Rx UTI. **Efficacy:** Possibly effective **Dose:** 300–400 mg bid in 6-oz juice qid; tincture 1/2–1 tsp up to 3×/d, tea 2–3 tsps of dried flowers/cup; creams apply topically 2–3×/d PO **W/P:** May ↑ kidney stones in some susceptible individuals, V **SE:** None known **Interactions:** May potentiate warfarin

Dong Quai (*Angelica polymorpha, sinensis*) Uses: Uterine stimulant; anemia, menstrual cramps, irregular menses, & menopausal Sx; anti-inflammatory, vasodilator, CNS stimulant, immunosuppressant, analgesic, antipyretic, antiasthmatic **Efficacy:** Possibly effective for menopausal Sx **Dose:** 3–15 g daily, 9–12 g PO tab bid. **W/P:** Avoid in PRG & lactation **SE:** D, photosens, skin CA **Interactions:** Anticoagulants (↑ INR w/ warfarin)

Echinacea (*Echinacea purpurea*) Uses: Immune system stimulant; prevention/Rx URI of colds, flu; supportive care in chronic Infxns of the resp/lower urinary tract **Efficacy:** Not established; may ↓ severity & duration of URI **Dose:** Caps 500 mg, 6–9 mL expressed juice or 2–5 g dried root PO **W/P:** Do not use w/ progressive systemic or immune Dzs (eg, TB, collagen–vascular disorders, MS); may interfere w/ immunosuppressive Rx, not OK w/ PRG; do not use > 8 consecutive wk; possible immunosuppression; 3 different commercial forms **SE:** N; rash **Interactions:** Anabolic steroids, amiodarone, MTX, corticosteroids, cyclosporine

Evening Primrose Oil **Uses:** PMS, diabetic neuropathy, ADHD **Efficacy:** Possibly for PMS, not for menopausal Sx **Dose:** 2–4 g/d PO **SE:** Indigestion, N, soft stools, HA **Interactions:** ↑ Phenobarbital metabolism, ↓ Sz threshold

Feverfew (*Tanacetum parthenium***)** **Uses:** Prevent/Rx migraine; fever; menstrual disorders; arthritis; toothache; insect bites **Efficacy:** Weak for migraine prevention **Dose:** 125 mg PO of dried leaf (standardized to 0.2% of parthenolide) PO **W/P:** Do not use in PRG **SE:** Oral ulcers, gastric disturbance, swollen lips, Abd pain; long-term SE unknown **Interactions:** ASA, warfarin

Fish Oil Supplements (Omega-3 Polyunsaturated Fatty Acid) **Uses:** CAD, hypercholesterolemia, hypertriglyceridemia, type 2 DM, arthritis **Efficacy:** No definitive data on ↓ cardiac risk in general population; may ↓ lipids & help w/ secondary MI prevention **Dose:** One FDA approved (see Lovaza, p 205); OTC 1500–3000 mg/d; AHA rec: 1 g/d **W/P:** Mercury contamination possible, some studies suggest ↑ cardiac events **SE:** ↑ Bleeding risk, dyspepsia, belching, aftertaste **Interactions:** Anticoagulants

Garlic (*Allium sativum***)** **Uses:** Antioxidant; hyperlipidemia, HTN; anti-infective (antibacterial, antifungal); tick repellant (oral) **Efficacy:** ↓ Cholesterol by 4–6%; soln ↓ BP; possible ↓ GI/CAP risk **Dose:** 2–5 g, fresh garlic; 0.4–1.2 g of dried powder; 2–5 mg oil; 300–1000 mg extract or other formulations = 2–5 mg of allicin daily, 400–1200 mg powder (2–5 mg allicin) PO **W/P:** Do not use in PRG (abortifacient); D/C 7 d pre op (bleeding risk) **SE:** ↑ Insulin/lipid/cholesterol levels, anemia, oral burning sensation, N/V/D **Interactions:** Warfarin & ASA (↓ plt aggregation), additive w/ DM agents (↑ hypoglycemia), CYP 3A4 inducer (may ↑ cyclosporine, HIV antivirals, oral contraceptives)

Ginger (*Zingiber officinale***)** **Uses:** Prevent motion sickness; N/V d/t anesthesia **Efficacy:** Benefit in ↓ N/V w/ motion or PRG; weak for post op or chemotherapy **Dose:** 1–4 g rhizome or 0.5–2 g powder PO daily **W/P:** Pt w/ gallstones; excessive dose (↑ depression, & may interfere w/ cardiac Fxn or anticoagulants) **SE:** Heartburn **Interactions:** Excessive consumption may interfere w/ cardiac, DM, or anticoagulant meds (↓ plt aggregation)

Ginkgo Biloba **Uses:** Memory deficits, dementia, anxiety, improvement Sx peripheral vascular Dz, vertigo, tinnitus, asthma/bronchospasm, antioxidant, premenstrual Sx (especially breast tenderness), impotence, SSRI-induced sexual dysfunction **Dose:** 60–80 mg standardized dry extract PO bid-tid **Efficacy:** Small cognition benefit w/ dementia; no other demonstrated benefit in healthy adults **W/P:** ↑ Bleeding risk (antagonism of plt-activating factor), concerning w/ anti-platlet agents (D/C 3 d pre op); reports of ↑ Sz risk **SE:** GI upset, HA, dizziness, heart palpitations, rash **Interactions:** ASA, salicylates, warfarin, antidepressants

Ginseng **Uses:** "Energy booster" general; also for pt undergoing chemotherapy, stress reduction, enhance brain activity & physical endurance (adaptogenic), antioxidant, aid to control type 2 DM; Panax ginseng being studied for ED **Efficacy:** Not established **Dose:** 1–2 g of root or 100–300 mg of extract (7% ginsenosides) PO tid **W/P:** w/ Cardiac Dz, DM, ↓ BP, HTN, mania, schizophrenia, w/ corticosteroids; avoid in PRG; D/C 7 d pre op (bleeding risk) **SE:** Controversial "ginseng abuse synd" w/ high dose (nervousness, excitation, HA, insomnia); palpitations, vag bleeding, breast nodules, hypoglycemia **Interactions:** Warfarin, antidepressants, & caffeine (↑ stimulant effect), DM meds (↑ hypoglycemia)

Glucosamine Sulfate (Chitosamine) and Chondroitin Sulfate
Uses: Osteoarthritis (glucosamine: rate-limiting step in glycosaminoglycan synth), ↑ cartilage rebuilding; *Chondroitin:* biological polymer, flexible matrix between protein filaments in cartilage; draws fluids/nutrients into joint, "shock absorption") **Efficacy:** Controversial **Dose:** Glucosamine 500 PO tid, chondroitin 400 mg PO tid **W/P:** Many forms come from shellfish, so avoid if have shellfish allergy **SE:** ↑ Insulin resistance in DM; concentrated in cartilage, theoretically unlikely to cause toxic/teratogenic effects **Interactions:** *Glucosamine:* None. *Chondroitin:* Monitor anticoagulant Rx

Kava Kava (Kava Kava Root Extract, *Piper methystium*) **Uses:** Anxiety, stress, restlessness, insomnia **Efficacy:** Possible mild anxiolytic **Dose:** Standardized extract (70% kavalactones) 100 mg PO bid-tid **W/P:** Hepatotox risk, banned in Europe/Canada. Not OK in PRG, lactation. D/C 24 h pre op (may ↑ sedative effect of anesthetics) **SE:** Mild GI disturbances; rare allergic skin/rash Rxns, may ↑ cholesterol; ↑ LFTs/jaundice; vision changes, red eyes, puffy face, muscle weakness **Interactions:** Avoid w/ sedatives, alcohol, stimulants, barbiturates (may potentiate CNS effect)

Melatonin Uses: Insomnia, jet lag, antioxidant, immunostimulant **Efficacy:** Sedation most pronounced w/ elderly pts w/ ↓ endogenous melatonin levels; some evidence for jet lag **Dose:** 1–3 mg 20 min before HS (w/ CR 2 h before hs) **W/P:** Use synthetic rather than animal pineal gland, "heavy head," HA, depression, daytime sedation, dizziness **Interactions:** β-Blockers, steroids, NSAIDs, benzodiazepines

Milk Thistle (*Silybum marianum*) Uses: Prevent/Rx liver damage (eg, from alcohol, toxins, cirrhosis, chronic hep); preventive w/ chronic toxin exposure (painters, chemical workers, etc.) **Efficacy:** Use before exposure more effective than use after damage has occurred **Dose:** 80–200 mg PO tid **SE:** GI intolerance **Interactions:** None

Red Yeast Rice Uses: Hyperlipidemia **Efficacy:** HMG-CoA reductase activity, naturally occurring lovastatin; ↓ LDL, ↓ triglycerides, ↑ HDL; ↓ secondary CAD events **Dose:** 1200–1800 mg bid **W/P:** CI w/ PRG, lactation; do not use w/ liver Dz, recent surgery, serious infection; may contain a mycotoxin, citrinin, can cause renal failure **Disp:** Caps 600–1200 mg **SE:** N, V, Abd pain, hepatitis, myopathy, rhabdomyolysis **Interactions:** Possible interactions many drugs, avoid w/ CYP3A4 inhibitors or EtOH **Notes:** Use only in adults; generic lovastatin cheaper

Resveratrol Uses: Cardioprotective, prevent aging; ? antioxidant **Efficacy:** Limited human research **W/P:** Avoid w/ Hx of estrogen responsive CA or w/

CYP3A4 metabolized drugs **Disp:** Caps, tabs 20–500 mg, skins of red grapes, plums, blueberries, cranberries, red wine **SE:** D/N, anorexia, insomnia, anxiety, jt pain, antiplatelet aggregation **Interactions:** Avoid w/ other antiplatelet drugs or anticoagulants; CYP3A4 inhibitor

Saw Palmetto (*Serenoa repens*)   **Uses:** Rx BPH, hair tonic, PCa prevention (weak 5α-reductase inhib like finasteride, dutasteride) **Efficacy:** Small, no sig benefit for prostatic Sx **Dose:** 320 mg daily **W/P:** Possible hormonal effects, avoid in PRG, w/ women of childbearing years **SE:** Mild GI upset, mild HA, D w/ large amounts **Interactions:** ↑ Iron absorption; ↑ estrogen replacement effects

St. John's Wort (*Hypericum perforatum*)   **Uses:** Mild–mod depression, anxiety, gastritis, insomnia, vitiligo; anti-inflammatory; immune stimulant/anti-HIV/antiviral **Efficacy:** Variable; benefit w/ mild–mod depression in several trials, but not always seen in clinical practice **Dose:** 2–4 g of herb or 0.2–1 mg of total hypericin (standardized extract) daily. Also 300 mg PO tid (0.3% hypericin) **W/P:** Excess doses may potentiate MAOI, cause allergic Rxn, not OK in PRG **SE:** Photosens, xerostomia, dizziness, constipation, confusion, fluctuating mood w/ chronic use **Interactions:** CYP 3A enzyme inducer; do not use w/ Rx antidepressants(especially MAOI); ↓ cyclosporine efficacy (may cause rejection), digoxin (may ↑ CHF), protease inhib, theophylline, OCP; potency varies between products/batches

Valerian (*Valeriana officinalis*)   **Uses:** Anxiolytic, sedative, restlessness, dysmenorrhea **Efficacy:** Probably effective sedative (reduces sleep latency) **Dose:** 2–3 g in extract PO daily bid added to 2/3 cup boiling H_2O, tincture 15–20 drops in H_2O, oral 400–900 mg hs (combined w/ OTC sleep product Alluna) **W/P:** Hepatotoxicity w/ long-term use **SE:** Sedation, hangover effect, HA, cardiac disturbances, GI upset **Interactions:** Caution w/ other sedating agents (eg, alcohol or prescription sedatives): may cause drowsiness w/ impaired Fxn

Yohimbine (*Pausinystalia yohimbe*) [Yocon, Yohimex]   **Uses:** Improve sexual vigor, Rx ED **Efficacy:** Variable **Dose:** 1 tab = 5.4 mg PO tid (use w/ physician supervision) **W/P:** Do not use w/ renal/hepatic Dz; may exacerbate schizophrenia/mania (if pt predisposed). α_2-Adrenergic antagonist (↓ BP, Abd distress, weakness w/ high doses), OD can be fatal; salivation, dilated pupils, arrhythmias **SE:** Anxiety, tremors, dizziness, ↑ BP, ↑ HR **Interactions:** Do not use w/ antidepressants (eg, MAOIs or similar agents)

(Adapted from Haist SA and Robbins JB. *Internal Medicine on Call.* 4th ed. New York, NY: McGraw-Hill;2005; and the FDA. http://dietarysupplements.nlm.nih.gov/dietary/index.jsp. Accessed July 2011.)

Unsafe Herbs With Known Toxicity

Agent	Toxicities
Aconite	Salivation, N/V, blurred vision, cardiac arrhythmias
Aristolochic acid	Nephrotox
Calamus	Possible carcinogenicity
Chaparral	Hepatotox, possible carcinogenicity, nephrotox
"Chinese herbal mixtures"	May contain ma huang or other dangerous herbs
Coltsfoot	Hepatotox, possibly carcinogenic
Comfrey	Hepatotox, carcinogenic
Ephedra/ma huang	Adverse cardiac events, stroke, Sz
Juniper	High allergy potential, D, Sz, nephrotox
Kava kava	Hepatotox
Licorice	Chronic daily amounts (> 30 g/mo) can result in increased K^+, Na/fluid retention w/ HTN, myoglobinuria, hyporeflexia
Life root	Hepatotox, liver CA
Pokeweed	GI cramping, N/D/V, labored breathing, increased BP, Sz
Sassafras	V, stupor, hallucinations, dermatitis, abortion, hypothermia, liver CA
Usnic acid	Hepatotox
Yohimbine	Hypotension, Abd distress, CNS stimulation (mania/& psychosis in predisposed individuals)

Source: Haist SA, Robbins JB. *Internal Medicine on Call.* 4th ed. New York, NY: McGraw-Hill; 2005.

Tables

TABLE 1
Local Anesthetic Comparison Chart for Commonly Used Injectable Agents

Agent	Proprietary Names	Onset	Duration	Maximum Dose mg/kg	Maximum Dose Volume in 70-kg Adult[a]
Bupivacaine	Marcaine	7–30 min	5–7 h	3	70 mL of 0.25% solution
Lidocaine	Xylocaine, Anestacon	5–30 min	2 h	4	28 mL of 1% solution
Lidocaine with epinephrine (1:200,000)		5–30 min	2–3 h	7	50 mL of 1% solution
Mepivacaine	Carbocaine	5–30 min	2–3 h	7	50 mL of 1% solution
Procaine	Novocaine	Rapid	30 min–1 h	10–15	70–105 mL of 1% solution

[a] To calculate the maximum dose if not a 70-kg adult, use the fact that a 1% solution has 10 mg/mL drug.

TABLE 2
Comparison of Systemic Steroids (See also p 259)

Drug	Relative Equivalent Dose (mg)	Relative Mineralo-corticoid Activity	Duration (h)	Route
Betamethasone	0.75	0	36–72	PO, IM
Cortisone (Cortone)	25	2	8–12	PO, IM
Dexamethasone (Decadron)	0.75	0	36–72	PO, IV
Hydrocortisone (Solu-Cortef, Hydrocortone)	20	2	8–12	PO, IM, IV
Methylprednisolone acetate (Depo-Medrol)	4	0	36–72	PO, IM, IV
Methylprednisolone succinate (Solu-Medrol)	4	0	8–12	PO, IM, IV
Prednisone (Deltasone)	5	1	12–36	PO
Prednisolone (Delta-Cortef)	5	1	12–36	PO, IM, IV

TABLE 3
Topical Steroid Preparations (See also p 260)

Agent	Common Trade Names	Potency	Apply
Alclometasone dipropionate	Aclovate, cream, oint 0.05%	Low	bid/tid
Amcinonide	Cyclocort, cream, lotion, oint 0.1%	High	bid/tid
Betamethasone			
Betamethasone valerate	Valisone cream, lotion 0.01%	Low	q day/bid
Betamethasone valerate	Valisone cream 0.01, 0.1%, oint, lotion 0.1%	Intermediate	q day/bid
Betamethasone dipropionate	Diprosone cream 0.05%	High	q day/bid
Betamethasone dipropionate	Diprosone aerosol 0.1%		
Betamethasone dipropionate, augmented	Diprolene oint, gel 0.05%	Ultrahigh	q day/bid
Clobetasol propionate	Temovate cream, gel, oint, scalp, soln 0.05%	Ultrahigh	bid (2 wk max)
Clocortolone pivalate	Cloderm cream 0.1%	Intermediate	q day–qid
Desonide	DesOwen, cream, oint, lotion 0.05%	Low	bid–qid
Desoximetasone			
Desoximetasone 0.05%	Topicort LP cream, gel 0.05%	Intermediate	q day–qid
Desoximetasone 0.25%	Topicort cream, oint	High	q day–bid
Dexamethasone base	Aeroseb-Dex aerosol 0.01%	Low	bid–qid
	Decadron cream 0.1%		
Diflorasone diacetate	Psorcon cream, oint 0.05%	Ultrahigh	bid/qid
Fluocinolone			
Fluocinolone acetonide 0.01%	Synalar cream, soln 0.01%	Low	bid/tid
Fluocinolone acetonide 0.025%	Synalar oint, cream 0.025%	Intermediate	bid/tid

302

Fluocinolone acetonide 0.2%	Synalar-HP cream 0.2%	High	bid/tid
Fluocinonide 0.05%	Lidex, anhydrous cream, gel, oint, soln 0.05%	High	bid/tid
	Lidex-E aqueous cream 0.05%		
Flurandrenolide	Cordran cream, oint 0.025% cream, lotion, oint 0.05%	Intermediate intermediate	bid/tid bid/tid
	tape, 4 mcg/cm²	Intermediate	q day
Fluticasone propionate	Cutivate cream 0.05%, oint 0.005%	Intermediate	bid
Halobetasol	Ultravate cream, oint 0.05%	Very high	bid
Halcinonide	Halog cream 0.025%, emollient base 0.1% cream, oint, soln 0.1%	High	q day/tid
Hydrocortisone			
Hydrocortisone	Cortizone, Caldocort, Hycort, Hytone, etc.—aerosol 1%, cream 0.5, 1, 2.5%, gel 0.5%, oint 0.5, 1, 2.5%, lotion 0.5, 1, 2.5%, paste 0.5%, soln 1%	Low	tid/qid
Hydrocortisone acetate	Corticaine cream, oint 0.5, 1%	Low	tid/qid
Hydrocortisone butyrate	Locoid oint, soln 0.1%	Intermediate	bid/tid
Hydrocortisone valerate	Westcort cream, oint 0.2%	Intermediate	bid/tid

(Continued)

TABLE 3 (continued)
Topical Steroid Preparations (See also p 260)

Agent	Common Trade Names	Potency	Apply
Mometasone furoate	Elocon 0.1% cream, oint, lotion	Intermediate	q day
Prednicarbate	Dermatop 0.1% cream	Intermediate	bid
Triamcinolone			
Triamcinolone acetonide 0.025%	Aristocort, Kenalog cream, oint, lotion 0.025%	Low	tid/qid
Triamcinolone acetonide 0.1%	Aristocort, Kenalog cream, oint, lotion 0.1% Aerosol 0.2-mg/2-sec spray	Intermediate	tid/qid
Triamcinolone acetonide 0.5%	Aristocort, Kenalog cream, oint 0.5%	High	tid/qid

TABLE 4
Comparison of Insulins (See also p 159)

Type of Insulin	Onset (h)	Peak (h)	Duration (h)
Ultra Rapid			
Apidra (glulisine)	< 0.25	0.5–1.5	3–4
Humalog (lispro)	< 0.25	0.5–1.5	3–4
NovoLog (aspart)	< 0.25	0.5–1.5	3–4
Rapid (regular insulin)			
Humulin R, Novolin R	0.5–1	2–3	4–6
Intermediate			
Humulin N, Novolin L	1–4	6–10	10–16
Prolonged			
Lantus (insulin glargine)	1–4	No peak	24
Levemir (insulin detemir)	1–4	No peak	24
Combination Insulins			
Humalog Mix 75/25 (lispro protamine/lispro)	< 0.25	Dual	Up to 10–16
Humalog Mix 50/50 (lispro protamine/lispro)	< 0.25	Dual	Up to 10–16
NovoLog Mix 70/30 (aspart protamine/aspart)	< 0.25	Dual	Up to 10–16
Humulin 70/30, Novolin 70/30 (NPH/regular)	0.5–1	Dual	Up to 10–16

Note: Do not confuse Humalog, NovoLog, Humalog Mix, and NovoLog Mix with each other or with other agents as serious medication errors can result.

TABLE 5
Oral Contraceptives (See also p 217)
[Note: 21 = 21 Active pills; 24 = 24 Active pills; Standard for most products is 28 [unless specified] = 21 Active pills + 7 Placebo[a]]

Drug (Manufacturer)	Estrogen (mcg)	Progestin (mg)	Content of Additional Pills (d = days)
Monophasics			
Alesse 21, 28 (Wyeth)	Ethinyl estradiol (20)	Levonorgestrel (0.1)	
Apri (Barr)	Ethinyl estradiol (30)	Desogestrel (0.15)	
Aviane (Barr)	Ethinyl estradiol (20)	Levonorgestrel (0.1)	
Balziva (Barr)	Ethinyl estradiol (35)	Norethindrone (0.4)	
Beyaz (Bayer)[b]	Ethinyl estradiol (20)	Drospirenone (3.0)[c]	0.451 mg levomefolate in all including 7 placebo
Brevicon (Watson)	Ethinyl estradiol (35)	Norethindrone (0.5)	
Cryselle (Barr)	Ethinyl estradiol (30)	Norgestrel (0.3)	
Demulen 1/35 21, 28 (Pfizer)	Ethinyl estradiol (35)	Ethynodiol diacetate (1)	
Demulen 1/50 21, 28 (Pfizer)	Ethinyl estradiol (50)	Ethynodiol diacetate (1)	
Desogen (Organon)	Ethinyl estradiol (30)	Desogestrel (0.15)	
Emoquette (Qualitest/Endo)	Ethinyl estradiol (30)	Desogestrel (0.15)	
Femcon Fe (Warner-Chilcott)	Ethinyl estradiol (35)	Norethindrone (0.4)	
Junel Fe 1/20, 21, 28 (Barr)	Ethinyl estradiol (20)	Norethindrone acetate (1)	75 mg Fe × 7 d
Junel Fe 1.5/30, 28 (Barr)	Ethinyl estradiol (30)	Norethindrone acetate (1.5)	75 mg Fe × 7 d
Kariva (Barr)	Ethinyl estradiol (20, 0, 10)	Desogestrel (0.15)	2 inert; 2 ethinyl estradiol (10)
Kelnor 1/35 (Barr)	Ethinyl estradiol (35)	Ethynodiol Diacetate (1)	
Lessina (Barr)	Ethinyl estradiol (20)	Levonorgestrel (0.1)	

306

Levlen 21, 28 (Bayer)	Ethinyl estradiol (30)	Levonorgestrel (0.15)
Levlite (Bayer)	Ethinyl estradiol (20)	Levonorgestrel (0.1)
Levora (Watson)	Ethinyl estradiol (30)	Levonorgestrel (0.15)
Loestrin 24 Fe (Warner-Chilcott)	Ethinyl estradiol (20)	Norethindrone (1)	75 mg Fe × 4 d
Loestrin Fe 1.5/30 21 28 (Warner-Chilcott)	Ethinyl estradiol (30)	Norethindrone acetate (1.5)	75 mg Fe × 7 d in 28 d
Loestrin Fe 1/20 21, 28 (Warner-Chilcott)	Ethinyl estradiol (20)	Norethindrone acetate (1)	75 mg Fe × 7d in 28 d
Loestrin 1/20 21 (Warner-Chilcott)	Ethinyl estradiol (20)	Norethindrone acetate (1)	
Loestrin 1.5/30 21 (Warner-Chilcott)	Ethinyl estradiol (20)	Norethindrone acetate (1.5)	
Lo/Ovral 21, 28 (Wyeth)	Ethinyl estradiol (30)	Norgestrel (0.3)	
Low-Ogestrel (Watson)	Ethinyl estradiol (30)	Norgestrel (0.3)	
Lutera (Watson)	Ethinyl estradiol (20)	Levonorgestrel (0.1)	
Microgestin 1/20 21, 28 (Watson)	Ethinyl estradiol (20)	Norethindrone acetate (1)	
Microgestin 1.5/30 21, 28 (Watson)	Ethinyl estradiol (30)	Norethindrone acetate (1.5)	
Microgestin Fe 1/20 21, 28 (Watson)	Ethinyl estradiol (20)	Norethindrone acetate (1)	75 mg Fe × 7 d in 28 d
Microgestin Fe 1.5/30 21, 28 (Watson)	Ethinyl estradiol (30)	Norethindrone acetate (1.5)	75 mg Fe × 7 d in 28 d
Mircette (Organon)	Ethinyl estradiol (20, 0, 10)	Desogestrel (0.15)	2 inert; 2 ethinyl estradiol (10)
Modicon (Ortho-McNeil)	Ethinyl estradiol (35)	Norethindrone (0.5)	
MonoNessa (Watson)	Ethinyl estradiol (35)	Norgestimate (0.25)	
Necon 0.5/35 (Watson)	Mestranol (35)	Norethindrone (0.5)	
Necon 1/50 (Watson)	Mestranol (50)	Norethindrone (1)	

307

(Continued)

TABLE 5 (continued)
Oral Contraceptives (See also p 217)
(Note: 21 = 21 Active pills; 24 = 24 Active pills; Standard for most products is 28 [unless specified] = 21 Active pills + 7 Placebo[a])

Monophasics

Drug (Manufacturer)	Estrogen (mcg)	Progestin (mg)	Content of Additional Pills (d = days)
Necon 1/35 (Watson)	Ethinyl estradiol (35)	Norethindrone (0.5)	
Necon 1/35 (Watson)	Ethinyl estradiol (35)	Norethindrone (1)	
Nordette 21, 28 (King)	Ethinyl estradiol (30)	Levonorgestrel (0.15)	
Norinyl 1/35 (Watson)	Ethinyl estradiol (35)	Norethindrone (1)	
Norinyl 1/50 (Watson)	Mestranol (50)	Norethindrone (1)	
Nortrel 0.5/35 (Barr)	Ethinyl estradiol (35)	Norethindrone (0.5)	
Nortrel 1/35 21, 28 (Barr)	Ethinyl estradiol (35)	Norethindrone (1)	
Ocella (Barr)	Ethinyl estradiol (30)	Drospirenone (3)[c]	
Ogestrel 0.5/50 (Watson)	Ethinyl estradiol (50)	Norgestrel (0.5)	
Ortho-Cept (Ortho-McNeil)	Ethinyl estradiol (30)	Desogestrel (0.15)	
Ortho-Cyclen (Ortho-McNeil)	Ethinyl estradiol (35)	Norgestimate (0.25)	
Ortho-Novum 1/35 (Ortho-McNeil)	Ethinyl estradiol (35)	Norethindrone (1)	
Ortho-Novum 1/50 2 (Ortho-McNeil)	Mestranol (50)	Norethindrone (1)	
Ovcon 35 21, 28 (Warner-Chilcott)	Ethinyl estradiol (35)	Norethindrone (0.4)	
Ovcon 35 FE (Warner-Chilcott)	Ethinyl estradiol (35)	Norethindrone (0.4)	75 mg Fe × 7 d in 28 d
Ovcon 50 (Warner-Chilcott)	Ethinyl estradiol (50)	Norethindrone (1)	
Ovral 21, 28 (Wyeth-Ayerst)	Ethinyl estradiol (50)	Norgestrel (0.5)	

Drug	Estrogen (mg)	Progestin (mcg)	Content of Additional Pills
Portia (Barr)	Ethinyl estradiol (30)	Levonorgestrel (0.15)	
Reclipsen (Watson)	Ethinyl estradiol (30)	Desogestrel (0.15)	
Safyral (Bayer)[b]	Ethinyl estradiol (30)	Drospirenone (3.0)	0.451 mg levomefolate in all including 7 placebo
Solia (Prasco)	Ethinyl estradiol (30)	Desogestrel (0.15)	
Sprintec (Barr)	Ethinyl estradiol (35)	Norgestimate (0.25)	
Sronyx (Watson)[d]	Ethinyl estradiol (20)	Levonorgestrel (0.1)	
Yasmin (Bayer)[d] [generic Ocella, Syeda, Zarah]	Ethinyl estradiol (30)	Drospirenone (3.0)[c]	
Yaz (Bayer) 28 day[d,e,f] [generics Gianvi, Loryna]	Ethinyl estradiol (20)	Drospirenone (3.0)	4 inert in 28 d
Zenchent (Watson)	Ethinyl estradiol (35)	Ethynodiol diacetate (0.4)	
Zovia 1/35 (Watson)	Ethinyl estradiol (35)	Ethynodiol diacetate (1)	

Drug	Estrogen (mg)	Progestin (mcg)	Content of Additional Pills

Multiphasics

Drug	Estrogen (mg)	Progestin (mcg)	Content of Additional Pills
Aranelle (Barr)	Ethinyl estradiol (35)	Norethindrone (0.5, 1, 0.5)	
Cesia (Prasco)	Ethinyl estradiol (25)	Desogestrel (0.1, 0.125, 0.15)	
Cyclessa (Organon)	Ethinyl estradiol (25)	Desogestrel (0.1, 0.125, 0.15)	
Enpresse (Barr)	Ethinyl estradiol (30, 40, 30)	Levonorgestrel (0.05, 0.075, 0.125)	
Estrostep (Warner-Chilcott)[e]	Ethinyl estradiol (20, 30, 35)	Norethindrone acetate (1)	
Estrostep Fe (Warner-Chilcott)[e]	Ethinyl estradiol (20, 30, 35)	Norethindrone acetate (1)	75 mg Fe × 7 d in 28 d

(Continued)

TABLE 5 (continued)
Oral Contraceptives (See also p 217)

(Note: 21 = 21 Active pills; 24 = 24 Active pills; Standard for most products is 28 [unless specified] = 21 Active pills + 7 Placebo[9]

Drug	Estrogen (mg)	Progestin (mcg)	Content of Additional Pills
Generess Fe (Watson) (Note: Chewable tablets)	Ethinyl estradiol (25)	Norethindrone acetate (0.8)	75 mg Fe × 4 d
Multiphasics			
Leena (Watson)	Ethinyl estradiol (35)	Norethindrone (0.5, 1, 0.5)	
Lessina (Watson)	Ethinyl estradiol (20)	Levonorgestrel (0.1)	
Lutera (Watson)	Ethinyl estradiol (20)	Levonorgestrel (0.1)	
Natazia (Bayer)[19]			
Necon 10/11 21, 28 (Watson)	Ethinyl estradiol (35)	Norethindrone (0.5, 1)	
Necon 7/7/7 (Watson)	Ethinyl estradiol (35)	Norethindrone (0.5, 0.75, 1)	
Nortrel 7/7/7 (Barr)	Ethinyl estradiol (35)	Norethindrone (0.5, 0.75, 1)	
Orsythia (Qualitest)	Ethinyl estradiol (20)	Levonorgestrel (0.1)	
Ortho-Novum 10/11 (Ortho-McNeil)	Ethinyl estradiol (35)	Norethindrone (0.5, 1)	
Ortho-Novum 7/7/7 21 (Ortho-McNeil)	Ethinyl estradiol (35, 35, 35)	Norethindrone (0.5, 0.75, 1)	
Ortho Tri-Cyclen 21, 28 (Ortho-McNeil)[c]	Ethinyl estradiol (25)	Norgestimate (0.18, 0.215, 0.25)	
Ortho Tri-Cyclen Lo 21, 28 (Ortho-McNeil)	Ethinyl estradiol (35, 35, 35)	Norgestimate (0.18, 0.215, 0.25)	
Previfem (Teva)	Ethinyl estradiol (35)	Norgestimate (0.25)	

310

Drug	Estrogen (mg)	Progestin (mcg)	Content of Additional Pills
Tilia Fe (Watson)	Ethinyl estradiol (20, 30, 35)	Norethindrone (1)	75 mg Fe × 7 d in 28 d
Tri-Legest (Barr)	Ethinyl estradiol (20, 30, 35)	Norethindrone (1)	
Tri-Legest Fe (Barr)	Ethinyl estradiol (20, 30, 35)	Norethindrone (1)	75 mg Fe × 7 d in 28 d
Tri-Levlen (Bayer)	Ethinyl estradiol (30, 40, 30)	Levonorgestrel (0.05, 0.075, 0.125)	
Tri-Nessa (Watson)	Ethinyl estradiol (35)	Norgestimate (0.18, 0.215, 0.25)	
Tri-Norinyl 21, 28 (Watson)	Ethinyl estradiol (35, 35, 35)	Norethindrone (0.5, 1, 0.5)	
Tri-Previfem (Teva)	Ethinyl estradiol (35)	Norgestimate (0.18, 0.215, 0.25)	

Multiphasics

Drug	Estrogen (mg)	Progestin (mcg)	Content of Additional Pills
Tri-Sprintec (Barr)	Ethinyl estradiol (35)	Norgestimate (0.18, 0.215, 0.25)	
Triphasil 21, 28 (Wyeth)	Ethinyl estradiol (30, 40, 30)	Levonorgestrel (0.05, 0.075, 0.125)	
Trivora 28 (Watson)	Ethinyl estradiol (30, 40, 30)	Levonorgestrel (0.05, 0.075, 0.125)	
Velivet (Barr)	Ethinyl estradiol (25)	Desogestrel (0.1, 0.125, 0.15)	

Progestin Only (aka "mini-pills")

Drug	Estrogen (mg)	Progestin (mcg)	Content of Additional Pills
Camila (Barr)	None	Norethindrone (0.35)	
Errin (Barr)	None	Norethindrone (0.35)	

(Continued)

TABLE 5 (continued)
Oral Contraceptives (See also p 217)

(Note: 21 = 21 Active pills; 24 = 24 Active pills; Standard for most products is 28 [unless specified] = 21 Active pills + 7 Placebo[a])

Drug	Estrogen (mg)	Progestin (mcg)	Content of Additional Pills

Progestin Only (aka "mini-pills")

Drug	Estrogen (mg)	Progestin (mcg)	Content of Additional Pills
Jolivette 28 (Watson)	None	Norethindrone (0.35)	
Micronor (Ortho-McNeil)	None	Norethindrone (0.35)	
Nor-QD (Watson)	None	Norethindrone (0.35)	
Nora-BE (Ortho-McNeil)	None	Norethindrone (0.35)	

Extended-Cycle Combination (aka COCP [combined oral contraceptive pills])

Drug	Estrogen (mg)	Progestin (mcg)	Content of Additional Pills
Jolessa (Barr) 91-d pack	Ethinyl estradiol (30)	Levonorgestrel (0.15)	7 inert
LoSeasonique (Duramed)	Ethinyl estradiol (20,10)	Levonorgestrel (0.1)	7(10 mcg ethinyl estradiol)
Lybrel (Wyeth) 28-d pack[b]	Ethinyl estradiol (20)	Levonorgestrel (0.09)	None
Quasense (Watson)	Ethinyl estradiol (30)	Levonorgestrel (0.15)	7 inert

312

			7 (10 mcg ethinyl estradiol)
Seasonique (Duramed) 91-d pack	Ethinyl estradiol (30)	Levonorgestrel (0.15)	7 inert
Seasonale (Duramed) 91-d pack	Ethinyl estradiol (30)	Levonorgestrel (0.15)	None
Extended-Cycle Combination, ascending dose			
Quartette (Teva) 91 d	Ethinyl estradiol 0.02 mg (42 d)	Levonorgestrel 0.15 mg (42 d)	None
	Ethinyl estradiol 0.025 mg (21 d)	Levonorgestrel 0.15 mg (21 d)	None
	Ethinyl estradiol 0.03 mg (21 d)	Levonorgestrel 0.15 mg (21 d)	None
	Ethinyl estradiol 0.01 mg (7 d)		None

Data from *The Medical Letter.* 2007;(1266); *Treat Guidel Med Lett.* 2010;(100); *The Medical Letter.* 2013;(1420) manufacturers, insert and Web sites as of July 5, 2013.

[a] The designations 21 and 28 refer to number of days in regimen available.

[b] Raises folate levels to help decrease neural tube defect risk with eventual pregnancy.

[c] Drospirenone containing pills have increased risk for blood clots compared to other progestins

[d] Avoid in patients with hyperkalemia risk.

[e] Also approved for acne.

[f] Approved for premenstrual dysphoric disorder (PMDD) in women who use contraception for birth control.

[g] First "four phasic" OCP. Varies doses of estrogen (estradiol valerate) with progestin (dienogest) throughout cycle with 2 inert pills at end of cycle: days 1–2: estradiol valerate 3 mg alone, days 3–7: estradiol valerate 2 mg/dienogest 2 mg; days 8–24: estradiol valerate 2 mg/d enogest 3 mg; days 25–26: estradiol valerate 1 mg alone; days 27–28: placebo.

[h] First FDA-approved pill for 365 d dosing.

313

TABLE 6
Oral Potassium Supplements (See also p 236)

Brand Name	Salt	Form	mEq Potassium/ Dosing Unit
Glu-K	Gluconate	Tablet	2 mEq/tablet
Kaon elixir	Gluconate	Liquid	20 mEq/15 mL
Kaon-Cl 10	KCl	Tablet, SR	10 mEq/tablet
Kaon-Cl 20%	KCl	Liquid	40 mEq/15 mL
K-Dur 20	KCl	Tablet, SR	20 mEq/tablet
KayCiel	KCl	Liquid	20 mEq/15 mL
K-Lor	KCl	Powder	20 mEq/packet
K-lyte/Cl	KCl/bicarbonate	Effervescent tablet	25 mEq/tablet
Klorvess	KCl/bicarbonate	Effervescent tablet	20 mEq/tablet
Klotrix	KCl	Tablet, SR	10 mEq/tablet
K-Lyte	Bicarbonate/ citrate	Effervescent tablet	25 mEq/tablet
Klor-Con/EF	Bicarbonate/ citrate	Effervescent tablet	25 mEq/tablet
K-Tab	KCl	Tablet, SR	10 mEq/tablet
Micro-K	KCl	Capsule, SR	8 mEq/capsule
Potassium Chloride 10%	KCl	Liquid	20 mEq/15 mL
Potassium Chloride 20%	KCl	Liquid	40 mEq/15 mL
Slow-K	KCl	Tablet, SR	8 mEq/tablet
Tri-K	Acetate/ bicarbonate and citrate	Liquid	45 mEq/15 mL
Twin-K	Citrate/gluconate	Liquid	20 mEq/5 mL

SR = sustained release.

Note: Alcohol and sugar content vary between preparations.

TABLE 7
Tetanus Prophylaxis (See also p 271)

History of Absorbed Tetanus Toxoid Immunization	Clean, Minor Wounds		All Other Wounds[a]	
	Td[b]	TIG[c]	Td[d]	TIG[c]
Unknown or < 3 doses	Yes	No	Yes	Yes
= 3 doses	No[e]	No	No[f]	No

[a] Such as, but not limited to, wounds contaminated with dirt, feces, soil, saliva, etc.; puncture wounds; avulsions; and wounds resulting from missiles, crushing, burns, and frostbite.

[b] Td = tetanus-diphtheria toxoid (adult type), 0.5 mL IM.
  • For children <7 y, DPT (DT, if pertussis vaccine is contraindicated) is preferred to tetanus toxoid alone.
  • For persons >7 y, Td is preferred to tetanus toxoid alone.
  • DT = diphtheria-tetanus toxoid (pediatric), used for those who cannot receive pertussis.

[c] TIG = tetanus immune globulin, 250 units IM.

[d] If only 3 doses of fluid toxoid have been received, then a fourth dose of toxoid, preferably an adsorbed toxoid, should be given.

[e] Yes, if >10 y since last dose.

[f] Yes, if > 5 y since last dose.

Data from Guidelines from the Centers for Disease Control and Prevention and reported in MMWR (MMWR, December 1, 2006; 55(RR-15):1-48).

TABLE 8
Oral Anticoagulant Standards of Practice (See also warfarin p 288)

Thromboembolic Disorder	INR	Duration
Deep Venous Thrombosis & Pulmonary Embolism		
Treatment of single episode		
Transient risk factor	2–3	3 mo
Idiopathic[a]	2–3	long-term
Recurrent systemic embolism	2–3	long-term
Prevention of Systemic Embolism		
Atrial fibrillation (AF)[b]	2–3	long-term
AF: cardioversion	2–3	3 wk prior; 4 wk post sinus rhythm
Mitral valvular heart dx[c]	2–3	long-term
Cardiomyopathy (usually ASA)[d]	2–3	long-term
Acute Myocardial Infarction		
High risk[e]	2–3 + low-dose aspirin	long-term
All other infarcts (usually ASA)[f]		

TABLE 8
Oral Anticoagulant Standards of Practice (See also warfarin p 288) (continued)

Thromboembolic Disorder	INR	Duration
Prosthetic Valves		
Bioprosthetic heart valves		
Mitral position	2–3	3 mo
Aortic position[g]	2–3	3 mo
Bileaflet mechanical valves in aortic position[h]	2–3	long-term
Other mechanical prosthetic valves[i]	2.5–3.5	long-term

[a] 3 mo if mod or high risk of bleeding or distal DVT; if low risk of bleeding, then long-term for proximal DVT/PE.

[b] Paroxysmal AF or ≥2 risk factors (age > 75, Hx, BP, DM, mod-severe LV dysfunction or CHF), then warfarin; 1 risk factor warfarin or 75–325 mg ASA; 0 risk factors ASA.

[c] Mitral valve Dz: rheumatic if Hx systemic embolism, or AF or LA thrombus or LA > 55 mm; MVP: only if AF, systemic embolism or TIAs on ASA; mitral valve calcification: warfarin if AF or recurrent embolism on ASA; aortic valve w/ calcification: warfarin not recommended.

[d] In adults only ASA; only indication for anticoagulation cardiomyopathy in children, to begin no later than their activation on transplant list.

[e] High risk = large anterior MI, significant CHF, intracardiac thrombus visible on TE, AF, and Hx of a thromboembolic event.

[f] If meticulous INR monitoring and highly skilled dose titration are expected and widely accessible, then INR 3.5 (3.0–4.0) w/o ASA or 2.5 (2.0–3.0) w/ ASA long-term (4 years).

[g] Usually ASA 50–100 mg; warfarin if Hx embolism, LA thrombus, AF, low EF, hypercoagulable state, 3 mo, or until thrombus resolves.

[h] Target INR 2.5–3.5 if AF, large anterior MI, LA enlargement, hypercoagulable state, or low EF.

[i] Add ASA 50–100 mg if high risk (AF, hypercoagulable state, low EF, or Hx of ASCVD).

Data from Antithrombotic and thrombolytic therapy: American College of Chest Physicians Evidence-Based Clinical Practice Guidelines (8th Edition). *Chest.* 2008;133(suppl 6):110S–112S.

TABLE 9
Antiarrhythmics: Vaughn Williams Classification

Class I: Sodium Channel Blockade

A. **Class Ia:** Lengthens duration of action potential (↑ the refractory period
   in atrial and ventricular muscle, in SA and AV conduction systems, and
   Purkinje fibers)
   1. Amiodarone (also classes II, III, IV)
   2. Disopyramide (Norpace)
   3. Imipramine (MAO inhibitor)
   4. Procainamide (Pronestyl)
   5. Quinidine
B. **Class Ib:** No effect on action potential
   1. Lidocaine (Xylocaine)
   2. Mexiletine (Mexitil)
   3. Phenytoin (Dilantin)
   4. Tocainide (Tonocard)
C. **Class Ic:** Greater sodium current depression (blocks the fast inward
   Na^+ current in heart muscle and Purkinje fibers, and slows the rate of ↑
   of phase 0 of the action potential)
   1. Flecainide (Tambocor)
   2. Propafenone

Class II: β-Blocker

D. Amiodarone (also classes Ia, III, IV)
E. Esmolol (Brevibloc)
F. Sotalol (also class III)

Class III: Prolong Refractory Period via Action Potential

G. Amiodarone (also classes Ia, II, IV)
H. Sotalol

Class IV: Calcium Channel Blocker

I. Amiodarone (also classes Ia, II, III)
J. Diltiazem (Cardizem)
K. Verapamil (Calan)

TABLE 10
Cytochrome P-450 Isoenzymes and Common Drugs They Metabolize, Inhibit, and Induce

Increased or decreased (primarily hepatic cytochrome P-450) metabolism of medications may influence the effectiveness of drugs or result in significant drug-drug interactions. Understanding the common cytochrome P-450 isoforms (eg, CYP2C9, CYP2D9, CYP2C19, CYP3A4) and common drugs that are metabolized by (aka "substrates"), inhibit, or induce activity of the isoform helps identify and minimize significant drug interactions.

CYP1A2

Substrates:	Acetaminophen, caffeine, cyclobenzaprine, clozapine, imipramine, mexiletine, naproxen, propranolol, theophylline
Inhibitors:	Amiodarone, cimetidine, most fluoroquinolone antibiotics, fluvoxamine, verapamil
Inducers:	Carbamazepine, charcoal-broiled foods, cruciferous vegetables, omeprazole, modafinil, tobacco smoking

CYP2C9

Substrates:	Most NSAIDs (including COX-2), glipizide, irbesartan, losartan, phenytoin, tamoxifen, warfarin
Inhibitors:	Amiodarone, fluconazole, isoniazid (INH), ketoconazole, metronidazole
Inducers:	Aprepitant, Barbiturates, rifampin

CYP2C19

Substrates:	Amitriptyline, clopidogrel, cyclophosphamide, diazepam, lansoprazole, omeprazole, pantoprazole, phenytoin, rabeprazole
Inhibitors:	Fluoxetine, fluvoxamine, isoniazid, ketoconazole, lansoprazole, omeprazole, ticlopidine
Inducers:	Barbiturates, carbamazepine, prednisone, rifampin

CYP2D6

Substrates:	**Antidepressants:** Most tricyclic antidepressants, clomipramine, fluoxetine, paroxetine, venlafaxine **Antipsychotics:** Aripiprazole, clozapine, haloperidol, risperidone, thioridazine **Beta-blockers:** Carvedilol, metoprolol, propranolol, timolol

(Continued)

TABLE 10
**Cytochrome P-450 Isoenzymes and Common Drugs
They Metabolize, Inhibit, and Induce (continued)**

CYP2D6 (continued)

	Opioids: Codeine, hydrocodone, oxycodone, tramadol
	Others: Amphetamine, dextromethorphan, duloxetine, encainide, flecainide, mexiletine, ondansetron, propafenone, selegiline, tamoxifen
Inhibitors:	Amiodarone, bupropion, cimetidine, clomipramine, doxepin, duloxetine, fluoxetine, haloperidol, methadone, paroxetine, quinidine, ritonavir
Inducers:	Dexamethasone, rifampin

CYP3A

(involved in the metabolism of > 50% of drugs metabolized by the liver)

Substrates:	**Anticholinergics:** Darifenacin, oxybutynin, solifenacin, tolterodine
	Benzodiazepines: Alprazolam, diazepam, midazolam, triazolam
	Calcium channel blockers: Amlodipine, diltiazem, felodipine, nifedipine, nimodipine, nisoldipine, verapamil
	Chemotherapy: Cyclophosphamide, erlotinib, ifosfamide, paclitaxel, tamoxifen, vinblastine, vincristine
	HIV protease inhibitors: Atazanavir, indinavir, nelfinavir, ritonavir, saquinavir
	HMG-CoA reductase inhibitors: Atorvastatin, lovastatin, simvastatin
	Immunosuppressive agents: Cyclosporine, tacrolimus
	Macrolide-type antibiotics: Clarithromycin, erythromycin, telithromycin, troleandomycin
	Opioids: Alfentanil, cocaine, fentanyl, methadone, sufentanil
	Steroids: Budesonide, cortisol, 17-β-estradiol, progesterone
	Others: Acetaminophen, amiodarone, carbamazepine, delavirdine, efavirenz, nevirapine, quinidine, repaglinide, sildenafil, tadalafil, trazodone, vardenafil
Inhibitors:	Amiodarone, amprenavir, aprepitant, atazanavir, ciprofloxacin, cisapride, clarithromycin, diltiazem, erythromycin, fluconazole, fluvoxamine, grapefruit juice (in high ingestion), indinavir, itraconazole, ketoconazole, nefazodone, nelfinavir, norfloxacin, ritonavir, saquinavir, telithromycin, troleandomycin, verapamil, voriconazole

(Continued)

TABLE 10
Cytochrome P-450 Isoenzymes and Common Drugs
They Metabolize, Inhibit, and Induce (continued)

CYP3A (continued)

Inducers:	Carbamazepine, efavirenz, glucocorticoids, modafinil, nevirapine, phenytoin, phenobarbital, rifabutin, rifapentine, rifampin, St. John's wort

Data from Katzung B, ed. *Basic and Clinical Pharmacology*. 12th ed. New York, NY: McGraw-Hill, 2012; *The Medical Letter*. July 4, 2004; 47; N Engl J Med. 2005;352:2211–2221. Flockhart DA, Drug Interactions: Cytochrome P450 Drug Interaction Table. Indiana University School of Medicine. http://medicine.iupui.edu/clinpharm/ddis/table.aspx. Accessed August 31, 2013.

TABLE 11
SSRIs/SNRIs/Triptans and Serotonin Syndrome

A life-threatening condition, when selective serotonin reuptake inhibitors (SSRIs) and 5-hydroxytryptamine receptor agonists (triptans) are used together. However, many other drugs have been implicated (see below). Signs and symptoms of serotonin syndrome include the following:

Restlessness, coma, N/V/D, hallucinations, loss of coordination, overactive reflexes, hypertension, mydriasis, rapid changes in BP, increased body temperature

Class	Drugs
Antidepressants	MAOIs, TCAs, SSRIs, SNRIs, mirtazapine, venlafaxine
CNS stimulants	Amphetamines, phentermine, methylphenidate, sibutramine
5-HT$_1$ agonists	Triptans
Illicit drugs	Cocaine, methylenedioxymethamphetamine (ecstasy), lysergic acid diethylamide (LSD)
Opioids	Tramadol, oxycodone, morphine, meperidine
Others	Buspirone, chlorpheniramine, dextromethorphan, linezolid, lithium, selegiline, tryptophan, St. John's wort

Management includes removal of the precipitating drugs and supportive care. To control agitation, the serotonin antagonists cyproheptadine can be used. When symptoms are mild, discontinuation of the medication or medications and the control of agitation with benzodiazepines may be needed. Critically ill patients may require sedation and mechanical ventilation as well as control of hyperthermia. (Ables AZ, Nagubilli R. Prevention, recognition, and management of serotonin syndrome. *Am Fam Physician*. May 1, 2010;81(9):1139–1142.)
MOAI = monoamine oxidase inhibitor.
TCA = tricyclic antidepressant.
SNRI = serotonin-norepinephrine reuptake inhibitors.

TABLE 12
Selected Multivitamin Supplements

This table lists common multivitamins available without a prescription, and most chains have generic versions. Many specialty vitamin combinations are available and are not included in this table. (Examples are B vitamins plus C; disease-specific supplements; pediatric and infant formulations; prenatal vitamins, etc.) A check (✓) indicates the component is found in the formulation; NA indicates it is not in the formulation. Details of the specific composition of these multivitamins can be found at www.eDrugbook.com or on the product site.

	Fat-Soluble Vitamins		Water-Soluble Vitamins[a]		Minerals[b]								Trace Elements[b]				Other
	A, D, E	K	C, B$_1$, B$_2$, B$_3$, B$_5$, B$_6$, B$_{12}$, Folate	Biotin	Ca	P	Mg	Fe	Zn	I	Se	K	Mn	Cu	Cr	Mo	
Centrum	✓	✓	✓	✓	✓	✓	✓	✓	✓	✓	✓	✓	✓	✓	✓	✓	
Centrum Performance	✓	✓	✓	✓	✓	✓	✓	✓	✓	✓	✓	✓	✓	✓	✓	✓	Lycopene Ginseng, Ginkgo
Centrum Silver	✓	✓	✓	✓	✓	✓	✓	NA	✓	✓	✓	✓	✓	✓	✓	✓	Lycopene
NatureMade Multi Complete	✓	NA	✓	NA	✓	NA	✓	✓	✓	✓	NA	NA	NA	NA	NA	NA	Lutein
NatureMade Multi Daily	✓		✓	✓	✓	NA	✓	✓	✓	✓	✓		✓	✓	NA		Lutein
NatureMade Multi Max	✓		✓	✓	✓	NA	✓	✓	✓	✓	✓	✓	✓	✓	NA	✓	
NatureMade Multi 50+	✓	✓	✓	✓	✓	NA	✓	NA	✓	✓	✓	✓	✓	✓	✓	✓	
One-A-Day 50 Plus	✓		✓	✓	✓	NA	✓	NA	✓	✓	✓	✓	✓	✓	✓	✓	Lutein

One-A-Day Essential	✓	NA		✓	NA			✓	NA	✓	✓	NA	✓	✓	NA	NA	NA	NA				
One-A-Day Maximum	✓	✓	NA	✓	✓	✓	✓	✓	NA	✓	✓	NA	✓	✓	NA	NA	NA	NA				
Therapeutic Vitamin	✓	✓	✓	✓	✓	✓	✓	✓	✓	✓	✓	✓	✓	✓	✓	NA	NA	NA				
Theragran-M Advanced Formula High Potency	✓	✓	✓	✓	✓	✓	✓	✓	✓	✓	✓	✓	✓	✓	✓	✓		lutein				
Theragran-M Premier High Potency	✓	✓	✓	✓	✓	✓	✓	✓	✓	✓	✓	✓	✓	✓	✓	✓	Lutein					
Theragran-M Premier 50 Plus High Potency	✓	✓	✓	✓	✓	NA	✓	✓	✓	low	✓	✓	✓	✓	✓	✓						
Therapeutic Vitamin + Minerals Enhanced	✓	✓	✓	✓	✓	✓	✓	✓	✓	✓	✓	✓	✓	✓	✓	✓						
Unicap M	✓	NA	NA	✓	✓	✓	✓	✓	✓	NA	✓	✓	✓	✓	✓	NA						
Unicap Senior	✓	NA	NA	✓	✓	✓	✓	✓	✓	low	✓	✓	✓	✓	✓	NA						
Unicap T	✓	NA	NA	NA	NA	NA	NA	✓	NA	low	✓	✓	✓	✓	✓	NA						

aVitamin B₁ = thiamine; B₂ = riboflavin; B₃ = niacin; B₅ = pantothenic acid; B₆ = pyridoxine; B₁₂ = cyanocobalamin.

bCa = calcium; Cr = chromium; Cu = copper; Fe = iron; Fl = fluoride; I = iodine; K = potassium; Mg = magnesium; Mn = manganese; Mo = molybdenum; P = phosphorus; Se = selenium; Zn = zinc.

TABLE 13
Influenza Vaccine Strains for 2013–2014 (See also pp 158–159)

The 2013–2014 trivalent influenza vaccine is made from the following three viruses:

- A/California/7/2009 (H1N1)pdm09-like virus;
- A(H3N2) virus antigenically like the cell-propagated prototype virus A/Victoria/361/2011;
- B/Massachusetts/2/2012-like virus.

It is recommended that quadrivalent vaccines containing two influenza B viruses contain the above three viruses and a B/Brisbane/60/2008-like virus.

Age	Brand Name Product	Dosage Form/Strength
6–35 mo	*Fluzone*	0.25 mL prefilled syringe
	Fluzone Quadrivalent	0.25 mL prefilled syringe
2–49 y	*FluMist Quadrivalent*	0.2 mL prefilled intranasal sprayer
≥ 36 mo	*Fluarix*	0.5 mL prefilled syringe
	Fluzone	0.5 mL prefilled syringe & single-dose vial; 5 mL multi-dose vial
	Fluarix Quadrivalent	0.5 mL prefilled syringe
	Fluzone Quadrivalent	0.5 mL prefilled syringe & single-dose vial
≥ 4 y	*Fluvirin*	0.5 mL prefilled syringe & 5 mL multi-dose vial
≥ 9 y[a]	*Afluria*	0.5 mL prefilled syringe & 5 mL multi-dose vial
≥ 18 y	*Flucelvax*	0.5 mL prefilled syringe
	FluLaval	5 mL multi-dose vial
18–49 y	*FluBlok*	0.5 mL single-dose vial
18–64 y	*Fluzone Intradermal*	0.1 mL prefilled microinjection system
≥ 65 y	*Fluzone High-Dose*	0.5 mL prefilled syringe

[a] Age indication per package labeling is ≥ 5 y; ACIP (www.cdc.gov/vaccines/acip) recommends *Afluria* not be used in children 6–8 y due to increased risk of febrile Rxn.

Index

Page numbers followed by *t* indicate tables.